The Charnoly Body
A Novel Biomarker of
Mitochondrial Bioenergetics

T0133864

Sushil Sharma
American International School of Medicine
89 Sandy Babb & Kitty Street
Guyana, South America

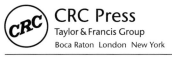

CRC Press
Taylor & Francis Group
Boca Raton London New York

CRC Press is an imprint of the
Taylor & Francis Group, an **informa** business
A SCIENCE PUBLISHERS BOOK

Cover credit: Cover illustration reproduced by kind courtesy of the author, Dr. Sushil Sharma

CRC Press
Taylor & Francis Group
6000 Broken Sound Parkway NW, Suite 300
Boca Raton, FL 33487-2742

First issued in paperback 2021

Version Date: 20181211

ISBN-13: 978-0-367-78029-6 (pbk)
ISBN-13: 978-1-138-55716-1 (hbk)

Library of Congress Cataloging-in-Publication Data

Names: Sharma, Sushil, Ph. D., D.M.R.I.T., author.
Title: The Charnoly body : a novel biomarker of mitochondrial bioenergetics / Sushil Sharma.
Description: Boca Raton, FL : CRC Press, Taylor & Francis Group, 2019. | "A Science Publishers book." | Includes bibliographical references and index.
Identifiers: LCCN 2018057446 | ISBN 9781138557161 (hardback)
Subjects: | MESH: Theranostic Nanomedicine--methods | Metallothionein--metabolism | Biomarkers--metabolism | Precision Medicine | Energy Metabolism
Classification: LCC QP552.M47 | NLM QT 36.5 | DDC 572/.68--dc23
LC record available at https://lccn.loc.gov/2018057446

Visit the Taylor & Francis Web site at
http://www.taylorandfrancis.com

and the CRC Press Web site at
http://www.crcpress.com

Acknowledgement

I extend heartiest gratitude to my respected late mother "Charnoly" who motivated me to work hard, face hardships, and be tolerant and patient during social, physical, mental, economical, and psychological crisises in life. It was indeed my mother who guided me to nursery school for the first time. I discovered "Charnoly body" as a doctoral student at the All India Institute of Medical Sciences (A.I.I.M.S.), New Delhi in 1982 when she was alive. I am also highly thankful to my friends, relatives, and professional colleagues who conferred their moral support and persuaded me to discover "Charnoly body".

My respected teacher, Prof. Christian De Duve from Belgium was awarded the Nobel Prize for his original discovery of lysosomes and peroxisomes in 1974. He was the one to introduce the term "autophagy." Last year, Prof. Yoshinori Ohsumi from Japan was awarded the Nobel Prize for elucidating the basic molecular mechanism of autophagy. I have been constantly following the footsteps of these legends to discover Charnoly body (CB) and its clinical significance in mitochondrial bioenergetics and intracellular detoxification (ICD) in chronic diseases during my doctoral and postdoctoral research.

I express my sincere thanks to google and the global scientific community for recognizing my original discovery of Charnoly body (CB) as a universal biomarker of physicochemical injury due to free radical-induced compromised mitochondrial bioenergetics (CMB) and charnolophagy as a basic molecular mechanism of intracellular detoxification (ICD) in the most vulnerable cells. Recently, I introduced charnolosome (CS) and disease-specific spatiotemporal (DSST) charnolosomics to develop novel charnolopharmacotherapeutics for the targeted, safe, and effective personalized theranostics of chronic diseases.

I express my sincere thanks to my mentors Dr. Baldev Singh, Dr. Krishnamurti Dakshinamurti, and Dr. Manuchair Ebadi for their moral support and encouragement during my professional and scientific career to discover CB as a novel biomarker of compromised mitochondrial bioenergetics (CMB) in progressive neurodegenerative diseases, cardiovascular diseases, and multidrug resistant malignancies as described elegantly in this book.

I sincerely hope that this manuscript will attract the global biomedical community due to its original, novel, and thought-provoking concepts and mechanisms to discover DSST charnolopharmacotherapeutics for the safe and effective evidence-based personalized theranostics (EBPT) of chronic diseases. Doctors, professors, researchers, basic scientists, nurses, and the public will enjoy going through its most interesting and motivating contents to enhance their basic knowledge regarding the mitochondrial bioenergetics (MB) and ICD in health and disease.

Sushil Sharma

American International School of Medicine
89 Sandy Babb & Kitty Street
Guyana, South America

Preface

Generally, therapeutic drugs have been designed and targeted to nucleic acid (DNA/RNA) and/or protein synthesis. There are only few drugs based on the mitochondrial bioenergetics (MB) and intracellular detoxification (ICD) in the pharmaceutical industry. This book describes CB as a pre-apoptotic biomarker of compromised mitochondrial bioenergetics (CMB) to develop novel charnolopharmacotherapeutics for the targeted, safe, and effective EBPT of chronic diseases. The book introduces for the first time charnolosomics and disease-specific spatio-temporal (DSST) charnolopharmacotherapeutics for the EBPT of chronic MDR diseases. This edition is an extension of my recently published books: Personalized Medicine (Beyond PET Biomarkers), Progress in PET RPs (Quality Control and Theranostics), and ZIKV Disease (Prevention and cure), Fetal Alcohol Spectrum Disorder (Concepts, Mechanisms, and Cure), and "Nicotinism and Emerging Role of Electronic Cigarettes" by Nova Science Publishers, New York, U.S.A.

It is well-established that free radicals are generated as a byproduct of oxidative phosphorylation in the electron transport chain during ATP synthesis in the mitochondria. The requirements of energy (ATP) are significantly elevated during DPCI in the most vulnerable cell. Thus, free radical-induced CMB induces CB formation involved in impaired ICD and cellular dysfunction. DPCI trigger CB formation as a pleomorphic, electron-dense, quasi-crystalline, multi-lamellar stack of degenerated mitochondrial membranes in the most vulnerable neural progenitor cells (NPCs) and cardiac progenitor cells (CPCs) derived from induced pluripotent cells (iPPCs) in the developing brain and heart, respectively, during the first trimester (gastrulation period) of pregnancy, which causes embryopathies in ZIKV, cytomegalovirus, rubella, and toxoplasma infections, and in nicotine addiction and fetal alcohol exposure. Various anesthetics, anti-epileptics, antidepressants, antipsychotics, and environmental pollutants can also induce charnolopathies, involving microcephaly and chronic diseases such as depression, diabetes, obesity, PD, and AD.

CB is a universal biomarker of cell injury whereas charnolophagy-induced CPS and CS formation serve as novel drug discovery targets to evaluate ICD in the oocyte during the pre-zygotic phase and in the NPCs, EPCs, CPCs, and OPCs, derived from iPPCs, during the post-zygotic phase of embryonic development.

DPCI compromise mitochondrial bioenergetics (MB) in the most vulnerable cells of the developing embryo, particularly during the first trimester of pregnancy (gastrulation period), causing charnolopathies involved in diversified embryopathies. Hence, drugs targeting MB by inhibiting CB formation, augmenting charnolophagy, and stabilizing CPS and CS will be promising charnolopharmacotherapeutics for the targeted, safe, and effective EBPT of chronic diseases, as described in this book.

Accumulation of CB at the junction of axon hillock impairs axoplasmic transport of various ions, enzymes, hormones, neurotrophic factors, neurotransmitters, and mitochondria to cause initially synaptic silence followed by synaptic atrophy, whereas accumulation of CS at the junction of axon hillock releases highly toxic mitochondrial metabolites including: cytochrome-C, iron, 8-OH, 2dG, 2,3, dihydroxy nonenal, acetaldehyde, ammonia, H_2O_2, GAPDH, and several other toxins to cause synaptic degeneration which induce cognitive impairments accompanied with early morbidity and mortality as noticed in FASD, autism, Down's syndrome, PD, AD, ALS, HD, and several other chronic diseases beyond the scope of this manuscript.

Non-specific induction of CB induces alopecia, myelosuppression, neurotoxicity, hepatotoxicity, GIT symptoms, nephrotoxicity, and infertility in MDR malignancies. Hence, drugs may be developed to prevent/inhibit CB formation and augment MB to enhance charnolophagy and CS exocytosis as a basic molecular mechanism of ICD to prevent or treat chronic diseases. Particularly, drugs may be developed to prevent CS destabilization, permeabilization, sequestration, and fragmentation by augmenting antioxidant drug delivery in the diseased organ. Although charnolostatic drugs will be clinically-beneficial to control acute diseased states, disease and organ-specific charnolocidals will be required for chronic MDR diseases as illustrated in this book.

The most unique feature of this edition is that it provides basic molecular mechanisms and the cure of chronic diseases by developing MB-based charnolopharmacotherapeutics as CB antagonists, charnolophagy agonists, and CS stabilizers. The book enhances our basic knowledge regarding safe and effective clinical management of chronic diseases by rejuvenating MB and microRNAs involved in ICD. The book motivates researchers to discover novel DSST charnolopharmacotherapeutics for the safe and effective EBPT of chronic diseases. The primary objective is to regulate MB at the transcriptional and translational level by preventing/inhibiting cell and tissue-specific free radical-induced CB formation involved in post-transcriptional microRNA deregulation.

The original concepts and mechanisms of charnolophagy, CPS, and CS as specific drug discovery targets of CMB for the clinical management of chronic diseases are presented for the first time in this book.

Antioxidants (glutathione, metallothioneins, CoQ_{10}, melatonin, selegiline, resveratrol, sirtuin, rutin, lycopene, and catechin) inhibit CB formation as free radical scavengers. Although, antioxidants can easily pass through blood brain barrier without inducing any adverse effects, their reduced potency necessitates bulk consumption. Hence, ROS-scavenging antioxidant-loaded nanoparticles (NPs) may be developed to enhance CNS drug delivery and augment charnolophagy for ICD as elegantly highlighted in this book.

This manuscript will serve as a text book for biomedical students and nurses, and a reference book for doctors, researchers, professors, and public. Women of reproductive age would like to read its most interesting and thought-provoking concepts for a better quality of life for their progeny. This book will attract the attention of old persons with CMB as well.

Basic biomedical students, researchers, M.D., Ph.D., D.Sc. students, doctors, teachers, and professors at the college and university level, and the public will be interested in studying the novel and thought-provoking contents of this book. Particularly, undergraduate, postgraduate, doctoral, and post-doctoral students, research associates, and research scientists will find this book interesting and motivating to discover novel therapeutic intervention for the safe and effective EBPT of fetal alcohol spectrum disorders (FASD), Zika viral (ZIKV) disease, AD, PD, major depression, diabetes, obesity, multiple drug addiction, schizophrenia, CVDs, and MDR malignancies.

This newly-released edition of "Charnoly body" by CRC Press, Boca Raton FL, U.S.A. will be interesting, easy to follow, and will facilitate the development of innovative DSST charnolopharmacotherapeutics based on MB for ICD to accomplish the ultimate-goal of targeted, safe, and effective EBPT of chronic diseases. Particularly, basic molecular mechanism(s) and concepts of CB formation, charnolophagy, and CS exocytosis/endocytosis in relation to post-transcriptional regulation of microRNAs promise to provide unique opportunities to discover safe and effective drugs for NDDs, CVDs, MDDs, MDR malignancies, and other chronic inflammatory diseases with currently limited success.

Sushil Sharma

Contents

Part-I General Introduction of Charnoly Body as a Novel
Theranostic Biomarker
(Basic Cellular and Molecular Biology)

Part-II Charnoly Body as a Drug Discovery
Biomarker Emerging Biotechnologies in Charnoly Body Research
(Personalized Theranostics)

Part-III Charnoly Body Molecular Pathogenesis
Clinical Significance of Disease-Specific Charnoly Body Formation and other Biomarkers in Chronic Diseases
(Recent Update on Evidence-based Personalized Theranostics)

Abbreviations

AAD	:	Alcohol Abuse Disorder
Alpha-SynMT$_{tko}$	:	Alpha-Synuclein-Metallothionein Triple Knock Out
Ach	:	Acetyl Choline
AD	:	Alzheimer's Disease
ADD	:	Average Daily Dose
ADHD	:	Attention Deficit Hyperactivity Disorder
ADI	:	Acceptable Daily Intake
ADNFLE	:	Autosomal Dominant Nocturnal Frontal Lobe Epilepsy
ADNI	:	Alzheimer's Disease Imaging Initiative
AGEP	:	Advanced Glycation Products
AHR	:	Aryl Hydrocarbon Receptor
AIS	:	Acute Ischmic Stroke
ALARA	:	As-Low-As-Reasonably-Achievable
ALI	:	Air-Liquid Interface
Alpha-Syn$_{ko}$	:	Syn Knock Out
ALS	:	Amyotrophic Lateral Sclerosis
AMPK	:	Adenosine Monophosphate (AMP)-Activated Protein Kinase
ANDS	:	Alternative Nicotine Delivery Systems
ANOVA	:	Analysis of Variance
ANS	:	Autonomic Nervous System
AOC	:	Area Under the Curve
AOPP	:	Advanced Oxidation Products (AOPP)
Apo E	:	Apolipoprotein E
ATR Index	:	Antidepressant Treatment Response Index
ATTUD	:	Association for the Treatment of Tobacco Use and Dependence
Avenic Cigarettes	:	Average Nicotine Cigarettes
Aβ	:	Amyloid-β
B[a]p	:	Benzo [a] Pyrene
BC	:	Biochemical Confirmation
BDDCS	:	Biopharmaceutics Drug Disposition Classification System
BDI	:	Beck Depression Inventory
BDNF	:	Brain Derived Growth Factor
BMI	:	Basal Metabolic Index
BOEs	:	Biomarkers of Exposure
BRITE-MD	:	Biomarkers for Rapid Identification of Treatment Effectiveness in Major Depression

CSF	:	Cerebrospinal Fluid
BSA	:	Bovine Serum Albumin
CAD	:	Cannabis Abuse Disorder
CAD	:	Cocaine Abuse Disorder
CAD	:	Coronary Artery Disease
CAP	:	Cholinergic Anti-Inflammatory Pathway
CB	:	(Charnoly Body: Multi lamellar stacks of electron dense degenerated mitochondrial membranes)
CBT	:	Cognitive-Behavioral Therapy
CCs	:	Combustible Cigarettes
CDC	:	Center for Disease Control and Prevention
CHARON	:	Chemical Analysis of Aerosol Online
CHD	:	Coronary Heart Disease
CHTP	:	Carbon-Heated Tobacco Product
CIPN	:	Chemotherapy-Induced Peripheral Neuropathy
CMB	:	Compromised Mitochondrial Bioenergetics
CMBEL	:	Compromised Mitochondrial Bioenergetic Levels (0–3)
CMV	:	Cytomegalovirus
CO	:	Carbon Monoxide
Complex-1	:	Ubiquinone NADH-Oxidoreductase
COPD	:	Chronic Obstructive Pulmonary Disease
CPS	:	Charnolophagosome
CPs	:	Charnolopharmaceutics
CRP	:	C-Reactive Protein
CS	:	Charnolosome
CS	:	Cigarette Smoking
CSE	:	Cigarette Smoke Extract
CSF	:	Cancer Slope Factor
CSF	:	Cerebrospinal Fluid
CT	:	Computerized Tomography
CTE	:	Chronic Traumatic Encephalopathy
CTLA4	:	Cytotoxic T-Lymphocyte Antigen 4
CVDs	:	Cardiovascular Diseases
DAD	:	Drug Abuse Disorder
DAergic	:	Dopaminergic
DAT	:	DA Transporter
DBS	:	Deep Brain Stimulation
DFX	:	Deferoxamine
DIP-EI/MS	:	Electron Ionization Mass Spectrometry by using a Direct Insertion Probe
DLB	:	Dementia with Lewy Body
DOM	:	Domoic Acid
DP	:	Decay Product
DPCI	:	Diversified Physico-Chemical Injuries
DSM	:	Diagnostic and Statistical Manual of Mental Disorders (IV)
DSST-CS	:	Disease-Specific Spatiotemporal Charnolosome
DTC	:	Disseminated Thyroid Carcinoma

E.M.	:	Electron Microscopy
EBC	:	Eye Blink Conditioning
EBPM	:	Evidence-Based Personalized Medicine
EBPT	:	Evidence-Based Personalized Theranostics
ELISA	:	Enzyme-Linked Immunosorbent Assay
FAPA	:	Flowing Atmospheric-Pressure Afterglow Plasma Ion Source
FAO	:	Fatty Acid Oxidation
[^{18}F]FAZA	:	1-(5-[^{18}F]Fluoro-5-Deoxy-α-D-Arabinofuranosyl)-2-Nitroimidazole
[^{18}F]-FdG	:	Fluorodeoxy Glucose
^{18}F-DOPA	:	^{18}F-Dihydroxyphenylaldehyde
^{18}F-FAZA	:	^{18}F-Fluoroazomycin-Arabinoside
^{18}F-FB-VAD-FMK	:	[^{18}F]4-Fluorobenzylcarbonyl-Val-Ala-Asp(OMe)-Fluoromethylketone
^{18}F-FMSIO	:	^{18}F-Fluoromisonidazole
fMRI	:	Functional Magnetic Resonance Imaging
FST	:	Forced Swimming Test
FTND	:	Fagerstrom Test for Nicotine Dependence
FTQ	:	Fonds de Solidarité
GAS	:	Goldberg Anxiety Scale
GATS	:	Global Adult Tobacco Survey
GD	:	Grave's Disease
GDS	:	Geriatric Depression Scale
GEE	:	Generalized Estimating Equations
GFP	:	Green-Fluorescence Protein
GIF	:	Growth Inhibitory Factor
Glut-1	:	Glucose Transporter-1
GO	:	Grave's Orbitopathy
GTS	:	Green Tobacco Sickness
GSD	:	Geometric Standard Deviations
GSH	:	Reduced Glutathione
GUI	:	Graphic User Interphase
GWAS	:	Genome Wide Association Studies
H_2O_2	:	Hydrogen Peroxide
6-OH-DA	:	6-Hydroxy Dopamine
HAM-D	:	Hamilton Scale of Depression
HD	:	Huntington's Disease
HDL	:	High Density Lipoprotein
HDL-C	:	High Density Lipoprotein-Cholesterol
HFD	:	High Fat Diet
HG	:	High Glucose
HIF-1α	:	Hypoxia-Inducible Factor-1α
Hinic Cigarettes	:	High Nicotine Cigarettes
HO-1	:	Heme Oxygenase-1
HONC	:	Hooked on Nicotine Checklist
Hp	:	Helicobacter Pylori
HPC	:	Hypoxic Preconditioning

HPHCs	:	Harmful and Potentially Harmful Constituents
HQ	:	Hazard Quotient
HRE	:	Hypoxia Response Element
HRMS	:	High-Resolution Mass Spectrometry
HSP	:	Heat Shock Protein
HSP-70	:	Heat Shock Protein-70
HSPs	:	Heat Shock Proteins
HS-SPME	:	Headspace Solid-Phase Micro-Extraction
5-HTTLPRP	:	Serotonin-Transporter-Linked Promoter Region Polymorphisms
IAQ	:	Indoor Air Quality
ICD	:	International Classification of Diseases
ICP-MS	:	Inductively-Coupled Plasma Mass Spectrometer
ICTL	:	Intracellular Toxicity Levels (0–3)
IDRS	:	Illicit Drug Reporting System
IL-10	:	Interleukin-10
IRS	:	Infrared Spectroscopy
IUR	:	Inhalation Unit Risk
KA	:	Kainic Acid
KRS	:	Kufor-Rakeb Syndrome
LADA	:	Latent Autoimmune Diabetes of Adulthood
LADD	:	Lifetime Average Daily Dose
LBs	:	Lewy Body
LC-MS	:	Liquid Chromatography-Tandem Mass Spectrometry
LCR	:	Life-Time Cancer Risk
LDCT	:	Lung Cancer Screening with Low-Dose Computed Tomography
LDL	:	Low Density Lipoprotein
LED	:	Light Emitting Diode
LOD	:	Limits of Detection
Lox	:	Lipoxygenase
LPB	:	Lipopolysaccharide Binding Protein
LPB	:	Lipoprotein Binding Protein
lp-ntPET	:	Linear Parametric Neurotransmitter PET
LPS	:	Lipopolysaccharides
LRP	:	Lung Resistance Related Protein
LSUT	:	Lung Screen Uptake Trial
MAD	:	Morphine Abuse Disorder
MB	:	Mitochondrial Bioenergetics
MCAO	:	Middle Cerebral Artery Occlusion
MCI	:	Mild Cognitive Impairment
MDD	:	Major Depressive Disorder
MDMA	:	Methylene Deoxy Methamphetamine
MDR	:	Multi Drug Resistance
MEAD	:	Methamphetamine Abuse Disorder
MEMS	:	Micro-Electromechanical Systems
MIC	:	Metabolism-Informed Care

MicroPET	:	Micro-Positron Emission Tomography
MIPs	:	Molecularly Imprinted Polymers
miRNA	:	microRNA
MMPs	:	Matrix Metalloproteinases
MNCs	:	Mononuclear Cells
MNWS	:	Minnesota Nicotine Withdrawal Scale
MOFs	:	Metal Organic Frameworks
MPP^+	:	1-Methyl, 4-Phenyl, Pyridinium Ion
MPTP	:	1-Methyl, 2-Phenyl, 1, 2, 3, 6-Tetrahydropyridine
MRE	:	Metal Response Element
MRI	:	Magnet Resonance Imaging
MRS	:	Magnetic Resonance Spectroscopy
MS	:	Multiple Sclerosis
MSA	:	Multiple System Atrophy
MT	:	Metallothionein
MT_{dko}	:	Metallothionein Double Gene Knockout
MTF-1	:	Metal Transcription Responsive Factor-1
MTG	:	MitoTracker Green
MTs	:	Metallothioneins
MT_{trans}	:	Metallothionein Transgenic
nAChR	:	Alpha-4 Nicotinic Acetylcholine Receptor
NAFLD	:	Nonalcoholic Fatty Liver Disease
NASH	:	Non-Alcoholic Steatohepatitis
NDDs	:	Neurodegenerative Disorders
Nef2	:	Nuclear Factor Erythroid 2-Related Factor
NIDA	:	National Institute on Drug Addiction
NIMH-RDCI	:	National Institute of Mental Health-Research Domain Criteria Initiative
NIOSH	:	National Institute for Occupational Safety and Health
nm	:	Nanometer
NMR	:	Nuclear Magnetic Resonance
NMR	:	Nicotine Metabolite Ratio
NNAL	:	4-(Methylnitrosamino)-1-(3-Pyridyl)-1-Butanol (A Pulmonary Carcinogen)
NNC	:	Normal Nicotine Content Cigarettes
NNCs	:	Normal Nicotine Content (NNC) Cigarettes (Nicotine: 1 Mg/Cigarette)
NNN	:	N-Nitrosonor Nicotine
NNK	:	4-(Methylnitrosamino)-1-(3-Pyridyl)-1-Butanone
NNN	:	N'-Nitrosonor Nicotine
NO	:	Nitric Oxide
NOS	:	Nitric Oxide Synthase
NPs	:	Nanoparticles
NR	:	Nuclear Reaction
NSAIDs	:	Nonsteroidal Anti-Inflammatory Drugs
OGD	:	Oxygen and Glucose Deprivation
$ONOO^-$	:	Peroxynitrite Ion

OPLS-DA	:	Orthogonal Projection to Latent Structures Discriminant Analysis
OSHA	:	Occupational Safety and Health Administration
OTC-NRT	:	Over the Counter-Nicotine Replacement
PA	:	Passive Avoidance
PAH	:	Polycyclic Aromatic Hydrocarbons
PAI	:	Plasminogen Activator Inhibitor-1
PAMAM	:	Poly (Amidoamine) Dendrimer
PC	:	Proxy Confirmation
PCA	:	Principal Component Analysis
PD	:	Parkinson's Disease
PEG	:	Poly Ethylene Glycol
Pegylation	:	Covalent Conjugation of Drug with PEG
PEL	:	Permissible Exposure Limit
PET	:	Positron Emission Tomography
PGAM1	:	Phosphoglycerate Mutase 1
PGLA	:	Poly (Lactic-co-glycolic) Acid
PIB	:	Pittsburg Compound-B
PKs	:	Pharmacokinetics
PLN	:	Polymer Lipid Nanoparticle
PLS-DA	:	Partial Least Squares-Discriminant Analysis
PM	:	Particulate Matter
PNs	:	Parkinsonian Neurotoxins
PNS	:	Peripheral Nervous System
POMS	:	Profile of Mood State
PPA	:	Point Prevalence of Abstinence
PROMIS®	:	Patient Reported Outcomes Measurement Information System
PT	:	Personalized Theranostics (individualized diagnosis and treatment simultaneously: particularly significant for highly proliferative malignant carcinomas where there is a limited time window for diagnosis as well as treatment)
PTPN22	:	Protein Tyrosine Phosphatase
PTR-ToF-MS	:	Proton-Transfer-Reaction Time-of-Flight Mass Spectrometer
PTSD	:	Post-Traumatic Stress Disorder
PTX	:	Paclitaxel
PUFA	:	Polyunsaturated Fatty Acids
PV/VG	:	Propylene Glycol/Vegetable Glycerin
PVD	:	Peripheral Vascular Disease
PWID	:	People Who Inject Drugs
[62]Cu-PTSM	:	^{64}Cu-Pyrualdehyde Bis-N-Methylthiosemicarbazone
QSPR	:	Quantitative Structure–Permeability Relationships
QSU	:	Questionnaire of Smoking Urges
RDS	:	Radioisotope Delivery System
REL	:	Recommended Exposure Limit
REM	:	Rapid Eye Movement
RES	:	Reticulo Endothelial System

RfC	:	Reference Concentration
RfD	:	Reference Dose
RhO_{mgko}	:	Mitochondial Genome Knock Out
RI	:	Reflection Index
RNS	:	Reactive Nitrogen Species
ROC	:	Receiver Operating Characteristic
ROI	:	Region of Interest
RONS	:	Reactive Oxygen and Nitrogen Species
ROS	:	Reactive Oxygen Species
RPs	:	Radiopharmaceuticals
RPU	:	Regular Psychostimulant Users
rtfMRI	:	Real Time Functional Magnetic Resonance Imaging
SAGE	:	Serial Analysis of Gene Expression
SHS	:	Secondhand Smoking
SI	:	Stiffness Index
SI	:	α-Synculein Index
SIDS	:	Sudden Infant Death Syndrome
SIN-1	:	3-Morpholinosydnonimine
SLE	:	Systemic Lupus Erythromatosus
SNP	:	Single Nucleotide Polymorphism
SOD	:	Superoxide Dismutase
SPD	:	Serious Psychological Distress
SPECT	:	Single Photon Emission Computerized Tomography
SR	:	Self-Reported
SRNT	:	Society for Research on Nicotine and Tobacco
SSRIs	:	Specific Serotonin Reuptake Inhibitors
ST	:	Smokeless Tobacco
STDS	:	Charnolosome: Spatio-Temporal Disease-Specific Charnolosome
STS-CPS	:	Spatio-Temporally-Specific Charnolopharmaceuticals
SUDs	:	Substance Use Disorders
α-Syn	:	α-Synculein
SI	:	α-Synculein Index (Nitrated α-Syn/Native α-Syn)
$α\text{-SynMT}_{tko}$ Mice	:	α-Synuclein Metallothioneins Triple Knockout Mice
^{68}Ga-TETA	:	^{68}Ga-Tetraazamacrocyclic-1,4,8,11-Tetraazacyclotetradecane-1,4,8,11-Tetraacetic Acid
TBI	:	Traumatic Brain Injury
Tg	:	Thyroglobulin
TG	:	Triglyceride
TGA	:	Thermogravimetric Analysis
THS	:	Tobacco Heating System
TIMPs	:	Tissue Inhibitors of Matrix Metalloproteinases
tMCAO	:	Transient Middle Cerebral Artery Occlusion
TMD	:	Total Mood Disturbance
TMRE	:	Tetramethylrhodamine Ethyl Ester
TNFα	:	Tumor Necrosis Factor-α
TP	:	Target Product

TP	:	Transformation Products
TRD	:	Treatment-Resistant Depression
TSNA	:	Tobacco Specific Nitrosamines
TSRH	:	Thyroid Stimulating Hormone Receptor
TUDs	:	Tobacco Use Disorders
UHPLC-QTOF-MS	:	Ultrahigh-Performance Liquid Chromatography-Quadrupole Time-of-Flight Mass Spectrometry
UN	:	Undernutrition
UPLC	:	Ultra-Performance Liquid Chromatography
US	:	Ultrasound
USPSTF	:	US Preventive Services Task Force
UV/VIS Analysis	:	Ultraviolet/Visible Analysis
VaD	:	Vascular Dementia
VEGF	:	Vasoendothelial Derived Growth Factor
VI	:	Vulnerability Index
VLDL	:	Very Low-Density Lipoproteins
VLNC	:	Very Low Nicotine Content Cigarettes
VOCs	:	Volatile Organic Compounds
WHO	:	Word Health Organization
WISDM	:	Wisconsin Inventory of Smoking Dependence Motives
wv/wv Mice	:	Homozygous Weaver Mutant Mice
wv/wv-MTs	:	Metallothioneins Over-Expressing Weaver Mice

Definitions

Vulnerable Cells. The cells derived from induced pluripotent stem cells and mesenchymal stem cells (such as neural progenitor cells, cardiac progenitor cells, endothelial progenitor cells, hepatic progenitor cells, renal progenitor cells, pulmonary progenitor cells, and osteogenic progenitor cells) particularly in the developing embryo are the most vulnerable to physicochemical injury.

Diversified Physicochemical Injury (DPCI). Physicochemical injury can occur due to severe malnutrition, toxic environmental exposure, and in response to microbial (bacteria, viral, and fungal) infection to cause mitochondrial oxidative and nitrative stress and triggers Charnoly body (CB) formation in the most vulnerable cell. **Note:** The term "diversified physicochemical injury (DPCI)" has been used in this book to represent malnutrition, toxic environmental exposure, and/or microbial (bacteria, viral and fungal) infection in the most vulnerable cell.

Charnoly Body (CB). Charnoly body is a pleomorphic, multi-lamellar, electron-dense, quasi-crystalline, inclusion body which is generated in the most vulnerable cell due to free radical-induced degeneration and condensation of the mitochondrial membranes. Free radicals ($\cdot$OH, NO$\cdot$, CO$\cdot$) are generated as a byproduct of mitochondrial oxidative phosphorylation in the electron transport chain. Free radical production is significantly augmented in DPCI. The energy (ATP) requirement is significantly increased during DPCI to eliminate CB as a basic molecular mechanism of ICD to sustain normal function in the most vulnerable cell. Free radicals cause degeneration of the mitochondrial membranes, which condense to form electron-dense penta or hepta-lamellar structures as an initial attempt to contain highly toxic mitochondrial metabolites such as cytochrome-C, 2,3-dihydroxy nonenal, 8-OH 2dG, acetaldehyde, H_2O_2, ammonia, GAPDH, monoamine oxidases (MAOs), TSPO (which serves as a cholesterol transport channel for the synthesis of steroid hormones to stabilize the mitochondrial and other intracellular membranes), and a canonical calcium channel (TRPC) protein. These proteins are delocalized during CB formation which disrupts intracellular homeostasis to initiate cellular demise. Hence, CB can serve as a universal pre-apoptotic biomarker of CMB.

Charnolosomics. A bioinformatic approach to analyze CB, CS, and charnolophagy biomarkers employing state of the art biotechnologies to evaluate mitochondrial bioenergetics (MB) and ICD for normal cellular function to accomplish the targeted, safe, and effective EBPT of chronic MDR diseases for a better quality of life.

Charnolophagy. An energy (ATP) driven phagocytosis of CB.

Charnolophagosome. A lysosome containing phagocytosed CB.

Charnolosome. An intracellular organelle following complete hydrolysis of CB by lysosomal enzymes.

Charnolopharmacotherapeutics. CB-targeted therapeutic drugs designed based on the CMB involving CB prevention or inhibition, charnolophagy induction, charnolophagosome (CPS)/charnolosome (CS) stabilization, and their exocytosis and endocytosis as a basic molecular mechanism of ICD for a normal cellular function.

Charnolophagy Index. A ratio of charnolophagy versus autophagy.

Charnolophagosome (CPS). A highly unstable and functionally-labile intracellular organelle which is formed following charnolophagy. It is electron-dense and almost 2.5 times larger than the size of a lysosome.

Charnolosome (CS). A CS is formed when the phagocytosed CB in the charnolophagosome is completely hydrolyzed by the lysosomal enzymes. It is a single layered, highly unstable, and functionally-labile intracellular organelle containing toxic mitochondrial metabolites.

CS Stability Index (CSSI). It is a ratio of stable charnolosome (CS_s) divided by stable charnolosome (CS_s) + permeable charnolosome (CS_{perm}) + sequestered charnolosome (CS_{seq}) + fragmented charnolosome (CS_{frag}), and can be quantitatively estimated by multiple fluorochrome flow cytometric analysis.

CS Body. A blebbing on the surface of a CS following a secondary or tertiary free radical attack due to lipid peroxidation during mitochondrial oxidative and ER stress. The CS body pinches off from the CS and fuses with the plasma membrane to synthesize the apoptotic body.

Charnolopathy. CB molecular pathogenesis.

Apoptotic Body. A blebbing on the surface of the plasma membrane following a tertiary or quaternary free radical attack. The fusion of CS body with the plasma membrane releases highly toxic mitochondrial metabolites as described above to cause phosphatidyl serine externalization and eventually release of intracellular constituents in the microenvironment to induce chronic MDR diseases as described systematically in this book.

Free Radicals. Free radicals are highly unstable, reactive oxygen and nitrogen species (including $\cdot OH$, $NO\cdot$, $CO\cdot$) which are formed in the mitochondria as a byproduct to oxidative phosphorylation in the electron transport chain. They cause lipid peroxidation of cellular membranes by inducing the structural and functional breakdown of polyunsaturated fatty acids (including: linoic acid, linolenic acid, and arachidonic acid).

Stages of Free Radical Attack. There are primarily four different stages of free radical attack: (i) Primary free radical attack, (ii) secondary free radical attack, (iii) tertiary free radial attack, and (iv) quaternary free radical attack. (i) Primary free radical attack is attenuated by endogenously-synthesized antioxidants such as glutathione, metallothioneins (MTs), heat shock proteins (HSPs), heat shock factor-α, thioredoxin, superoxide dismutase (SOD), and catalase. (ii) Secondary free radical attack requires endogenously synthesized antioxidants as well as naturally-produced antioxidants such as polyphenols (resveratrol), lycopene, sirtuins, rutins, catechin, and flavonoids to maintain ICD and sustain intra-mitochondrial homeostasis. (iii) Tertiary free radical attack requires endogenously-synthesized antioxidants, naturally synthesized antioxidants as describe above, and pharmacological antioxidants such as all B vitamins, Vitamin-A, D, E, probucol, edaravone, statins (simvastatin, atorvastatin), and several others in the pharmaceutical industry. (iv) Quaternary free radical attack is difficult to attenuate and cannot be prevented by all the above three sources of antioxidants. In general, quaternary free radical attack is associated with degenerative and proinflammatory apoptosis which cause chronic MDR diseases.

Charnolopharmaceuticals. CB-targeted pharmaceutical agents for the safe and effective EBPT of chronic MDR diseases such as malignancies.

Charnolopharmacology. CB-targeted mitochondrial bioenergetics-based therapeutic drugs with well-established pharmacokinetics (PKs), pharmacodynamics (PDs), and pharmacogenomics, beneficial effects, and adverse effects.

Charnoloscopy. A microscopic (usually confocal, atomic force, and TEM) evaluation of CB, charnolophagy, charnolophagosome, CS, and its exocytosis/endocytosis as a basic molecular mechanism of ICD.

Charnolostatic. An agent which inhibits CB formation.

Charnolocidal. An agent which eliminates CB in a physicochemically-injured cell.

Charnolomimetic. An agent which augments CB formation.

Charnologenetics. Genetically-linked CB formation.

Charnolopharmacogenomics. Genomic changes associated with pharmacological induction or inhibition of CB.

CB-PET RPs. These PET RPs are based on CB-induced CMB and primarily targeted to label CB, CPS, and CS, in addition to detecting charnolophagy (CB-autophagy) and CS exocytosis/endocytosis. Disease-specific CB-PET radioligands will be clinically significant for early differential diagnosis of progressive NDDs, CVDs, and cancer. CB, CPS, and CS can be isolated by differential ultracentrifugation in sucrose-density gradient, purified by MACs separation, and characterized by multifluorochrome flow cytometery with a sorting facility for the safe and effective EBPT of MDR diseases.

CB Epigenetics. Methylation of mitochondrial DNA at the N-4 position of cytosine and acetylation of histones at lysine residues.

α-Synuclein Index. A ratio of nitrated α-synuclein versus native α-synuclein.

Detection of CS. A CS can be detected by employing two fluorescent imaging probes including (i) mitotracker, and (ii) lysotracker. The cells or tissues can be labeled with these fluorochromes. The mitotracker can determine the number of mitochondria and the lysotracker can determine the number of lysosomes. The mitochondria and lysosomes can be distinguished based on the red and green fluorescence respectively. These digital images are merged to localize yellow fluorescence-labeled CS. A CS exhibits yellow fluorescence because it has both lysosomal enzymes as well as metabolites of mitochondria. Moreover, CS are rich in the mtDNA oxidation product, 8-OH 2dG, and plasma membrane oxidation product, 2,3 dihydroxy nonenal, which can be determined by labeling cells with fluorescently-labelled specific antibodies. In addition to tissues and cultured cells, circulating CS biomarkers including 8-OH, 2dG, and 2, 3 dihydroxy nonenal can be estimated from the saliva, serum, plasma, blood, urine, hair, and toenail samples to quantitatively assess CB-based mitochondrial bioenergetics (MB). Various biomarkers of CS can also be determined by performing multiplex ELISA, antibody microarrays, cDNA microarray, and microRNA microarrays.

Introduction

Christian de Duve, the Nobel Laureate from Belgium, discovered lysosomes and introduced the term "Autophagy". He was awarded the shared Nobel Prize for Physiology or Medicine in 1974, along with Albert Claude and George E. Palade for describing the structure and function of organelles (lysosomes and peroxisomes) in biological cells. Recently, the Nobel Prize in Physiology or Medicine was awarded to Prof. Yoshinori Ohsumi from Japan for discovering the basic molecular mechanisms of Autophagy (2016). I discovered "Charnoly body" (CB) as a pre-apoptotic biomarker of CMB in the developing undernourished (UN) rat cerebellar Purkinje neurons and introduced "charnolophagy" (CB autophagy) which occurs by lysosomal activation due to free radical overproduction during physicochemical injury in the most vulnerable cells.

The CB is a universal biomarker of cell injury, whereas charnolophagy is a novel drug discovery target to evaluate CMB and ICD in health and disease. Charnolosome (CS) is a byproduct of CB and is implicated in the molecular pathogenesis of chronic illnesses. Hence, novel charnolopharmacotherapeutics can be developed by analyzing DSST combinatorial and correlative charnolosomics to accomplish the targeted, safe, and effective EBPT of NDDs, CVDs, and MDR malignancies for a better quality of life. By definition CB is a pleomorphic, electron-dense, multilamellar, quasi-crystalline, pre-apoptotic, universal biomarker of physico-chemical injury which is formed in the most vulnerable cell due to free radical-induced down-regulation of MB. Malnutrition, environmental toxins, heavy metal ions Hg^{2+}, Pb^{2+}, Cd^{2+}, Ni^{2+}, polychlorobiphenyls (PCBs), and microbial (bacteria, virus, and fungus) infections induce CB formation in the most vulnerable cells (like NPCs, CPCs, and EPCs, derived from iPPCs) due to free radical-induced mitochondrial degeneration. Nutritional rehabilitation, physiological Zn^{2+}, and MTs prevent CB formation as potent free radical scavengers and boosters of the MB. MTs and several other antioxidants prevent CB formation and augment charnolophagy during the acute phase and stabilize and facilitate CS exocytosis during the chronic phase as a basic molecular mechanism of ICD to prevent disease progression and remain healthy. Hence, CB, charnolophagy, and CS are novel drug discovery biomarkers and targets for NDDs, CVDs, MDR malignancies, and several other infectious and non-infectious diseases.

This book introduces the original discovery of CB as a universal biomarker of cell injury and CS as a novel drug development target of CMB. A CS is formed after charnolophagy in the most vulnerable cell in response to DPCI as an immediate and early attempt of ICD to remain healthy. This discovery opens a brand-new era of charnolomics and DSST charnolopharmacotherapeutics including CB agonists/antagonists, charnolophagy agonists/antagonists, and CS exocytosis enhancers, inhibitors, and stabilizers for the targeted, safe, and effective EBPT of NDDs (AD, PD, drug addiction, MDDs, and schizophrenia), CVDs, MDR malignancies, and numerous proinflammatory diseases beyond the scope of this book. Identification of CB contributes to understand the cellular, molecular, and genetic basis of conception and infertility, delayed eye conditioning response in fetal alcohol syndrome (FAS), drug addiction, PD, AD, HD, ALS, MS, aging, environmental neurotoxicity, CVDs, MDR malignancies, and numerous chronic inflammatory diseases. The book also describes origin, development, maturation, and degradation of CB and CS and their theranostic significance in health and disease.

It is important to emphasize that mitochondrial repair, rejuvenation, regeneration, and synthesis are constantly required to sustain normal MB and ICD. The accumulation of CBs in the most vulnerable cell triggers apoptotic cell death and eventually, morbidity and mortality due to release of highly toxic substances such as Cyt-C, iron, 8-hydroxy, 2 deoxy guanosine (as mitochondrial DNA oxidation product), 2,3, dihydroxy nonenal (as a byproduct of lipid peroxidation), glyceraldehyde phosphate dehydrogenase (GAPDH), acetaldehyde, H_2O_2, ammonia, lactic acid, Bax, caspase-3, and apoptosis-inducing factor (AIF) which induce further degeneration in chronic diseases. No other intracellular organelle and its metabolites are as toxic as compared to the mitochondrial metabolites in the structurally and functionally-labile CS. Hence, their disposal, particularly in chronic diseases, remains a significant challenge in MDR diseases. The condensation of free radical-induced degenerated mitochondrial membranes to form CB is an initial and early attempt to contain highly toxic Cyt-C, which is loosely and non-covalently attached to the inner mitochondrial membrane. The Cyt-C can be easily delocalized and scattered in the cell in response to any physico-chemical injury. Hence, CB formation is an immediate and early attempt to maintain ICD by condensing degenerated mitochondrial membranes in the most vulnerable cell during DPCI.

As CB is a nonfunctional intracellular inclusion, it is phagocytosed by a lysosome to form a charnolophagosome (CPS). The CPS is transformed to CS when the phagocytosed CB is hydrolyzed by the lysosomal enzymes. The CS is subsequently exocytosed by an energy (ATP)-driven process as a basic molecular mechanism of ICD as a secondary attempt to remain healthy. Thus, a physico-chemically-injured cell initially attempts to prevent CB formation and subsequently augments charnolophagy and CS exocytosis to remain free from toxins of mitochondrial metabolism to remain structurally and functionally-intact. Accumulation of CBs in the perinuclear regions can impair microRNAs-mediated signal transduction at the transcriptional and translational level to induce chronic diseases, and at the junction of the axon hillock, impairs the axoplasmic transport of ions, neurotransmitters, neurotropic factors (insulin like growth factor-1: IGF-1, and brain-derived neurotrophic factor: BDNF), enzymes, and mitochondria to cause initially synaptic silence during acute phase, followed by synaptic atrophy and synaptic degeneration during chronic phase of disease progression. Similarly, accumulation and destabilization of CB or CS at the junction of axon hillock releases toxic substances of mitochondrial metabolism to cause synaptic degeneration and early cognitive impairments in learning, intelligence, memory, and behavior. The CS destabilization and permeabilization can also induce atherosclerotic plaque rupture as noticed in coronary artery diseases and hemorrhagic stroke patients. Therefore, drugs may be developed to inhibit CB formation and augment charnolophagy during acute phase and stabilize CS and augment its exocytosis during chronic phase in NDDs and CVDs, and vice versa for the safe and effective EBPT of MDR malignancies. A nonspecific induction of CB formation in hyper proliferating cells during cancer chemotherapy causes adverse effects including: alopecia, myelosuppression, GIT symptoms, cardiovascular toxicity, neurotoxicity, infertility and selective degeneration of highly proliferating cells and organs rich in mitochondria. Hence, drugs may be developed to induce cancer stem cell-specific CB formation to cure MDR malignancies, chronic inflammations, and infections.

Natural abundance and genetic susceptibility of mtDNA qualify CB as an early, unique, and sensitive universal biomarker of clinical significance. Indeed, a balanced diet and moderate exercise alleviate clinical symptoms of various chronic diseases by activating anti-inflammatory, antioxidant, and antiapoptotic metal (Zn^{2+})-binding proteins. Particularly, MTs prevent CB formation and its interconversion to CS, inflammasome, apoptosome, necroapoptosome, and metallosome, and are involved in the etiopathogenesis of NDDs, CVDs, and MDR malignancies. Recently, I reported that nutritional rehabilitation, physiological Zn^{2+}, and MTs confer theranostic potential as potent free radical scavengers and mitochondrial protective agents. Hence, a balanced diet rich in antioxidants and moderate exercise can alleviate clinical symptoms of pro-inflammatory and apoptotic events in chronic diseases. MTs as potent antioxidants and free radical scavengers induce charnolophagy, CS stabilization, and CS exocytosis as a basic molecular mechanism of ICD to prevent chronic diseases as highlighted in this book.

It is now well-established that translocation of MTs in the nucleus is implicated in storing, buffering, and sequestering Zn^{2+} ions. MTs-mediated release of Zn^{2+} regulates transcriptional activation of genes and triggers microRNA synthesis involved in DNA cell cycle, cell growth, proliferation, migration, differentiation, and development through the induction of AgNOR. The AgNOR induction in the nucleolus enhances ribosomal formation for protein synthesis on the rough endoplasmic reticulum (RER) depending on the extent of Zn^{2+}-induced transcriptional activation of microRNAs during induction/repression of mitochondrial and nuclear genes. Free radical-induced destabilization of CS releases toxic mitochondrial metabolites and inhibits protein synthesis involved in normal growth and development by inhibiting AgNOR and by preventing poly-ribosomal assembly on the RER membranes as observed in developing UN rat cerebellar Purkinje neurons and in chronic patients of cancer, drug addiction, AD, and aging as described in this book.

The origin, development, maturation, and degradation of CB facilitates further understanding the cellular, molecular, and genetic basis of ZIKV-induced microcephaly, FASD in new born infants, and Guillain Barre Syndrome (GBS) in adults as described in detail in my recently published books "ZIKV Disease; Prevention & Cure" and Fetal Alcohol Spectrum Disorders: Concepts, Mechanisms, and Cure, Nova Science Publishers, New York, U.S.A. This book elucidates the basic molecular mechanism of depression, drug addiction, and progressive NDDs such as: PD, AD, MS, HD, ALS, environmental neurotoxicity, infertility, drug addiction, alcoholism, aging, CVDs, and many other MDR diseases (including malignancies with special reference to free radicals-induced CMB and induction of DSST charnolopathies).

The mtDNA is a highly sensitive, GC-rich, intron-less, transmitted exclusively through the female germ line, double-stranded, circular molecule of 16569 bp and contains 37 genes coding for two rRNAs, 22 tRNAs, and 13 polypeptides, which remains in a hostile microenvironment of free radicals, generated as a byproduct of oxidative phosphorylation in the electron transport chain. Hence, genetic and epigenetic modification occur more readily in the mtDNA as compared to nuclear DNA. The DNA methylating molecule, S-adenosyl methionine (SAM) is synthesized in the mitochondria by methionine and ATP in the presence of an enzyme, methyl transferase to cause mtDNA methylation at N-3 position of the cytosine residue to induce epigenetic changes. The mtDNA is oxidized to synthesize 8-OH, 2dG, which may be estimated from the serum, plasma, CSF, amniotic fluid, saliva, tear, toe nails, hair, and urine samples along with estimation of cytosine, methyl cytosine, and hydroxymethyl cytosine to clinically evaluate epigenetic changes as well as mtDNA oxidation simultaneously by microtiter colorimetric ELISA, immunoblotting, RT-PCR, cDNA microarray, antibody microarrays, flow cytometry, capillary electrophoresis, next generation sequencing, LC-MS analysis, and surface plasmon resonance (SPR) spectroscopy as described systematically in this book.

It is important to emphasize that soon after fertilization, CB formation occurs in the middle piece of the spermatocyte due to down-regulation of MB in the oocyte. The paternal CB in the oocyte is eliminated soon after the conception by energy (ATP)-driven lysosomal-dependent charnolophagy. Subsequently, CS is eliminated by ATP-dependent exocytosis as a basic molecular mechanism of ICD for the normal growth, proliferation, and development of an embryo. Mother Nature has provided between 22–75 spirally-arranged and condensely-packed mitochondria in the middle piece for sperm motility and translocation of paternal nuclear DNA to hybridize with the oocyte nuclear DNA during fertilization. However, a considerable amount of energy (ATP) is required for charnolophagy and CS exocytosis. Hence, an oocyte has as many as 200,000 to 600,000 mitochondria, which also participate in the normal growth and development of the fetus during the post-zygotic phase in addition to their involvement in paternal charnolophagy and CS exocytosis to prevent zygote death which can occur in severe malnutrition, nicotine addiction, binge drinking, severe microbial (bacteria, virus, fungus) infection, and in response to certain drugs and environmental neurotoxins.

As the number of mitochondria (usually > 1000) are more compared to the lysosomes in a cell, charnolophagy is compromised in severe malnutrition, microbial infections, aging, progressive NDDs, CVDs, and cancer. These deleterious events pose a significant challenge in ICD and may trigger denaturation/aggregation of intracellular proteins in chronic MDR diseases as illustrated systematically in this book. In addition, I have proposed the charnolophagy index as a sensitive biomarker to quantitatively assess ICD. CB formation occurs in chronic NDDs, CVDs, and drug addiction, where it induces early aging, morbidity, and mortality by augmenting the microRNA-induced apoptotic signaling cascade. However, CB formation is attenuated due to induction of genes (particularly MTs, cmyc, P[53], HSPs, and heat shock factor-α) involved in cellular immortalization in MDR malignancies in cancer stem cells. Hence, it is logical to assume that *"Life begins and ends with CB"*, because "functionally-efficient mitochondrial bioenergetics sustains our health; whereas CMB triggers CB formation involved in charnolophagy as a basic molecular mechanism of ICD or apoptotic cell death due the release of highly toxic mitochondrial metabolites to induce acute or chronic diseases." Although, microRNAs are quite stable, the release of toxic substances from free radical-induced destabilized CS inhibits their post-transcriptional activity, and significantly influences their normal function in a physico-chemically-injured cell. The CS destabilization is characterized by permeabilization and sequestration during the acute phase, and fragmentation during the chronic phase of the disease progression.

The basic molecular mechanism of ICD by charnolophagy is compromised due to DPCI and in chronic MDR diseases in the most vulnerable cells.

Free radicals are produced as a byproduct of oxidative phosphorylation during ATP synthesis in the electron transport chain in the mitochondria. Thus, any physico-chemical injury to a cell poses a tremendous physiological burden of energy (ATP) requirement by the mitochondria to maintain ICD. During DPCI, the mitochondria are destroyed by their own free radicals due to lipid peroxidation and mtDNA oxidation, accompanied with structural and functional breakdown of polyunsaturated fatty acids (PUFA: linoic acid, linolinic acid, and arachidonic acid) in the plasma membrane and Cyt-C release. In addition, free radicals induce proteases to cause proteolysis, lipases to cause lipolysis, and nucleases to cause DNA fragmentation resulting in apoptosis and/or necrosis.

A degenerating CS is potentially harmful, particularly when it starts releasing iron, Cyt-C, GAPDH, heme iron, ammonia, acetaldehyde, H_2O_2, 2.3 dihydroxy noncnal, 8-OH, 2dG, and peptides like apoptosis-inducing factor (AIF), caspase-3, Bax and Bid due to CPS induction and CS destabilization. CB formation also occurs in a normally aging cell due to CMB in response to free radical-induced down-regulation of the mitochondrial genome and microRNAs, triggering molecular pathogenesis. However, this natural process of mitochondrial degeneration is very slow and occurs primarily in very old age. We confirmed these findings in cultured mitochondrial genome knock out (RhO_{mgko}) human DArgic (SK-N-SH, and SH-SY5Y) neurons as *in vitro* experimental models of stroke, PD, AD, drug addiction, MDD, and aging. The charnolophagy index was increased as a function of increasing concentrations of 1-methyl, 4-phenyl, 1, 2, 3, 6 tetrahydropyridinium (MPP^+) treatment in the DAergic cell lines in culture. The charnolophagy index was proportional to the α-synuclein index, involved in neurodegenerative α-synucleinopathies.

Indeed! CB, charnolophagy, charnolophagy index, CPS, CS, and CS bodies as excellent drug discovery targets and biomarkers to develop novel charnolopharmacotherapeutics are now well established, published, and quoted in several international journals of high impact factor. Hence, further systematic studies along this direction will go a long way in the targeted, safe, and effective EBPT of various NDDs, CVDs, and MDR malignancies as elegantly described in this book.

CB Discovery

I was conducting basic research on developing normal (N) and undernourished (UN) rat cerebellar Purkinje neurons employing neurochemical, electrophysiological, neuromorphological, and neuropharmacological studies at the light and electron microscopic level as a Research Officer and Ph.D. student, in the Department of Neurology at the A.I.I.M.S., New Delhi (India) during the early eighties. At the ultrastructural level, I discovered peculiar, pleomorphic, quasi-crystalline, multi-lamellar, electron-dense membrane stacks of degenerated mitochondrial membranes in the developing UN rat cerebellar Purkinje neuron dendrites and synaptic terminals possessing maximum number of highly susceptible mitochondria. Subsequently, I named these pleomorphic structures as "Charnoly bodies (CBs)" as a token of love, respect, and appreciation to my late mother "Charnoly".

This book describes the clinical significance of CB in accomplishing the EBPT of progressive NDDs, CVDs, and cancer. The book describes particularly free radical-induced CB formation, charnolophagy, and CS destabilization as biomarkers of microRNA down-regulation and novel DSST charnolopharmacotherapeutics for the targeted, safe, and effective EBPT of chronic MDR diseases, involving mitochondrial oxidative and ER stress, inflammation, and apoptosis.

The most unique feature of this book is that it presents a novel concept of DSST charnolosomics which can be accomplished with cDNA, antibody, and nanoparticle probes employing state-of the art biotechnologies (such as LC-MS, fluorescent multiplex ELISA, capillary electrophoresis, flow cytometry, next generation sequencing, magnetic resonance spectroscopy, and SPR spectroscopy) to determine the MB implicated in ICD for normal cellular function and homeostasis to remain healthy. Correlative and combinatorial bioinformatics of DSST charnolosomic microarrays in combination with conventional omics employing genomics, proteomics, metabolomics, metallomics, and lipidomics microarray analysis can provide precise information to accomplish the targeted, safe, and effective EBPT of progressive NDDs, CVDs, and chronic MDR malignancies for a better quality of life.

In earlier studies, I described the clinical significance of α-synuclein index (SI) in the differential diagnosis of progressive neurodegenerative α-synucleinopathies. This book introduces systematically-described the original discovery of CB as a universal biomarker of cellular injury and novel concepts of charnolophagy index and CS stability index (CSSI) for the EBPT of chronic MDR diseases, such as AD, PD, stroke, ALS, HD, MS, MDDS, schizophrenia, multiple drug addiction, CVDs, and cancer. More specifically, it describes the clinical significance of CB, charnolophagy, and CS-labelled NPs and radiotracers to quantitatively assess the MB, microRNAs, and ICD and to discover novel DSST charnolopharmacotherapeutics for the safe and effective EBPT of MDR diseases with currently limited therapeutic options.

This book is divided in three major parts: Part-I General introduction of CB which describes its basic cellular and molecular biology; Part-II Emerging biotechnology in CB research; and Part-III Clinical significance of DSST, CB, and CS in EBPT.

The primary objective of presenting this unique manuscript is to motivate, guide, and inspire young budding scientists to work hard and think rationally without any reservation and/or hesitation. Sometimes your guides, mentors, teachers, and professional colleagues may ignore your hard-earned original research work as happened with Alexander Fleming during his original discovery of Penicillin. So, we should not be scared that we are alone in this venture. Several others have already undergone through hardships and accomplished difficult tasks and several others are ready to experience similar social, physical, mental, economical, and psychological stresses, irrespective of their profession.

Any invention, innovation, and/or discovery passes through different phases of ignorance, straight-forward rejection, frustration, professional jealousy, laughter, serious consideration, and eventually national and international recognition as a function of time. Let me share with you the following nice words Professor Luis

Pasteur said on his 70th birthday which was being celebrated at the National level in France: "*Future will belong to those who have suffered for humanity*". Luis Pasteur suffered for humanity even though he did not receive a Nobel Prize like Professor Robert Koch, Madam Marie Currie, and Alexander Fleming.

CB is formed as an early pre-apoptotic biomarker in the most vulnerable cell due to free radical-induced CMB and is a universal biomarker of DPCI. CB, charnolophagy, and CS were also discovered in the cultured human DArgic (SK-N-SH and SH-SY5Y) neurons due to $\Delta\Psi$ collapse and mtDNA down-regulation in RhO_{mgko} neurons as a cellular model of aging.

Based on the original discovery of CB in the developing UN Purkinje neurons of the rat cerebellar cortex and in the intrauterine domoic acid exposed developing mice, a novel concept of charnolopharmacotherapeutics was introduced as described in my several manuscripts and books.

This book describes the clinical significance of CB as a novel biomarker of CMB in chronic diseases. The development of drugs based on CB-based CMB promises to have either minimum or no adverse effects and an increased therapeutic index with acceptable margin of safety. Hence, DSST-CB agonists/antagonists, charnolophagy agonists/antagonists, CPS and CS stabilizers/destabilizers, and CB sequestrates/desequestrates are introduced for the safe and effective treatment of progressive NDDs, CVDs, cancer, and infectious diseases (including: ZIKV, cytomegalovirus, and rubella virus) for the first time in this book.

This manuscript provides an original and unique approach to treat chronic intractable diseases and will serve as a "Text Book" for biomedical students (M.D., M.Sc., Ph.D., D.Sc.), nurses, and other healthcare professionals; and "Reference Book" for doctors, researchers, professors, and public. All universities, medical schools, and public libraries across the globe will be interested in going through the original, thought-provoking, motivating concepts, and basic molecular mechanisms of charnolopathies and CB-based charnolopharmacotherapeutics as described elegantly in this book.

This book confers original thought-provoking basic concepts and mechanisms to explore further in the multidisciplinary areas of EBPT. The book is not simply based on the conventional wisdom and existing literature evidence as it has a significant component of nonconventional wisdom and highlights lacunae in our existing knowledge regarding basic molecular mechanisms of diversified charnolopathies involved in chronic diseases and potential theranostic strategies of targeting CMB-based CB formation, charnolophagy, and CS exocytosis for ICD to remain healthy.

CB molecular pathogenesis occurs primarily in three major phases. Phase-1: synaptic silence involving mild cognitive impairment (MCI); Phase-2: synaptic atrophy involving early morbidity; and Phase-3: synaptic degeneration involving early mortality as noticed in cerebral palsy, Down's syndrome, progeria, AD, PD, ALS, MS, HD, schizophrenia, multiple drug addiction, and MDDs.

The book also explains how the nonspecific induction of CB formation causes alopecia, myelosuppression, and GIT abnormalities in MDR malignancies, and evaluates how drugs may be developed to prevent/inhibit CB formation and augment MB to enhance charnolophagy as a basic molecular mechanism of ICD. More specifically, it describes how novel drugs may be developed to prevent CS destabilization, permeabilization, sequestration, and/or fragmentation. Although charnolostatic drugs for the treatment of chronic intractable diseases will be clinically-beneficial to control acute disease states, charnolocidals will be required for chronic MDR diseases particularly for the immunocompromised and aging patients.

While going through the interesting and thought-provoking concepts and mechanisms involved in disease progression/regression, the readers will enhance their basic knowledge regarding charnolophagy, CPS, CS, and ICD in relation to down-regulation of microRNA-mediated post-transcription of genes involved in DNA cell cycle, proliferation, migration, differentiation, and development to remain healthy. The book also provides the molecular mechanism of CB formation, charnolophagy, and CS as novel drug discovery targets in chronic inflammatory diseases (CIDs) including; depression, AD, PD, FASD, MDDs, schizophrenia, chronic drug addiction, infectious disease, CVDs, and MDR malignancies.

The concepts and mechanisms described are original, interesting, thought-provoking, and will motivate young scientists, doctors, and other health care professionals to explore further in this clinically-significant and challenging area to discover novel charnolopharmacotherapeutics for a better quality of life. Novel charnolopharmacotherapeutics and the crucial role of genomics, microRNA, and epigenomics in sustaining MB by CB prevention/inhibition, charnolophagy induction to maintain ICD, and CS stabilization are original and clinically-significant for the prevention and/or treatment of CIDs. Hence, drugs augmenting MB by inhibiting CB formation, augmenting charnolophagy during the acute phase, and inhibiting CB formation and CS destabilization during the chronic phase will be promising for the EBPT of CIDs, as elegantly described in this book.

It is well-established that antioxidants (glutathione, MTs, CoQ_{10}, melatonin, selegiline, polyphenols (resveratrol), flavonoids, sirtuin, rutin, lycopene, and catechin) inhibit CB formation as free radical scavengers. Although they can pass through the blood brain barrier readily, their reduced potency necessitates bulk consumption. Hence, ROS-scavenging antioxidant-loaded NPs may be developed to improve CNS delivery to enhance MB and charnolophagy in CIDs. MTs provide neuroprotection by regulating Zn^{2+}-mediated transcriptional regulation of genes involved in microRNA synthesis implicated in normal or abnormal growth, proliferation, differentiation, development, and invasion. MTs also inhibit MAOs activation, and TRPC and TSPOs delocalization to prevent CB formation and CS destabilization by augmenting (a) lysosome-sensitive CB (LSCB) formation during acute phase and (b) by preventing lysosome-resistant CB (LRCB) formation during the chronic phase of disease progression. Particularly, this book provides emerging concepts of MB, genomics, and epigenomics of CIDs with ROS scavenging antioxidant loaded NPs to accomplish EBPT of chronic MDR diseases.

It is well-known that brain regional induction of MAO-A and MAO-B-specific CBs induces the down-regulation of monoaminergic (NE-ergic, 5HT-ergic, and DA-ergic) neurotransmission to cause cognitive impairments in CIDs. This book presents MB-based CB prevention/inhibition, charnolophagy induction, and CS stabilization for executing normal microRNAs-mediated post-transcriptional regulation of disease-specific genes as potential therapeutic targets for the safe and effective treatment of CIDs. Particularly, malnutrition, FASD, ZIKV disease, AD, PD, CVDs, and MDR malignancies are described as DSST charnolopathies and the development of novel charnolopharmacotherapeutics for their targeted, safe and effective cure.

This book augments the existing knowledge and wisdom regarding CIDs and their safe and effective clinical management by targeting CB-induced CMB. The CMB is characterized by down-regulation of mitochondrial membrane potential ($\Delta\Psi$ collapse), formation of megapores, influx of calcium ions due to TRPCs, MAOs, and TSPO delocalization, membrane fragmentation, aggregation, and condensation to trigger CB formation and induce charnolophagy, followed by CPS and CS destabilization involved in degenerative apoptosis and chronic intractable diseases.

More specifically, this book describes the original discovery of CB and its origin and life cycle, classification of CB, and maternal and paternal CB formation during conception, CB formation and its elimination during normal embryonic growth and development, classification of CB based on structure and genetic susceptibility; MAO-A and MAO-B-specific CB formation and its therapeutic significance; inducers of CB formation including (a) drugs, (b) environmental toxins, (c) microbial infections, and (d) life style; prevention of CB formation by antioxidants such as sirtuins, rutins, resveratrol, (e) diet and exercise; charnolophagy and its clinical significance. Furthermore, it illustrates CPS and its clinical significance; CB in health and disease (basic concepts and mechanisms); therapeutic potential of MTs as CB antagonists in obesity, hippocampal CB formation in MDDs, epilepsy, and AD; medio basal-hypothalamic CB formation in bulimia; transcriptional regulation of CB formation, genetics, and epigenetics of CB formation; CB as a universal biomarker of cell injury; CB formation in the hippocampus and medio-basal hypothalamus in dementia and obesity; CB as a novel therapeutic target of drug discovery; clinical significance of charnolophagy in personalized theranostics; early detection of CS biomarkers and their clinical significance; charnolosomics in EBPT; and DSST circulating CS biomarkers and their clinical significance in EBPT. In addition, cancer stem cell specific CS vs normal CS; cancer stem cell-specific CS biomarkers vs normal CS biomarkers; disease-specific cellular and circulating CS biomarkers; charnolopharmacotherapeutics as charnolophagy agonist/antagonists; and future prospect of CB-based research in novel drug discovery and EBPT are described in detail.

Although, it is generally believed that only maternal fetal alcohol abuse can induce diversified embryopathies in the developing fetus, I have now evidence to suggest that chronic ethanol abuse by both parents can induce deleterious consequences in the developing embryo. The original discovery of CB formation, charnolophagy, CPS formation, and CS exocytosis at the ultrastructural level provide scientific evidence to propose that both paternal as well as maternal mitochondria participate in the normal fertilization and subsequent growth and development of an embryo during the postzygotic phase.

Recently, I reported that intrauterine ethanol exposure causes apoptosis of the most vulnerable NPCs, derived from iPPCs via CB formation. Generally, two types of CBs are formed during fetal alcohol exposure (FAE): (a) lysosome-sensitive CB formation (LSCB) during the acute phase and (b) lysosome-resistant CB (LRCB) formation during the chronic phase. The LSCB is subjected to charnolophagy as an efficient basic molecular mechanism of ICD. Following charnolophagy, the lysosome becomes almost 2.5 times enlarged, electron-dense, and can be easily distinguished from the normal lysosomes. An abnormally enlarged lysosome, possessing phagocytosed CBs is classified as CPS. When CB is hydrolyzed in the CPS, it is named as CS. The CS is a relatively more unstable and toxic intracellular organelle as compared to CPS and is eliminated by exocytosis. Intrauterine ethanol and/or nicotine exposure can inhibit or impair charnolophagy, induce CPS destabilization/sequestration, and inhibit CS exocytosis to trigger charnolopathies, involved in diversified embryopathies. Thus, microbial infections and drugs of abuse (nicotine and alcohol) compromise zygote detoxification and trigger charnolopathies, involved in diversified embryopathies including microcephaly and other congenital anomalies. These basic molecular events are highly crucial for the ICD, cell proliferation, differentiation, and normal development of the fetus during the intrauterine life.

Based on two types of monoamine oxidases (i.e., MAO-A, and MAO-B) on the outer mitochondrial membranes and their heterogeneous micro-distribution in the brain, I have proposed two types of CBs: that is, (i) MAO-A and (ii) MAO-B-specific CB formation in response to toxins, which can cause down-regulation of NE-ergic, 5HT-ergic, and DA-ergic neurotransmission, respectively, involved in sensorimotor and cognitive impairments, and chronic intractable diseases such as PD, AD, ALS, HD, MS, MDDs, drug addiction, and schizophrenia. This book promotes existing knowledge by introducing novel concepts, mechanisms, and the cure of diversified charnolopathies/embryopathies with DDST charnolopharmacotherapeutics. The deleterious consequences of DPCI are described right from the pre-conceptional stage. The DSST-MB of both spermatocytes and oocytes, and toxins-induced CB formation, compromised charnolophagy, CS destabilization, and microRNAs down-regulation are unique, and are described for the prevention and/or cure of chronic diseases by antioxidants and novel charnolopharmacotherapeutics.

Although, several concepts, mechanisms, and potential therapeutics have been introduced recently in the healthcare arena to overcome the deleterious consequences of chronic intractable diseases, I have now proposed a novel concept of charnolopharmacology, that is, based on DSST-CMB and charnolopathies in the most vulnerable developing and aging cells. Hence, drugs inhibiting CB formation and/or augmenting charnolophagy as a basic molecular mechanism of ICD during the acute phase, and stabilizing CPS, and preventing CB and CPS/CS sequestration during the chronic phase will have promising therapeutic potential in NDDs, CVDs, and cancer. The book is primarily focused on conferring novel preventive and theranostic strategies for the clinical management of chronic intractable diseases such as FAS, AD, PD, CVDs, and MDR malignancies with deleterious consequences and how to prevent or treat them by developing safe and effective DSST charnolopharmacotherapeutics for a better quality of life.

The number of mitochondria (usually > 1000) is more than lysosomes in a cell, hence charnolophagy as a primary molecular mechanism of ICD is compromised in severe malnutrition, aging, chronic and progressive NDDs, CVDs, and in MDR malignancies. The primary highlights of this book are as follows:

(i) Functionally-efficient MB keeps us healthy whereas free radical-induced CMB triggers CB formation involved in either charnolophagy or apoptotic cell death due the release of toxic substances from the degenerating mitochondria.

(ii) Mitochondrial repair, rejuvenation, and regeneration is constantly required to maintain intracellular bioenergetics for ICD to remain healthy.

(iii) CB formation is triggered due to CMB. The CB is a highly unstable, pre-apoptotic, pleomorphic, multi-lamellar (usually penta or heptalemellar), quasi-crystalline, electron-dense stack of primarily degenerated mitochondria, that is formed in a highly vulnerable cell (such as NPCs and CPCs, derived from iPPCs) due to free radical-induced oxidative and nitrative stress.

(iv) Accumulation of CBs triggers apoptotic cell death and eventually morbidity and mortality form degenerating mitochondrial membranes, proteins, and DNA.

 (v) Degenerating mitochondria are potentially harmful particularly when they start releasing toxic substances such as Cyt-C, iron, acetaldehyde, acetone, H_2O_2, ammonia, heme iron, and other proteins like Bax, Bid, caspase-3, and AIF due to CB sequestration, inducing apoptosis to cause cell death as occurs in normal aging due to the down-regulation of the MB. These findings were confirmed in mitochondrial genome knock out (RhO_{mgko}) cells as an *in vitro* model of aging.

(vi) This book describes the origin, development, maturation, and degradation of CB and its clinical significance in NDDs, CVDs, and cancer in addition to chronic MDR infections. The appearance and disappearance of CB is a reversible process as it can be regulated by microRNA-mediated nuclear or mitochondrial gene manipulation. The CB formation is eliminated by nutritional rehabilitation as we discovered in developing UN rat Purkinje neurons. CB formation does not occur under normal physiological conditions and is eliminated efficiently by lysosomes, as an energy (ATP)-driven process called "charnolophagy" to represent CB autophagy as a basic molecular mechanism of ICD. The persistence of CB in any vulnerable cell is potentially harmful as it can lead to progressive NDDs, CVDs, and cancer.

(vii) Recently, I proposed that CB can be utilized as an early, sensitive, and universal biomarker of cell injury. I also proposed charnolostatic drugs for acute cell injury and charnolocidal drugs for the prevention and treatment of chronic NDDs and CVDs, and charnolomimetic drugs for the safe and effective treatment of cancer. Nonspecific induction of CB is involved in alopecia, GIT distress, and myelosuppression in MDR malignancies. Hence, drugs may be developed to prevent CB formation in the follicle for the hair growth and regeneration. Further investigations in this direction will go a long way in the safe and effective clinical management of chronic intractable MDR diseases (Sharma and Ebadi 2014a).

(viii) To make this book more interesting particularly for the young biomedical students and scientists, I have written in very simple and straight-forward language. In addition to biomedical students and paramedical professionals, the book will be of considerable interest for the general-public, accomplished and well-experienced biomedical scientists, doctors, professors, nurses, and researchers.

Rationale of Mitochondrial Vulnerability. (i) Mitochondria serve as constant source of energy (ATP) in a cell and maintain the intracellular homeostasis and detoxification. (ii) Free radicals are generated in the mitochondria as a byproduct of oxidative phosphorylation during ATP synthesis in the electron transport chain. (iii) Mitochondrial membranes are highly rich in PUFA (linoic acid linolinic acid, and arachidonic acid), which render them highly vulnerable to free radical-induced lipid peroxidation. (iv) The mtDNA is GC-rich, which renders it highly susceptible to oxidation at guanosine and methylation at the cytosine moiety to induce genetic and epigenetic modifications. (v) The mtDNA is non-helical, intron-less, and remains in a hostile microenvironment of free radicals ($\cdot$OH, NO$\cdot$, CO$\cdot$). (vi) Mitochondria contain highly toxic metabolites such as Cyt-C, GAPDH, 8-OH, 2dG, 2, 3 dihydroxy nonenal, acetaldehyde, acetone, ammonia, and H$_2$O$_2$. The release of these toxic substance can induce spontaneous apoptosis and/or necrosis to trigger chronic MDR diseases. Hence, CB formation is an immediate and early attempt of ICD to contain highly toxic mitochondrial metabolites in a physico-chemically-injured cell.

CB is an immediate early and most sensitive pre-apoptotic biomarker of CMB. DPCI and many drugs enhance CB formation in the most vulnerable cells such as NPCs, CPCs, EPCs, and OPCs, derived from iPPCs cells to induce microcephaly, craniofacial abnormalities, and other embryopathies in FASD victims. CB formation, charnolophagy, CPS, and CS can serve as early, pre-apoptotic biomarkers of CMB and can be detected at a much earlier stage of disease progression as intracellular neuronal inclusions in NDDs and other chronic diseases. Natural abundance of mitochondria and genetic and epigenetic susceptibility of mtDNA qualify CB as an early, unique, and sensitive universal biomarker of clinical significance.

The most important events in CB molecular pathogenesis are the efficient induction of energy-driven charnolophagy (CB autophagy) and CS exocytosis as a basic molecular mechanism of ICD. The CS is structurally and functionally highly labile intracellular organelle and is readily destabilized by free radical attack. The destabilized CS releases highly toxic mitochondrial metabolites through permeabilization, sequestration, and fragmentation depending on the frequency and intensity of free radical attack which disrupts microRNA-mediated transcriptional regulation of genes involved in normal cell growth, DNA cell cycle, proliferation, differentiation, and development. Glutathione and MTs provide structural and functional stability to CS by maintaining intracellular sanitation and normal post-transcriptional regulation of microRNAs. Hence, CB and microRNA-based biomarkers can be utilized to differentially diagnose and effectively treat preclinical stages of progressive NDDs (such as PD, AD, drug addiction, schizophrenia, and MDDs), CVDs, and MDR malignancies (Sharma 2016, 2017, 2018).

Free radicals are generated as a byproduct of mitochondrial oxidative phosphorylation in the electron transport chain; CB is the byproduct of primary free radical-induced CMB. Charnolophagy is a byproduct of ATP-dependent lysosomal autophagy of CB, whereas CS is a byproduct of phagocytosed CB when it is completely hydrolyzed by the lysosomal enzymes; CS body is the byproduct of secondary free radical-induced CS destabilization due to lipid peroxidation; Apoptotic body is the byproduct of CS body destabilization; Apoptosis is a byproduct of apoptotic body disintegration; NDDs and CVDs are byproducts of degenerative apoptosis; and MDR malignancy is a byproduct of inhibited apoptosis. Hence, DSST charnolopharmacotherapeutics can be developed to inhibit cancer stem cell specific CS destabilization involved in malignant transformation of nonproliferating cells. DPCI-induced cortisol release augments CB formation, whereas MTs, IGF-1, and BDNF inhibit hippocampal CB formation, augment charnolophagy, CS stabilization, and exocytosis (involved in post-transcriptional regulation of microRNAs) to prevent early morbidity and mortality in neurodegenerative α-synucleinopathies such as PD, AD, HD, ALS, and MS, schizophrenia, drug addiction, and MDDs.

Compensation-effect doctrine states that accumulated mtDNA mutations in the cell must reach a certain set threshold before they have a negative effect on cellular function from mtDNA (Chen et al. 2013). However, accumulation of aberrant mtRNA transcribed from mtDNA mutations negatively influences cellular function through complex internal and external mitochondrial pathways, and might be a significant cause of aging and aging-associated diseases due to CB formation, impaired charnolophagy, and CS destabilization, leading to down-regulation of microRNA-mediated post-transcriptional regulation of genes involved in DNA cell cycle, cell proliferation, differentiation, development, and malignant transformation (Sharma 2017).

TEM analysis revealed that ER stress occurs primarily in the dendritic regions and in the growth cones, where active protein synthesis takes place; whereas the mitochondrial oxidative stress and CB formation occurs more frequently at the synaptic region of developing UN rat Purkinje neurons to induce initially synaptic silence, followed by synaptic atrophy, and eventually synaptic degeneration depending on the frequency and intensity of free radical-induced CS destabilization, involving permeabilization, sequestration, and fragmentation, respectively.

The mitochondrial and ER-stress inhibits AgNOR to disrupt nucleolar synthesis of ribosomes required for the protein synthesis (particularly mitofusion, involved in the synthesis and repair of mitochondria) during DPCI. E.R. stress was noticed primarily in the dendrites and growth cones, whereas the mitochondrial oxidative stress occurred primarily in the synaptic terminals during DPCI in the most vulnerable cell. Thus, CB formation in the synaptic region can induce synaptic silence, synaptic atrophy, and eventually synaptic degeneration, depending on the free radical-induced CS permeabilization, sequestration, and/or fragmentation to cause mild cognitive impairment (MCI) during the acute phase, and morbidity and mortality during the chronic phase, respectively in NDDs, CVDs, and MDR malignancies.

MTs provide neuroprotection by preventing and/or inhibiting CB formation during the acute phase, and by augmenting charnolophagy and stabilizing CS during the chronic phase by serving as potent free radical scavengers in MDR diseases. MTs also provide ubiquinone (CoQ_{10})-mediated neuroprotection by inhibiting CB formation, augmenting charnolophagy, preventing CS destabilization, and by augmenting CS exocytosis as a basic molecular mechanism of MB, ICD, and post-transcriptional regulation of microRNAs for health and prolongevity (Sharma 2016, 2017, 2018). Brain regional down-regulation of MTs-induced Zn^{2+} homeostasis in aging is involved in mitochondrial degeneration, CB formation, CS destabilization, and impaired CS exocytosis to trigger neurodegenerative apoptosis due to impaired microRNA-mediated post-transcriptional activity in early cognitive impairment, morbidity, and mortality (Sharma et al. 2013; Sharma 2016; Sharma 2016; Sharma 2017). Free radicals-induced CS destabilization triggers epigenetic modifications and disrupts microRNA-mediated post-transcriptional regulation of genes involved in DNA cell cycle, proliferation, differentiation, and development. Hyper-methylation of the promoter region of IGF-1 gene causes insulin-resistant (Type-2) diabetes; hyper methylation of the promoter region of VEGF gene causes stroke; hyper methylation of the promoter regions of nicotinic acetyl choline receptor (nAChR) gene is involved nicotinism and multiple drug addiction, whereas hyper methylation of the promoter region of leptin gene in the medio-basal hypothalamic region causes bulimia and obesity.

Two main hypotheses have been proposed in the etiopathogenesis of AD. These are (a) amyloid-β (Aβ-1-42) hypothesis and (b) mitochondrial hypothesis. According to amyloid-β hypothesis, AD occurs due to abnormal accumulation of Aβ-1-42 in the senile plaques in the cortical ribbon. This hypothesis was confirmed by detecting Aβ-1-42 in the autopsy AD samples using Congo-Red and by immunohistochemical analyses using specific Aβ-1-42 antibody in the senile plaques of AD patients. The senile plaques can be detected *in vivo* by performing ^{18}F-PiB (^{18}F-Florbetapir) PET neuroimaging in AD patients. The Aβ-1-42 hypothesis was further confirmed by observing the progression of neurobehavioral symptoms with neurodegeneration and cognitive impairment proportional to the number of amyloid-β 1-42 containing senile plaques. It is now believed that the truncated form of Aβ-1-42 is particularly involved in the etiopathogenesis of AD. Nevertheless, several AD patients do not exhibit amyloid-β senile plaques in their brain yet exhibit progressive cholinergic and other neurodegeneration as a function of time due to free radical-induced CMB and lipid peroxidation of the mitochondrial membranes by structural and functional breakdown of PUFA. The MB can be evaluated *in vivo* by performing ^{18}FdG PET neuroimaging. AD patients exhibit distinct loss of glucose metabolism in the fronto-temporal regions, ventriculomegaly, and hippocampal atrophy accompanied with trans-callosal and cerebral atrophy due to the induction of CB molecular pathogenesis early in life. Hence, fluid biomarkers such as 8-OH, 2DG, lactate, glutamate, choline, and N-acetyl aspartate (NAA), acetate, ammonia, and H_2O_2 can be estimated as rudiments of CB formation. Platelets, lymphocytes, buccal cells, and skin cells can be cultured and used to examine ΔΨ collapse using sensitive fluorescent indicator, dihydrofluorescein, JC-1, or rhodamine to assess MB and CB molecular pathogenesis at an earlier stage of disease progression as described in this book.

CB formation in the hippocampal region causes AD, in the NS-DAergic region causes PD, and in the medio-basal hypothalamic region causes bulimia and obesity. CB formation may also be utilized as an early and sensitive biomarker of neurodegeneration in MDDs. Nonspecific induction of CB formation in MDR malignancies, causes GIT distress, myelosuppression, alopecia, pulmonary fibrosis, cardiovascular and renal damage, and infertility (Sharma et al. 2013; Sharma 2014; Li et al. 2014). Hence, DSST novel CB antagonists may be developed as natural or synthetic antioxidants, anti-inflammatory, and anti-apoptotic agents to prevent CB formation and its inhibition during acute phase, charnolophagy agonists during the intermediate phase, and CB/CS sequestration inhibitors as intracellular detoxifiers during chronic phase as safe and effective theranostics in NDDs and CVDs, and vice versa for the EBPT of MDR malignancies.

It remains unknown whether epigenetic changes in the mtDNA and microRNAs can modify CB molecular pathogenesis involving charnolophagy and CS pharmacodynamics in chronic diseases. Hence, drugs may be developed to inhibit CB formation and augment microRNAs-mediated post-transcription in progressive NDDs and CVDs and vice versa for the EBPT of MDR malignancies. Hence, charnolophagy seems more appropriate to describe "CB autophagy and CS exocytosis" as a basic molecular mechanism of ICD. The clinical management of patients can be improved by utilizing DSST charnolopharmacotherapeutics involving CB prevention/inhibition, charnolophagy induction, CS stabilization, and CS-exocytosis for normal microRNA-mediated post-transcriptional regulation of mitochondrial and nuclear genes involved in growth, proliferation, differentiation, and development. Hence, multimodality imaging employing novel NPs and RPs targeting DSST-CMB, CB, charnolophagy, and CS stabilization and exocytosis will be highly beneficial in pharmaceutical industries and research organizations for novel drug discovery.

It is envisaged that a combination of omics biotechnology along with microRNA profiling; *"Mouse Avatar"* and co-clinical trials of CMB, CB, charnolophagy, and DSST-CS-targeted charnolopharmacotherapeutics will revolutionize the drug development industry and EBPT of NDDs, CVDs, cancer, and other chronic inflammatory diseases.

Unfortunately, conventional chemotherapeutic drugs used for the treatment of cancer trigger generalized apoptosis of nonspecific hyper proliferating cells. Consequently, we encounter several undesirable adverse effects. Nonspecific induction of CB in the hyper-proliferating cells causes alopecia, myelosuppression, GIT symptoms, cardiovascular degeneration, neurotoxicity, renal impairments, and infertility during cancer chemotherapy. Hence, drugs may be developed to augment cancer stem cell-specific CB formation to eradicate MDR malignancies with minimum or no adverse effects. Nutritional rehabilitation, physiological Zn^{2+}, and MTs prevent CB formation by acting as potent free radical scavengers. Accumulation of CBs at the junction of axon hillock may impair axoplasmic transport of various ions, neurotransmitters, enzymes, neurotrophic factors (such as BDNF, IGF-1, and NGF-1), and mitochondria at the synaptic terminals to cause synaptic atrophy. The release of toxic substances from the destabilized CS due to increased permeabilization, sequestration, and fragmentation at the junction of axon hillock or in the synaptic terminals can induce initially synaptic silence followed by progressive NDDs, such as; PD, AD, ALS, HD, MS, stroke, depression, schizophrenia, and chronic drug addiction due to endogenous toxins-induced synaptic sequestration and synaptic degeneration. Hence, novel drugs may be developed to inhibit CB formation, induce charnolophagy, and prevent CS destabilization in NDDs and CVDs and vice versa for the personalized theranostics of MDR malignancies.

Soon after the conception, paternal CB must be phagocytosed by the maternal lysosomes in the oocyte by charnolophagy as a basic molecular mechanism of ICD; otherwise it could have deleterious effects on the zygote and may induce abortion, anencephaly, microcephaly, cyclopia, craniofacial anomalies, still birth, and abortion; as observed in FAS, chronic nicotine and toxins exposure, and microbial (ZIKV, cytomegalovirus, and rubella virus) infections. Many pharmacological agents used in routine clinical practice including anesthetics, antidepressants, antipsychotics, HMG-CO-A reductase inhibitors (statins), ACE inhibitors, and anti-epileptic drugs can also induce microcephaly due to free radical-induced CB formation and CS destabilization (involved in microRNAs-mediated post-transcriptional down-regulation of genes) in the NPCs and CSs derived from iPPCs in the embryo to cause developmental charnolopathies (also named as embryopathies).

CB formation is significantly influenced by inducers and microenvironment and is spatio-temporally and transcriptionally-regulated by microRNAs in healthy aging, whereas; it becomes uncontrolled in NDDs, CVDs, inflammatory diseases, cancer, and in microbial infections. Malnutrition, toxins (nicotine and ethanol) and microbial (ZIKV, cytomegalovirus, rubella) infection induce CB formation and CS destabilization to cause developmental charnolopathies, involved in diversified embryopathies, including microcephaly. The CB, CPS, and CS are stored in the meconium during embryonic development under normal physiological conditions. In general, CB, CPS, and CS are subjected to hepatic metabolism through systemic circulation and after phase-1 (through cytochrome-P450) and phase-2 (through glucronidation, sulphatation, acetylation) metabolism for renal and fecal clearance.

CB can be classified depending on the type of MAO on the outer mitochondrial membrane. The neuronal mitochondria in the dorsal raphe and periaqueductal gray regions are rich in MAO-A, and are involved in the oxidation of NE and 5-HT at the synaptic terminals to modulate pain, perception, and depression; whereas mitochondria in the striatal neurons are rich in MAO-B. Thus, MAO-A-specific CB is formed in the dorsal raphe and PAG, whereas MAO-B-specific CB is formed in the striatum due to loss of monoaminergic neurotransmission as a function of disease and/or aging. The MAO-B specific CB formation can be prevented by selegiline, rasagiline, safinamide, and moclobemide to delay the requirement of L-DOPA therapy in PD. Selegiline induces MTs to provide neuroprotection in AD and PD by preventing free radical-induced CB formation and CS destabilization involved in apoptotic neurodegeneration. MTs as potent free radical scavengers also augment charnolophagy and CS exocytosis to boost MB, microRNA-modulated epigenetics, and maintain ICD for normal health and well-being. Premature degradation of CPS or CS membranes releases toxic substances such as: Cyt-C, iron, caspase-3, Bax, Bak, and AIF to cause craniofacial or other abnormalities depending on which iPPCs are involved and/or destroyed during FASD and multiple drug addiction. Similar pathological changes may occur during CB sequestration, when it is inefficiently phagocytosed and/or becomes lysosomal-resistant. A CPS is transformed to CS when the phagocytosed CB is completely hydrolyzed by the lysosomal (proteases, lipases, nucleases) enzymes. The CS is exocytosed by an energy (ATP)-driven process as a basic molecular mechanism of ICD to prevent chronic diseases and remain healthy.

Prolonged retention of CS in a cell results in the formation of CS bodies due to secondary or tertiary free radical attack during the chronic phase of disease progression. The CS bodies fuse with the plasma membrane to cause phosphatidyl serine externalization and the formation of apoptotic bodies by membrane blebbing. The apoptotic bodies eventually rupture to release toxic apoptogenic substances to further disseminate apoptosis in the neighboring cells. The exocytosed CS can also be endocytosed by the neighboring cells to cause MDR malignancies if a cancer stem cell-specific CS (CSscs) is endocytosed by the neighboring or remote nonproliferating cells.

Malignancies may develop by endocytosis of the circulating cancer stem cell-specific CS in a specific tissue of the human body. The CSscs is drug-resistant because it is rich in antiapoptotic proteins such as MTs, glutathione, BCl_2, HSP-70, and P^{53} which provide immortalization in a non-proliferative cell where it is endocytosed. Hence, drugs may be developed to prevent and/or eliminate CSscs formation, and/or inhibit induction of CS bodies involved in malignant transformation and chronic MDR diseases.

Accumulation of CB at the junction of axon hillock blocks the normal axoplasmic transport of various ions, neurotransmitters, hormones, neurotrophic factors (IGF-1,

BDNF), and mitochondria in the terminal end bulbs to cause synaptic atrophy; whereas the accumulation of structurally and functionally-destabilized CS causes the release of toxic substances of mitochondrial metabolism to cause synaptic degeneration, involved in early morbidity and mortality due to cognitive impairments in learning, intelligence, memory, and behavior (Sharma 2016, 2017). Hence, fusion imaging with ^{18}F or ^{11}C-labelled CB, charnolophagy, and/or CS biomarkers along with a specific PET-RPs for brain regional DAeric, cholinergic, 5-HT-ergic, GABAergic neurotransmission will provide a precise understanding and will establish the exact interaction between CMB, charnolophagy, CS stabilization, and brain regional neurotransmission, which is either compromised or impaired in NDDs and other chronic diseases due to down-regulation of microRNAs-mediated post-transcriptional regulation of genes involved in the DNA cell cycle, cell proliferation, differentiation, migration, and development. Further studies in this direction will provide the precise molecular mechanism of ICD and its exact significance in regulating brain regional neurotransmission in health and disease. The distinct advantage of antioxidants derived from functional foods is that these can pass through the blood brain barrier (BBB) without inducing adverse effects unlike presently-available antidepressants, antipsychotic, anti-histaminergic, cholinesterase, and NMDA receptor antagonists used in the treatment of AD and other NDDs.

Motivation to Discover CB

Once Luis Pasteur said "*luck always favors the prepared mind*" which is true to achieve success in any discipline and in every walk of life. Original scientific achievements are no exceptions. Let me describe some of my early life experiences which persuaded me to discover CB during my professional and scientific career as a biomedical student. There was increased prevalence of protein calorie malnutrition in India, South Africa, and China in young developing children during the early seventies when I started my career in biomedical sciences. There was no birth control and early childhood morbidity and mortality was quite prevalent. Relatives, friends, and the husband of a lady who lost her child would console by persuading her to reproduce another child within next year. In addition to ignorance and poverty, the child neglect, physical abuse, and psychological abuse was at maximum. Parents in remote villages were reluctant to send their children to school because they wanted them to work in their farms. The U.S. President John F. Kennedy was very kind to send milk powder and biscuits to poor children of Indian villages. Hot milk and biscuits were distributed to children in villages during lunch time as an incentive to attend the primary school. In addition to my early childhood memories, I observed deleterious signs and symptoms of children suffering from kwashiorkor and marasmus (types of malnutrition) which inspired, motivated, and encouraged me to discover something new for the welfare of humanity. These events inspired me to discover "Charnoly body" when I was a doctoral student at the All India Institute of Medical Sciences, New Delhi (India). Subsequently, I decided to continue my research on the effect of undernutrition in the developing brain. I was also interested in culturing neurons under glucose and serum-deprived conditions in a petri dish to evaluate the direct effect of various antiepileptic drugs *in vitro* and in N and UN rats because epilepsy and malnutrition were very common in those days in India. By trypsinization of the developing cerebellum from the young developing pups, I could purify Purkinje neurons along with their structurally-intact synaptic terminals (Sharma and Ebadi 2014).

While serving as a Research Officer at the All India Institute of Medical Sciences, New Delhi (India), I met Dr. Baldev Singh who was the Emeritus Professor in the Department of Neurology and Physiology. Working along with intelligent doctors, neurologist, physiologist, and particularly with Dr. Baldev Singh was really challenging, thrilling, and an exciting experience, aiding my early professional and scientific development. He graciously agreed to guide me in my Ph.D. research project on the developing UN rat brain. I met Dr. GFX David who was the officer in-charge of the transmission and scanning electron microscope labs. Soon he became my very good friend and invited me to organize National Training Programs on Sophisticated Equipments as a Faculty Member. I processed brain samples obtained from the developing N and UN rats for T.E.M. analyses in addition to my regular electrophysiological experiments on these animals. One day, I was lucky to discover multilamellar electron dense membrane stacks in the developing Purkinje neurons of 15 days UN rats, which I named as CBs as a token of love, respect, and appreciation to my mother. I was quite convinced that these multi-lamellar electron membrane stacks (penta, hepta) are originating from the degenerating mitochondrial membranes during severe malnutrition due to free radical-induced lipid peroxidation. I wrote to my parents that I have discovered something new which I named as "Charnoly body" (abbreviation: CB).

I became curious and started counting the number of CBs in the UN Purkinje neurons. In the beginning my interest was restricted to only determining the number of mitochondria in the N and UN rat Purkinje neurons. But later, I realized that these electron dense membrane stacks (CBs) are formed by the degeneration of mitochondria due to nutritional stress. In severely UN animals, the mitochondria were depolarized, swollen, and degenerated to form penta or hepta lamellar structures. When I showed T.E.M. pictures of CB to my mother, she bowed before them and said *"Look how beautiful they are"*. My first paper appeared in the Journal of Neurological Sciences where I described their unknown origin, without any clinical significance. My mentor, Dr. Baldev Singh encouraged me by saying, *"Although I do not know what is happening and neither, I am a neuromorphologist, all I can say is that there is something interesting going on in these developing UN neurons about which we do not know at this moment"*.

In 1982, I was invited to Paris for the 3rd World Congress on Nuclear Medicine and Biology in the Invention and Innovation Session for my original discovery of an electro-microinjector for intra-neuronal microinjection to determine the influence of mitochondrial-targeted RPs and NPs, on CB formation or inhibition. Based on the original discovery of CB, I was awarded the Merck (German) Gold Medal in the Neurological Society of India Conference held in December 1984 at Varanasi (Kashi). In September 1985, I was invited to serve as a chairman in the 13th world congress of Neurology in Hamburg, where I presented this work in more detail. Subsequently, I was invited to Calgary for the 13th International Congress of Biometeorology on September 1993, where I presented my research on the CB life cycle, which was later published in the conference proceedings. In this lecture, I highlighted that malnutrition, environmental neurotoxins including Kainic acid (KA), Domoic acid

(DOM), and microbial (bacteria, virus, and fungal) infection induce apoptosis in the hippocampal CA-3 and dentate gyrus by CB formation to cause dementia, as noticed in AD. Subsequently, I was invited to present my original discovery on CB as a sensitive biomarker in Nanomedicine in the First International Conference on Translational Nanomedicine, and in the 12th International Congress on Drug discovery on July 25–27, 2013 in Boston. I presented CB as a universal biomarker and highlighted its clinical significance as a pre-apoptotic biomarker of cell injury for novel drug discovery. Recently, I was invited to deliver a speech on "CB as Novel Biomarker in Chronic Drug Addiction" in the 4th International Conference on Drug Addiction and Therapy in Orlando, FL, U.S.A. on August 3–5, 2015 and at the Harvard Medical School in September 22–25, 2016, I delivered a lecture on CB as a novel biomarker of nutritional stress in AD. I was again invited to deliver a lecture on "Antioxidant-Charnolosome Interaction in Health and Disease" at the Harvard Medical School in the 20th International Conference on Functional Foods in Health & Disease, September 22–25, 2017.

I had an opportunity to observe severely malnourished kwashiorkor and marasmus children in my village, which persuaded me to conduct basic research on developing UN brain. Particularly, clinical cases of severe malnutrition motivated me to conduct further research in this direction. These interesting cases are described below:

Case-1. This was a rich family of two truck drivers who had a single wife. No doubt they were rich, but illiterate and so was their wife. Usually their every evening was spent on heavy drinking after long routes of driving a heavy truck. Their wife was severely anemic, weak, and frail. During pregnancy, she was neglected and was treated like a sex object by both these truck drivers. Her condition deteriorated further during pregnancy particularly when she gave birth to a severely malnourished female child. The truck drivers did not like her giving birth to a female child, because a female child was considered a liability and burden to society in those days in their family. The young lady was psychologically demoralized and suffered from not only anemia and depression, but also lactation failure. Consequently, her female child was reduced to a skeleton and suffered from mixed symptoms of marasmus and kwashiorkor, characterized by loss of weight, stunted growth, folded dry skin and face like an old person, peripheral edema, and extremely thin abdominal skin. She could not even cry and suffered from severe diarrhea and dehydration. One day, her mother decided to dispose this severely malnourished child in a toilet sink when an old lady saw her committing this sin. She rushed to the scene and shouted at this young lady, "What are you doing?" The lady replied in a choking voice: "My husbands do not like female child in their family". I do not have milk in my breast and am suffering from severe depression and weakness. I cannot take care of my child who is almost dying in agony, and I can't see her suffering like this". The old lady gave her sincere advice like a big mother. "Look! Am I not a woman? Are you not a woman? If our parents would have done the same merciless job of killing us right after birth, we would not have been on this earth any more. It is a sin to do these types of heinous acts". Both the young lady and the old lady started weeping bitterly. In those days, I was staying with my friend who was our university photographer in a remote village about 3 Kilometer away from our university. He knew that I am conducting research on developing UN animals and perhaps he trusted my intellectual abilities. He brought me to this house where this weak and frail female child was at the verge of her death. I notice that she was suffering from severe malnutrition and instructed her mother to prepare a feed under strict hygienic conditions. It was a simple formula of cow's milk, glucose, two to three lemon and multivitamin drops, supplemented with iron and folate. I also instructed her parents that they were also born by a female who was their mother to emphasize the significance of a female child. In addition, I gave example of almighty Goddess "Durga" and "Mrs. Indira Gandhi", who was the Prime Minister of India in those days. So, they agreed to purchase at least a small bottle of multivitamin drops for their miserably-dying child on the following day. Within 25 days, nutritional rehabilitation conferred a new life to this child. The edema and the folded skin dissappeared and hair started growing. There was no frequent diarrhea. The child regained coordination of muscular activity as shown in Fig. 1. There was a natural smile on her face as well as on the face of her parents. This experience made me believe that we are living on this earth only because of *"mitochondrial bioenergetics (MB)"* which is derived from the food we consume. By this time, I had learned from my biochemistry classes that mitochondria through oxidative phosphorylation synthesize ATP to provide energy. Particularly during vulnerable periods of brain development, protein calorie restriction has deleterious consequences on learning, intelligence, memory, and behavior due to the depletion of argyrophilic nucleolar organizer (AgNOR) involved in ribosome production and eventually protein (mitofusin) synthesis at the rough endoplasmic reticulum (RER) to synthesize and repair mitochondria and prevent CB formation implicated in progressive neurodegeneration as described elegantly in this book.

Usually body weight and chest to encephalic ratio (circumference) are determined to assess the severity of nutritional stress in developing malnourished children. On moral and ethical grounds, CB formation cannot be studied in the developing UN children. However, clinical manifestations of the deleterious effects of nutritional stress in the malnourished children motivated me to discover the physiological and pharmacological significance of MB in developing UN rats, which led to the discovery of CB formation as a universal pre-apoptotic biomarker of oxidative stress due to severe mitochondrial injury. Hence, CB formation in experimental animals and brain/body weight ratio in developing children may be used as novel biomarkers of nutritional stress and rehabilitation (or degeneration and regeneration) (Source:

Fig. I (A-B)

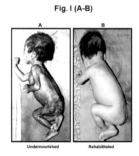

Fig. 1: Undernourished child (A) Clinical manifestations of 2.5-month old protein malnourished female child due to lactation failure in mother presenting folded skin, loss of muscle tone, neuromuscular degeneration, peripheral edema, loss of hair, and face like an old person. (B) The same child after 25 days of nutritional rehabilitation with cow's milk formula exhibiting alleviation of clinical symptoms, coordination of muscular activity, reappearance of muscle tone, and hair growth.

Author's original findings). From: Sharma, S. and M. Ebadi. 2014. Recent studies have shown that skeletal muscles from aging mice exhibit low levels of miR-434-3p and high levels of eIF5A1 involved in sarcopenia, as noticed in this child during severe malnutrition (Pardo et al. 2017).

Case-2. I noticed a male child suffering from marasmus due to his mother's unemployment, loneliness, lactation failure, and father's divorce in my village. The local doctor had already declared that this child will die in couple of days and refused to treat him. One day the doctor asked his mother if her malnourished child was still alive. His mother brought this dying child to me. I simply gave her strict instructions of sanitation and prepared a formula in cow's milk containing glucose, few drops of multivitamins, and lemon juice. Within 15 days, this child had a new life and was fully recovered within 3 weeks.

Brain Sparing Hypothesis. Since the brain weight was not affected significantly in protein calorie malnutrition (PCM) compared to body weight, some investigators proposed a brain sparing hypothesis, which mislead researchers in those days. However, later it was confirmed that, the developing brain, in fact, is most vulnerable to the deleterious consequences of malnutrition. This was based on neuromorphological studies at the light and E.M. level, neurochemical analysis of enzymes, neurotransmitters, and hormones. However, EEG findings were largely inconclusive unless the developing child was severely malnourished during the lactation phase. My own electrophysiological and morphological studies on developing N and UN rat Purkinje neurons confirmed that the brain sparing hypothesis is misleading and brain weight criteria was not appropriate to assess the nutritional status of the developing child. However, the ratio of the brain weight to body weight was significantly high in the UN rats as compared to their well-fed normal litter mates. The EEG of the UN rats exhibited considerable background inhibition with dominance of delta activity and lethargic behavior. Penicillin or kainic acid-induced seizure activity of prolonged duration was observed in UN animals. Although, the intensity of seizure discharge was reduced, they exhibited reduced seizure thresholds of prolonged duration in response to penicillin, KA, and DOM-induced seizures of hippocampal origin. Although, developing UN rats did not exhibit overt clinical symptoms of epilepsy; the seizure thresholds were significantly reduced in these animals. They also exhibited delayed neuronal recovery in response to antiepileptic treatment with intra-rectal sodium valproate (Shrama et al. 1987; Sharma et al. 1990). The latency of response was increased, whereas the duration, frequency, and amplitude of response were significantly reduced, and these animals were easily fatigued upon repeated peripheral electrical stimulation. Subsequently, it was confirmed that electrical fatigue is occurring in the developing UN animals due to significantly impaired MB and CB formation in the developing neurons (Sharma et al. 1986; Sharma et al. 1987). I published this research in the Indian Journal of Medical Research, Journal of Neurological Sciences, Journal of Neuroscience, Epilepsia, Journal of Neural Transmission, and in the Annals of New York Academy of Science.

I got interested in determining the number of mitochondria in the Purkinje neurons of developing N and UN rats employing E.M. examination. My presumption was that the UN animals had a reduced number of mitochondria as compared to N animals, or perhaps there could be only reduced functional activity of mitochondria.

A significant difference in the ^{14}C-glucose utilization between N and UN rat cerebellar vermis Purkinje neurons was observed from where electrical activity was recorded. At the ultrastructural level, the mitochondria appeared swollen and blotted with electron dense inclusions and increased Ca^{2+}. Their membranes were stacked together to form condensed multilamellar penta and heptalamellar structures. Instead of counting their number, I got interested in their subcellular and molecular pathology, which led to the discovery of charnolophagy, CPS, and CS and its exocytosis and endocytosis as a basic molecular mechanism of ICD. The number of these electron dense membrane stacks (CBs) increased as a function of nutritional stress. In fact, in 30 days UN rats, these multi-lamellar stacks were phagocytosed by lysosomes, which was named as "charnolophagy".

When I showed these findings to my doctoral committee members, they simply ignored and rejected these findings except for Dr. Baldev Singh and Dr. Subimal Roy who encouraged and motivated me to explore further along this direction. Particularly, Dr. GFX David encouraged me by saying: "*Mr. Sharma, if you have prepared a successful model of undernutrition and your electrophysiological results are accurate and making sense and the same animals you are subjecting to E.M. evaluation; you are bound to get neuromorphological differences as well. Moreover, these days researchers are demonstrating significant differences between N and UN animals even at the light microscopic level, then why you should not have differences at the E.M. level? In my opinion these observations are genuine and true. Unfortunately, we do not know their exact clinical significance at this moment*".

My guide, Dr. Baldev Singh introduced me to two eminent professors Dr. Parab Dastur from the Department of Pathology Bombay and Dr. Shastry from the National Institute of Science, Bangalore. Dr. Sastry only appreciated my observations and told that he was not an electron microscopist. But Dr. Parab Dastur said: "*Definitely these multilamallar stacks are not artifacts. Neither I can make any further comment on their origin and clinical significance*"; but he made a very important statement which will encourage and motivate young investigators. "*Observations are always true; interpretation may or may not be. What is more important is that you should: work hard, believe in yourself, and should have perseverance*".

These electron dense membrane stacks were not observed in the axons because axons are devoid of mitochondria. If that is so, then from where do we get mitochondria in the synaptic terminals? The synaptic terminals cannot synthesize mitochondria as they do not have regional protein synthesizing machinery. The mitochondria are synthesized in the cell body near the nucleus because out of 2000 proteins required for the mitochondriogenesis, only 13 are synthesized by the mtDNA for the electron transport chain and oxidative phosphorylation. The remaining proteins required to generate the electron transport chain of enzyme complexes (I–V) are synthesized by the nuclear DNA. The mitochondria are transported at the synaptic terminals by proximodistal axoplasmic transport through axons. The microtubules in the axons serve as molecular rail grids for the transport of mitochondria from the cell soma to the synaptic terminals.

Since we require continuous mitochondrial energy (ATP) during neurotransmitter release for interneuronal communication and cognitive and motor performance, we need a continuous supply of mitochondria, enzymes, neuro-transmitters, and neurotropic factors for the synthesis, storage, and release of the neurotransmitters, physiologically-normal synaptic terminals for proper neurocybernatics and cognitive performance. However, CB formation can occur at the synaptic terminals to cause cognitive impairments associated with impairments in learning, intelligence, memory, and behavior, and early morbidity and mortality.

CB Definition

CB is a highly pleomorphic, unstable, pre-apoptotic, multi-lamellar (usually penta or heptalamellar), quasicrystalline, electron-dense membrane stack that is formed in the most vulnerable cell due to free radical-induced mitochondrial oxidative and nitrative stress of DPCI. CB is formed in response to any physicochemical injury in the most vulnerable cell (including NPCs, CPCs, derived from iPPCs in the developing embryo) due to free radical-induced CMB and down-regulation of the mitochondrial genome due to DPCI as a basic molecular mechanism of ICD during the acute phase for normal cellular function to remain healthy.

Basic Knowledge about CB

(i) Matter can neither be created nor destroyed, although it may transform from one form to the other.

(ii) Similar moleculars tend to associate, whereas dissimilar moleculars tend to dissociate.

(iii) Molecular association induces wound healing, whereas molecular dissociations results in wound progression depending on the inducers and microenvironment in its vicinity.

(iv) Mitochondrial bioenergetics is compromised as a function of increase in intracellular toxicity due to DPCI.

(v) CB formation, charnolophagy, and CS exocytosis are immediate and initial attempts to contain highly toxic metabolites of mitochondrial metabolism for ICD.

(vi) Novel charnolopharmacotherapeutics targeting CB inhibition, augmenting charnolophagy, CS stabilization, and exocytosis will be clinically beneficial for the safe and effective EBPT of NDDs, CVDs, and MDR malignancies.

A TEM picture illustrating CB molecular pathogenesis is presented in Fig. 2 (upper panel). Severe protein malnutrition triggers the formation of small sized mitochondria without cristae. These nonfunctional mitochondria aggregate to synthesize electron-dense membrane stacks (also named as CBs). The damaged mitochondria behave as destabilized CS and release toxic mitochondrial metabolites to cause plasma membrane perforations (arrow). The condensation of multilamellar electron-dense membrane stacks form penta or heptalamellar units to synthesize a mature CB, which is phagocytosed by lysosome and ATP-driven charnolophagy to form structurally and functionally labile CS (lower panel). The structural and functional destabilization of CS triggers non-DNA-dependent apoptotic cell death involved in MDR disease.

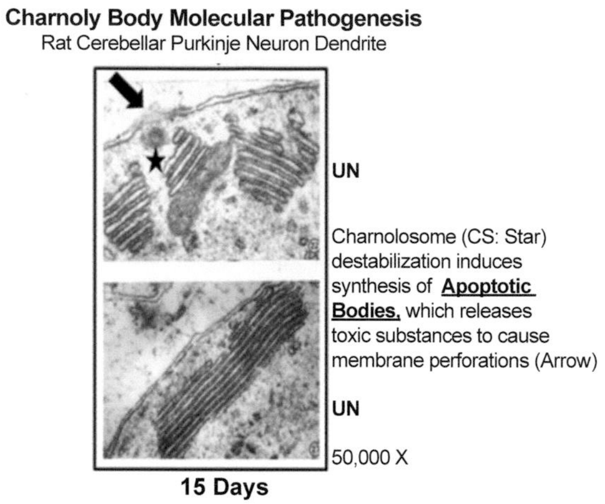

Charnoly Body Molecular Pathogenesis
Rat Cerebellar Purkinje Neuron Dendrite

UN

Charnolosome (CS: Star) destabilization induces synthesis of **Apoptotic Bodies,** which releases toxic substances to cause membrane perforations (Arrow)

UN

50,000 X

15 Days

Fig. 2: Charnoly body molecular pathogenesis in 15 days UN rat cerebellar Purkinje neuron.

Charnolosome (CS)

A CS is an intracellular organelle which is formed by phagocytosis of "CB" by a lysosome (also named as CB autophagy or "charnolophagy"). A CS is eliminated by energy (ATP)-driven exocytosis as a basic molecular mechanism of ICD during the chronic phase of disease progression. The degenerated mitochondria condense to form pleomorphic, multilamellar, electron-dense membrane stacks (CBs) as noticed in Fig. 3 (Left panel). Charnolophagy (CB autophagy) is induced by free radical-induced lysosomal activation to synthesize CPS, which is transformed to CS when the phagocytosed CB is hydrolyzed by the lysosomal enzymes as a basic molecular mechanism of ICD (Fig. 3: right panel).

Charnolophagy Index. (charnolophagy/autophagy) is a novel biomarker to quantitatively assess the molecular pathogenesis of CB in health and disease.

Charnolosome Stability Index (CSSI). The CS stability index (CSSI) can be determined by taking a ratio of stable CS divided by the sum of stable CS, permeable

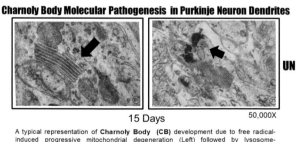

Charnoly Body Molecular Pathogenesis in Purkinje Neuron Dendrites

UN

15 Days   50,000X

A typical representation of **Charnoly Body (CB)** development due to free radical-induced progressive mitochondrial degeneration (Left) followed by lysosome-dependent **Charnolophagy** (Right) to form a highly toxic **Charnolosome** (CS) which is involved in **apoptotic neurodegeneration** in the developing undernourished rat cerebellar Purkinje neurons.

Fig. 3: A TEM picture illustrating CB formation in the Purkinje neuron of developing UN rat cerebellar cortex due to free radicals-induced mitochondrial oxidative and nitrative stress.

CS, sequestered CS, and fragmented CS in the most vulnerable physico-chemically-injured cell, as shown in the following equation:

$$CSSI = CS_n/CS_n + CS_{perm} + CS_{seq} + CS_{frag}$$

where: CS_n = Stable CS; CS_{perm} = permeabilized CS; CS_{seq} = sequestered CS; CS_{frag} = fragmented CS. At least five different types of CSs can be isolated and characterized by flow cytometry equipped with sorting facility.

The E.R. stress is noticed primarily in the dendrites and growth cones, whereas the mitochondrial oxidative stress occurs primarily in the cytoplasm and at the synaptic terminals during DPCI in the most vulnerable cell. Hence, CB formation in the synaptic terminals can induce synaptic silence, synaptic atrophy, and eventually synaptic degeneration depending on the frequency and intensity of free radical-induced CS permeabilization, sequestration, and/or fragmentation to trigger diversified charnolopathies. These charnolopathies induce MCI during the acute phase, and morbidity and mortality during the chronic phase in MDR diseases, including malignancies.

Mitochondrial Morphology During Severe Nutritional Stress and Physicochemical Injury. Usually mitochondria appear as elliptical double-layered membranous structures at the ultrastructural level. During DPCI, they are transformed into pleomorphic structures to induce CB formation. We observed small sized mitochondria devoid of cristae in the most vulnerable developing rat Purkinje neuronal dendrites and growth cones during severe nutritional stress. These structurally and functionally-impaired mitochondria are unable to synthesize ATP because the Cyt-C and the electron transport chain are delocalized. The impaired mitochondria did not transform to CB and behaved directly as CS. Some of these small-sized, destabilized, and primitive mitochondria released toxic substances to cause membrane perforations in the absence of CB formation and charnolophagy. In the absence of mtDNA, AgNOR, mitofusin, and structurally and functionally intact protein synthesizing machinery; they behaved as destabilized CS, released toxic substances through permeabilization, sequestration, and fragmentation, and triggered apoptosis depending on the severity of malnutrition or physico-chemical insult as noticed in cancer, CVDs, and NDDs including: stroke, traumatic brain injury (TBI), AD, PD, MDDs, drug addiction, schizophrenia, and aging, as illustrated in the following pictorial diagram.

Free radicals induce endoplasmic reticular stress (ERS) to cause ribosomal delocalization and inhibition of protein synthesis. Free radicals directly inhibit the AgNOR, involved in the synthesis of ribosomes in the nucleolus to shut down protein (mitofusin) synthesis at the transcriptional level. Free radicals also disrupt microRNA-mediated post-transcriptional regulation of genes and induce gene silencing. Thus, free radical-induced charnolopathies and ERS are primarily involved in the down-regulation of normal microRNA-mediated post-transcriptional regulation of genes implicated in the DNA cell cycle, proliferation, migration, differentiation, and development for normal health and well-being as illustrated in Fig. 4.

Usually, methionine enters in the mitochondria, where it is transformed to s-adenosyl methionine (SAM) in the presence of ATP. SAM is translocated in the nucleus and donates $-CH_3$ group to synthesize methyl cytosine or hydroxymethyl cytosine at the N-4 position. These epigenetic changes occur more frequently in the mtDNA as compared to the nuclear DNA because the mtDNA is naked, uncoiled, intron-less,

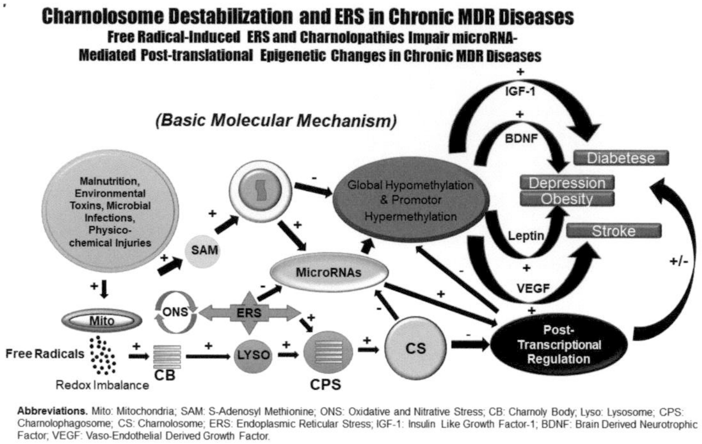

Fig. 4: Charnolosome (CS) destabilization and ERS in chronic MDR diseases. A systematic diagram illustrating that malnutrition, environmental toxins, microbial (bacteria, viral, and fungal) infections, and diversified physico-chemical injuries (DPCI), induce mitochondrial oxidative stress and redox imbalance due to free radical overproduction.

and GC rich. Moreover, the mtDNA remains in a hostile microenvironment of free radicals, being generated persistently as a byproduct of oxidative phosphorylation. Whereas, the nuclear DNA is supercoiled and compactly arranged with structural and functional support of histones and protamines. Histones and protamines maintain helicity and protect cytosines from being readily methylated by SAM. Therefore, any epigenetic change occurring at the supercoiled nuclear DNA level, initially requires histone acetylation at the lysine residues to uncoil the double-helical nuclear DNA. Free radical-induced ERS and charnolopathies disrupt microRNA-mediated regulation of genes. Destabilization of CS releases highly toxic mitochondrial metabolites to cause disruption of the microRNA-mediated post-transcriptional regulation of genes involved in normal growth, proliferation, differentiation, and development.

In general, global hypomethylation and hyper-methylation of the promotor regions of IGF-genes are involved in insulin-resistant (Type-2) diabetes, in the BDNF gene is involved in major depression, in the leptin gene is involved in obesity, and in the VEGF gene is involved in the molecular pathogenesis of AIS. The mitochondrial redox imbalance and ERS disrupt normal microRNA-mediated post-transcriptional regulation of genes involved in normal signal transduction during AIS in humans as well as in experimental animals. The AIS can be induced by middle cerebral artery occlusion (MCAO) in experimental animals. MCAO triggers hyper-methylation of the VEGF promoter and global hypo-methylation to cause stroke due to induction of proinflammatory and apoptotic signal transduction. Endogenous as well as exogenous antioxidants may prevent these deleterious changes by scavenging free radicals to a certain extent. Unfortunately, the mitochondrial and ERS-induced microRNA disruption occur more frequently due to limited bioavailability of exogenous as well as endogenous antioxidants at the site of physicochemical injury due to glucose and O_2 depletion during AIS. Generally, an antioxidant drug edaravone is prescribed to stroke patients to scavenge free radicals with a limited success. Hence, regional microinjections of anti-inflammatory and antiapoptotic microRNA sequences may have some promise in the safe and effective clinical management and better prognosis of stroke patients. In addition, bone marrow-derived stem cells can confer antioxidant, anti-inflammatory, antiapoptotic, and proangiogenic potential through the release of VEGF from the EPCs, involved in neovascularization during post-stroke recovery, as illustrated in following pictorial diagram.

Primary free radical attack causes mitochondrial oxidative and nitrative stress and degeneration due to lipid peroxidation. The fragmented mitochondrial membranes condense to form electron-dense, multi-lamellar, quasicrystalline stacks (named as Charnoly body and abbreviated as CB). CB is phagocytosed by energy (ATP)-dependent phogocytosis (named as charnolophagy) to form a CPS. A. CPS is transformed to CS when the entire phagocytosed CB in the lysosome is hydrolyzed by the lysosomal enzymes. B. A secondary free radical attack induces CS condensation in the perinuclear region. C. A tertiary free radical attack induces CS sequestration to release toxic mitochondrial metabolites. D. A quaternary free radical attack causes CS fragmentation to release toxic mitochondrial metabolites. A comprehensive list of these toxic metabolites is presented in this book, which can be used as CS biomarkers for their identification and characterization employing a combinatorial and correlative bioinformatic approach. E. The above molecular pathological changes in CS dynamics can be prevented or inhibited by endogenous or exogenous antioxidants. The antioxidants as free radical scavengers stabilize CS and facilitate their exocytosis as a basic molecular mechanism of ICD. In addition, antioxidants such as MTs, HSPs, HIF-1α, and BCl-2 prevent CS condensation, permeabilization, sequestration and fragmentation to provide cytoprotection in chronic MDR diseases. Antioxidants also prevent free radical-induced disruption in microRNA-mediated post-transcriptional regulation of genes and epigenetic changes involved in DNA cell cycle, cell division, proliferation, differentiation, and development for normal cellular function as presented in Fig. 5.

As described earlier, it is only the mother's mitochondria that the child inherits. That is why the developing fetus is severely influenced by maternal drug abuse including alcohol, contraceptive pills, antiepileptic drugs, anesthetic agents, and environmental toxins as compared to paternal DNA. However, it is now believed that epigenetic changes even in the paternal nuclear DNA can influence the growth and development of the fetus. Recently, I reported that paternal mitochondria are phagocytosed by charnolophagy during conception in the oocyte during conception. I introduced the term "charnolophagy" to describe CB autophagy.

CB Life Cycle. Just like the life cycle of a human being, primarily 4 major phases of CB life cycle were discovered. (i) origin, (ii) development, (iii) maturation, (iv) degradation (charnolophagy) (Sharma et al. 2013a; Sharma et al. 2013b; Sharma and Ebadi 2014; Sharma 2015, 2016, 2017). CB, charnolophagy, CPS, CS, and CS body were identified at the TEM level, with promising targets for developing DSST charnolopharmacotherapeutics for the safe and effective EBPT of chronic MDR diseases. The structurally-intact synaptic terminal has normal shape and size with round and dense appearance, whereas the degenerated synaptic terminal is swollen, club-shaped, and have cloudy appearance due to the CB formation and impaired axoplasmic transport. Synaptic degeneration in the Purkinje neurons is responsible for impaired and/or delayed motor learning in nutritionally-stressed and delayed eye blink conditioning in intrauterine fetal alcohol-exposed developing children.

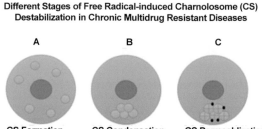

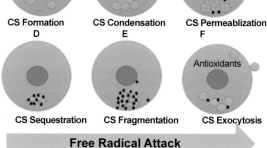

Fig. 5: A pictorial diagram illustrating different stages of free radical-induced CS destabilization following CB formation and charnolophagy in the most vulnerable cell.

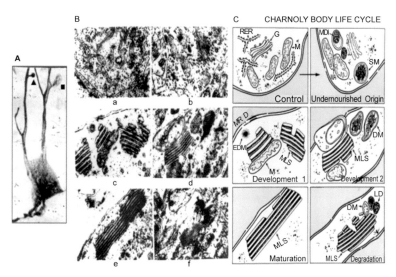

Fig. 6: Analysis of rat Purkinje neuron cytomorphology in developing rat cerebellar Purkinje neurons. Panel A. Analysis of rat Purkinje neuron cytomorphology. Left panel A: A light microscopic picture of a Purkinje neuron isolated from 30 days undernourished rat cerebellar cortex, exhibiting a structurally-intact (▲ left) and a degenerated synaptic terminal (■ right).

CB life cycle is systematically presented in Fig. 6 (upper right panel-B). E.M. pictures illustrating CB life cycle in the developing UN rat cerebellar Purkinje neurons. a. Normal rat cerebellar Purkinje neuron dendrite with normal appearing Golgi apparatus, RER, and elliptical mitochondria with well-defined cristae during 15 days of postnatal life. b. The mitochondria and Golgi body become swollen and start aggregating in 15 days UN rats. c. Subsequently, the mitochondrial membranes are degenerated and fragmented. The degenerated mitochondrial membranes are transformed into electron-dense membrane stacks. d. The mitochondria are fused with the electron-dense membrane stacks in the basal region to maintain their structural and functional integrity. CB can also translocate towards the damaged region of the plasma membrane to repair degenerating desmosomes to preserve the structural and functional integrity of the plasma membrane. The swollen mitochondria fuse with the already existing immature CB. e. The electron–dense membrane stacks become independent ultra-structural units to form pentalamellar or hepta-lamellar units (named as mature CB). The mature CB serves as membrane reserve during nutritional stress. A fully mature CB appears as multi-lamellar, electron-dense, penta-lamellar, or hepta-lamellar independent units. f. These multi-lamellar ultra-structural units are eliminated by ATP-dependent charnolophagy due to increased lysosomal enzyme activity to meet the energy demands of the neuron during chronic undernutrition. The desmsomes are relatively more resistant to the deleterious effects of the free radical-induced lipid peroxidation as seen in the above TEM picture (Source: Author's original findings).

L.M and E.M. Analysis of Rat Purkinje Neuron Cytomorphology. A light microscopic picture of an isolated Purkinje neuron from 30 days UN rat cerebellar cortex exhibited a structurally-intact (▲ left) and a degenerated synaptic terminal (■ right). The structurally intact synaptic terminal has normal shape and size with round and dense appearance, whereas degenerated synaptic terminal is swollen, club-shaped, with cloudy appearance due to CB formation and impaired axoplasmic transport. Synaptic degeneration in the Purkinje neurons may be responsible for impaired and/or delayed motor learning in nutritionally-stressed and delayed eye blink conditioning in intrauterine fetal alcohol-exposed developing children.

CB appears to form a bridge between apoptosis and neurodegeneration; it is a transitory phase as nutritional rehabilitation can eliminate CB formation by efficient charnolophagy as noticed in 80 days rehabilitated UN rats. The swollen mitochondria fuse with the already existing immature CB as illustrated in the middle right panel. These electron-dense membrane stacks become independent ultra-structural units to form penta or hepta-lamellar units as mature CB. The mature CB seem to serve as membrane reserve during nutritional stress. A fully mature CB appears as multi-lamellar, electron-dense, penta-lamellar, or hepta-lamellar independent units depending on the brain-region specific vulnerability of the neurons. During severe nutritional stress, lysosomal activation induces charnolophagy. However, in permanently damaged neurons, these multi-lamellar electron-dense CBs may participate in further neurodegenerative process.

Recently, we reported that antioxidant Zn^{2+}-binding low molecular weight proteins, MTs, inhibit CB formation as potent free radical scavengers, which are significantly reduced in the hippocampal regions of AD patients and thus induce further degeneration by formation of amyloid-β plaques in AD and Lewy body in PD patients. Whether CBs can synthesize ATP by oxidative phosphorylation and if these membranes have structurally and functionally intact electron transport system to synthesize ATP remains unknown. Our studies suggest that CB may be transformed into functional mitochondria during nutritional rehabilitation (Source: Sharma's original findings). From: Sharma, S. and M. Ebadi. 2014. The Charnoly Body as a

Universal Biomarker of Cell Injury. Biomarkers in Genomic Med. 6: 89–98 (Elsevier Publishers) [With Permission].

CB Formation and Infertility. Particularly, spatio-temporal chronobiology of CB and charnolophagy are very important to understand the basic molecular mechanism of successful fertilization. Soon after conception, the paternal mitochondria are degenerated to form CB. The paternal CB is recognized as a foreign nonfunctional intracellular inclusion and is eliminated by charnolophagy by the oocyte. Charnolophagy occurs efficiently to prevent structural and/or functional damage to the nuclear membrane and DNA. The paternal mtDNA is also destroyed during the prezygotic phase of fertilization. Any delay in charnolophagy during fertilization due to DPCI can destroy the zygote and induce premature abortion. Hence, spatio-temporal chronobiology of CB formation, charnolophagy, and CS exocytosis in the oocyte are very important and crucial events for the successful conception and normal embryonic development. The microenvironment in the cytoplasmic compartment of the oocyte is primarily acidic with many lysosomes to facilitate charnolophagy (highly essential for the normal growth and development of an embryo), as described in detail in my recently published book "Fetal Alcohol Spectrum Disorder" Concepts, Mechanisms and Cure" by Nova Science Publishers New York, U.S.A. During cell division, mitochondrial fusion occurs, whereas during growth and development mitochondrial fission occurs for the growth and survival of the developing embryo. During fertilization, the vibratile movements of the spermatocyte tail occurs due to the condensed mitochondrial battery in the middle piece which provides required energy (ATP) for sperm motility and successful fertilization.

To sustain the normal MB, CB formation should be prevented and if at all it is formed due to any specific or nonspecific reasons; it must be eliminated efficiently by "charnolophagy", which is highly crucial for the normal growth and development of the fetus. That is why the number of lysosomes is significantly increased in the developing UN brain to eliminate CB and degenerating E.R. and mitochondrial membranes as a basic molecular mechanism of ICD. However, when CBs cannot be eliminated due to certain proteins being resistant to lysosomal enzyme degradation such as α-synuclein, parkin, ubiquitin, amyloid-β, huntingtin, fractine, and SOD, it triggers neurotoxicity and cell death due to apoptosis in progressive NDDs such as AD, PD, HD, ALS, drug addiction, depression, and aging to cause CB formation in Lewy bodies, amyloid bodies, or in other intraneuronal inclusions. Hence, CB formation, charnolophagy, and CS-exocytosis are immediate and early basic molecular events of ICD to remain healthy.

Rationale of CB Formation

We have recently reported CB as a universal biomarker of physico-chemical injury because its formation occurs in response to DPCI in the most vulnerable cell (particularly in the NPCs and CPCs, derived from the iPPCs). CB formation is an initial and immediate early attempt to maintain ICD from iron, Cyt-C, ammonia, acetaldehyde, acetone, H_2O_2, and GAPDH localized on the inner mitochondrial membrane (Sharma et al. 2013a; Sharma et al. 2013b; Sharma and Ebadi 2014). Particularly, Cyt-C is highly toxic and can scatter all over the cell during a free radical attack. In addition, iron participates in the Fenton reaction to synthesize highly toxic ONOO⁻ from ·OH and NO· radicals. ONOO⁻ ions not only induce oxidative but also nitrative stress to enhance α-synuclein index and DNA oxidation to synthesize 8-OH, 2dG which causes disruption in the normal epigenetic changes (histone acetylation and DNA methylation) and microRNA, involved in the transcriptional regulation of genes involved in cell growth, proliferation, migration, differentiation, and development. Entry of Cyt-C, 8-OH-2dG, 2,3, dihydroxy nonenal, and GAPDH, along with free radicals in the nucleus enhances DNA damage. Hence, the formation of condensed multilamellar membrane stacks in the form of CB is to primarily contain Cyt-C and other highly toxic mitochondrial metabolites. Moreover, Cyt-C is non-covalently attached with the inner mitochondrial membrane and can easily delocalize MAOs, TRPCs, TSPOs, and StAR to induce pro-inflammatory as well as apoptotic signal transduction involved in progressive neurodegeneration.

CS Destabilization Causes Dendritic Pruning and Synaptic Degeneration. The frequency of CB formation and hence CS increased as a function of severity and duration of nutritional stress or toxic exposure. The incidence of CS formation was significantly increased in the developing rat cerebellar Purkinje neuron dendrites. The dendrites exhibited immature developmental characteristics. The CS is highly labile and exhibits pleomorphic electron-dense appearance. The CS releases highly toxic mitochondrial metabolites to inhibit protein synthesis in the dendrites. The sequestration of intranuclear CS is involved in the down-regulation of AgNOR that manufactures ribosomes depending on MTs-mediated Zn^{2+}-induced transcriptional regulation of genes involved in microRNAs synthesis during the DNA cell cycle, cell division, proliferation, migration, development, and differentiation. The inhibition of ribosomal synthesis is responsible for delayed or the absence of protein synthesis required for normal dendritic growth and synaptogenesis. In addition, local release of toxic substances from the CS inhibits protein synthesis to cause dendritic pruning. A free ribosomal pool was observed in the UN rat Purkinje neuron dendrites. Hence, it will be clinically significant to stabilize CS by endogenous and/or exogenous antioxidants for the normal growth and development of the brain. DPCI can also induce CS destabilization by permeabilization, sequestration, and disintegration due to free radical overproduction. Free radicals induce lipid peroxidation to cause structural and functional degradation of PUFA in the plasma membranes to cause CS membrane blebbings. The CS membrane blebs are named as CS bodies. The CS bodies fuse with the nuclear membrane or plasma membrane to cause the formation of apoptotic bodies. The apoptotic bodies are highly labile, thin walled membranous structures and are readily disintegrated to release intracellular constituents to cause non-nuclear DNA-dependent cellular demise. Hence, drugs can be developed to prevent CB formation and augment charnolophagy during the acute phase, and stabilize and contain CS dynamics during the chronic phase of DPCI.

Intracellular, extracellular, and circulating CS can participate in dendritic pruning and synaptic degeneration to cause impaired or delayed sensory motor learning accompanied with impaired cognitive performance in learning, intelligence, memory, and behavior as noticed in FAS, ZIKV diseases, rubella virus infection, and cytomegalovirus infection in addition to intrauterine exposure to toxic heavy metal ions (Pb, Hg, Cd, Ni), antidepressants, anti-psychotics, anti-epileptic drugs, nicotine, alcohol, and anesthetic agents. Several new-born infants do not exhibit overt clinical symptoms of microcephaly, because of the well-built physical status, robust immune system and nutritional status of a western woman during pregnancy. Although CB formation occurs in the developing NPCs of these pregnant women, it is very efficiently phagocytosed by energy-driven charnolophagy and exocytosed in the systemic circulation. Hence, the toxic metabolites of the circulating CS are primarily involved in dendritic pruning, synaptic silence, synaptic atrophy, and eventually synaptic degeneration without any overt clinical symptoms of craniofacial anomalies. This is reflected as impaired cognitive performance of new-born children from alcohol and/or nicotine abusing western women with or without exposure of environmental toxins and/or microbial infections. Antioxidants such as glutathione, MTs, SOD, and catalase are induced simultaneously as cyto-protective agents in the most vulnerable cells as potent free radical scavengers to prevent microcephaly.

CS-Antioxidants Interaction in Health and Disease

The primary objective of this book is to describe a novel hypothesis of CS-antioxidant interaction in health and disease. This study was performed on gene-manipulated rat and mouse models *in vivo*, and in cell culture models *in vitro* employing TEM, SEM, confocal microscopy, digital fluorescence imaging microscopy, molecular biology methods, and molecular imaging employing [18]FdG and ^{18}F-DOPA as biomarkers of DAergic neurotransmission, and mitochondrial bioenergetics respectively by microPET neuroimaging utilizing microPET manager for the data acquisition in list mode and AsiPro for constructing sinograms and generating 3D molecular images to authenticate antioxidant-mediated cytoprotection in health and disease.

As described above, CS bodies are formed by free radical-induced budding of structurally-labile CS membranes. CS bodies coalesce with the plasma membrane to form apoptotic bodies, which induce membrane permeabilization and release cytosolic constituents to cause non-nuclear DNA-induced apoptosis (cellular demise). Antioxidants such as glutathione and MTs provide structural and functional stability to CS membranes by serving as potent free radical scavengers and facilitate charnolophagy and CS exocytosis as a basic cellular and molecular mechanism of intranuclear, intracellular, extracellular, and systemic detoxification to prevent chronic illnesses. CS endocytosis as well as endonucleosis induce MDR malignancies, whereas CS exocytosis is involved in the ICD to remain healthy and prevent further degenerative changes. Non-specific induction of CS and its structural degradation is involved in GIT symptoms, alopecia, myelosuppression, neurotoxicity, hepatoxicity, and nephrotoxicity in MDR malignancies. Hence, cancer stem cell-specific charnolo-mimetics and CS inducers may be developed to eradicate MDR malignancies with minimum or no adverse effects and vice versa for the clinical management of various CVDs and NDDs. Moreover, charnolophagy as well as CS exocytosis by the oocyte following conception are highly intricate, spatio-temporally-regulated events involved in the normal development of the embryo during post-zygotic phase. Thus, CS-antioxidant interaction is primarily involved in almost every aspect of health and disease, which has been described in detail in this book.

A DSST destabilization of CS is involved in progressive NDDs, such as: epilepsy, AD, PD, HD, ALS, MDDs, MS, multiple drug addiction, and schizophrenia. There are primarily 4 different regions (A: dendritic region; B: perinuclear region; C: junction of the axon hillock; and D: the synaptic region), where free radical-induced CB is transformed by energy (ATP)-dependent lysosomal-mediated charnolophagy to form a CS as illustrated in Fig. 7.

The CS is structurally and functionally highly labile intracellular organelle. The DSST destabilization of CS occurs in response to primary, secondary, and/or tertiary free radical attack. The CS destabilization is represented by (i) permeabilization, (ii) sequestration, and/or (iii) fragmentation depending on the intensity and frequency of free radical-induced physicochemical insult. A. Presence of free-radical-mediated destabilized CS in the dendritic region releases highly toxic substances to cause inhibition in protein synthesis due to mitochondrial as well as ER oxidative stress resulting in direct inhibition of AgNOR involved in ribosomal synthesis and eventually protein synthesis. These deleterious events are involved in dendritic pruning as observed in DPCI to induce microcephaly and other craniofacial abnormalities as noticed in FASD, chronic tobacco smoking, and ZIKV infection during pregnancy. B. The presence of destabilized CS in the perinuclear region induces (a) epigenetic changes in the mitochondrial and nuclear DNA and (b) disruption in the microRNA-mediated post-transcriptional regulation of genes involved in DNA cycle, cell proliferation, differentiation, and development. C. The accumulation of CB/CS at the junction of axon hillock inhibits normal axoplasmic transport of various enzymes, neurotransmitters, hormones, ions, neurotrophic factors (BDNF, IGF-1, VEGF), and mitochondria to initially cause synaptic silence during acute phase, followed by

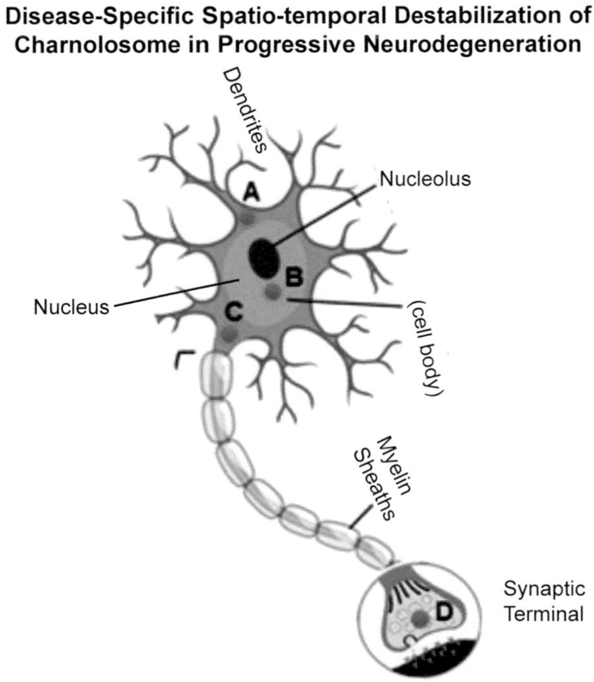

Disease-Specific Spatio-temporal Destabilization of Charnolosome in Progressive Neurodegeneration

Fig. 7: A pictorial diagram illustrating disease-specific spatio-temporal destabilization of *CS* involved in progressive *NDDs*.

synaptic atrophy and synaptic degeneration during chronic phase of disease progression. D. The presence of CS in the synaptic terminal can induce similar neurodegenerative changes, but more frequently as compared to the CS at the junction of axon hillock to cause early morbidity and mortality. Early events in CS destabilization at the synaptic terminal are accompanied with ionic disturbances involving excito-neurotoxicity as observed in intractable epilepsy, AD, PD, HD, ALS, MDD, chronic drug addiction and schizophrenia. Hence, novel DSST charnolopharmacotherapeutics may be developed to prevent and/or inhibit CB formation during acute phase and stabilize CS during chronic phase of disease progression for the safe and effective EBPT of these patients. Mitochondrial as well as ERS occur primarily in the dendritic regions and in the growth cones because these are rich in RER, essential for protein synthesis during brain development. Particularly NPCs and CSs (derived from iPPCs) are highly vulnerable to free-radical-induced ERS and mitochondrial oxidative stress; whereas mitochondrial oxidative stress occurs primarily in the synaptic region, where requirement of energy (ATP) is highly crucial and constantly needed for the normal brain regional neurocybernetics to maintain normal cognitive function. Any impairment in the synaptic transmission due to the release of toxic metabolites from destabilized CS can induce impairments in learning, intelligence, memory, and behavior to cause early morbidity and mortality, as noticed in chronic MDR patients.

The Mitochondrial Disorders and CB

Up to 4,000 children per year are born in the U.S.A. with some form of mitochondrial disease (The Mitochondrial and Metabolic Disease Center). It has been estimated that ~ 1 in 4,000 children will develop mitochondrial disease by the age of 10 years. Because mitochondrial disorders contain numerous variations and subsets, some mitochondrial disorders are rare. The average number of births per year among women at risk for transmitting mtDNA disease is estimated ~ 150 in the UK and 800 in the US (Gorman et al. 2015).

The first pathogenic mutation in mtDNA was identified in 1988, from that time to 2016, around 275 other disease-causing mutations have been identified (Claiborne et al. 2016). The most significant persons who suffered from mitochondrial disease include: Mattie Stepanek suffered from dysautonomic mitochondrial myopathy. He was a poet, peace advocate, and motivational speaker who died at age 13. Rocco Baldelli was a coach and former center fielder in Major League Baseball who had to retire at age 29 due to "mitochondrial channelopathy". Charlie Gard a British boy suffered from mtDNA depletion syndrome.

The mitochondria generate > 90% of ATP required to sustain life and support organ function. They are found in almost every cell of the human body except erythrocytes, and convert food molecules into the ATP for most cellular functions. The mitochondrial diseases are caused by mitochondrial dysfunction. The mtDNA produces its own mRNA, tRNA, and rRNA. These organelles possess their own ribosomes, called mitoribosomes. When a person has mitochondrial disease, these organelles do not produce sufficient ATP required for cell growth, development, and survival. The most significant parts of the body affected are those that have the highest energy demands: brain, muscle, liver, heart and kidney, when these systems are affected, mitochondrial diseases are usually progressive. Thus, CMB in these organs could be life-threatening. Although, certain therapeutic CS-antioxidant interactions can ease some of the symptoms or slow down the progression of mitochondrial diseases, none can absolutely cure them.

The mammalian mitochondrial genome is transmitted through the maternal germ line. The human mtDNA is a double-stranded, circular molecule of 16569 bp and contains 37 genes coding for two rRNAs, 22 tRNAs, and 13 polypeptides. The *CB* is formed in the most vulnerable cell in response to any physicochemical injury-induced free radical overproduction due to CMB and down-regulation of the mtDNA. Mitochondrial diseases are ($\sim$ 15% of the time) caused by mutations in the mtDNA that affect mitochondrial function (DiMauro and Davidzon 2005). Other mitochondrial diseases are caused by mutations in genes of the nuclear DNA, whose gene products are imported into the mitochondria (mitochondrial proteins) and acquired mitochondrial conditions. The neuromuscular diseases are named as mitochondrial myopathies including: (a) mitochondrial myopathy; (b) diabetes mellitus and deafness (DAD); (c) Leber's hereditary optic neuropathy (LHON); (d) Leigh syndrome, subacute sclerosing encephalopathy; (e) Neuropathy, ataxia, retinitis pigmentosa, and ptosis (NARP); (f) myoneurogenic gastrointestinal encephalopathy (MNGIE). Extranuclear inheritance (also known as cytoplasmic inheritance) is a form of non-Mendelian inheritance (Correns 1909).

Signs and Symptoms of Mitochondrial Diseases. Typical symptoms of mitochondrial diseases include stunted growth, loss of muscle coordination, muscle weakness, visual problems, hearing problems, learning disabilities, heart disease, liver disease, kidney disease, GIT disorders, respiratory disorders, neurological disorders, autonomic dysfunction and dementia as noticed in chronic nicotine and alcohol abuse. The body, and each mutation, is modulated by other genome variants; the mutation that in one individual may cause liver disease might in another person may cause a CNS disorder. The severity of the specific defect may also vary among different individuals due to disease-specific CB formation. Minor defects cause only "*exercise intolerance*", with no serious illness or disability. Defects often affect the operation of the mitochondria and tissues more severely, leading to multi-system diseases. Generally, mitochondrial diseases are worse when the defective mitochondria are present in the muscles, cerebrum, or nerves, because these cells consume more energy than most other cells in the body (Finsterer 2007). Although mitochondrial diseases vary in presentation from person to person, several major clinical conditions have been defined, based on the most common phenotypic features, symptoms, and signs associated with a mutation that tend to cause them. Whether ATP depletion or ROS are responsible for the observed phenotypic consequences remains unknown. However, it will be promising to develop DSST charnolopharmacotherapeutics for the targeted, safe, and effective EBPT of patients with mitochondrial disorders (such as diabetes, AD, MDDs, schizophrenia, bulimia, and Obesity).

Causes of Mitochondrial Disorders. It is now well established that mitochondrial disorders may be caused by mutations (acquired or inherited) in mtDNA, or in nuclear genes that code for mitochondrial components involving CB molecular pathogenesis. They may also be the result of acquired mitochondrial dysfunction due to adverse effects of DPCI. Nuclear DNA has two copies per cell (except for spermatocytes and oocytes), one copy being inherited from the father and the other from the mother. However, mtDNA is inherited from the mother and each mitochondrial organelle contains between 2–10 mtDNA copies. During cell division, the mitochondria segregate randomly between the two new cells and make more copies, normally reaching 500 mitochondria per cell. As mtDNA is copied when mitochondria proliferate, they can accumulate random mutations, also named as heteroplasmy. If only a few of the mtDNA copies inherited from the mother are defective, mitochondrial division may cause most of the defective copies resulting in just one of the new mitochondria. Mitochondrial disease may become clinically apparent once the number of affected mitochondria reaches a certain level; this phenomenon is named as "*threshold expression*".

Mutations in the mtDNA occur due to the lack of the error checking capability that nDNA possesses. Hence, mtDNA disorders may occur relatively quite often. Defects in enzymes that control mtDNA replication (all of which are encoded for by genes in the nDNA) may also cause mtDNA mutations. Most mitochondrial function and biogenesis is controlled by nDNA. Human mtDNA encodes 13 proteins of the respiratory chain, while ~ 1,500 proteins of mitochondria are nuclear-encoded. Defects in nuclear-encoded mitochondrial genes are associated with numerous diseases, including anemia, dementia, hypertension, lymphoma, retinopathy, seizures, and neurodevelopmental disorders (Scharfe et al. 2009). A study explored the role of mitochondria in insulin resistance among the offspring of patients with type 2 diabetes (Petersen et al. 2004). Other studies showed that the mechanism may involve the interruption of the mitochondrial signaling in body cells (intramyocellular lipids). Another study demonstrated that this partially downregulates the genes that produce mitochondria (Parish and Peterson 2005).

Examples of Mitochondrial Diseases. Representative mitochondrial diseases include: mitochondrial myopathy, diabetes mellitus and deafness (DAD). This combination at an early age can be due to mitochondrial disease. DAD can be found together for other reasons; such as Leber's hereditary optic neuropathy (LHON) accompanied with visual loss in young adulthood. This eye disorder characterized by progressive loss of central vision due to degeneration of the optic nerves and retina, affects 1 in 50,000 people in Finland. Leigh syndrome, subacute sclerosing encephalopathy alter normal development. The disease usually begins late in the first year of life, although onset may occur in adulthood; a rapid decline in function occurs and is marked by seizures, impaired consciousness, dementia, and ventilatory failure. Neuropathy, ataxia, retinitis pigmentosa, and ptosis (NARP) as noticed in dementia. Myoclonic epilepsy with ragged red fibers (MERRF) are clumps of defected mitochondria that accumulate in the subsarcolemmal region of the muscle fiber. These patients have short stature; hearing loss; lactoacidosis; and exercise intolerance. Mitochondrial myopathy, encephalomyopathy, lactoacidosis, stroke-like symptoms (MELAS), and mtDNA depletion; mitochondrial neurogastrointestinal encephalomyopathy (MNGIE) are also disorders of CMB. Although Friedreich's ataxia can affect the mitochondria, it is not associated with mitochondrial proteins.

Mechanisms of Mitochondrial Diseases. The effective unit for the body energy is referred to as the daily glycogen generation capacity, and is used to compare the mitochondrial output of healthy individuals to that of afflicted or chronically glycogen-depleted individuals (Lorini and Ciman 1962; Mitchell Michelakis 2007). This value is slow to change, as it takes between 18–24 months to complete a full cycle (Michelakis 2007). The glycogen synthesis capacity is determined by the functional levels of the mitochondria in all cells of the human body (Stacpoole 1998); however, the relation between the energy generated by the mitochondria and the glycogen capacity is very loose and is mediated by many biochemical pathways. Most of the mitochondrial energy (ATP) is consumed by the brain and is not easily measurable.

Diagnosis of Mitochondrial Disorders. Mitochondrial diseases are detected by analyzing muscle samples, where the presence of these organelles is highest (40%). The most common tests for the detection of these diseases are: *(a) Southern blot analysis to detect deletions or duplications; (b) PCR and mutation analysis; and (c) DNA Sequencing* (Stacpoole 1998).

Treatment of Mitochondrial Disorders. Treatment options are currently limited. Usually, vitamins are prescribed, though the evidence for their effectiveness is not established (Marriage et al. 2003). Pyruvate was proposed in 2007 as a treatment option (Tanaka et al. 2007); N-acetyl cysteine reverses several experimental models of mitochondrial dysfunction (Frantz and Wipf 2010).

Gene Therapy Prior to Conception. Spindle transfer, where the nuclear DNA is transferred to another healthy oocyte leaving the defective mtDNA behind, is a potential therapeutic intervention that has been carried out in monkeys (Ghosh 2009; Tachibana et al. 2009). Using a similar pronuclear transfer technique, healthy DNA was transplanted in oocytes from women with mitochondrial disease into the eggs of women donors who were unaffected (Boseley 2010; Craven et al. 2010). In such cases, ethical questions were raised regarding biological motherhood, since the child received genes and gene regulatory molecules from two different women. Hence, using genetic engineering to produce babies free of mitochondrial disease remains controversial and raises ethical issues (UK urged to permit IVF procedure to prevent fatal genetic diseases); (Three Parent Baby Laws 2015). A male baby was born in Mexico in 2016 from a mother with Leigh syndrome using spindle transfer (Hamzelou 2016). In 2012, a public consultation was launched in the UK to explore the ethical issues (Sample 2012). Human genetic engineering was used to allow infertile women with genetic defects in their mitochondria to have children (Genetically altered babies born 2001). In June 2013, the UK government developed legislation that would legalize the 'three-person IVF' procedure as a treatment to fix or eliminate mitochondrial diseases that are passed on from mother to child. The procedure could be offered once regulations had been established (The Human Fertilization and Embryology 2015; Knapton 2014). Embryonic mitochondrial transplant and protofection were proposed as a treatment for inherited mitochondrial disease, and allotopic expression of mitochondrial proteins as a treatment for mtDNA mutation. Currently, human clinical trials are underway at GenSight Biologics (ClinicalTrials.gov # NCT02064569) and at the University of Miami (ClinicalTrials.gov # NCT02161380) to examine the safety and efficacy of mitochondrial gene therapy in Leber's hereditary optic neuropathy.

Correlation Between Brain Regional MRS and Circulating CS Biomarkers

There are several circulating CS biomarkers which can be estimated and correlated with brain regional MRS analyses of lactate, Cr/PCr ratio, and N-acetyl-aspartate (NAA) to evaluate FASD-induced CMB. Other CS biomarkers include acetate, acetone, ammonia, and H_2O_2, and LDH, phosphatidyl serine (PS), MTs, glutathione, CoQ_{10}, NADH oxidase (NOX), cyclocygenase (Cox), thioredoxine, caspases (caspase-3, caspase-9), HSPs, HIF, and P^{53}. These CS biomarkers can be estimated to establish the therapeutic potential of novel charnolopharmacotherapeutics for the targeted, safe, and effective EBPT of FASD and numerous other disorders. In addition, S-adenosyl methionine (SAM) and folate can be estimated to assess FASD-induced epigenetic modulation. Various *in vivo* PET neuroimaging biomarkers including ^{18}FdG and ^{18}F-Florbetapir (PIB) have been introduced. More specifically, PET imaging biomarkers representing reduced fronto-temporal ^{18}FdG uptake, increased ^{11}C or ^{18}F-PIB uptake, ^{11}C-PBR-28 to measure 18 kDa translocator protein (TSPO), a biomarker of inflammation, and 3-D MRI can be employed for assessing ventriculomegaly and MRS for the estimation of $Cr/CrPO_4$ as high energy phosphorylated metabolites and NAA to assess neuronal injury for the early, safe, and effective clinical management of FASD and AD (Sharma 2017; Sharma and Lippincott 2017). It will require rigorous IRB and radiation safety approval for the afore-mentioned PET imaging biomarkers to assess the exact MB and CS dynamics in developing infants. Another viable option will be to conduct these experiments on animal models of FASD and/or use cell culture, 3D embryoid bodies, and cerebral organoids. Moreover, it will be essential to follow up FASD victims for at-least 6–8 years after their birth. The afore-mentioned PET biomarkers can be estimated *in vivo*, employing multi-modality molecular imaging with PET, SPECT, CT, and MRI to provide precise 5D information regarding CB formation, charnolophagy, and CS pharmacodynamics to quantitatively assess functional deficit in brain regional MB for the safe and effective EBPT of MDR diseases. Moreover, multimodality molecular neuroimaging can quantitatively assess the therapeutic potential of newly developed charnolopharmacotherapeutics for a better quality of life for FASD and other victims of multiple drug addiction.

Limitations of Estimating Circulating CS Biomarkers

The estimation of afore-mentioned circulating CS biomarkers will not provide precise localization of chronic drug (nicotine, alcohol)-induced brain regional neurodegenerative apoptosis. The circulating CS will also not provide precise information regarding their exact origin from a tissue (brain, liver, muscle, heart, kidney, etc.). It will be a challenging task to pinpoint which specific circulating CS biomarker has originated from which specific brain region and its exact theranostic significant in chronic MDR diseases. Hence, a comprehensive analyses of brain region-specific CS biomarkers will be required to establish peripheral CS theranostic biomarkers for the safe and effective clinical management of chronic MDR diseases. Ethanol-induced brain regional (hippocampal) CB formation causing neurodegenerative apoptosis can be precisely estimated by multi-modality fusion imaging with PET, SPET, MRI, CT, and ultrasound, which will have promising future prospect to discover therapeutically-beneficial charnolopharmacotherapeutics for an early prevention and/or treatment of MDR diseases. However, radiation safety issues will remain a significant challenge in these versatile biotechnologies particularly for the pediatric population.

Inflammasome vs Charnolosome

It is now well-established that inflammasome is linked to atherosclerosis, periodic fever syndromes, vitiligo, Crohn's disease, gout, asbestosis, silicosis, AD, and periodontitis. Endometriosis has been related with IL-1β and another NLR, Nlrp7, was correlated with myometrial invasion in human endometrial cancer tissue.

Recently, Bullon and Navarro (2017) highlighted that endometriosis remains a significant challenge to treat. There is a dire need to develop novel therapeutic strategies based on pathophysiological mechanisms targeting the etiologic and pathogenic processes involved. These investigators proposed inflammosome as a novel pathogenic mechanism in endometriosis. Inflammasome is a multiprotein complex and is a key regulator of the innate and adaptive host response that surveys the cytosol and other compartments into the cell. It is involved in the early detection and responds to the presence of pathogen-associated molecular patterns named DAMPs and PAMPs respectively, and is demonstrated in several cells, particularly in immune cells of the myeloid lineage and epithelial cells in tissues with mucosal surfaces.

Four inflammasome are: Noll like receptors (NLR) proteins Nlrp1b, Nlrp3, Nlrc4, and Nlrp6, as well as in melanoma 2. They activate the production of IL-1β and IL-18 that induce a host response such as pyroptosis, a proinflammatory cell death, and the secretion of cytokines and growth factors. Hence, inflammasome may be crucial in the future development for endometriosis therapy.

Ferreira et al. (2017) recently reported that an intricate interaction between innate and adaptive immune cells is crucial for an effective immune response during disease, infection, and vaccination. This interaction is primarily performed by dendritic cells (DCs), which are antigen presenting cells with the potential to translate innate into adaptive immunity. They recognize and uptake antigens, migrate to lymphoid tissues, and activate naïve T-cells. The DCs have germline encoded pattern recognition receptors (PRR) that recognize conserved pathogen associated molecular patterns (PAMPs) or danger associated molecular patterns (DAMPs). While some PRRs like Toll-like receptors (TLRs) recognize PAMPs and DAMPs at the cell surface and in endosomal/lysosomal compartments, others, such as NOD-like receptors (NLRs), act as cytosolic sensors. NLRs activation through recognition of PAMPs and DAMPs leads to the assembly of signaling inflammasome as regulators of caspase 1, the enzyme responsible for the proteolytic cleavage of precursors' pro-IL-1β and pro-IL-18 into their active form.

A study was performed recently to determine how inflammasomes are related to maturation, migration, antigen presenting function and dendritic cells (DCs)' ability to fine-tune adaptive immune responses. It is now well established that in danger/infectious scenarios NLR and TLR synergize to expand DCs' maturation, migration, antigen presenting function, and adaptive immune system activation. However, in the absence of a danger scenario, and without TLR engagement, inflammasome activation stimulates an immunosuppressive profile on DCs. Thus, activation of the inflammasome in DCs should not be viewed in isolation but rather considering its interconnections with the various PPR-driven pathways. Due to the increasing evidences of inflammasome involvement in multiple inflammatory and immune diseases, this information is highly significant since precise inflammasome pharmacological targeting could lead to clinical utility through targeted therapies.

It is currently recognized that the inflammasome functions as a platform of pro-inflammatory cytokine production such as IL-1β and IL-18. Under certain conditions, however, the inflammasome produces effects such as induction of cell death, pyroptosis, and cell metabolism alterations. Recently, Conley et al. (2017) reported several types of inflammasomes in mammalian cells. The most widely studied is the inflammasome containing NOD-like receptor with pyrin domain 3 (NLRP3), as a molecular mechanism of chronic degenerative diseases. Many activators or risk factors exert their actions through the activation of the NLRP3 inflammasome to produce functional changes in different cells including inflammatory, metabolic, or survival responses. Several molecular signaling pathways mediate the activation of the NLRP3 inflammasome, and are related to the modifications in K^+ efflux, increased lysosome leakage and activation of cathepsin B, or enhanced ROS production. In the kidney, inflammation promotes the progression of glomerular sclerotic pathologies resulting in end-stage renal disease (ESRD). NLRP3 inflammasome activation may trigger glomerular inflammation and other cell damages, contributing to the onset of glomerular injury and ESRD. The inflammasome activation not only occurs in immune cells, but also in endothelial cells and podocytes in the glomeruli. There is now evidence of NLRP3 inflammasome activation and related molecular mechanisms in renal glomeruli. The possible canonical and non-canonical effects of inflammasome activation and its implication in the development of different glomerular diseases have been proposed.

Autophagy, Inflammasome, and Charnolopathies. The molecular crosstalk between inflammation and autophagy is an emerging field of research that is essential for the understanding of cellular homeostasis and how these processes influence pathological conditions. de Lavera et al. (2017) recently described the relationship between autophagy and inflammasome activation. They discussed that mitochondria play a crucial role in both cellular processes (i.e., autophagy as well as inflammasome activation). There are primarily 3 phases of free radical-induced attack to CS. A primary free radical attack (PFA) to CS triggers induction of CS bodies rich in pro-inflammatory cytokines and are named as inflammasome. The inflammosome participates in the progression of inflammation. A secondary free radical attack (SFA) to CS triggers the formation of apoptosomes. The apoptosome is rich in caspases and AIF. A tertiary free radical attack (TFA) to CS triggers the formation of necrosome involved in the necrosis of a cell. A stem cell-specific CS is primarily involved in MDR malignant transformation through the induction of inflammosome, apoptosome, and necrosome, during the primary, secondary, and tertiary phase of free radical attack, respectively. The translocation of inflammasome, apoptosome, and necrosome from stem cell specific CS (SC_{scs}) during DPCI-induced free radical attack is involved in MDR malignanat transformation. It is proposed that inflammasome and autophagy modulate each other by common inhibitory mechanisms that are controlled by different input pathways. Thus, inflammasome components coordinate autophagy and autophagy regulates inflammasome activation, making the balance between both processes crucial in cellular homeostasis. A pictorial representation of interplay between inflammasome, autophagy, and mitochondrial damage, leading to CB formation, charnolophagy, and CS exocytosis as a basic molecular mechanism of ICD for normal cellular function to remain healthy is systematically presented in the following pictorial diagram. DPCI induce mitochondrial degeneration to cause CB formation which is an immediate and early pre-apoptotic event. Hence, disease induction and its prevention, depends on the severity of free radical attack as illustrated in Fig. 8.

Generally, primary free radical attack is readily attenuated by endogenously synthesized mitochondrial antioxidants including SOD, catalase, HSP-70, thioredoxin, HIF-1α, MTs, and glutathione. Secondary free radical attack can be inhibited or attenuated by endogenous as well as exogenously-synthesized antioxidant therapeutic agents such as MAO-Is (trenylcypromine, phenelzine, semithiocarbazide, selegiline, rasagiline, moclobemide, safinamide, linezolid) and naturally available antioxidants such as sirtuins, rutins, LSDs, resveratrol, lycopene, and catechin. Tertiary free radical attack cannot be prevented and/or attenuated by endogenously and exogenously synthesized, and naturally-available antioxidants. Chronic intoxication of a vulnerable cell due to primary, secondary, or tertiary free radical attack enhances CS destabilization to synthesize highly labile CS bodies, which fuse with the plasma membranes to cause the formation of apoptotic bodies. The apoptotic bodies burst to release highly toxic mitochondrial metabolites to cause disease progression. In fact, the structural and functional destabilization of cancer stem cell-specific CS bodies is involved in MDR malignancies. To prevent and/or inhibit tertiary and quaternary free radical attack (TFA) involved primarily in MDR malignancies and other chronic diseases, we need to develop DSST charnolopharmacotherapeutics including: CB antagonists, charnolophagy agonists, CS stabilizers, and CS exocytosis enhancers as intracellular detoxifiers to remain healthy.

Pathophysiology of CS in Health and Disease. The CS bodies from the CS derived cancer stem cells and other cells also contain three subcellular organelles including: (i) apoptosomes, (ii) inflammasomes, and (iii) necrosomes. An apoptosome is composed of all the molecular biomarkers of apoptosis including: caspases (particularly

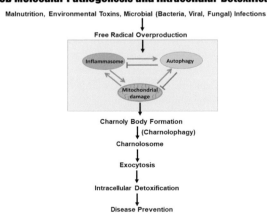

Fig. 8: A systematic diagram illustrating free radical hypothesis of CB formation and charnolophagy as a basic molecular mechanism of ICD for disease prevention.

caspase-3) and AIF. The caspase-3 induces PARP cleavage to trigger inter-nucleosomal DNA fragmentation to cause program cell death (Apoptosis). Inflammasomes are important regulators of caspase 1, the enzyme responsible for the proteolytic cleavage of precursors' pro-IL-1β and pro-IL-18 into their active form. Inflammasome is a multiprotein complex and is a key regulator of the innate and adaptive host response that surveys the cytosol and other compartments into the cell. It is involved in the immediate detection and responds to the presence of DAMPs and PAMPs respectively, and has been demonstrated in several cells, mainly on immune cells of the myeloid lineage and epithelial cells in tissues with mucosal surfaces. An inflammasome is involved in the induction of proinflammatory cytokines such as IL1β, IL-6, TNFα, and NFκβ. These proinflammatory cytokines induce progressive degenerative changes, involving pyroptosis. A necrosome is involved in cellular necrosis and is induced by free radical-induced intracellular injury. Thus, depending on the extent of free radicals-induced attack, inflammosome, apoptosome, charnolosome, and/or necrosomes are synthesized in a biological system. In general, (i) primary free radical attack induces pro-inflammatory response due to CS destabilization, (ii) secondary free radical attack induces apoptosome activation and apoptosis, and (iii) tertiary free radical attack induces necrosome to induce cellular necrosis. During necrosis, DNA fragmentation occurs randomly, and these fragments are of heterogenous sizes. We notice a ladder of internucleosomal fragments of 180–200 bp during apoptosis, whereas necrotic cells exhibit a smear in the DNA agarose gel electrophoresis.

Charnolopharmacotherapeutics in Osteoporosis Treatment. Osteoporosis, a bone disease resulting in the loss of bone density and microstructure quality, is often associated with fragility fractures, and the latter imposes enormous burden on the patient and society. Osteoporosis is common among post-menopausal women due to estrogen deficiency. During osteoporosis, osteoclastic activity is significantly elevated, and osteoblasts are down-regulated. The osteoclasts are rich in lysosomes containing acid phosphatases, whereas osteoblasts are rich in alkaline phosphatase (ALP) involved in cell proliferation, development, and differentiation. The mitochondria are rich in ALP because their pH is 8.0 as compared to the cytoplasmic pH of 7.2. The acid phosphatase is localized in the lysosomes as these organelles have acidic pH 4–4.5. The lysosomal activity of osteoclasts is responsible for bone resorption. The mitochondrial survival becomes significantly challenging in an acidic environment of lysosomes; hence these are destroyed due to CB formation, involved in various pro-inflammatory, pro-apoptotic, and pro-necrotic events during osteoporosis. Moreover, CS is destabilized and/or disintegrated in an acidic microenvironment to trigger pathological events in chronic diseases including, osteoporosis. Although there are several different treatments available for osteoporosis such as hormone replacement therapy, bisphosphonates, denosumab, and parathyroid hormone, concerns have been raised regarding the side effects of their chronic use. Hence, search for alternative natural compounds could circumvent the limitations of the currently available therapy. Recently, Wang et al. (2017) reviewed current literature on natural compounds that might have therapeutic potential for osteoporosis. These researchers included following search terms: bone resorption, bone density, osteoporosis, postmenopausal, osteoporosis, or bone density conservation agents, and any of the terms related to traditional, herbal, natural therapy, natural health, diet, or phytoestrogens. All the compounds and herbs were naturally bioactive or were used in herbal medicine attenuated osteopenia or osteoporosis *in vivo* or *in vitro*, through mechanisms including: estrogen-like activity, antioxidant and anti-inflammatory properties, or by modulating the key signaling pathways in the pathogenesis of osteoporosis. These researchers provided perspective for a complementary anti-osteoporotic treatment option and prevention strategy for osteoporosis or osteolytic bone disorders. Hence, it will be promising to develop osteoblast CB antagonists, charnolophagy agonists, CS stabilizers, and CS exocytosis enhancers to prevent and/or cure pre or postmenopausal osteoporosis with novel DSST charnolopharmacotherapeutics.

Drug Target Validation Methods in Malaria. It has been recognized that the validation of drug targets in malaria and other human diseases remains a significant challenge. In many cases, highly specific small molecular tools to inhibit a proteins function *in vivo* are unavailable. Moreover, the use of genetic tools in the analysis of malarial pathways is challenging. These issues result in difficulties in modulating a hypothetical drug target's function *in vivo*. Recently, Meissner et al. (2017) highlighted that the current strategies to identify a protein's function *in vivo* remains limited and there is a dire need for expansion. Novel approaches are required to support target validation in the drug discovery process. Oligomerization is the natural assembly of multiple copies of a single protein into one object and this self-assembly is present in more than half of all protein structures. Thus, oligomerization plays a crucial role in the generation of functional biomolecules. A key feature of oligomerization is that the oligomeric interfaces between the individual parts of the final assembly are highly specific. However, these interfaces have not yet been explored to delineate biochemical pathways *in vivo*. These investigators described the current state of the antimalarial biotechnology as well as the potentially-druggable malarial pathways. A specific focus was drawn to exploit oligomerization surfaces in drug target validation. It has been proposed that as an alternative to the conventional methods, protein interference assay (PIA) can be utilized for specific distortion of the target protein function and pathway assessment *in vivo*.

Phytometabolites Targeting the Warburg Effect in Cancer Cells. It is known that phytometabolites are functional elements derived from plants and most of them exhibit therapeutic potential such as anti-cancer, anti-inflammatory, and anti-oxidant effects. Phytometabolites exert their anti-cancer effect by targeting multiple signaling pathways (Hasanpourghadi et al. 2017). One of the remarkable phenomena targeted by phytometabolites is the Warburg effect, which describes "that cancer cells exhibit an increased rate of glycolysis and aberrant redox activity compared to normal cells, which promotes further cancer development and progression". Some phytometabolites could target metabolism-related enzymes (e.g., hexokinase, pyruvate kinase M2, and HIF-1) in cancer cells, with little or no harm to normal cells. Since hyper-proliferation of cancer cells is fueled by higher cellular metabolism, phytometabolites targeting these metabolic pathways can create synergistic crosstalk with induced apoptotic pathways and sensitize cancer cells to chemotherapy. These investigators discussed specific phytometabolites that target the Warburg effect and molecular mechanism that leads to tumor growth suppression.

Thioredoxin Binding Protein and Function of Thioredoxin. It has been shown that thioredoxin-interacting protein (TXNIP), also known as thioredoxin binding protein-2, interacts negatively, and regulates the expression and function of thioredoxin (TXN).

Alhawiti et al. (2017) recently reported that TXNIP has attracted considerable attention due to its diversified functions impacting several aspects of energy metabolism. TXNIP acts as an important regulator of glucose and lipid metabolism through pleiotropic actions including regulation of β-cell function, hepatic glucose production, peripheral glucose uptake, adipogenesis, and substrate utilization. Overexpression of TXNIP in animal models induce apoptosis of pancreatic β-cells, reduce insulin sensitivity in peripheral tissues like skeletal muscle and adipose, and decrease energy expenditure. On the contrary, TXNIP deficient animals are protected from diet induced insulin resistance and type 2 diabetes. Consequently, targeting TXNIP may offer novel therapeutic opportunity and TXNIP inhibitors could be a novel therapeutic tool for the treatment of diabetes mellitus. These investigators summarized the current state of our understanding of TXNIP biology and its role in metabolic regulation and raised questions that could help to exploit TXNIP as a therapeutic target. It is now proposed that TXNIP inhibitors may prevent CB molecular pathogenesis by augmenting charnolophagy and by stabilizing CS in chronic MDR diseases such as insulin-resistant (Type-2) diabetes.

Structural Basis for the Inhibition of Cyclin-Dependent Kinases. Levin et al. (2017) recently reported that cyclin-dependent kinases (CDKs) comprise an important protein family for the development of drugs for the treatment of cancer but there is also potential for the development of drugs for NDDs and diabetes. Since the early 1990s, studies have been carried out on CDKs, to determine the structural basis for the inhibition of this protein target. These investigators reviewed recent studies focused on CDKs. They focused on understanding the structural basis for inhibition of CDKs, relating structures, and ligand-binding information. Crystallography was applied to elucidate > 400 CDK structures. Most of these structures are complexed with inhibitors. They used this information to describe the structural features determining the inhibition of this enzyme and elucidated the structures of CDK 1, 2, 4–9, 12, 13, and 16. Analysis of these structures with different competitive inhibitors indicated some common features that could be used for the development of specific CDK inhibitors, such as a pattern of hydrogen bonding and the presence of halogen atoms in the ligand structure. Based on this study, these investigators suggested that by combining the structural and functional information, a pattern of intermolecular hydrogen bonds is important for inhibitor specificity. In addition, machine learning techniques have shown improvements in predicting binding affinity for CDKs.

Charnolopharmacotherapeutics of Neonatal and Adult Epilepsy

Electrophysiologically, epilepsy is characterized by sudden episodes of spike and wave activity followed by paroxysmal burst discharge activity in the EEG records of a patient. Computerized EEG analysis demonstrates relative dominance of delta (Δ: 0.5–3 Hz) and (Θ: 4–7 Hz) and reduction in the alpha (α: 8–12 Hz) and beta (β: 12–20 Hz) spectral frequencies. Neuro-pharmacologically, epilepsy is characterized by a significant brain regional reduction in the GABA-ergic neurotransmission and increase in the glutamatergic neurotransmission. Enhanced glutamate release causes neuro-excitotoxicity due to activation of its receptors, primarily AMPA and kainate receptors. Increased glutamate release is also accompanied with increased intra-cellular calcium $[Ca^{2+}]_i$, influx, which causes depolarization of the mitochondrial membranes. The energy (ATP) requirements are significantly increased during electrical seizure discharge activity in an epileptic patient. Free radicals (reactive oxygen species: ROS) are generated in excess as a byproduct of oxidative phosphorylation during the electron transport chain in the mitochondria during epileptic attack. Overproduction of free radicals is primarily involved in the degeneration of sensitive mitochondrial membranes to trigger CB formation, charnolophagy, and CS destabilization, which releases highly toxic mitochondrial metabolites to induce progressive neurodegeneration, as observed in chronic epileptic patients. We reported selective degeneration of hippocampal CA-3 and dentate gyrus regions of the developing mice which were exposed to DOM during their intrauterine life due to CB formation in the NPCs derived from iPPCs during embryonic development to cause symptoms of AD (Dakshinamurti et al. 1993).

Primarily three stages of free radical-induced attack are involved inducing CMB and CB pathogenesis in an epileptic patient. These include; (i) primary free radical attack; (ii) secondary free radical attack; and (iii) tertiary free radical attack. A quaternary free radical attack can induce the spontaneous death of an individual due to uncontrolled CB-mediated neurodegenerative apoptosis, which can occur following exposure to highly toxic nerve gases (Soman) used in chemical wars. A brief description of free radical-induced attacks on the mitochondrial membranes involved in CB molecular pathogenesis is presented in this book. Seizure-induced primary, secondary, and tertiary free radical attacks result in CMB to cause mitochondrial membrane fragmentation. The fragmented mitochondrial membranes condense to synthesize electron-dense multilamellar (pentalamellar or heptalamellar) intracellular inclusions to cause CB formation.

Different Stages of Free Radical Attack

The different stages of free radical attack can be classified as follows:

(i) CB formed during the acute early stage of the free radical attack is called as the primary free radical attack. The primary free radical attack usually occurs during the acute early phase of disease progression.

(ii) CB formed during the immediate early phase of epileptogenesis is usually phagocytosed readily by the lysosomes as a basic molecular mechanism of ICD. A CPS is formed when CB is phagocytosed by a lysosome. This energy (ATP)-driven intricate process of CB phagocytosis is designated as charnolophagy. A CPS is transformed to CS, when the phagocytosed CB is hydrolyzed by the lysosomal enzymes. A CS is a structurally highly labile single-membrane bound intracellular organelle and is exocytosed by energy (ATP)-driven process. The exocytosis of CS occurs efficiently during acute stages of the free radical attack as a basic molecular mechanism of ICD. Various endogenously-synthesized antioxidants such as SOD, catalase, cysteine, glutathione, MTs, and heat shock proteins (HSPs) serve as free radical scavengers to stabilize CS membranes and prevent the further degeneration of plasma membranes, which facilitate their exocytosis as a basic molecular mechanism of ICD during an acute epileptic attack. A secondary free radical attack (SFA) can be attenuated by the afore-mentioned endogenously-synthesized antioxidants as well as exogenously synthesized antioxidant prescription drugs.

(iii) A tertiary free radical attack (TFA) severely compromises the MB and increases the frequency of CB formation, impairs charnolophagy, and destabilizes CPS as well as CS membranes to release highly toxic mitochondrial metabolites and triggers progressive neurodegeneration, as noticed in intractable drug-resistant temporal lobe epilepsy. Hence, antiepileptic drugs may be developed to enhance brain regional MB by preventing CB formation, augmenting charnolophagy, by preventing CS destabilization, and by augmenting its exocytosis as a basic molecular mechanism of ICD to remain healthy.

We reported that accumulation of CB at the junction of axon hillock prevents and/ or slows down the normal axoplasmic transport of various enzymes, neurotransmitter, hormones, neurotrophic factors (such as NGF-1, IGF-1, BDNF), and mitochondria in the synaptic terminals to cause their atrophy (Sharma and Ebadi 2014). Synaptic atrophy causes slow neurodegeneration of the CNS, whereas accumulation of CS at the junction of the axon hillock and its destabilization and permeabilization releases highly toxic mitochondrial metabolites (including: Cyt-C, iron, 8-OH, 2dG, 3,4 dihydroxy nonenal, mono amine oxidases, ammonia, acetaldehyde, and H_2O_2, cholesterol, Ca^{2+}, and 18 KDa (TSPO) protein to induce progressive NDDs. Axoplasmic transport of these highly toxic substances causes synaptic degeneration, resulting in early morbidity and mortality as noticed in epilepsy, PD, AD, ALS, MS, HD, MDD, schizophrenia, and chronic drug addiction. CS-destabilization-induced synaptic degeneration in the hippocampal CA-3 and dentate gyrus regions is involved in impaired brain regional neurocybenetics and early cognitive impairments, represented by diversified learning, intelligence, memory, and neurobehavioral deficits in epileptic and AD patients. The synaptic depletion of BDNF also causes severe depression among epilepsy, AD, and MDD patients. Hence, it is highly significant to augment and stabilize the brain regional MB of epileptic patients to prevent CB formation, augment charnolophagy, and CS exocytosis as a basic molecular mechanism of ICD to prevent further seizure attacks and remain healthy. Free radicals-induced CS destabilization is characterized by three different phases:

Phase-I CS permeabilization causes slow release of afore-mentioned toxic substances of mitochondrial metabolism to cause synaptic silence leading to mild cognitive impairment (MCI); **Phase-2** CS sequestration causes excessive release of toxic substances to trigger early morbidity; whereas **Phase-3** CS fragmentation causes synaptic degeneration to trigger early mortality due to progressive neurodegeneration. Hence, further studies in this direction will go a long way for the safe and effective EBPT of not only epilepsy but also several other chronic diseases of known and unknown etiopathogenesis. The readers may enjoy learning more about CB molecular pathogenesis by listening to some of my video presentations in the YouTube at the following Web Sites:

1. A podcast on "Emerging Biomarkers in Alzheimer's Disease (Recent https://www.youtube.com/watch?v=nXHdXqJ1Ang Year: April 2017).

2. Podcast: Translational Multimodality Neuroimaging | - WordPress.com https://benthamsciencepublishers.wordpress.com/.../podcast-translational-multimodalit. Web: http://www.eurekaselect.com/150882 Year: May: 2017.

3. 4th International Conference and Exhibition on Addiction Research and Therapy, Aug 3–5, 2015. Orlando, FL, U.S.A. Title: Charnoly Body as a Novel Biomarker in Drug Addiction. https://www.youtube.com/watch?v=9mcu1LuTbKs Year: Aug: 2015.

4. Adolescent Brain Maturation - Video abstract: 39776 - YouTube https://www.youtube.com/watch?v=xnJViXuY120 Year: Aug. 2013.

5. Metallothioneins and Nanomedicine - Video abstract: 42019 - YouTube https://www.youtube.com/watch?v=VIq-MZG1zoM Year: Sep. 2013.

Antioxidants Inhibit CB Formation

Various antipsychotic drugs induce Parkinsonism, whereas antiparkinsonian drugs induce schizophrenia due to brain regional CB formation, implicated in progressive NDDs. Antioxidants inhibit CB formation to prevent and/or inhibit neurodegeneration. Hence, pharmacological agents preventing or inhibiting CB formation and/or augmenting charnolophagy will be beneficial in the effective clinical management of neurodegenerative and other diseases as presented in Fig. 9.

The concentration of glycosylated hemoglobin is increased in chronic diabetes. This increase occurs as a function of severity of illness and is reduced with antidiabetic (meformin or pioglitazone) treatment. Glycosylated hemoglobin compromises the MB by down-regulating the $\Delta\Psi$ and mt-DNA, and increased synthesis of oxidation product, 8-OH, 2dG, resulting in CB formation and apoptosis. These deleterious changes due to free radical overproduction cause progressive neurodegeneration in diabetes and AD. Functional foods (rich in antioxidants, i.e., reseveratrol, lycopenes, catechin, sirtuis, rutins, flavinoids, and polyphenols) and anti-diabetic drugs prevent CB formation and hence, confer therapeutic benefit in diabetes as well as AD as illustrated in Fig. 10.

MTs inhibit CB formation by serving as free radical scavengers and vice versa. MAOIs such as selegiline and rasagiline inhibit apoptosis by augmenting MTs and by

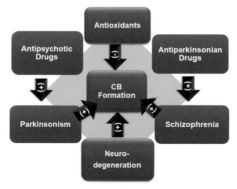

Fig. 9: Various antipsychotic drugs induce Parkinsonism, whereas antiparkinsonian drugs induce schizophrenia due to brain regional CB formation, implicated in progressive neurodegenerative disorders.

Glycosylated Hemoglobin Facilitates CB Formation

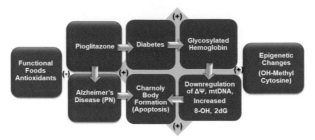

Fig. 10: A schematic flow diagram illustrating that chronic diabetes induces glycosylation of hemoglobin.

MTs Inhibit CB Formation to Prevent AD

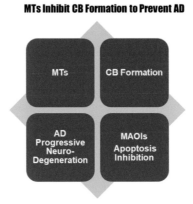

Fig. 11: A schematic flow diagram illustrating MTs-mediated inhibition of CB formation.

preventing CB formation. MAOIs induce MTs to prevent CB-triggered apoptosis to provide neuroprotection in diabetes and AD as illustrated in Fig. 11.

MT_{trans} mice were lean and agile, whereas MT_{dko} mice were obese and lethargic. MT_{dko} mice were also highly susceptible to 1-methyl, 4-phenyl, 1,2,3,6 tetrahydropyridine (MPTP)-induced Parkinsonism as illustrated in Fig. 12.

In Vivo Multimodality Neuroimaging

Recently high-resolution, noninvasive, multimodality *in vivo* molecular imaging with PET, SPECT, CT, and MRI, employing fusion algorithms has revolutionized EBPT. However, the novel discovery of specific RPs for the accurate diagnosis and effective treatment of progressive NDDs such as AD, PD, drug addiction, and other cognitive impairments remains a significant challenge. Recently, Sharma et al. (2017) highlighted the theranostic significance of multimodality fusion neuroimaging for the determination of: pharmacokinetics and pre-clinical development of RPs; *in vivo* monitoring of stem cell transplantation therapy; nicotinic acetylcholine receptors (nAChRs) investigations; regional cerebral blood flow and glucose metabolism in cognitively-impaired subjects employing multimodality noninvasive PET, CT,

MTs as CB Antagonists in Obesity

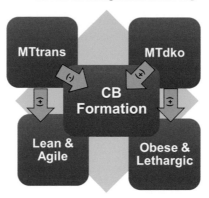

Fig. 12: A flow diagram illustrating the therapeutic potential of MTs as CB antagonists in obesity. (+) Activation; (–) Inhibition (Sharma et al. 2004; Sharma and Ebadi 200; Sharma and Ebadi 2013; Sharma and Ebadi 2014).

In vivo Multimodality Neuroimaging

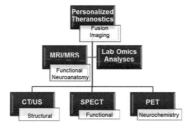

Fig. 13: *In vivo* and noninvasive, multimodality molecular imaging can be employed to determine the exact functional genomics and personalized theranostic significance of disease-specific spatiotemporal CB in health and disease.

MRI/MRS, and SPECT imaging. Recent advances in multimodality imaging employing computer-based fusion algorithms are illustrated in Fig. 13 with a primary emphasis on nanoSPECT/CT, PET-CT, and PET-MRI in experimental animals. Multimodality imaging is being performed to detect CNS infections using ^{99m}Tc-HMPAO SPECT and ^{18}F-FDG PET/CT. Furthermore, limitations of the individual neuroimaging system, body movements due to cardiorespiratory activity, and co-registration of multimodality neuroimaging data are significant challenges. Multimodality neuroimaging is clinically-significant because it emphasizes the importance of complementary imaging for theranostic applications and minimizes the inherent limitations of an individual neuroimaging approach. However, it may increase the radiation dose to a susceptible pediatric population. Future developments in specific RPs with minimum radiation exposure will facilitate early differential diagnosis, prevent, slowdown, and/or cure NDDs, CVDs, and cancer. Eventually, conventional and functional neuroimaging, combined with clinical, lab and—omics analyses will facilitate accomplishing EBPT by developing novel CB, charnolophagy, and CS targeted PET-RPs, as described in one of the chapters of this book.

Clinical Significance of CB

Various disease-specific spatio-temporal (DSST) charnopharmacotherapeutics including: (i) mtDNA targeted CB/CPS/CS agonists/antagonists; (ii) MB-targeted CB/CPS/CS agonists/antagonists; (iii) cytochrome-P-450 rejuvinators/protectants; (iv) CS exocytosis agonists/antagonists; and (v) CS endocytosis agonists/antagonists can be developed to accomplish EBPT of chronic MDR diseases with currently limited therapeutic success, including: NDDs, CVDs, and MDR malignancies.

References

Alhawiti, N.M., S.A. Mahri, M.A. Aziz, S.S. Malik and S. Mohammad. 2017. TXNIP in Metabolic Regulation: Physiological Role and Therapeutic Outlook 18: 1095–1103.

Boseley, S. 2010. Scientists reveal gene-swapping technique to thwart inherited diseases. London, Guardian.

Bullon, P. and J.M. Navarro. 2017. Inflammasome as a key pathogenic mechanism in endometriosis. Curr Drug Targets 18: 997–1002.

Chabenne, A., C. Moon, C. Ojo, A. Khogali, B. Nepal and S. Sharma. 2014. Biomarkers in fetal alcohol syndrome (Recent Update). Biomarkers and Genomic Med 6: 12–22.

Committee on the Ethical and Social Policy Considerations of Novel Techniques for Prevention of Maternal Transmission of Mitochondrial DNA Diseases; Board on Health Sciences Policy; Institute of Medicine. 2016. Claiborne, Anne, English, Rebecca and Kahn, Jeffrey (eds.). Mitochondrial Replacement Techniques: Ethical, Social, and Policy Considerations. National Academies Press.

Conley, S.M., J.M. Abais, K.M. Boini and P.L. Li. 2017. Inflammasome activation in chronic glomerular diseases. Curr Drug Targets 18: 1019–1029.

Craven, L., H.A. Tuppen, G.D. Greggains, S.J. Harbottle, J.L. Murphy, L.M. Cree, A.P. Murdoch, P.F. Chinnery, R.W. Taylor, R.N. Lightowlers, M. Herbert and D.M. Turnbull. 2010. Pronuclear transfer in human embryos to prevent transmis. Z. Indukt. Abstamm. Vererbungsl sion of mitochondrial DNA disease. Nature 465: 82–85.

Correns, C. 1909. Vererbungsversuche mit blass(gelb)grünen und buntblättringen Sippen bei *Mirabilis jalapa*, *Utrica pilulifera* und *Lunaria annua*. pp. 291–329.

Dakshinamurti, K., S.K. Sharma and M. Sundaram. 1991. Domoic acid induced seizure activity in normal rat. Neurosci Lett 127: 193–197.

Dakshinamurti, K., S.K. Sharma, M. Sundaram and T. Watanabe. 1993. Hippocampal changes in developing postnatal mice following intra-uterine exposure to domoic acid. J Neurosci 13: 4486–4495.

de Lavera, I., A.D. Pavon, M.V. Paz, M. Oropesa-Avila et al. 2017. The connections among autophagy, inflammasome and mitochondria. Curr Drug Targets 18: 1030–1038.

DiMauro, S. and G. Davidzon. 2005. Mitochondrial DNA and disease (PDF). Department of Neurology, Columbia University Medical Center. Retrieved March 20, 2013.

Ferreira, I., J. Liberal, J.D. Martins, A. Silva, B.M. Neves and M.T. Cruz. 2017. Inflammasome in dendritic cells immunobiology: implications to diseases and therapeutic strategies. Curr Drug Targets 18: 1003–1018.

Finsterer, J. 2007. Hematological manifestations of primary mitochondrial disorders. Acta Haematol 118: 88–98.

Frantz, M.C. and P. Wipf. 2010. Mitochondria as a target in treatment. Environ Mol Mutagen 51: 462–475.

Genetically altered babies born. BBC News 2001-05-04.

Ghosh, P. 2009. Genetic advance raises IVF hopes By Pallab Ghosh. BBC News, Science Correspondent. UK.

Gorman, G.S., J.P. Grady, Y. Ng, A.M. Schaefer, R.J. McNally, P.F. Chinnery, P. Yu-Wai-Man, M. Herbert, R.W. Taylor, R. McFarland and D.M. Turnbull. 2015. Mitochondrial donation—how many women could benefit? New England Journal of Medicine 372: 150130091413004.

Hamzelou, J. 2016. Exclusive: World's first baby born with new "3 parent" technique. New Scientist.

Hasanpourghadi, M., C.Y. Looi, A.K. Pandurangan, G. Sethi, W.F. Wong and M.R. Mustafa. Phytometabolites targeting the warburg effect in cancer cells: a mechanistic review. Current Drug Target 18: 1086–1094.

Jagtap, A., S. Gawande and S. Sharma. 2015. Biomarkers in vascular dementia 6 (A Recent Update). Biomarkers and Genomic Med 7: 43–56.

Knapton, S. 2014. 'Three-parent babies' could be born in Britain next year. The Daily Telegraph Science News.

Levin, N.M.B., V.O. Pintro, M.B. de Avila, B.B. de Mattos and W.F. De Azevedo Jr. 2017. Understanding the structural basis for inhibition of cyclin-dependent kinases. New Pieces in the Molecular Puzzle 18: 1104–1111.

Lorini, M. and M. Ciman. 1962. Hypoglycaemic action of Diisopropylammonium salts in experimental diabetes. Institute of Biochemistry, University of Padua, September 1962. Biochemical Pharmacology 11: 823–827.

Marriage, B., M.T. Clandinin and D.M. Glerum. 2003. Nutritional cofactor treatment in mitochondrial disorders. J Am Diet Assoc 103(8): 1029–38.

Meissner, K.A., S. Lunev, Y.-Z. Wang, M. Linzke, F. de Assis Batista, C. Wrenger and M.R. Groves. 2017. Drug Target Validation Methods in Malaria - Protein Interference Assay (PIA) as a Tool for Highly Specific Drug Target Validation. 18: 1069–1085.

Michelakis, E. 2007. A mitochondria-K^+ channel axis is suppressed in cancer and its normalization promotes apoptosis and inhibits cancer growth. University of Alberta 11: 37–51.

Mitchell, P. 1978. David Keilin's respiratory chain concept and its chemiosmotic consequences (PDF). Nobel Institute.

Petersen, K.F., S. Dufour, D. Befroy, R. Garcia and G.I. Shulman. 2004. Impaired mitochondrial activity in the insulin-resistant offspring of patients with type 2 diabetes. New England Journal of Medicine 350: 664–671.

Sample, I. 2012. Regulator to consult public over plans for new fertility treatments. The Guardian. London.

Scharfe, C., H.H. Lu, J.K. Neuenburg, E.A. Allen, G.C. Li, T. Klopstock, T.M. Cowan, G.M. Enns and R.W. Davis. 2009. Rzhetsky, Andrey (ed.). Mapping gene associations in human mitochondria using clinical disease phenotypes. PLoS Comput Biol 5(4): e1000374.

Sharma, S., K. Dakshinamurti and W. Selvamurthy. 1993. Effect of environmental neurotoxins on the developing brain. Biometeriology 2: 447–455.

Sharma, S., E. Carlson and M. Ebadi. 2003. The neuroprotective actions of selegiline in inhibiting 1-methyl, 4-phenyl, pyridinium ion (MPP$^+$)-induced apoptosis in dargic neurons. J Neurocytology 32: 329–343.

Sharma, S. and M. Ebadi. 2013. Antioxidant Targeting in Neurodegenerative Disorders. Ed. I. Laher, Springer Verlag, Germany, Chapter 85, pp. 1–30.

Sharma, S., A. Rais, R. Sandhu, W. Nel and M. Ebadi. 2013. Clinical significance of metallothioneins in cell therapy and nanomedicine. International Journal of Nanomedicine 8: 1477–1488.

Sharma, S., C.S. Moon, A. Khogali, A. Haidous, A. Chabenne, C. Ojo, M. Jelebinkov, Y. Kurdi and M. Ebadi. 2013. Biomarkers of Parkinson's disease (Recent Update). Neurochemistry International 63: 201–229.

Sharma, S. 2014. Beyond Diet and Depression (*Volume-1*). Book Nova Sciences Publishers, New York, U.S.A.

Sharma, S. 2014. Beyond Diet and Depression (*Volume-2*). Book Nova Science Publishers, New York, U.S.A.

Sharma, S. 2014. Molecular pharmacology of environmental neurotoxins. *In*: Kainic Acid: Neurotoxic Properties, Biological Sources, and Clinical Applications. Nova Science Publishers. New York. pp. 1–47.

Sharma, S. 2014. Nanotheranostics in evidence based personalized medicine. Current Drug Targets 15: 915–930.

Sharma, S. and M. Ebadi. 2014. The *charnoly body* as a universal biomarker of cell injury. Biomarkers and Genomic Medicine 6: 89–98.

Sharma, S. and M. Ebadi. 2014. Significance of metallothioneins in aging brain. Neurochemistry International 65: 40–48.

Sharma, S., B. Nepal, C.S. Moon, A. Chabenne, A. Khogali, C. Ojo, E. Hong, R. Goudet, A. Sayed-Ahmad, A. Jacob, M. Murtaba and M. Firlit. 2014. Psychology of craving. Open Jr of Medical Psychology 3: 120–125.

Sharma, S. 2015. Alleviating Stress of the Soldier & Civilian. Nova Science Publishers, New York. U.S.A.

Sharma, S. 2015. Monoamine Oxidase Inhibitors: Clinical Pharmacology, Benefits, & Adverse Effects. Nova Science Publishers, New York. U.S.A.

Sharma, S., S. Gawande, A. Jagtap, R. Abeulela and Z. Salman. 2015. Fetal alcohol syndrome; prevention, diagnosis, & treatment. *In*: Alcohol Abuse: Prevalence, Risk Factors. Nova Science Publishers, New York, U.S.A.

Sharma, S. 2016. Personalized Medicine (Beyond PET Biomarkers) Nova Science Publishers. New York. U.S.A.

Sharma, S. 2016. Pet RPs for personalized medicine. Curr Drug Targets 17: 1894–1907.

Sharma, S. 2016. Progress in PET RPs (Quality Control & Theranostics). Nova Science Publishers. New York. U.S.A.

Sharma, S., J. Choga, V. Gupta et al. 2016. Charnoly body as novel biomarker of nutritional stress in Alzheimer's disease. Functional Foods in Health and Disease 6: 344–377.

Sharma, S. 2017. Translational multimodality neuroimaging. Current Drug Targets 18: 1039–1050.

Sharma, S. 2017. *ZIKV* Disease (Prevention and Cure). Nova Science Publishers, New York, U.S.A.

Sharma, S. 2017. Fetal Alcohol Spectrum Disorders (Concepts, Mechanisms, and Cure). Nova Science Publishers, New York, U.S.A.

Sharma, S. 2017. Translational Multimodality Neuroimaging. 18: 1039–1050.

Sharma, S. and W. Lippincott. 2017. Emerging biomarkers in Alzheimer's disease (Recent Update). Current Alzheimer Research 14 (in press).

Sharma, S.K., U. Nayar, M.C. Maheshwari and G. Gopinath. 1986. Ultrastructural studies of P-cell morphology in developing normal and undernourished rat cerebellar cortex. Electrophysiological Correlates Neurology India 34: 323–327.

Sharma, S.K., U. Nayar, M.C. Maheshwari and B. Singh. 1987. Effect of undernutrition on developing rat cerebellum: Some electrophysiological and neuromorphological correlates. J Neurol Sciences 78: 261–272.

Sharma, S.K., W. Selvamurthy, M. Behari, M.C. Maheshwari and T.P. Singh. 1987. Computerized EEG analysis of Penicillin induced seizure threshold in developing rats. Ind J Med Res 86: 775–782.

Sharma, S.K. 1988. Nutrition and Brain Development. Published in the Proceedings of the First World Congress of Clinical Nutrition. New Delhi (India) pp. 5–8.

Sharma, S.K., W. Selvamurthy, M.C. Maheshwari and T.P. Singh. 1990. Kainic acid induced epileptogenesis in developing normal and undernourished rats—A computerized EEG analysis. Ind Jr Med Res 92: 456–466.

Sharma, S.K., M. Behari, M.C. Maheshwari and W. Selvamurthy. 1990. Seizure susceptibility and intra-rectal Sodium Valproate induced recovery in developing undernourished rats. Ind J Med Res 92: 120–127.

Sharma, S.K. and K. Dakshinamurti. 1992. Seizure activity in Pyridoxine-deficient adult rats. Epilepsia 33: 235–247.

Sharma, S.K. and K. Dakshinamurti. 1993. Suppression of domoic acid-induced seizures by 8-(OH)-DPAT. J Neural Transmission 93: 87–89.

Sharma, S.K., U. Nayar, M.C. Maheshwari and B. Singh. 1993. Purkinje cell evoked unit activity in developing undernourished rats. J Neurol Sci 116: 212–219.

Sharma, S.K., W. Selvamurthy and K. Dakshinamurti. 1993. Effect of environmental neurotoxins in the developing brain. Biometeorology 2: 447–455.

Sparks, L.M., H. Xie, R.A. Koza, R. Mynatt, M.W. Hulver, G.A. Bray and S.R. Smith. 2005. A high-fat diet coordinately downregulates genes required for mitochondrial oxidative phosphorylation in skeletal muscle. Diabetes 54: 1926–1933.

Stacpoole, P.W., G.N. Handerson, Z. Van and M.O. James. 1998. Clinical pharmacology and toxicology of dichloroacetate. University of Florida. Environmental Health Perspectives 106: 989–994.

Tachibana, M., M. Sparman, H. Sritanaudomchai, H. Ma, L. Clepper, J. Woodward, Y. Li, C. Ramsey, O. Kolotushkina and S. Mitalipov. 2009. Mitochondrial gene replacement in primate offspring and embryonic stem cells. Nature 461: 367–372.

Tanaka, M., Y. Nishigaki, N. Fuku, T. Ibi, K. Sahashi and Y. Koga. 2007. Therapeutic potential of pyruvate therapy for mitochondrial diseases. Mitochondrion 7: 399–401.

The Human Fertilization and Embryology (Mitochondrial Donation) Regulations 2015 No. 572

Three parent baby law is 'irresponsible' says Church of England ahead of vote". London: The Telegraph. 2015-04-30.

UK government backs three-person IVF. BBC News. 27 June 2013.

UK urged to permit IVF procedure to prevent fatal genetic diseases; Three Parent Baby Laws 2015 UK urged to permit IVF procedure to prevent fatal genetic diseases; Three Parent Baby Laws 2015.

Wang, T., Q. Liu, W. Tjhioe, J. Zhao, A. Lu, Ge. Zhang, R.X. Tan, M. Zhou, J. Xu and H.T. Feng. 2017. Therapeutic Potential and Outlook of Alternative Medicine for Osteoporosis. 18: 1051–1068.

Concluding Remarks

Charnoly body (CB) is formed in the most vulnerable cell such as, NPCs, EPCs, OPCs, and CPCs, derived from iPPCs in DPCI including severe malnutrition (undernutrition/over-nutrition), toxic exposure (environmental toxins/drugs), and in response to microbial (bacteria, virus, and fungal) infections due to free radicals-induced CMB and depletion of energy (ATP). The frequency of CB formation depends on the severity of the DPCI. In general, protein malnutrition induces ER stress, whereas protein calorie malnutrition (PCM) induces mitochondrial stress to cause CB formation, charnolophagy, and CS destabilization. Particularly, PCM in the developing brain induces both ER as well as mitochondrial oxidative stress. Nutritional stress can be categorized as (i) minor, (ii) moderate, and severe, depending on the intensity and frequency of free radicals generated during nutritional stress or in any other DPCI. Minor nutritional stress delays, moderate nutritional stress impairs, whereas, severe nutritional stress inhibits neuronal development, resulting in mild cognitive impairment (MCI), early morbidity, and mortality, respectively. The development of dendrites, growth cones, and synapses is significantly diminished in malnutrition. The dendrites in UN rat cerebellar Purkinje neurons were devoid of RER due to the inhibition of AgNOR in the nucleolus and release of toxic substances from the destabilized CS. Hence, we observed only lipid droplets in the Purkinje cell body and dendrites, and plasma membrane perforations due to CS body fusion with the plasma membrane to form structurally and functionally-destabilized apoptotic bodies. The breakdown of apoptotic bodies induced non-DNA dependent neurodegenerative apoptosis. In addition, the structural and functional integrity of the plasma membrane was severely compromised in chronic PCM due to down-regulation of protein synthesizing machinery, resulting in the absence of tubulin synthesis involved in tubulinogenesis in the cytoplasm as well as in the axons is delayed, impaired, or inhibited. CB is phagocytosed by lysosomes to form a CPS. A CPS is transformed to CS, when the phagocytosed CB is hydrolyzed by the lysosomal enzymes. A subsequent free radical attack causes CS destabilization, accompanied with permeabilization, sequestration, and/or fragmentation to release highly toxic mitochondrial metabolites. These toxic metabolites induce ER stress by inhibiting AgNOR, involved in ribosomal synthesis. The ribosomes are translocated from the nucleolus to the cytosol and are involved in protein (mitofusin) synthesis on the RER. The protein, mitofusin, is involved in the synthesis and repair of mitochondria to regain its bioenergetics. The MB is impaired in chronic MDR diseases, which compromises ICD for normal cellular function and homeostasis. Thus, free radical-induced CPS or CS destabilization is involved in NDDs. The conversion of CPS to CS is a highly crucial step during ICD and requires adequate energy (ATP) from the mitochondria. However, free radical-induced CMB triggers mitochondrial as well as ER membrane stress to cause CB formation. In the absence or denaturation of lysosomal enzymes during severe malnutrition, toxic exposure, microbial (bacteria, virus, fungus) infections, and/ or in response to other DPCI, free radicals induce further structural and functional breakdown of PUFA (linoic acid, linolenic acid, and arachidonic acid) in the labile CS membrane to induce permeabilization, sequestration, and/or fragmentation resulting in release of highly toxic mitochondrial metabolites in the cell. Concomitant lipid peroxidation of multilamellar electron dense membrane stacks of CB within CS also triggers structural and functional breakdown of PUFA, leaving several proteins in a hostile microenvironment of mitochondrial toxins and free radicals. These unprotected proteins are subsequently denatured by direct exposure of free radicals as well as by toxic metabolites of the degenerated mitochondria. The degenerated proteins aggregate to form nonfunctional intracellular inclusions. Thus, free radical-induced DSST-CS destabilization is involved in the aggregation of α-synuclein to form Lewy body in PD, amyloid β1-42 to form senile plaques in AD, Huntingtin to form HD, prion proteins in prion's diseases, SOD in ALS, Frederictin in Fredrick ataxia, Nigri bodies in Rabies viral diseases, and in several other NDDs. Hence, DSST-CS stabilizers can be developed to prevent and/or slowdown the progression of afore-mentioned and other chronic MDR diseases. Particularly, development of novel DSST charnolopharmacothetapeutics in the prevention and/or inhibition of CB and charnolophagy induction will be clinically significant during acute phase; whereas, prevention/inhibition of CPS/CS destabilization and induction of CS exocytosis will be therapeutically beneficial during chronic phase of disease progression. Future studies in this direction promise to confer the targeted, safe, and effective EBPT of NDDs, CVDs, and MDR malignancies as described elegantly in this book.

The circulating destabilized CS induces immunosuppression by augmenting systemic toxicity. The circulating destabilized CS, slowly (through permeabilization) or rapidly (through sequestration and fragmentation) releases toxic metabolites of degenerated mitochondria and inhibits normal phagocytic function of macrophages to enhance systemic toxicity. It has been noticed that as many as 30% post-stroke patients die because of bacterial, viral, or fungal pneumonia. Moreover, an antibiotic, minocycline, used as an anti-inflammatory agent in these patients causes further immunosuppression. All these events (including circulating CS destabilization and antibiotics) render post-stroke patients highly vulnerable to pneumonia due to immunodeficiency. Hence, CS stability particularly in post-stroke and other patients with NDDs and aging becomes highly crucial for their health and well-being.

The structurally-intact neurotubules (microtubules) were present in the nourished and were absent or distorted in the UN cerebellar Purkinje neurons. Neurotubules confer cytoskeletal support and serve as molecular-rail grids for the normal axoplasmic flow of various enzymes, neurotransmitters, hormones, neurotrophic factors, and mitochondria at the synaptic terminals. Twisted neurotubules were observed in the UN rat cerebellar Purkinje neurons, which can impair normal axoplasmic flow of afore-mentioned substances at the synaptic terminals to cause cognitive impairments as noticed in NDDs. The axoplasmic flow is also impaired by accumulation of CB, CPS, or CS at the junction of the axon hillock. A free ribosomal pool was observed in the absence of ER in minor to moderate UN Purkinje neurons and their dendrites. The mitochondria, ER membranes, and Golgi body were hypertrophied in the developing

UN rat Purkinje cells dendrites. The Golgi body is involved in processing proteins. Particularly conjugation of lipids with proteins, synthesizes lipoproteins (involved in myelin synthesis), and conjugation of carbohydrates with proteins synthesizes glycoproteins (involved in microtubules synthesis). Thus, synthesis of lipoprotein as well glycoproteins was delayed, impaired, or inhibited depending on the severity of nutritional stress which directly or indirectly influenced myelinogenesis and synaptogenesis. These deleterious events induce structural and functional breakdown of dendrites, axons, and synaptic terminals resulting in impaired brain regional neurocircuitry. Thus, brain regional neurotubulinogenesis, growth cones, dendritic development, axonogenesis, myelinogenesis, and synaptogenesis are compromised due to CB aggregation and CS destabilization depending on the severity of malnutrition or physicochemical insult, resulting in early morbidity and mortality as noticed in severe malnutrition and progressive NDDs including AD and aging.

We observed the stunted growth of axons and loss of arborization due to afore-mentioned deleterious molecular events at the cellular and subcellular level in the developing UN Purkinje neurons, resulting in delayed, impaired, and/or no development of sensorimotor learning in the experimental rats and UN children. Hence, DSST charnolomics can be developed by utilizing cDNA, antibody, and fluorescent NPs. Modern biotechnology (LC-MS, fluorescent multiplex ELISA, capillary electrophoresis, flow cytometry, magnetic resonance spectroscopy, and SPR spectroscopy) can be utilized to estimate various CS biomarkers as described in this book. Furthermore, the charnolosomic data derived from CS-microarrays can be correlated and confirmed with conventional omic biomarkers by analyzing genomic, proteomic, metabolomic, metallomic, and lipidomic analysis. Studies along this direction will provide unique opportunities to accomplish long-quested goal of targeted, safe, and effective personalized theranostics of NDDs, CVDs, and chronic MDR malignancies. A combinatorial and correlative strategy to analyze the omics data employing translational bioinformatics will pave the way to precise information regarding mitochondrial bioenergetics, CB molecular pathogenesis, and ICD for normal cellular functional and homeostasis to remain healthy. Important charnolosomic biomarkers include: (i) mitochondrial biomarkers, (ii) CB biomarkers, (iii) charnolophagy biomarkers, and (iv) CS biomarkers (CS is a byproduct of CB following its phagocytosis by lysosome). Thus, mitochondrial bioenergetics implicated in ICD in health and disease can be precisely determined by developing novel DSST charnolosomic microarrays. These data will be highly beneficial for the precise assessment of molecular pathogenesis involved in CB formation, charnolophagy induction/inhibition, Charnolophagy index induction/inhibition, CS destabilization/ stabilization, and CS exocytosis/endocytosis for the targeted, safe, and effective evaluation of disease progression/regression and personalized EBPT.

CB as a universal biomarker of cell injury elucidates various aspects of cell biology, molecular biology, molecular genetics/epigenetics, molecular pharmacology, and molecular pathogenesis of progressive NDDs, CVDs, MDR malignancies, and several proinflammatory diseases involved in early morbidity and mortality. Hence, future development of novel DSST charnolopharmacotherapeutics improvising DSST charnolomic bioinformatics will provide better strategies for the targeted, safe, and effective EBPT of chronic NDDs, CVDs, MDR malignancies, and other pro-inflammatory diseases for a better quality of life, as described in this book.

Part-I
General Introduction of Charnoly Body as a Novel Theranostic Biomarker
(Basic Cellular & Molecular Biology)

CHAPTER-1

Free Radical-induced Compromised Mitochondrial Bioenergetics Triggers Charnoly Body Formation

INTRODUCTION

It is now well-established that the energy requirement of a cell is significantly increased during DPCI in the most vulnerable cells. These deleterious events induce ER and mitochondrial oxidative stress to accelerate ATP synthesis. Free radicals are generated as a byproduct of mitochondrial oxidative phosphorylation during ATP synthesis in the electron transport chain. Free radicals are highly unstable reactive oxygen and nitrogen species (such as $\cdot OH$, $CO\cdot$, and $NO\cdot$). Particularly, $ONOO^-$ ions are highly deleterious and are synthesized by the Fenton reaction from $\cdot OH$ and $NO\cdot$ in the presence of iron. $ONOO^-$ ions not only induce oxidative but also nitrative stress to cause degeneration of mitochondrial membranes. Thus, free radical-induced CMB triggers CB formation to prevent dissemination of highly toxic mitochondrial metabolites as an initial attempt of ICD. CB is eliminated from the intracellular compartment by an ATP-driven charnolophagy (CB autophagy), resulting in the formation of a CPS. The CPS is subsequently transformed to CS when the phagocytosed CB is hydrolyzed by the lysosomal enzymes.

This chapter describes 4 different stages of free radical attack (including primary, secondary, tertiary, and quaternary), general biomarkers of ICD, specific biomarkers of CMB (including CB, charnolophagy, CPS, and CS), therapeutic potential of antioxidants during different stages of free radical attack, different stages of intracellular toxification/detoxification, and free radical-induced CB molecular pathogenesis during acute and chronic physicochemical injury in the most vulnerable cell. The chapter also describes the theranostic potential of MTs as potent free radical scavengers, CB antagonists, charnolophagy agonists, and CS stabilizers to prevent cellular and molecular injury in chronic MDR diseases.

Different Stages of Free Radical Attack. There are primarily 4 different stages of free radical attack: (a) primary free radical attack (PFA), (b) secondary free radical attack (SFA), (c) tertiary free radical attack (TFA), and (d) quaternary free radical attack (QFA). Intracellular degeneration depends on the acute or chronic exposure to free radical-induced lipid peroxidation and neuronal injury. ROS-induced lipid peroxidation involves structural and functional degradation of PUFA from the plasma membrane to cause initially enhanced permeabilization followed by perforations of labile CS membranes. During PFA, down-regulation of $\Delta\Psi$ occurs, resulting in the formation of a megapore due to TRPC delocalization. A lot of Ca^{2+} enters inside the mitochondria along with water through the mitochondrial megapore. As a result, the mitochondria become swollen and eventually get fragmented and their membranes are disseminated in the cell. The SFA is associated with disintegration and condensation of the degenerated mitochondrial membranes to form electron-dense membrane stacks triggering CB formation, charnolophagy, and CS exocytosis for ICD. The most frequent events which occur during SFA are CB formation, charnolophagy induction, and CS exocytosis as a basic molecular mechanism of ICD. During TFA, CS destabilization, CS formation, and translocation in the plasma membranes induces the synthesis of apoptotic bodies due to the uncontrolled release of highly toxic mitochondrial metabolites resulting in non-DNA dependent apoptotic degeneration.

Although the nDNA remains preserved during CB formation, charnolophagy, and CS exocytosis due to its double-helical structure with noncoding introns and protective histones and protamines, the mtDNA is highly labile because it is intron-less, GC-rich, and remains in a hostile microenvironment of free radicals generated as a byproduct of oxidative phosphorylation. Hence, it is readily oxidized to synthesize highly toxic 8-OH, 2dG, which can induce impairments in the genetic and epigenetic mechanisms of a cell. The other important metabolite which is synthesized during the free radical-mediated attack is 2, 3 dihydroxy nonenal, which is also involved in CB molecular pathogenesis, and is formed due to the degeneration of mitochondrial membranes. Thus, lipid peroxidation, mtDNA oxidation, and epigenetic modifications occur more readily in the mitochondria as compared to other intracellular organelles.

Biomarkers of ICD. It is important to highlight that CB formation is an initial attempt to contain highly toxic substances of mitochondrial metabolism in a stressed cell in response to DPCI. Particularly, Cyt-C is highly toxic and is attached non-covalently with the inner mitochondrial membrane. It is easily delocalized during mitochondrial degeneration. Hence, condensation of the fragmented mitochondrial membranes, triggering CB formation prevents the uncontrolled release of highly toxic substances as an initial attempt of ICD to alleviate CMB in chronic MDR diseases. Various potential biomarkers of ICD have been proposed. The most important event in ICD is CB autophagy (also named as charnolophagy). While charnolophagy and CS exocytosis is involved in ICD, charnolophagy inhibitors or antagonists, and CS exocytosis inhibitors or antagonists are involved in cellular degeneration due to non-DNA-dependent apoptosis, whereas, CScsc formation is involved in invading nonproliferating cells due to induction of antiapoptotic proteins such as MTs, BCl_2, HSPs, HIF, SOD, catalase, P^{53}, cmyc, and retinoblastoma genes, involved in cell immortalization and malignant transformation. Hence, endocytosis of CScsc in a nonproliferating cell is involved in MDR malignant transformations. The basic molecular mechanisms of ICD is compromised in a cancer cell. In the process of

ICD, a stressed cell over-expressing antioxidant genes is involved in MDR malignant transformation.

Biomarkers of Compromised Mitochondrial Bioenergetics. There are primarily 4 main biomarkers of CMB. These include: (i) CB, (ii) CPS, (iii) CS, and (iv) CS body.

Therapeutic Outcome of Antioxidants in Response to Different Stages of a Free Radical Attack. Generally, ICD of a cell is governed by the MB. A cell with CMB is incapable of sustaining ICD and vice versa. DPCI can induce primary, secondary, tertiary, and/or quaternary free radical attack depending on the frequency and intensity of injury to the most vulnerable cell. For example, lung epithelial cells in response to chronic nicotine exposure can induce lung carcinoma. The PFA can be inhibited and/or attenuated by endogenously-synthesized antioxidants such as: glutathione, SOD, catalase, MTs, HPP-70, BCl-2, and P[53]. The SFA can be attenuated by exogenous antioxidants such as: resveratrol, rutins, sirtuins, vitamin-E, D, A, probucol, statins, and edaravone) and PUFA (linoic acid, linolinic acid, and archidonic acid), and omega-3 fatty acids [(eicosapentaenoic acid (EPA) and docosahexaenoic acid (DHA)] to prevent or inhibit CB formation, enhance charnolophagy, and augment CPS and CS exocytosis as a basic molecular mechanism of ICD. During TFA, the chances of mitochondrial membrane recovery are minimized and/or eliminated due to CS destabilization, CS body formation, CS membrane permeabilization, and blebbing. The CS membranes or their bodies fuse with the plasma membrane to form apoptotic bodies, which can easily burst to release highly toxic substances of mitochondrial metabolism and induce non-DNA-dependent cellular demise. A QFA can induce spontaneous cellular demise due to accelerated induction of CB formation, inhibition of charnolophagy, destabilization of CPS and CS, and prevention of CS exocytosis as a basic molecular mechanism of ICD. The QFA can induce sudden infant death syndrome (SIDS), still birth, or abortion as noticed in the developing fetus of smoking, binge drinking, and/or ZIKV infected pregnant women. Likewise, QFA is involved in sudden death following a massive heart attack or AIS in adults.

Stages of Intracellular Toxification/Detoxification. Primarily, 4 stages of intracellular toxification/detoxification are proposed. The intracellular toxification/detoxification depends on the intensity and frequency of the free radical attack. A free radical-induced attack can be divided in 4 different stages.

 (i) Primary Free Radical Attack (PFA)
 (ii) Secondary Free Radical Attack (SFA)
 (iii) Tertiary Free Radical Attack (TFA)
 (iv) Quaternary Free Radical Attack (QFA)

The PFA is usually accompanied with the down-regulation of MB due to $\Delta\Psi$ collapse, which causes the formation of megapores on the mitochondrial membrane due to downregulation of the Ca^{2+} channel protein, TRPC. This is followed by Cyt-C, TSPO (18 kDa), MAOs, and TRPC delocalization. The intra-mitochondrial Ca^{2+} ions are increased to induce ionic imbalance and accumulation of lot of water, resulting in the induction of mega-mitochondriogenesis, which causes degeneration of the membranes due to ROS ($\cdot$OH, NO$\cdot$)-induced lipid peroxidation. Lipid peroxidation triggers structural and functional breakdown of PUFA and omega-3 fatty acids to cause fragmentation of mitochondrial membranes. These fragmented membranes release highly toxic iron, Cyt-C, 8-OH, 2dG, 2,3 dihydroxy nonenal, acetaldehyde, ammonia, and H_2O_2 to trigger microRNA-mediated apoptotic signal transduction. The condensation of fragmented mitochondrial membranes occurs to form multi-lamellar, electron-dense membrane stacks to maintain intracellular sanitation. Thus, condensation of degenerated mitochondrial membrane to form CB is an immediate and early attempt of ICD for normal cellular function to remain healthy. CB is subsequently phagocytosed by ATP-dependent lysosomal activation. This process is called as charnolophagy. CPS is synthesized as a result of charnolophagy. Thus, a lysosome containing a phagocytosed CB is named as CPS. The CPS is transformed to CS, when the phagocytosed CB is hydrolyzed by the lysosomal enzymes such as: hydrolases, lipases, proteases, and nucleases. The CS is then exocytosed by an energy-driven process as a basic molecular mechanism of ICD. The PFA is thus controlled by an intricate CB detoxification process. Subsequently, regeneration of new mitochondria initiates as the cell is detoxified by charnolophagy and CS exocytosis. If charnolophagy and CS exocytosis is impaired, the mitochondrial synthesis and regeneration is disrupted due to inhibition in the protein synthesis on the RER membranes. Endogenous antioxidants such as: glutathione, MTs, SOD, and catalase prevent CB formation as potent free radical scavengers. However, this attempt becomes futile during SFA and TFA. The endogenously-synthesized antioxidants stabilize CS and facilitate charnolophagy in addition to free radical scavenging. However, the endogenous antioxidants-induced mitochondrial defense system is significantly compromised during SFA, which occurs due to further down-regulation of the MB. During SFA, CB becomes highly resistant to charnolophagy as the lysosomal enzymes are unable to execute charnolophagy at this stage. The SFA can also induce CPS and CS permeabilization due to lipid peroxidation of their highly labile single-layered plasma membrane. Following deleterious events can occur during SFA:

(i) Accumulation of CB at the junction of the axon hillock can impair the normal axoplasmic transport of various ions, enzymes, neurotransmitters, hormones, proteins, neurotropic factors (such as BDNF, NGF-1, and IGF-1), and mitochondrial axoplasmic transport from the cell body to the terminal end bulb, resulting in progressive synaptic atrophy.

(ii) Release of toxic substances from the permeabilized, destabilized, and degenerated CPS or CS at the junction of the axon hillock can cause synaptic terminal degeneration to induce impaired brain regional neuro-cybernetics and eventually cognitive impairments resulting in learning, memory, intelligence, and behavioral deficits, accompanied with early morbidity and mortality as noticed in ZIKV-induced embryopathies, following intrauterine exposure to ethanol, insulin-resistant type-2 diabetes, and in AD.

SFA can be attenuated to a certain extent by endogenous (glutathione, MTs, SOD, catalase) antioxidants as well as by exogenous antioxidants, administered in the form of drugs or obtained from natural sources such as: resveratrol, polyphenols, sirtuis, rutins, catechin, and lycopenes. Naturally available fruits and vegetables are rich in these antioxidants.

TFA is accompanied with a disintegration of CPS and CS which occurs due to free radical-induced lipid peroxidation and triggers apoptotic neurodegeneration, causing early morbidity and mortality as noticed in PD, AD, ALS, MDD, schizophrenia, and chronic drug addiction. Thus, MB is governed by the frequency and intensity of a free radical attack, which can induce repairable or irreparable damage to execute either cell survival or cellular demise. The endogenous as well as exogenous antioxidants can attenuate free radical-induced mitochondrial degeneration, CB formation, and enhance charnolophagy and CS exocytosis to remain healthy. QFA may also induce spontaneous apoptosis due to the uncontrolled release of highly toxic mitochondrial metabolites from the destabilized CS.

Major Highlights

Different Stages of ICD

(i) **Primary Attempt**: Maintaining the MB by endogenously synthesized antioxidants.

(ii) **Secondary Attempt**: CB formation by endogenously-synthesized antioxidants and naturally-available antioxidants.

(iii) **Tertiary Attempt**: Induction of charnolophagy, CS stabilization, CS exocytosis by endogenously-synthesized antioxidants, naturally-available antioxidants, and synthetic antioxidant drugs.

ICD during Acute and Chronic Injury to the Most Vulnerable Cell

(i) Primary ICD is characterized by CB formation.

(ii) Secondary ICD involves charnolophagy, CPS stabilization, CS formation.

(iii) Tertiary ICD is represented by CS Exocytosis.

(iv) Quaternary ICD involves detoxification of all 7 forms of CS including systemic CS through hepatic and renal clearance.

CHAPTER-2

Free Radical-induced Molecular Pathophysiology of Charnoly Body and Charnolosome

INTRODUCTION

Recently, we described various stages of CB life cycle to elucidate its molecular pathogenesis in progressive NDDs, including stroke, epilepsy, PD, AD, vascular dementia, HD, MS, ALS, schizophrenia, MDDs, drug addiction, ZIKV disease, FASD, and in nicotinism (Sharma et al. 2013a; Sharma et al. 2013b; Sharma and Ebadi 2014; Sharma et al. 2014; Sharma 2015; Sharma et al. 2015; Sharma et al. 2016; Sharma 2017a; Sharma 2017b). We also reported that CB is generated in the most vulnerable cell in response to severe DPCI due to free radicals-induced oxidative and nitrative stress to the mitochondrial membranes (Sharma 2017a; Sharma et al. 2017b). The mitochondrial membranes are degenerated by free radicals due to lipid peroxidation, which results in the structural and functional breakdown of PUFA. The aggregation and condensation of the degenerated mitochondrial membranes to form CB is an initial attempt to contain highly toxic mitochondrial metabolites such as Cyt-C, which is noncovalently and loosely bond to the inner mitochondrial membranes and can easily disseminate within the cell. The Cyt-C is highly toxic to the mtDNA as well as nuclear DNA, and initiates degenerative apoptosis. In addition, release of other toxic substances, such as AIF-1, 2,3 dihydroxynonenal (a mitochondrial membrane oxidative product), and 8-OH, 2dG (as a DNA oxidative product) can significantly impact microRNA-mediated post-transcriptional activity of genes involved in DNA cell cycle, cell growth, proliferation, differentiation, migration, and development. Hence, the acute step of ICD is energy (ATP)-dependent charnolophagy to maintain intracellular sanitation. A CPS is formed through energy (ATP)-driven CB phagocytosis by the lysosomes. The CPS is transformed to CS, when the phagocytosed CB is hydrolyzed by the lysosomal enzymes. The CS is a single-layered, structurally and functionally labile and can be easily destabilized following subsequent exposure to a free radical attack. The destabilization of CS is represented by permeabilization, sequestration, or fragmentation, depending on the intensity and frequency of free radicals generated and the severity of DPCI. The CS releases highly toxic mitochondrial metabolites (acetaldehyde, H_2O_2, and ammonia) to trigger spontaneous apoptosis due to the formation of CS bodies and their fusion with the plasma membranes. Hence, CS is efficiently exocytosed by energy (ATP)-dependent process to sustain ICD.

This chapter describes free radical-induced CS pathophysiology, molecular biomarkers of CMB, and CB-induced microcephaly in ZIKV disease and FASD, in addition to mitochondrial molecular dynamics and charnolopathy in chronic MDR diseases.

Free Radical-induced CS Molecular Pathogenesis. Free radicals are synthesized as a byproduct of mitochondrial oxidative phosphorylation. The requirement of energy (ATP) is significantly increased during DPCI in the most vulnerable cells such as NPCs derived from iPPCs. The most significant free radicals are CO·, ·OH, and NO·. In the presence of iron, ·OH and NO· trigger Fenton reaction to synthesize $ONOO^-$ ions, which induce not only oxidative but also nitrative stress particularly in the most sensitive mtDNA. The mtDNA is highly vulnerable because it is nonhelical, intron-less, directly exposed to a hostile microenvironment of free radicals, and devoid of histones and protamines. Moreover, mtDNA is GC-rich, which renders it highly vulnerable to epigenetic changes involving DNA methylation at the N-4 position of the cytosine residue and oxidation at the guanosine residue to synthesize highly toxic 8-OH, 2dG. The oxidation of mtDNA occurs to synthesize 8-OH, 2dG (which can be estimated in the saliva, peripheral blood, serum, plasma, and urine samples of a patient). The PFA triggers induction of CS bodies, highly rich in pro-inflammatory cytokines and are named as inflammasomes. The inflammosomes participate in the progression of inflammation. The SFA to a CS triggers the formation of apoptosomes. The apoptosomes are rich in caspases and AIF. The TFA triggers the formation of necrosomes. These intracellular organelles are involved in the necrosis of a cell, whereas a CS_{scs} is involved in MDR malignancies through induction of inflammosome, apoptosome, and necrosome, during primary, secondary, and tertiary phases of a free radical attack, respectively. Thus, translocation of inflammasomes, apoptosomes, and necrosomes from the SC_{scs} during free radical attack is involved in MDR malignancies.

Mitochondrial Dynamics and Charnolopathy in Chronic MDR Diseases. A healthy life style, proper diet, and moderate exercise enhance mitochondrial regeneration, rejuvenation, repair, reunion, and replacement under normal physiological conditions; whereas, DPCI increase the requirement of energy ATP through accelerated oxidative phosphorylation. Free radicals are generated as a byproduct of oxidative phosphorylation in the electron transport chain. Free radicals are highly reactive and unstable oxygen and nitrogen species (ROS and RNS) which induce lipid peroxidation to cause structural and functional breakdown of PUFA in the mitochondrial membranes. These degenerated membranes are aggregated to form pleomorphic electron-dense membrane stacks to generate CBs as a basic molecular mechanism of ICD. CBs are recognized as nonfunctional intracellular inclusions and are immediately phagocytosed by energy (ATP)-driven chranolophagy (CB autophagy). Following charnolophagy, a CPS is formed, which is transformed to CS when the phagocytosed membranes are hydrolyzed by the lysosomal enzymes. The

CS is structurally and functionally labile organelle and is exocytosed by an energy (ATP)-dependent mechanism as a secondary step of ICD. During SFA and TFA, the lipid peroxidation of the CS membranes induces the formation of CS bodies. CS bodies are pinched off from the parent CS and are fused with the plasma membranes to form apoptotic bodies. The apoptotic bodies release toxic mitochondrial metabolites due to free radical-induced ruptured plasma membranes. These toxic substances induce the progressive degeneration of neighboring cells to cause NDDs, CVDs, and MDR malignancies. The endocytosis of apoptotic body from a SCscs in the nonproliferating cell induces malignant transformation.

CB Induction and Microcephaly. As described in this chapter, DPCI including but not limited to malnutrition (overnutrition, undernutrition, and malabsorption), environmental toxins (heavy metal ions, and polychloro biphenyl: PCB), microbial (bacterial, virus, and fungal) infections, and pharmacological agents (anesthetics, antidepressants, antipsychotics) drugs of abuse (alcohol, tobacco, morphine, heroin, cocaine, opiates, amphetamine, METH, and methylene deoxy methamphetamine: MDMA), and antiepileptic drugs (phenytoin, sodium valproate, carbamazepine) induce CB formation in the most vulnerable NPCs, CPCs, EPCs, and OPCs derived from iPPCs, to cause early morbidity and mortality due to apoptosis, which may also induce microcephaly or other developmental embryopathies; hence these are contraindicated during pregnancy.

References

Chabenne, A., C. Moon, C. Ojo, A. Khogali, B. Nepal and S. Sharma. 2014. Biomarkers in fetal alcohol syndrome (Recent Update). Biomarkers and Genomic Medicine 6: 12–22.
Jagtap, A., S. Gawande and S. Sharma. 2015. Biomarkers in Vascular Dementia (A Recent Update). 7: 43–56.
Sharma, S., C.S. Moon, A. Khogali, A. Haidous, A. Chabenne, C. Ojo, M. Jelebinkov, Y. Kurdi and M. Ebadi. 2013a. Biomarkers of Parkinson's disease (Recent Update). Neurochemistry International 63: 201–229.
Sharma, S. and M. Ebadi. 2013b. Antioxidant Targeting in Neurodegenerative Disorders. Ed. I. Laher, Springer Verlag. Germany. Chapter 85, pp. 1–30.
Sharma, S., A. Rais, R. Sandhu, W. Nel and M. Ebadi. 2013c. Clinical significance of metallothioneins in cell therapy and nanomedicine. International Journal of Nanomedicine 8: 1477–1488.
Sharma, S. 2014. Molecular pharmacology of environmental neurotoxins. In Kainic Acid: Neurotoxic Properties, Biological Sources, and Clinical Applications. Nova Science Publishers. New York. pp. 1–47.
Sharma, S. 2014. Nanotheranostics in evidence based personalized medicine. Current Drug Targets 15: 915–930.
Sharma, S. and M. Ebadi. 2014. Charnoly body as a universal biomarker of cell injury. Biomarkers and Genomic Med 6: 89–98.
Sharma, S. and M. Ebadi. 2014. Significance of metallothioneins in aging brain. Neurochemistry International 65: 40–48.
Sharma, S., B. Nepal, C.S. Moon, A. Chabenne, A. Khogali, C. Ojo, E. Hong, R. Goudet, A. Sayed-Ahmad, A. Jacob, M. Murtaba and M. Firlit. 2014. Psychology of craving. Open Jr of Medical Psychology 3: 120–125.
Sharma, S., S. Gawande, A. Jagtap, R. Abeulela and Z. Salman. 2015. Fetal alcohol syndrome; prevention, diagnosis, & treatment. In Alcohol Abuse: Prevalence, Risk Factors. Nova Science Publishers, New York, U.S.A.

Sharma, S., J. Choga, V. Gupta, P. Doghor, A. Chauhan, F. Kalala, A. Foor, C. Wright, J. Renteria, K.E. Theberge and S. Mathur. 2016. Charnoly body as a novel biomarker of nutritional stress in Alzheimer's disease. Functional Foods in Health and Disease 6: 344–377.

Sharma, S. and W. Lippincott. 2017. Emerging biomarkers in Alzheimer's disease (Recent Update). Current Alzheimer Research 14 (in press).

Sharma, S. 2017a. *ZIKV* Disease, Prevention and Cure. Nova Science Publishers, New York, U.S.A.

Sharma, S. 2017b. Fetal Alcohol Spectrum Disorder. Concepts, Mechanisms, and Cure. Nova Science Publishers, New York, U.S.A.

Sharma, S. 2017c. Charnolosome-antioxidants interaction in health and disease. Conference: 22nd International Conference on Functional Foods, At Harvard Medical School, Boston, Mass, U.S.A. (Invited lecture). Sep 22.

CHAPTER-3

Charnoly Body as a Novel Biomarker of Cell Injury

INTRODUCTION

In earlier studies, we discovered multi-lamellar, electron-dense membrane stacks in the developing UN rat Purkinje neurons (Sharma et al. 1986; Sharma et al. 1987; Sharma et al. 1993). Subsequently, these peculiar structures were identified in the hippocampal CA-3 and dentate gyrus neurons of intra-uterine KA and DOM-exposed mice; and were named as "CBs" (Sharma et al. 1993; Dakshinamuti et al. 1993; Sharma 2013). Hippocampal microinjection of 5-HT$_{1A}$ receptor agonist, 8-hydroxy-DPAT in the dentate gyrus inhibited DOM-induced seizures in male adult rats (Sharma and Dakshinamurti 1993). Later, we reported that stress-induced free radical overproduction may cause CB formation in the hippocampal neurons due to degeneration of mitochondria in PD, AD, drug addiction, and depression (Sharma et al. 2014). Nutritional rehabilitation, Zn^{2+}, and MTs inhibit CB formation in the rat brain (Sharma et al. 2013). Recently, we reported that MTs inhibit CB formation and provide ubiquinone (CoQ$_{10}$)-mediated neuroprotection by serving as potent free radical scavengers (Sharma and Ebadi 2014). MTs are low molecular weight, cysteine-rich, Zn^{2+}-binding proteins and are induced in nutritional stress and in response to NPs toxicity (Sharma et al. 2013). MTs regulate Zn^{2+}-mediated transcriptional activation of genes and microRNA-mediated post-transcription involved in DNA cell cycle, growth, proliferation, differentiation, and development may serve as early and sensitive biomarkers of NDDs, CVDs, and cancer (Sharma et al. 2013; Sharma and Ebadi 2013).

This chapter highlights the clinical significance of CB as a universal mitochondrial biomarker of cell injury; whereas, nutritional rehabilitation, physiological Zn^{2+}, and MTs as CB antagonists and CS stabilizers confer neuroprotection.

In earlier studies, we confirmed that parkinsonian neurotoxins: salsolinol, 1-benzyle TIQ, rotenone, and drugs of abuse: MPTP, cocaine, METH, and MDMA trigger CB formation by down-regulating ubiquinone (NADH) oxidoreductase (complex-1; a rate limiting enzyme in oxidative phosphorylation) in human DArgic (SK-N-SH and SH-S-Y5Y) neurons; whereas a MAO-B inhibitor, selegiline, prevents MPP$^+$-induced mitochondrial degeneration and CB formation by augmenting MTs induction (Sharma and Ebadi 2014). A Ca^{2+} channel regulatory protein, TRPC-1 also prevented MPP^+-induced complex-1 inhibition and apoptosis in cultured human DAergic (SH-S-Y5Y) neurons (Bollimuntha et al. 2005).

Translocation of MTs in the mitochondria and nucleus during oxidative and/or nitrative stress occurs as a basic molecular mechanism of intracellular defense. Peroxynitrite ($ONOO^-$) ions are generated by Fenton reaction in the presence of Fe^{3+}, $NO^.$, an $.OH$ radicals as a byproduct of oxidative phosphorylation. These ions induce oxidative and nitrative stress. MTs attenuate $ONOO^-$-induced DNA damage whereas α-synuclein nitration facilitate Lewy body (LB) formation during PD progression (Sharma and Ebadi 2003; Sharma et al. 2004). We discovered α-synuclein index (SI) as a ratio of nitrated α-synuclein vs native α-synuclein. Therefore, SI may be used as early and sensitive biomarker of CB/LB pathogenesis in the submandibular gland of PD patients.

The accumulation of CBs at the junction of the axon hillock may inhibit axoplasmic transport of ions, enzymes, neurotransmitters, growth factors, and mitochondria at the synaptic terminals; resulting in sensorimotor impairments in PD, AD, and depression. Therefore, drugs may be developed to inhibit CB formation, augment charnolophagy, and prevent CS destabilization in the highly vulnerable hippocampal neurons. We suggested that $\Delta\Psi$, 8-OH, 2dG synthesis, and SI may be determined by confocal microscopy, flow cytometry, and comet assay as early rudiments of CB formation to evaluate the therapeutic potential of drugs in cell culture. EM studies may be performed subsequently to authenticate CB formation *in vivo*. This unique approach can save lot of time, money and energy of pharmaceutical industry interested in developing novel drugs or NPs for the safe and effective EBPT of NDDs, CVDs, and cancer.

It is now known that cancer stem cells remain in their niches and induce malignancies upon stimulation. MTs are induced in MDR malignancies due to inhibition of CB formation and induction of anti-apoptotic genes. Nonspecific induction of CB with presently-available anticancer and anti-infective drugs causes alopecia, neurotoxicity, myelo-suppression, hepatotoxicity, nephrotoxicity, GIT symptoms, neurotoxicity, and infertility. Therefore, drugs may be developed to augment cancer stem cell specific CB formation for the safe and effective EBPT of MDR malignancies with minimum or no adverse effects. Furthermore, CB formation may also be used as an early and sensitive biomarker in drug addiction, depression, diabetes, obesity, pain, and other chronic diseases.

We performed series of experiments on mitochondrial genome knock out (RhO_{mgko}) cells in culture and MTs gene-manipulated mice to confirm our original hypothesis: "*MTs provide ubiquinone (CoQ$_{10}$)-mediated neuroprotection by inhibiting CB formation, augmenting charnolophagy, and by stabilizing highly-labile CS, as potent free radical scavengers.*"

CB Formation in RhO$_{mgko}$ Cells. We prepared mitochondrial genome knock out (RhO_{mgko}) cells by selectively knocking out the mitochondrial genome to mimic the cellular model of aging. Dulbecco's modified Eagle's medium (DMEM), containing high glucose, glutamine, pyruvate, and sodium bicarbonate was supplemented with 5 ng/L of ethidium bromide as a DNA intercalating agent was used to culture human dopaminergic (SK-N-SH) cells for 6–8 weeks. At this minimum concentration of ethidium bromide, mtDNA is down-regulated, whereas the nuclear DNA remains structurally and functionally intact. Although, RhO_{mgko} cells become de-differentiated, they do not lose their potential to divide and remain viable. Nevertheless, RhO_{mgko} cells are highly susceptible to MPP^+, rotenone, and salsolinol-induced mitochondrial degeneration and augment CB formation without any significant influence on the nDNA. Depending on the metabolic activity, a cell may have as many as 1000 (a neuron), or 600,000 (an oocyte) or more mitochondria and each one has its own double-stranded, intron-less 34 Kb, highly sensitive, GC-rich, naked DNA. Some of the mitochondria may be devoid of DNA. A spermatocyte has anywhere, between 22–75 condensed mitochondria, arranged spirally in the middle piece. Adipocytes have a minimum number of mitochondria, whereas erythrocytes have no mitochondria. That is why erythrocytes have a reduced life span of only 110 days. It has been estimated that 40% of the heart, 20% of the liver, and 15% of the brain is composed of mitochondria. The mtDNA damage occurs at an early stage of NDDs or CVDs because it remains constantly under the direct influence of free radicals, generated as a byproduct of oxidative phosphorylation (Sharma and Ebadi 2014). Brain is the most significant organ which requires continuous and maximum supply of energy (ATP). It is rich in lipids, hence highly susceptible to a free radical attack. Free radicals induce oxidation of the mtDNA to synthesize 8-OH-2dG. Hence, significantly increased levels of 8-OH, 2dG in the serum and urine samples is an early indication of mtDNA damage in NDDs. CoQ_{10} as well as the rate limiting enzyme complex (ubiquinone-NADH oxido-reductase: complex-1) are significantly reduced in the RhO_{mgko} cells as observed in AD, PD, and aging. Transfection of RhO_{mgko} cells with ubiquinone-NADH-oxido-reductase (complex-1) gene increased CoQ_{10} and ATP synthesis, suggesting that NDDs occur due to CMB and down-regulation of the mitochondrial genome, involving CB molecular pathogenesis. It is important to emphasize that almost every mammalian cell possesses mitochondria as power-houses of intracellular bioenergetics. Hence, we can expect CB formation in any cell having mitochondria. However, we cannot expect CB formation in the erythrocytes, bacteria, and viruses as those are devoid of mitochondria. Hence, they can be used as controls to determine the frequency of CB formation in the most vulnerable cells as a basic molecular mechanism of ICD during any physicochemical injury, particularly in the CNS.

CB Formation in Gene-Manipulated Mice. We developed α-synuclein metallothioneins triple knockout (α-Syn-MT_{tko}) mice. These genotypes exhibit 40% mortality, body tremors, and typical Parkinsonian symptoms. The brain regional CoQ_{10} as well as complex-1 activity were significantly reduced in these animals. Therefore, we developed a highly sensitive procedure to detect CoQ_{10} from the brain samples of these rare animals (Sharma and Ebadi 2004).

Homozygous weaver mutant (wv/wv) mice exhibit progressive nigrostriatal, hippocampal, and cerebellar damage as noticed in PD, AD, and drug addiction, respectively. MTs are significantly down-regulated and these genotypes exhibit typical symptoms of multiple drug addiction, morbidity, and early mortality.

To further authenticate the therapeutic potential of MTs as CB antagonists in progressive NDDs such as PD, AD, and drug addiction, we developed MTs over-expressing weaver mutant (wv/wv-MTs) mice by crossbreeding MTs transgenic males with wv/wv females as male wv/wv mice remain sterile. The wv/wv-MTs mice exhibit attenuation of body tremors and serve as an animal model of drug rehabilitation. By performing *in vivo* microPET neuroimaging with [18]FdG and ^{18}F-DOPA, and by estimating CoQ_{10} and complex-1 activity, we established that MB is significantly improved in wv/wv-MTs mice as compared to control (C57BL/6J) mice, further supporting our original hypothesis that MTs provide neuroprotection by augmenting the MB and by inhibiting CB molecular pathogenesis (Sharma et al. 2013; Sharma and Ebadi 2014).

CB as Universal Biomarker. CB is a pleomorphic, multi-lamellar, electron dense structure of degenerated mitochondrial membranes that is formed in DPCI due to free radical overproduction in a highly vulnerable cell. Hence, CB formation is a transitory phase between pre-apoptosis and neurodegeneration. In general, CB formation occurs in highly vulnerable and hyper-proliferative cells in response to DPCI. The CB formation can be induced by nutritional deprivation in developing postnatal rat cerebellar Purkinje neurons, in intrauterine KA and DOM-exposed mice hippocampal CA-3 and dentate gyrus neurons, in mitochondrial complex-1 inhibitors (rotenone, MPP^+, and salsolinol)-exposed gene-manipulated mice, and in cultured human dopaminergic (SK-N-SH and SH-Y-5Y) neurons in response to glucose and O_2 deprivation. Particularly, CB formation can be induced by selectively knocking out the mitochondrial genome encoding the rate-limiting enzyme complex (complex-1: ubiquinone-NADH oxido-reductase) in SK-N-SH and SHY-5Y cells in culture. In addition, α-synuclein-MT_{tko} mice and wv/wv-MTs mice can be used for further investigations on charnolophagy and CS stabilization/destabilization. Hence, CB, CPS, and CS are universal biomarkers of cell injury as described in this chapter.

Recently, we highlighted the clinical significance of MTs, ubiquinone, $\Delta\Psi$, mtDNA oxidation product (8-OH-2-dG), SI, charnolophagy, charnolophagy index, and microRNAs as novel biomarkers for the early detection of CB formation and diagnosis of neurodegenerative α-synucleinopathies. We also reported that MTs inhibit CB formation as potent free radical scavengers. Hence, these sensitive biomarkers of CMB may facilitate exploring further the clinical significance of charnolophagy and CS dynamics in health and disease and in the safe and effective EBPT of chronic MDR diseases (Sharma et al. 2016; Sharma 2017).

Accumulation of CB at the junction of the axon hillock may inhibit the axoplasmic transport of ions, neurotransmitters, neurotropic factors (NGF-1, BDNF, and IGF-1), and mitochondria in AD and aging patients with severe depression and memory loss due to synaptic atrophy, whereas release of toxic substances from free radical-induced destabilized CS at the axon hillock can induce spontaneous synaptic silence, sequestration, and degeneration to cause early morbidity and mortality. Hence, CB formation in the aging brain might be responsible for the impaired brain regional neurotransmission to cause morbidity and mortality. Delayed motor learning in postnatal developing UN rats occurs due to CB formation. Inadequate mitochondrial supply may lead to sensorimotor impairments as observed in neurodegenerative α-synucleinopathies including AD and PD. Hippocampal atrophy is typically noticed in AD and depression. CB formation, particularly in the Zn^{2+} containing hippocampal neurons occurs due to MT-3 deficiency in AD (Kang and Gleason 2013; Pipatpiboon et al. 2013). In fact, CB formation in the vulnerable hippocampal neurons triggers depression. Hence, CB formation can be prevented by MTs induction, physiological Zn^{2+}, and by nutritional rehabilitation. MT-3 inhibits CB formation to prevent hippocampal damage in AD patients. MTs inhibit CB formation by serving as free radical scavengers and prevent senile dementia by boosting brain regional (hippocampal) MB. Hence, drugs or antioxidants may be developed to inhibit

CB formation, augment charnolophagy, and stabilize and excytose CS to prevent progressive neurodegeneration in PD, AD, ALS, schizophrenia, and MDDs.

Depression is the most predominant comorbidity factor in progressive NDDs, CVDs, chronic inflammatory diseases, postoperative patients, post-traumatic stress syndrome, war-wounded soldiers, space explorers, and cancer patients. Hippocampal neurons are selectively destroyed in MDDs due to BDNF depletion and CB formation. PUFA and omega-3 fatty acids (DHA, and EPA) inhibit CB formation and augment mitochondrial regeneration to enhance hippocampal neurogenesis, promoting antidepressant action. In addition, MTs may be induced by diet and moderate exercise. Future studies in this direction will improve the quality of life of particularly older subjects with chronic diseases like AD, PD, MDDs, drug addiction, and schizophrenia.

Recently, it was discovered that the fat-1 transgenic mouse, which has increased levels of DHA in the brain (because it can convert n-6 to n-3 fatty acids), exhibits increased hippocampal neurogenesis, suggesting a mechanism by which n-3 fatty acids could influence depression and mood. Hence, omega-3 Fatty acids may help prevent and treat depression by their effects on neurogenesis in the hippocampus by inhibiting CB formation. Because DHA can be obtained through diet, increasing DHA intake in depressed patients or those at high risk for depression may be one way of clinically-managing depression and helping those who have not been able to achieve remission via pharmacological interventions.

Studies were conducted to test the hypothesis that vildagliptin prevents insulin resistance, brain mitochondrial dysfunction, and learning and memory deficit caused by high fat diet (HFD) (Jacobson et al. 2011; Pintana et al. 2013). In HFD rats, neuronal insulin resistance and brain mitochondrial dysfunction were evident with impaired learning and memory. Vildagliptin prevented insulin resistance by restoring long-term depression and neuronal IR phosphorylation, IRS-1 phosphorylation, Akt/PKB-ser phosphorylation, and improved brain MB and cognitive function. Vildagliptin also restored neuronal IR function, increased glucagon-like-peptide levels, and attenuated the impaired cognitive function caused by HFD. Hence, preventing CB formation by nutritional rehabilitation, physiological Zn^{2+}, and MTs induction particularly during aging is highly significant to enjoy healthy aging, whereas unhealthy life-style choices including: alcohol intake, cigarette smoking, high-fat and salt-rich diet, or malnutrition, due to ignorance and poverty may cause morbidity and early mortality by CMB, implicated in CB molecular pathogenesis. Furthermore, by augmenting cancer stem cell-specific CB formation, we can treat MDR malignancies with minimum or no adverse effects. Hence, drugs may be developed to enhance cancer stem cell-specific CB formation for novel therapeutic interventions for the safe and effective EBPT of cancer.

Charnolophagy. The terms autophagy, endophagy, and cytophagy, have been used to explain the basic molecular mechanism of self-destruction during nutritional, toxins, and/or oxidative stress in the most vulnerable cell. During severe malnutrition, the cell starts consuming its own proteins from mitochondria, ER membranes, Golgi bodies, at the cost of protein-rich diet. Therefore, CB autophagy is more accurately explained as charnolophagy. Chronolophagy occurs when a significant proportion of CB is phagocytosed by lysosomal activation due to free radical over production, oxidative stress, and increased intracellular acidity during nutritional stress and/or toxin exposure. Hence, the term, charnolophagy may be utilized to describe specifically degenerated mitochondrial autophagy (more specifically CB autophagy) in progressive NDDs of aging. By quantitative analyses, we observed that the incidence of CB formation is practically eliminated after 80 days of nutritional rehabilitation, suggesting that CB is recycled during nutritional rehabilitation. CB is a pleomorphic and transitory phase between malnutrition and rehabilitation. During sever nutritional stress, CBs are either phagocytosed or agglomerated with other synaptic proteins such as α-synuclein to form neuronal inclusions at an early stage of neurodegeneration. A further research may resolve this highly significant yet intriguing issue. Above all, natural abundance of mitochondria and genetic susceptibility of mtDNA and microRNAs qualify CB as a universal biomarker of cell injury and apoptosis.

CB formation is triggered in the most vulnerable cell such as NPCs, derived from an iPPCs due to CMB in response to DPCI. The appearance and disappearance of CB is a reversible process as it can be regulated by microRNA-mediated nuclear or mitochondrial gene manipulation. The CB formation is eliminated by nutritional rehabilitation as we discovered in experimental animals. Under physiological conditions, CB formation should not occur in any cell to live a normal healthy life. Usually, CB is eliminated by lysosomes by "charnolophagy" as a basic molecular mechanism of ICD. The persistence of CB in any cell is usually harmful and can lead to progressive NDDs, CVDs, and cancer. Recently, we proposed that CB can be used as an early, sensitive, and universal biomarker of cell injury as it has tremendous EBPT significance (Sharma and Ebadi 2014a). We also proposed charnolostatic and charnolocidal drugs for the prevention and treatment of chronic NDDs and CVDs, and specific charnolomimetics for the effective treatment of cancer. Nonspecific induction of CB is implicated in alopecia, GIT distress, and myelosuppression in MDR malignancies. Hence, drugs may be developed to prevent CB formation in the hair follicles for the normal hair growth and regeneration. Further investigations in this direction will be beneficial for the safe and effective personalized theranostics of chronic MDR diseases.

Postnatal Undernutrition, Body Weight vs Brain Weight. We studied the effect of undernutrition on the electrophysiological and neuromorphological parameters of the developing rat brain. Undernutrition was induced by increasing the litter size from 8 to 16 pups and simultaneously restricting the mother's dietary intake of protein casein to 50% of her daily requirement, while normal animals were reared in the litters of 8 and their mothers were fed diet *ad libitum*. Lactating mothers in both experimental groups received high protein containing 25% casein (Widdowson and McCance 1957). Cerebellar tissue was processed for the E.M. analysis as described in our earlier publications (This experimental model was preferred because the rat cerebellar Purkinje neurons develop post-natally and are highly vulnerable to the deleterious effects of postnatal undernutrition) (Sharma et al. 1986; Sharma et al. 1987; Sharma et al. 1993; Sharma et al. 2003).

The ratios of brain weight and body weights of 5–30 days developing N and UN rats were determined. At any given postnatal age, this ratio was significantly high in the UN rats as compared to N rats, suggesting that brain weight vs body weight ratio may be used as a biomarker of severity of nutritional stress to qualitatively and quantitatively assess the CMB. The brain to body weight ratio reduced as a function of nutritional rehabilitation. Severely UN rats exhibited significantly high brain to body weight ratio proportional to the frequency of CB formation in the developing

UN rats. Hence, CB formation and brain/body weight ratio may be used as novel biomarkers of nutritional stress and rehabilitation or neurodegeneration vs neuro-regeneration. CB formation was discovered in the Purkinje neurons of 15–30 days old postnatal rats which is the most critical period of cerebellar development and any nutritional and/or toxic insult during this critical period of cerebellar development can induce CB molecular pathogenesis in these highly vulnerable, metabolically-active mitochondria-rich neurons. CB formation in the developing cerebellar Purkinje neurons was associated with electrophysiological deficits in the UN rat brain. In addition, hippocampal and hypothalamic CB formation was reported in MDDs and eating disorders (anorexia and bulimia) respectively (Sharma 2015).

Experimental Observations in Developing Rat Brain. Electrophysiological and neuromorphological studied were conducted to correlate and confirm the origin of CB as a result of CMB in the developing UN brain. Spontaneous unit activity of Purkinje neurons including (i) extracellular, intracellular, and evoked unit activity, (ii) mossy fiber evoked responses, and (iii) morphological studies at the light and EM level of the cerebellar cortex were performed to correlate and confirm studies on CB formation and its clinical significance. Electrophysiological investigations were carried out in the N and UN rats during 5th postnatal day to 30 days of postnatal life. UN rats were studied at 5 different age groups namely 5th, 10th, 15th, 20th, and 30th days. In the normal rats, the postnatal development of the spontaneous unit activity of Purkinje neurons was first established from 5th day to 21st day of postnatal life. The mean firing frequency of simple spikes increased as the age advanced making up a value of 37 spikes/sec in adult rats, whereas intracellular unit activity increased from 12 spikes/sec to 25 spikes/sec in N and from 11 spikes per/sec to 19 spikes/sec in the UN rats. As the age advanced, not only the firing frequency of simple and complex spikes of Purkinje cells increased, the pattern of firing changed; and the duration of spikes also decreased from 5 mSec to 1 mSec by the 20th postnatal day. In the UN rats, the mean firing frequency of the Purkinje neurons was lower; and the duration of spikes was prolonged as compared to their normal age-matched controls.

The postnatal development of the MFR was first established in young developing N rats during first 20 days of postnatal life, by stimulating the sciatic nerve ipsilaterally and picking up the MF responses from the anterior vermis. The MFR activity could be recorded on the 10th postnatal day and thereafter. During maturation, the MFR showed a gradual shortening in latency and the duration of response, while the number of functional components increased with advancing age. The stimulus threshold to elicit the MFR also reduced as the age advanced. In the UN animals, evoked MFR exhibited a prolongation of latency, reduction in the number of functional components, and the increased duration of the MFR with typical immature developmental characteristics, when compared to their age-matched controls in all the age groups studied. Even the stimulus threshold required to elicit MFR was comparatively higher in the UN animals as compared to N controls. A typical phenomenon of electrical fatigue was observed in the UN animals in the Purkinje neuron evoked unit activity and the MFR at relatively higher stimulus intensity and at higher stimulus frequencies due to CMB involving CB molecular pathogenesis (Sharma et al. 1987).

Usually, patients with MDDs are subjected to electroconvulsive therapy (ECT) when the pharmacotherapy remains ineffective. ECT is required to activate the neurons to increase their responsiveness to external stimuli. Usually, lower stimulus intensities increased MFR linearity; the medium stimulus intensity did not alter the response, whereas higher stimulus intensities reduced the MFR in UN animals. The augmentation of the MFR was observed at higher stimulus intensities and at higher stimulus frequencies in UN animals, suggesting that these electrophysiological deficits occur due to CMB involving CB molecular pathogenesis in the developing Purkinje neurons, which is responsible for delayed or impaired synaptic neurotransmission and sensorimotor development in UN children.

We conducted neuromorphological studies at light and E.M. levels. At light microscopic level, the persistence in the external granular layer, the reduced molecular layer thickness, apical accumulation of the cytoplasm in the Purkinje neurons, and increased granular cell packing density in the internal granular layer were the most significant findings in the UN rat cerebelli. At the E.M. level, the Purkinje cell cytoplasm exhibited a free ribosomal pool, immature developmental characteristics of RER, and increased incidence of lysosomes and electron-dense membrane stacks (CBs) at 15–30 days of postnatal life. These morphological deficits at the ultra-structural level reduced the Purkinje neurons' electrical activity (required for motor learning) in undernutrition. These studies indicated that undernutrition severely impacts the maturation of neurons. Immature developmental characteristics of the brain regional neurocircuitry in undernourished animals was responsible for the prolongation of electrical conduction times, increased latent periods, and abnormalities in the response pattern in term of reduced frequency, amplitude, and waveforms. These electrophysiological changes correlated with the neuromorphological deficits at the LM and E.M. levels. The frequency of CB formation was proportional to the severity of nutritional stress. Nutritional rehabilitation of 80 days eliminated (via charnolophagy; as a basic molecular mechanism of ICD) almost all CBs from the developing 30 days UN rats as ΔT and ΔE approached to zero during nutritional rehabilitation (Sharma and Ebadi 2014a).

Hippocampal and PFC Atrophy in Depression. Recently, Ota and Duman (2013) reported atrophy of neurons and structural alterations in the limbic brain regions, including prefrontal cortex (PFC) and hippocampus, in brain imaging and postmortem studies of depressed patients. They demonstrated that prolonged negative stress can induce changes comparable to those seen in MDD, through dendritic retraction and decreased spine density in PFC and hippocampal CA3 pyramidal neurons. Interestingly, these studies suggested that environmental and pharmacological manipulations, including antidepressant medication, exercise, and diet, can block or even reverse molecular changes induced by stress, providing a functional link between these factors and susceptibility to MDD, as described in my recently published books "Beyond Diet and Depression, Alleviating stress of the Soldier and Civilian, and the Therapeutic Potential of Monoamine Oxidase inhibitors (MAOI)". I have discussed various environmental and pharmacological factors, as well as the contribution of genetic polymorphisms, involved in the regulation of neuronal morphology and plasticity in MDD and preclinical stress models in these books. Particularly, the pro-depressive changes induced by stress and their reversal by antidepressants, exercise, and diet have been noticed. These *in vivo* experimental studies on the MB were further confirmed by developing mitochondrial genome knock out human DArgic (Rho$_{mgko}$) neurons as a cellular model of progressive neurodegeneration as noticed in the aging brain. The RhO$_{mgko}$ neurons were highly susceptible to MPP$^+$ neurotoxicity as compared to control neurons. Transfection of RhO_{mgko} neurons with the gene encoding complex-1 enhanced neuritogenesis, prevented CB formation, and increased CoQ_{10} levels (Sharma et al. 2004). To further confirm that MTs provide neuroprotection by inhibiting CB formation, augmenting charnolophagy, and by stabilizing CS, the following experimental genotypes were raised: (a) control mice, (b) metallothioneins transgenic (MT_{trans}), and (c) metallothioneins double gene knock out (MT_{dko}) mice. Following 10 mg/kg body weight i.p. treatment for 7 days, the MT_{dko} mice were completely immobilized, whereas MT_{trans} mice could still walk with their erect tail and stiff legs, confirming that MTs provide mitochondrial neuroprotection by preventing CB formation and by serving as potent free radical scavengers. Although no overt neurobehavioral abnormality was observed in MT_{dko} mice, these genotypes were mildly obese (particularly females) and lethargic. They were also highly susceptible to mitochondrial inhibitors and CB inducers, whereas MT_{trans} mice were lean, agile, and genetically-resistant to Parkinonian neurotoxins such as rotenone, MPTP, METH, and salsolinol (Sharma et al. 2004).

Basic Mitochondrial Events in Health and Disease. There are primarily 5 basic mitochondrial events which can happen at the subcellular level under normal and pathological conditions in a living system: (i) mitochondrial fission; (ii) mitochondrial fusion; (iii) CB formation; (iv) charnolophagy; and (v) CB sequestration. In addition, CS de-stablilization can also participate in apoptotic neurodegeneration. CB formation is based on the basic principle "*similar molecules associate, whereas dissimilar molecules dissociate.*" CB formation occurs when a cell faces abnormal physicochemical challenge involving overproduction of free radicals. Mitochondrial fission and fusion are normal physiological events which occur when the structural and functional integrity of the mitochondrial membranes as well as mtDNA remains intact, whereas CB formation, charnolophagy, CB sequestration, and CS destabilization and/or permeabilization are pathological events and occur when $\Delta\Psi$ collapse occurs and the mitochondrial membranes and mtDNA are either destroyed or becomes nonfunctional due to CMB. We confirmed these findings by developing the RhO_{mgko} neurons as a cellular model of aging as described above (Sharma et al. 2004). In general, charnolophagy occurs during the acute phase when CB is phagocytosed as a basic molecular mechanism of ICD by CPS and CS formation. During the chronic phase, the sequestration of lysosomal resistant CB releases toxic substances such as Cyt-C, iron, Ca^{2+}, acetaldehyde, CO, H_2O_2, ammonia, Bax, and Bak, and AIF to induce progressive neurodegeneration and atherosclerotic plaque rupture. Hence, drugs may be developed to inhibit CB formation during acute phase to prevent depression and by developing charnolophagy agonists and CS stabilizers to treat NDDs and other degenerative diseases and vice versa for the eradication of MDR malignancies.

Neurotoxins in Developing N and UN Brain. An environmental neurotoxin "Domoic acid" (amnesic shellfish poison, DOM) is a rigid structural analog of excitatory amino acids, KA and glutamate. Accidental ingestion of DOM in some blue mussels caused its toxicity and fatal emergencies in Montreal, Canada. Quantitative estimation of DOM and its isomers from sea food and body fluids was made by Zhao et al. (1997) using capillary electrophoresis, while microtiter receptor assay was developed by performing glutamate receptors by Van Dolah et al. (1997). Using competitive ELISA, Osada et al. (1997) estimated DOM levels in the sea food (Osada et al. 1995).

Similarly, a competitive ELISA was developed from human body fluids by Smith and Kitt (1994). Such methods for quantitative estimation of DOM from different biological sources helped to assess the safety and toxicity of DOM and provided evidence of its natural abundance. Dom has been used extensively to further elucidate the basic molecular mechanism of spatio-temporal disease-specific CB, CS, and apoptosis and their possible prevention by pharmacological or dietary interventions. We reported hippocampal CB formation and apoptosis due to DOM exposure and its association with cardiac arrhythmia, stroke, epilepsy, AD, and depression (Sharma and Dhalla 2001). Since both KA as well as DOM induce hippocampal CB formation and selective apoptosis in the CA3 and dentate gyrus neurons as observed in AD and depression; these environmental neurotoxins and sea food contaminants could be used to study the basic cellular, molecular, and genetic basis of sensorimotor impairments and depression in the future.

Recently, we reported the molecular pharmacology of various environmental neurotoxins with special reference to KA and DOM to elucidate the basic molecular mechanism of neurodegeneration particularly in AD, PD, and depression (Sharma et al. 2014). The KA and DOM models were used to examine the effect of various anti-epileptic agents in developing N and UN rats. Experimental epilepsy was induced in developing N, UN, and subsequently rehabilitated rats, by locally injecting graded doses of KA (an environmental neurotoxin from an algae, Digenia simplex) in the right frontal cortex. Frequency and power spectral analysis of EEG was performed to assess the progressive changes in the computerized EEG during KA or DOM-epileptogenesis. UN animals were highly susceptible to seizure discharge. They exhibited frequent tonic-clonic discharge and had frequent episodes of clinical seizures even after temporary neuronal recovery. Generalization of seizure discharge activity occurred at lower doses of KA in UN rats and these animals exhibited considerable background electrical inhibition even in their basal EEG records. Increases in δ and θ and decrease in α and β frequencies were observed in the compressed spectral array (CSA) of UN animals. Delayed neuronal recovery with reduced background EEG and marked electro-silence in response to intra-rectal sodium valproate was observed in the UN animals due to CMB, implicated in CB molecular pathogenesis. Nutritionally-rehabilitated animals exhibited partial neuronal recovery as was evident from their body weight gain and elimination of CBs in the Purkinje neurons. Spike frequency, spike amplitude, and neuronal recovery times were not significantly different between N and UN animals at lower doses of KA (7.5–60 ng) whereas, at higher doses (120–500 ng), marked differences were observed in these parameters. The relative dominance of low frequency rhythm particularly in response to either local KA or DA in the hippocampal CA-3 or dentate gyrus regions of UN rats, indicated CMB. The ^{3}H-Glycine uptake was significantly higher in the hippocampus and spinal cord and lower in the cerebellum in the UN rats than N rats indicating that undernutrition can significantly influence the response to various pharmacological agents (Sharma et al. 1990).

Further studies were performed to examine the neurotoxic effects of KA as well as DOM in the developing rat cerebral cortex and mice hippocampus employing computerized EEG, neurochemical, and NMR analyses. KA as well as DOM produced reductions in α and β and increases in δ and θ EEG frequencies. A reverse trend was noticed following antiepileptic treatment. DOM enhanced KCl-induced glutamate release from the rat hippocampal slices and increased $[Ca^{2+}]_i$ in NG-108/15 cells. HPLC and NMR analyses revealed a typical reduction in GABA and increase in glutamate levels in DOM-treated mice hippocampus. DOM-induced dose and time-dependent induction of proto-oncogenes (c-fos and c-jun) was inhibited following prophylactic or therapeutic antiepileptic treatment with sodium valproate, pyridoxine, 5-α pregnan-3 α-ol-20-one, nimodipine, or 8-(OH)-DPAT. High energy phosphorylated metabolites were not significantly affected with the sub-convulsive doses of DOM. However, reductions in N-acetyl aspartate (NAA) and phosphocreatine (PCr) and ATP were observed with direct exposure of DOM to NG-108/15 cells in culture. CB formation in the developing UN hippocampal and Purkinje neurons was enhanced in intrauterine KA or DOM-exposed mice. MRI revealed a progressive increase in the T_2 intensities following a sub-convulsive dose of DOM at the level of hippocampus, which was confirmed histologically as CA3 and dentate gyrus; however the CA1 layer remained preserved. In general, environmental neurotoxins enhanced glutamate release, Ca^{2+} influx and proto-oncogenes expression to accelerate neuronal apoptosis via CB formation which increased the after-hyperpolarization (AHP) duration of developing neurons particularly during severe nutritional stress due to increased $[Ca^{2+}]_i$ overloading and mitochondrial degeneration (Dakshinamurti et al. 1993; Sharma and Dakshinamurti 1993; Sharma et al. 1993; Sharma and Ebadi 2014).

Neuroprotective Effect of 8-OH-DPAT. Microinjections of DOM in the hippocampal CA-3 and dentate gyrus regions induced generalized electrical seizure discharge activity, characterized by spike and waves followed by intermittent burst discharges. Computerized EEG analysis exhibited typical reduction in α and β and increase in δ and θ activities during DOM neurotoxicity which was attenuated by microinjections of a 5-HT1A receptor agonist, 8-hydroxy, di L propylamino tetraline (8-OH-DPAT), and augmented by antagonist, spiroxatrine, in the contralateral hippocampal CA-3 region. Neuronal recovery following 8(OH)-DPAT administration was accompanied with reductions in δ and θ and increase in α and β EEG rhythms, suggesting that activation of serotonergic mechanisms in the CNS has neuroprotective actions (Sharma and Dakshinamurti 1993). Furthermore, Fedotova and Ordyan (2010) studied the effect of chronic administration of 5-HT(1A)-receptor agonist 8-OH-DPAT (0.05 mg/kg s.c.) or antagonist NAN-190 (0.1 mg/kg i.p.) for 14 days on anxious-depressive-like behavior of female rats during the estrous cycle. Chronic administration of NAN-190 produced an anxiogenic effect, while its administration during the proestrus phase induced an anxiolytic effect. 8-OH-DPAT had no effect on anxiety level; but produced a pronounced anti-depressive effect irrespective of the phase of the estrous cycle. In their previous study, Fedotova (2006) examined the influence of the chronic administration of 8-OH-DPAT (0.05 mg/kg, s.c.) and NAN-190 (0.1 mg/kg, i.p.) alone or in combination with 17β-estradiol (0.5 μg/animal, i.m.) for 14 days on the depressive behavior and the monoamine level in the hippocampus of adult ovariectomized (OVX) female rats. This model of depression was confirmed under the Porsolt test conditions. Chronic administration of 8-OH-DPAT produced an antidepressant effect in OVX rats. 8-OH-DPAT in combination with 17β-estradiol potentiated the antidepressant action. The antidepressant effect of 8-OH-DPAT in OVX rats was correlated with the restoration of NE-ergic, 5-HT-ergic, and DA-ergic neurotransmission in the hippocampus, indicating a close interaction between the ovarian hormonal system and the cerebral 5-HTergic system in the etiology of depression. Furthermore, Montgomery et al. (1991) examined the effect of 8-OH-DPAT (0–300 µg/kg), and Buspirone (0–3.0 mg/kg), on variable-interval, threshold-current self-stimulation of rat lateral hypothalamus. Buspirone produced a prolonged depression, whereas the effects of 8-OH-DPAT were biphasic: 3.0 µg/kg produced a sustained enhancement of response while higher doses (100–300 µg/kg) produced a short-lasting depression. This biphasic pattern corroborated previously reported effects of 8-OH-DPAT on food intake and on other behaviors. Furthermore, threshold-current self-stimulation was highly sensitive to alterations in DA-ergic neurotransmission but relatively insensitive to changes in 5-HT. Thus, the facilitating effect of low-dose 8-OH-DPAT seems most plausibly interpretation in terms of enhanced DA-ergic neurotransmission. This could be brought about by $5HT_{1A}$-mediated inhibition of 5-HT release and disinhibition of DAergic neurotransmission. Depression of self-stimulation by higher doses of 8-OH-DPAT may reflect the activity of 8-OH-DPAT at postsynaptic 5-HT receptors, with consequent inhibition of DAergic transmission. Suppression of response after buspirone may reflect the action of this compound as a partial agonist at postsynaptic 5-HT receptors, and/or its effects on other systems. In a similar study, Sapronov et al. (2006) studied the effect of chronic (14 days) 8-OH-DPAT (0.05 mg/kg, s.c.) and NAN-190 (0.1 mg/kg, i.p.) alone or in combination with the acetylcholinesterase inhibitor galantamine (1.0 mg/kg, i.p.) on depression and anxiety in old (24 months) male rats with dementia of Alzheimer's type. The combined administration of 8-OH-DPAT with galantamine resulted in pronounced antidepressant and anxiolytic action, indicating that 8-OH-DPAT provides neuroprotection from glutamate-induced excitotoxicity by inhibiting CB molecular pathogenesis in the hippocampal CA-3 and dentate gyrus neurons.

Several terms have been used to describe autophagy such as endophagy, cytophagy, endoparasitism as an ICD mechanism during severe nutritional or environmental toxins stress due to free radical overproduction. The number of lysosomes is significantly increased in the developing UN Purkinje neurons. Lysosomes are involved in the phagocytosis of degenerated mitochondria. However, Mother Nature has provided more number of mitochondria to sustain cellular bioenergetics as compared to lysosomes. Therefore, during oxidative and nitrative stress of malnutrition or toxins, lysosomes are increased to phagocytose intracellular CBs to a certain extent. Hence, charnolophagy is a rare phenomenon as compared to transfomation of CB to functional mitochondria during nutritional rehabilitation.

In my opinion, charnolophagy is appropriate term to describe CB autophagy. I have discussed how to prevent CB formation for maintaining healthy nervous system and cardiovascular system; and induce it in cancer stem cells to eradicate MDR malignancies with minimum or no side effects. Hence, CB formation has a direct clinical significance in health and disease. Moreover, natural abundance of mitochondria and increased sensitivity of the mitochondrial genome qualifies CB as a universal pre-apoptotic biomarker of cell injury and can have tremendous clinical applications in biomedical field particularly in developing novel antioxidant-loaded NPs for mitochondrial protection and hence disease control. Any physiological and/or pharmacological intervention augmenting MTs can inhibit CB formation, enhance charnolophagy, and stabilize CS to prevent progressive NDDs and CVDs. For example, balanced diet and moderate exercise can augment MTs to inhibit CB formation in the most vulnerable cells in our body. I have explained the therapeutic potential of nutritional rehabilitation, physiological Zn^{2+}, antioxidants, and MTs in preventing and/or inhibiting CB formation to provide benefit to a patient suffering from chronic illness.

Induction of CB early or late in life at the junction of the axon hillock can block the axoplasmic transport of various ions, neurotransmitters, enzymes, neurotropic factors, and mitochondria at the synaptic terminals, to cause synaptic atrophy involved in cognitive impairments in learning, intelligence, memory, and behavior. The degeneration of synaptic terminals is responsible for several chronic diseases such as PD, AD, HD, ALS, MS, Fredrick ataxia, and several other diseases involving inter-neuronal and intra-neuronal accumulation of inclusions bodies, such as Hirano bodies, Lafora bodies, Merinesco bodies, Lewy bodies, Pick bodies, amyloid-β-42 bodies, etc. Hence drugs may be developed to prevent nonspecific accumulation of CBs at the junction of the axon hillock and in the perinuclear region to treat chronic NDDs effectively. In general, the secondary or tertiary free radical attack is associated with CS destabilization, permeabilization, and disintegration at the junction of axon hillock, which causes a massive release of highly toxic mitochondrial metabolites to trigger synaptic degeneration and consequently impairments in cognitive performance resulting in early morbidity and mortality. Nonspecific induction of CB formation in highly proliferative cells can induce various adverse effects of anticancer chemotherapy including GIT symptoms (nausea, vomiting, diarrhea, dehydration, alkalosis, paralysis, coma, and death), myelosuppression (anemia, neutropenia, and thrombocytopenia), alopecia, cardiotoxicity (myocardial infarction), neurotoxicity, and infertility during treatment of MDR malignancies.

It is now well-established that cancer stem cells are difficult to eradicate because they are genetically-resistant to CB formation due to induction of several anti-apoptotic genes involved in regulating the MB. These anti-apoptotic genes tend to immortalize the cell because of several genetic and epigenetic causes including impaired synthesis of microRNAs, DNA methylation, and histone acetylation. Particularly, nuclear and mtDNA methylation and acetylation has been implicated in the cell growth, division, proliferation, differentiation, and organogenesis. However, various environmental neurotoxins and drugs of abuse (cocaine, METH, morphine, and ethanol) can induce impairments in the DNA methylation at N3 position of the cytosine and histones acetylation at lysine residues to cause changes in the gene expression at the post-translational level and can be noticed in response to early childhood nutritional stress, anesthetic agents, antiepileptic agents, and ethanol (FAS). It is important to point out that these epigenetic changes (DNA methylation) are very easy to induce in the mtDNA as compared to the nDNA, because the mtDNA is GC-rich, intron less, and remains in a hostile microenvironment of free radicals which are constantly synthesized as a byproduct of oxidative phosphorylation in the electron transport chain during ATP synthesis, whereas, the nDNA is double helical coil with introns and exons and histones and protamines which provide structural and functional stability to the nDNA and maintain its supercoiled helicity. Moreover, nDNA repair mechanisms are more efficient as compared to mtDNA. The histone acetylation at the lysine residues occurs first to uncoil the nDNA. The uncoling of the nDNA by histone acetylation at lysine residues exposes the cytosine residues of the nDNA to be methylated. Hence, drugs or agents may be developed to induce cancer stem cell-specific CB formation to eradicate MDR malignancies with minimum or no adverse effects. Further detailed epidemiological studies on mtDNA are needed to determine the exact role of epigenetic changes including DNA methylation and histone acetylation during CB formation and elimination in health and disease.

Sucrose Density Gradient Centrifugation to Isolate CS. The CS layer can be derived and isolated from the sucrose gradient. The majority of CSs are present in between the lowermost nuclear layer and the mitochondrial layer as these are denser than the lysosomes. The lysosomes are lighter than the mitochondria followed by the ribosomal layer, which remains at the top of the density gradient as illustrated in the diagram. A pictorial diagram illustrating a typical sucrose density gradient, to purify and isolate CS-rich layer is presented in Fig. 14.

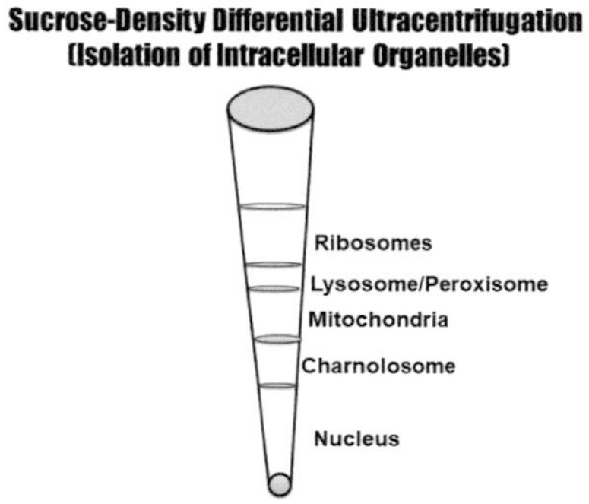

Sucrose-Density Differential Ultracentrifugation
(Isolation of Intracellular Organelles)

Ribosomes
Lysosome/Peroxisome
Mitochondria
Charnolosome
Nucleus

Fig. 14: Sucrose density differential centrifugation (isolation of intracellular organelles).

Spatio-Temporal Classification of CS. At least 7 different types of CSs have been reported depending on their spatio-temporal microdistribution inside or outside the cell. These include: (i) intranuclear CS, (ii) perinuclear CS, (iii) intramitochondrial CS, (iv) peri-mitochondrial CS, (v) intracellular CS, (vi) extracellular CS, and (vii) circulating CS. The spatio-temporal microdistribution of CS determines the deleterious clinical consequences of intrauterine nicotine and ethanol during pregnancy. Release of toxic substances from the intranuclear CS can induce prezygotic death and abortion; from the perinuclear CS is responsible for the still birth and cyclopia; from the intra-mitochondrial CS is involved in microcephaly and craniofacial abnormalities, from the perimitochondrial CS is involved in cleft pellet, cleft lip, and loss of philtrum; from the intracellular CS is involved in micro-opthalmia and microganathia; from the extracellular CS is involved in visual and auditory impairments in addition to cognitive impairments in learning, intelligence, memory, and behavior; from the circulating or systemic CS is involved in dendritic pruning, synaptic synaptic atrophy, and synaptic degeneration accompanied with loss of cognitive performance, early morbidity, and early mortality without any craniofacial abnormalities. A pictorial diagram illustrating a spatio-temporal classification of CS during intrauterine exposure to ethanol is presented in Fig. 15.

Toxic CS Metabolites. The toxic metabolites are originated from the mitochondrial metabolism. These include but are not limited to Cyt-C, acetaldehyde, ammonia, H_2O_2, iron, AIF, caspase-3, and Bax/Bak, 8-OH, 2dG, 2,3 dhydroxynonenal, monoamine oxidases, TSPO (18 kDa), cholesterol, Ca^{2+}, and tetrahydroisoquinolines (TIQs). All

Spatiotemporal Charnolosome Classification

Intranuclear CS	• Prezygotic Death • Abortion
Perinuclear CS	• Still Birth • Cyclopia
Intra-mitochondrial CS	• Microcephaly • Craniofacial Abnormalities
Peri-mitochondrial CS	• Cleft Pellet, Cleft Lip, • Loss of Philtrum
Intracellular CS	• Microopthalmia • Microganathia
Extracellular CS	• Visual Impairment • Auditory Impairment
Systemic CS	• Dendritic Pruning • Synaptic Degeneration, Cognition (LIMB)

Fig. 15: Spatiotemporal charnolosome (CS) classification.

Toxic Charnolosome Metabolites

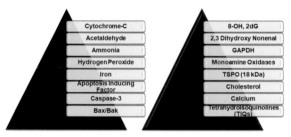

Cytochrome-C	8-OH, 2dG
Acetaldehyde	2,3 Dihydroxy Nonenal
Ammonia	GAPDH
Hydrogen Peroxide	Monoamine Oxidases
Iron	TSPO (18 kDa)
Apoptosis Inducing Factor	Cholesterol
Caspase-3	Calcium
Bax/Bak	Tetrahydroisoquinolines (TIQs)

Fig. 16: Toxic charnolosome metabolites.

these toxic metabolites of degenerated mitochondria are released near the CS to cause impaired growth and development. These toxic metabolites also inhibit the expression of genes involved in cell growth, proliferation, differentiation, and development at the transcriptional and translational level. A brief list of toxic CS metabolites is presented in this pictorial diagram as presented in Fig. 16.

Mitochondrial Dynamics and Charnolopathy in Chronic MDR Diseases. Healthy life style, proper diet, and moderate exercise enhance mitochondrial regeneration, rejuvenation, repair, reunion, and replacement under normal physiological conditions; whereas, malnutrition, environmental toxins (including drugs of abuse), and microbial (bacteria, virus, fungal) infections enhance the requirement of energy (ATP) through accelerated oxidative phosphorylation. Free radicals are highly reactive oxygen and nitrogen species (ROS and RNS) which induce lipid peroxidation to cause structural and functional breakdown of PUFA in the mitochondrial membranes. These degenerated membranes are aggregated to form pleomorphic electron-dense membrane stacks to generate CBs as a basic molecular mechanism of ICD. CBs are recognized as nonfunctional intracellular inclusions and are phagocytosed by energy (ATP)-driven charnolophagy (CB autophagy). Following charnolophagy, a CPS is formed, which is transformed to CS when the phagocytosed membranes are completely hydrolyzed by the lysosomal enzymes. The CS is structurally and functionally highly labile organelle and is exocytosed by an energy (ATP)-dependent mechanism as a secondary major step of ICD. During SFA and TFA, lipid peroxidation of the CS membranes induces the formation of CS bodies. The CS bodies are pinched off from the parent CS and are fused with the plasma membranes triggering the formation of apoptotic bodies. The apoptotic bodies release highly toxic mitochondrial metabolites due to rupture of plasma membranes. These toxic metabolites cause progressive degeneration of neighboring cells to cause NDDs, CVDs, including MDR malignancies if an apoptotic body from a CS_{scs} is endocytosed by a nonproliferating cell in the body. A pictorial diagram illustrating MB in health and disease is presented in Fig. 17.

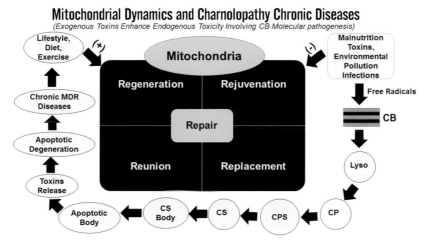

Fig. 17: Mitochondrial dynamics and charnolopathy in chronic diseases.

References

Bollimuntha, S., B. Singh, S. Shavali, S. Sharma and M. Ebadi. 2005. TRPC-1-mediated inhibition of MPP⁺ toxicity in human SH S-Y5Y neuroblastoma cells. J Biol Chem 280: 2132–2140.

Chabenne, A., C. Moon, C. Ojo, A. Khogali, B. Nepal and S. Sharma. 2014. Biomarkers in fetal alcohol syndrome. Biomarkers and Genomic Medicine 6: 12–22.

Dakshinamurti, K., S.K. Sharma, M. Sundaram and T. Watanabe. 1993. Hippocampal changes in developing postnatal mice following intra-uterine exposure to domoic acid. J Neurosci 13: 4486–4495.

Fedotova, Y.O. and N.E. Ordyan. 2010. Effects of 8-OH-DPAT and NAN-190 on anxious-depressive-like behavior of female rats during the estrous cycle. Bull Exp Biol Med 150(2): 165–167.

Jacobson, S.W., M.E. Stanton, N.C. Dodge, M. Pienaar, D.S. Fuller, C.D. Molteno, E.M. Meinties, H.E. Hoyme, L.K. Robinson, N. Khaole and J.L. Jacobson. 2011. Impaired delay and trace eye blink conditioning in school-age children with fetal alcohol syndrome. Alcohol Clin Exp Res 35: 250–264.

Kang, J.X. and E.D. Gleason. 2013. Omega-3 fatty acids and hippocampal neurogenesis in depression. CNS Neurol Disord Drug Targets 12: 460–465.

Montgomery, A.M., I.C. Rose and L.J. Herberg. 1991. 5-HT1A agonists and dopamine: the effects of 8-OH-DPAT and buspirone on brain-stimulation reward. J Neural Transm Gen Sect 83: 139–148.

Ota, K.T. and R.S. Duman. 2013. Environmental and pharmacological modulations of cellular plasticity: role in the pathophysiology and treatment of depression. Neurobiol Dis 57: 28–37.

Pintana, H., N. Apaijai, N. Chattipakorn and S.C. Chattipakorn. 2013. DPP-4 inhibitors improve cognition and brain mitochondrial function of insulin-resistant rats. J Endocrinol 218: 1–11.

Pipatpiboon, N., H. Pintana, W. Pratchayasakul and S.C. Cahttipakorn. 2013. DPP4-inhibitor improves neuronal insulin receptor function, brain mitochondrial function and cognitive function in rats with insulin resistance induced by high-fat diet consumption. Eur J Neurosci 37: 839–849.

Sapronov, N.S., I.O. Fedotova and N.A. Losev. 2006. Optimizing effect of the combined administration of 8-OH-DPAT and galantamine on depression—anxiety behavior in old rats with dementia of Alzheimer's type. Eksp Klin Farmakol 69(3): 10–13.

Sharma, S., W. Selvamurthy and K. Dakshinamurti. 1993. Effect of environmental neurotoxins in the developing brain. Biometeorology 2: 447–455.

Sharma, S. and M. Ebadi. 2003. Metallothionein attenuates 3-morpoholinosydnonimone (SIN-1)-induced oxidative and nitrative stress in DArgic neurons. Antioxidants and Redox Signaling 5: 251–264.

Sharma, S., E. Carlson and M. Ebadi. 2003. The neuroprotective actions of selegiline in inhibiting 1-methyl, 4-phenyl, pyridinium ion (MPP$^+$)-induced apoptosis in DArgic neurons. J Neurocytology 32: 329–343.

Sharma, S., M. Kheradpezhou, S. Shavali, H. EI Refaey, J. Eken, C. Hagen and M. Ebadi. 2004. Neuroprotective actions of coenzyme Q_{10} in Parkinson's disease. Methods in Enzymology 382: 488–509.

Sharma, S., A. Rais, W. Nel, R. Sandhu and M. Ebadi. 2013. Clinical significance of metallothioneins in cell therapy and nanomedicine. International Journal of Nanomedicine 8: 1477–1488.

Sharma, S., C.S. Moon, A. Khogali, A. Haidous, A. Chabenne, C. Ojo, M. Jelebinkov, Y. Kurdi and M. Ebadi. 2013. Biomarkers of Parkinson's disease (Recent Update). Neurochemistry International 63: 201–229.

Sharma, S. 2013. Charnoly body as a sensitive biomarker in nanomedicine. Proceedings of the International Translational Nanomedicine Conference. Boston, July 26–28 (Invited Speaker).

Sharma, S., B. Nepal, C.S. Moon, A. Chabenne, A. Khogali, C. Ojo, F. Hong, R. Goudet, A. Sayed-Ahmad, A. Jacob, M. Murtaba and M. Firlit. 2014. Psychology of craving. Open Jr of Medical Psychology 3: 120–125.

Sharma, S. and M. Ebadi. 2014. Antioxidants as potential therapeutics in neurodegeneration. pp. 1–30. *In*: Laher, I. (ed.). System Biology of Free Radicals and Antioxidants. Springer Verlag. Germany, Chapter 85.

Sharma, S. and M. Ebadi. 2014. Significance of metallothioneins in aging brain. Neurochemistry International 65: 40–48.

Sharma, S.K., U. Nayar, M.C. Maheshwari and G. Gopinath. 1986. Ultrastructural studies of P-cell morphology in developing normal and undernourished rat cerebellar cortex. Neuromorphological Correlates Neurology, India 34: 323–327.

Sharma, S.K., U. Nayar, M.C. Maheshwari and B. Singh. 1987. Effect of undernutrition on developing rat cerebellum: Some electrophysiological and neuromorphological Correlates. J Neurol Sciences 78: 261–272.

Sharma, S.K., U. Nayar, M.C. Maheshwari and B. Singh. 1993. Purkinje cell evoked unit activity in developing undernourished rats. J Neurol Sci 116: 212–219.

Sharma, S.K. and K. Dakshinamurti. 1993. Suppression of Domoic acid-induced seizures by 8-(OH)-DPAT. J Neural Transmission 93: 87–89.

Sharma, S.K. and M. Ebadi. 2004. An improved method for analyzing coenzyme Q homologues and multiple detection of rare biological samples. J Neurosci Methods 137: 1–8.

Widdowson, E.M. and R.A. McCance. 1957. Effect of a low-protein diet on the chemical composition of the bodies and tissues of young rats. Br J Nutr 11(2): 198–206.

CHAPTER-4

Charnoly Body as a Novel Biomarker of Compromised Mitochondrial Bioenergetics

INTRODUCTION

As described in earlier chapters, free radicals are generated as a byproduct of mitochondrial oxidative phosphorylation in the electron transport chain. The requirement of energy (ATP) is significantly increased during severe malnutrition, in response to environmental toxicity (heavy metal ions: Pb, Cd, Ni, Hg, polychlorobiphenyl; PCBs), and during microbial (bacteria, virus, fungus) infection in the most vulnerable cells such as NPCs, derived from iPPCs (Sharma 2017a, 2017b). The most common free radicals, produced as a byproduct of oxidative phosphorylation, are, ·OH and NO· radicals. ·OH and NO· radicals in the presence of iron participate in the Fenton reaction and produce $ONOO^-$ ions. $ONOO^-$ ions are highly devastating, as these ions induce oxidative as well as nitrative stress to cause progressive NDDs (Ebadi and Sharma 2003; Sharma and Ebadi 2003). We reported that CoQ_{10} provides neuroprotection as an anti-inflammatory and antiapoptotic agent in PD by attenuating mitochondrial complex-1 downregulation and NFkβ activation in the NS-DAergic neurons (Ebadi et al. 2004). Furthermore, CoQ_{10} confers neuroprotection by attenuating iron-induced apoptosis in cultured human DAeric (SK-N-SH) cells (Kooncumchoo et al. 2006).

In this chapter, 4 different stages of a free radical attack, i.e., (i) primary, (ii) secondary, (iii) tertiary, and (iv) quaternary, are described to elucidate CB molecular pathogenesis and its prevention by enhancing the MB to sustain ICD for normal cellular function and homeostasis to remain healthy.

Stages of Intracellular Toxification/Detoxification. The intracellular toxification/detoxification can be described primarily in 4 different stages. The intracellular toxification/detoxification depends on the intensity and frequency of a free radical attack in response to DPCI.

(i) Primary Free Radical Attack (PFA)

(ii) Secondary Free Radical Attack (SFA)

(iii) Tertiary Free Radical Attack (TFA)

(iv) Quaternary Free Radical Attack (QFA)

The PFA is usually accompanied with the down-regulation of MB because of $\Delta\Psi$ collapse, which causes formation of mega-pores on the mitochondrial membrane due to the downregulation of the Ca^{2+} channel protein, TRPC. This is followed by TSPO (18 kDa) cholesterol ion channel protein, MAOs, and TRPC (calcium channel regulating protein) delocalization. The intra-mitochondrial Ca^{2+} is significantly increased, which induces ionic imbalance to accumulate water inside the mitochondria. As a result, mega-mitochondriogenesis is initiated, which induces degeneration of the membranes due to ROS-induced lipid peroxidation. ROS-induced lipid peroxidation induces structural and functional breakdown of PUFA to cause fragmentation of the mitochondrial membranes. The extent of intracellular degeneration depends on the acute or chronic exposure to free radical-induced lipid peroxidation and neuronal injury. ROS-induced lipid peroxidation causes initially enhanced permeabilization followed by perforations of mitochondrial membranes. SFA is associated with disintegration followed by condensation of the degenerated mitochondrial membranes to trigger CB formation, charnolophagy, and CS exocytosis for ICD.

During TFA, CS formation, CS destabilization, and translocation on the plasma membranes causes the formation of apoptotic bodies due to the uncontrolled release of highly toxic mitochondrial metabolites resulting in non-DNA dependent apoptotic degeneration (Sharma 2017c). Although nDNA remains preserved during CB formation, charnolophagy, and CS exocytosis, the mtDNA is easily oxidized to synthesize highly toxic 8-OH, 2dG, which can impair genetic and epigenetic mechanisms (Sharma et al. 2016). The other important metabolite which is synthesized during the free radical-induced lipid peroxidation is 2,3 dihydroxy nonenal, which is formed due to degeneration of mitochondrial membranes involved in CB formation. A pictorial diagram illustrating primarily three major stages of a free radical attack in a cell is presented in Fig. 18.

Accumulation of CB at the junction of axon hillock can impair the normal axoplasmic transport of various ions, enzymes, neurotransmitters, hormones, proteins, neurotropic factors (such as BDNF, NGF-1, and IGF-1), and mitochondria from the

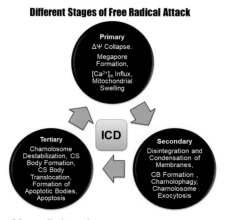

Fig. 18: Different stages of free radical attack.

cell body to the terminal end bulb, resulting in progressive synaptic atrophy. The release of toxic substances from the permeabilized, destabilized, and degenerated CPS or CS at the junction of the axon hillock induce terminal degeneration, resulting in impaired brain regional neuro-cybernetics and eventually cognitive loss involving learning, intelligence, memory, and behavioral deficits. These deleterious changes trigger early morbidity and mortality due to synaptic degeneration as noticed in AD patients. The SFA can be attenuated to a certain extent by endogenous (glutathione, MTs, SOD, catalase) antioxidants as well as by exogenous antioxidants, administered as pharmacotherapeutic agents or derived from natural sources such as: resveratrol, polyphenols, sirtuis, rutins, catechin, and lycopenes. Fruits and vegetables are rich in these antioxidants. However, these are not highly potent, hence, need to be consumed in bulk quantities. The TFA is accompanied with a disintegration of CPS and CS which occurs due to further lipid peroxidation and induces apoptotic neurodegeneration causing early morbidity and mortality, as noticed in chronic drug addiction. QFA can induce irreversible damage to the mitochondrial membranes, mtDNA, and triggers CB formation and neurodegenerative apoptosis accompanied with SIDS, still birth and/or abortion as noticed in the developing fetuses of binge-drinking and/or tobacco-smoking pregnant women. Thus, the endogenous as well as exogenous antioxidants can attenuate free radical-induced mitochondrial degeneration, augment MB, trigger CB formation, enhances charnolophagy and CS exocytosis as illustrated in Fig. 19.

Mitochondrial Bioenergetics and ICD. The MB is governed by spatiotemporal frequency and intensity of a free radical attack, which may induce repairable or irreparable damage in our body to execute either cell survival or cellular demise. In general, DPCI enhance free radical overproduction due to mitochondrial oxidative and nitrative stress. Free radicals induce CMB by causing $\Delta\Psi$ collapse, megapore formation, and increased intra-mitochondrial Ca^{2+} influx to cause water and electrolyte imbalance due to TRPC, TSPO (18 KDa), and MAOs delocalization from the outer mitochondrial membrane. Consequently, mitochondria become swollen and fragmented. The fragmented mitochondrial membranes condense to form multi-lamellar CBs. CBs are phagocytosed by lysosomes to form CPS. The CPS is transformed to CS, when the phagocytosed CB is hydrolyzed by the lysosomal enzymes. The CS is exocytosed as a basic molecular mechanism of ICD. Hence,

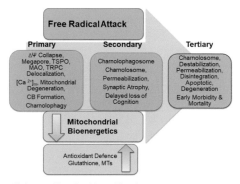

Fig. 19: Stages of intracellular toxification/detoxification.

CS exocytosis is highly crucial for the health and well-being of a biological system. Endogenous antioxidants such as MTs, glutathione, SOD, and catalase may provide protection during the acute phase, whereas exogenously-administered antioxidants as free radical scavengers may be required during the chronic phase to prevent and-or inhibit CB formation, augment charnolophagy, and stabilize CS to preserve MB and sustain ICD. A pictorial diagram illustrating a functional relationship between MB and ICD is presented in Fig. 20.

Major Detoxification Sites. There are primarily 7 major sites of detoxification in a biological system. These include: (a) intranuclear, (b) perinuclear, (c) intra-mitochondrial, (d) peri-mitochondrial, (e) intracellular, (f) extracellular, and (g) systemic. These sites must to be detoxified for the health and well-being of a living system. DPCI enhance oxidative phosphorylation, free radical overproduction, mitochondrial degeneration, CB formation, charnolophagy, CS formation and destabilization to compromise MB and may pose a significant challenge in ICD, required for normal cellular function to remain healthy. Particularly, systemic detoxification is clinically-significant to prevent and/or eradicate MDR malignancies because the circulating CSscs is involved in the malignant transformation of non-proliferating cells. Their transfection induces cellular immortalization during malignancy. A pictorial diagram illustrating the 7 major sites of detoxification is presented in Fig. 21.

Intracellular Pathophysiology of CB (Acute Phase). Acute exposure to DPCI induce mitochondria to synthesize increased ATP, required for ICD. Free radicals are generated as a byproduct of oxidative phosphorylation in the electron transport chain. Free radicals induce lipid peroxidation to cause structural and functional degradation of PUFA in the plasma membranes. As consequence, membranes are disintegrated and condensed to form multi-lamellar structures to form CBs. CBs are efficiently eliminated by ATP-driven lysosomal-dependent charnolophagy to form a highly unstable CPS. The CPS is transformed to CS, when the phagocytosed CB is hydrolyzed. The CS is subsequently exocytosed as a basic molecular mechanism of ICD for health and well-being. Intracellular pathophysiology of CB (Acute Phase) is presented in Fig. 22.

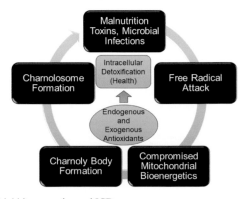

Fig. 20: Mitochondrial bioenergetics and ICD.

Major Sites of Detoxification

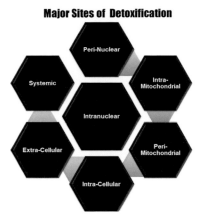

Fig. 21: Major sites of detoxification.

Intra-Cellular Pathophysiology of Charnoly Body
Acute Phase

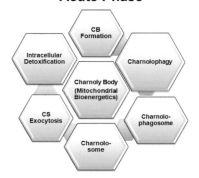

Fig. 22: Intracellular pathophysiology of charnoly body (Acute phase).

Intracellular Pathophysiology of CB (Intermediate Phase). During the intermediate phase, charnolophagy and/or CS formation may be either delayed, impaired, or inhibited. The lysosome-resistant CB can accumulate in the perinuclear region to cause impaired transcriptional and translational regulation of microRNA and genes involved in normal growth, proliferation, differentiation, and development. The accumulation of CB at the junction of the axon hillock can cause impaired axoplasmic flow of various ions, enzymes, neurotransmitters, hormones, growth factors (BDNF, NGF-1), and mitochondria to cause synaptic atrophy. Slowly and steadily-induced synaptic atrophy causes delayed neurodegeneration as observed in PD, AD, drug addiction, MDD, schizophrenia, and aging as illustrated in Fig. 23.

Intracellular Pathophysiology of CB (Chronic Phase). During the chronic phase, CB becomes lysosome-resistant and disrupts charnolophagy. The failure of charnolophagy during the chronic phase involves CPS and CS destabilization, resulting in the release of highly toxic mitochondrial metabolites (including: iron, Cyt-C, acetaldehyde, acetone, ammonia, H_2O_2, 8-OH, 2dG, 2,3 dihydroxy-nonenal, AIF, and caspase-3). The axoplasmic transport of toxic metabolites induces synaptic degeneration to

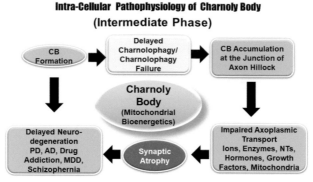

Fig. 23: Intracellular pathophysiology of charnoly body (Intermediate phase).

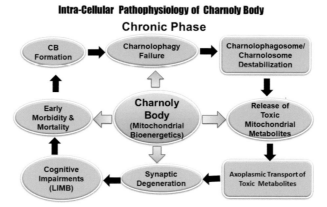

Fig. 24: Intracellular pathophysiology of charnoly body (Chronic phase).

cause cognitive impairments resulting in impaired learning, intelligence, memory, and behavior, leading to early morbidity and mortality as observed in DPCI, which compromise MB to trigger CB formation, charnolophagy failure, CS destabilization, and intracellular toxicity involved in progressive NDDs. A pictorial diagram illustrating the chronic phase of free radicals-induced neurodegeneration in the most susceptible cells during the chronic phase is presented in Fig. 24.

Biomarkers of ICD. The most important event during ICD is charnolophagy (also named as CB autophagy). While charnolophagy and CS exocytosis are involved in ICD; charnolophagy inhibitors or antagonists, and CS exocytosis inhibitors or antagonists are involved in cellular degeneration due to non-DNA-dependent apoptosis. CC_{scs} formation is involved in malignant transformation of nonproliferating cells. The endocytosis of CS_{csc} is involved in malignant transformation. A pictorial diagram illustrating potential biomarkers of ICD is presented in Fig. 25.

Biomarkers of CMB. There are primarily 4 types of biomarkers of CMB. These include: CB, CPS, CS, and CS body. A pictorial diagram of these biomarkers is presented in Fig. 26.

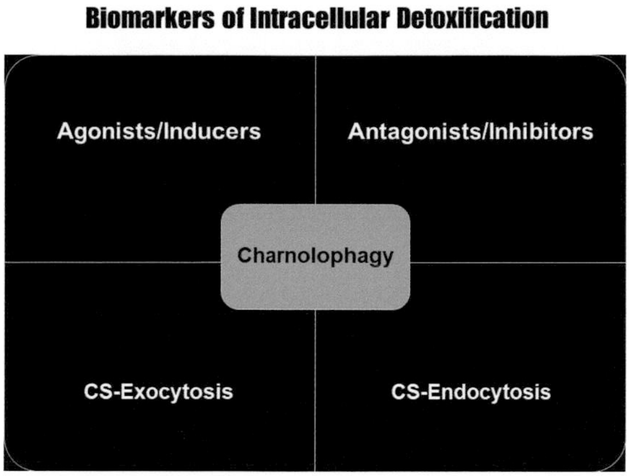

Biomarkers of Intracellular Detoxification

Agonists/Inducers	Antagonists/Inhibitors
Charnolophagy	
CS-Exocytosis	CS-Endocytosis

Fig. 25: Biomarkers of ICD.

Biomarkers of Intracellular Mitochondrial Bioenergetics

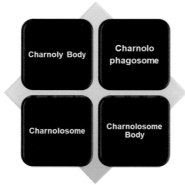

Fig. 26: Biomarkers of intracellular mitochondrial bioenergetics.

Therapeutic Outcome of Antioxidants During Different Stages of Free Radical Attack. The MB determines the ICD of a cell. A cell with a CMB is incapable of sustaining ICD and vice versa. Endogenous antioxidants such as: glutathione, SOD, catalase, MTs, HPP-70, BCl-2, and P53 can inhibit or attenuate PFA. SFA can be recovered or attenuated by exogenous antioxidants such as: resveratrol, rutins, sirtuins, vitamin-E, D, A, probucol, PUFA, and omega-3 fatty acids to prevent or inhibit CB formation, enhance charnolophagy, and augment CPS and CS exocytosis as a basic molecular mechanism of ICD. During TFA, the chances of mitochondrial membrane recovery are minimized and/or eliminated which is accompanied by CS destabilization, CS body formation, CS membrane permeabilization, and blebbing. The CS bodies fuse with the plasma membrane to form apoptotic-bodies, which release highly toxic mitochondrial metabolites to cause non-DNA-dependent cellular demise as illustrated in Fig. 27.

QFA can induce spontaneous cellular demise due to accelerated induction of CB formation, inhibition of charnolophagy, destabilization of CPS and CS, and prevention

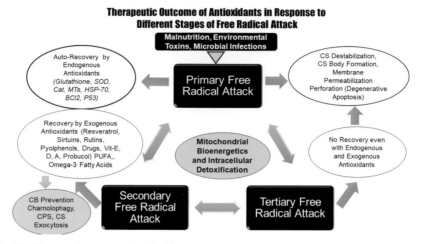

Therapeutic Outcome of Antioxidants in Response to Different Stages of Free Radical Attack

Fig. 27: Therapeutic outcome of antioxidants in response to different stages of free radical attack.

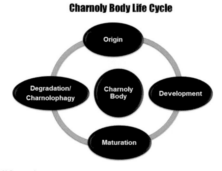

Charnoly Body Life Cycle

Fig. 28: Charnoly body life cycle.

of CS exocytosis as a basic molecular mechanism of ICD. QFA can induce SIDS, still birth, or abortion as noticed in the developing fetus of smoking, bing drinking, and/or ZIKV infected pregnant women.

CB Life Cycle. The CB life cycle can be divided in four major phases including (i) origin, (ii) development, (iii) maturation, and (iv) degradation or charnolophagy. CB is formed as a result of free radicals-induced down-regulation of MB. A pictorial diagram illustrating different phases of CB life cycle are presented in Fig. 28. CB appears as a multi-lamellar, electron-dense, stacks of degenerated mitochondrial membranes in the most vulnerable cell due to DPCI and is eliminated by energy (ATP) driven lysosome-dependent charnolophagy as a basic molecular mechanism of ICD.

Free Radicals-induced CB Molecular Pathogenesis. There is a limit beyond which lysosomes can not eradicate CB from the intracellular compartment. It depends primarily on the frequency of CB formation in the most vulnerable cell in response to DPCI and pre-existing MB. Hence, the frequency and size of CB depends on the vulnerability of a cell, number of mitochondria, severity of malnutrition, toxic exposure, and intensity of microbial infection. When a small-sized CB is subjected to charnolophagy, it is eliminated by lysosomal enzymes. However, a large CB is partially eliminated due to a limited number of lysosomes in a cell. The partial elimination of CB occurs when its size is abnormally enlarged, or the frequency of its formation significantly increases the capacity of a cell to eliminate it through charnolophagy. Hence, in chronic diseases, CB is either partially eliminated or becomes resistant to lysosomal hydrolysis, resulting in the formation of intracellular aggregates of denatured proteins due to the toxic release of mitochondrial metabolites. The CS destabilization due to a free radical attack induces the formation of CS bodies. The CS bodies are pinched off to fuse with the plasma membrane. The fusion of CS bodies with the plasma membrane causes phosphatidylserine externalization and ballooning to form apoptotic bodies, which release highly toxic substances to cause membrane perforations and cellular demise. The release of highly toxic mitochondrial metabolites from destabilized CS in the most vulnerable cell also triggers denaturation of proteins to cause accumulation of intracytoplasmic inclusions such as Lewy body, amyloid body, Hirano body, Merinesco body, Pick body, and Lofora body. Thus, ICD through CB formation, charnolophagy induction, and CS exocytosis depends on the intensity and severity of a free radical attack and genetic susceptibility of a cell. The release of highly toxic metabolites from the degenerating CS during TFA causes membrane perforations as presented in Fig. 29.

Ethanol-induced Oxidative Stress Causes Craniofacial Abnormalities in FASD by CB Formation, Charnolophagy, and CS Destabilization. In general, ethanol enhances ROS production and depletes antioxidants from cells. A concomitant depletion in the intracellular antioxidants and increase in ROS are involved in the oxidative stress to trigger CB formation. Antioxidants such as glutathione and MTs serve as potent free radical scavengers to maintain the antioxidant defense to escape from the deleterious effects of FASD. However, depletion of antioxidant defense in FASD triggers CB formation, charnolophagy, and CS destabilization. The release of apoptogenic substances from the destabilized CS is primarily involved in the degeneration of the NPCs, derived from the iPPCs to cause microcephaly and other craniofacial abnormalities. A systematic diagram illustrating the influence of intrauterine ethanol exposure on the developing embryo is presented in Fig. 30.

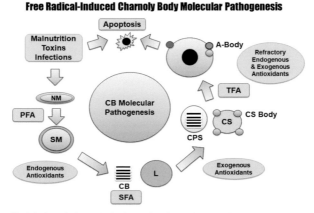

Fig. 29: Free radical-induced charnoly body molecular pathogenesis.

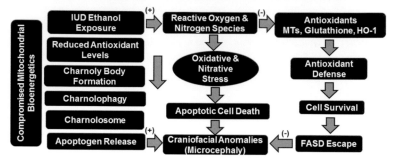

Ethanol-Induced Oxidative and Nitrative Stress Causes Craniofacial Abnormalities Through CB Formation, Charnolophagy, and Charnolosome Destabilization

Fig. 30: Ethanol-induced oxidative and nitrative stress causes craniofacial abnormalities through CB formation, charnolophagy, and charnolosome destabilization.

Charnoly Body Induction and Microcephaly

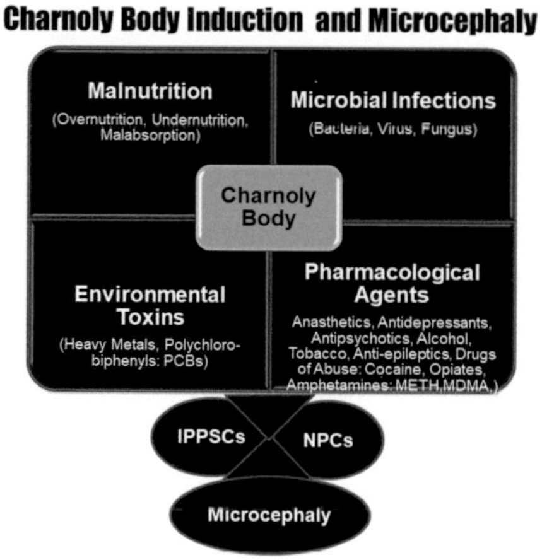

Fig. 31: Charnoly body induction and microcephaly.

CB Induction and Microcephaly. Generally, DPCI including malnutrition (overnutrition, undernutrition, and malabsorption), environmental toxins (heavy metal ions, and polychloro biphenyl: PCB), microbial (bacterial, virus, and fungal) infections, and pharmacological agents (anesthetics, antidepressants, antipsychotics, ethanol, nicotine, antiepileptic drugs, cocaine, opiates, amphetamine, METH, and MDMA) induce CB formation in the most vulnerable NPCs derived from iPPCs to cause early morbidity and mortalities due to apoptosis, which may induce microcephaly. A pictorial diagram illustrating DPCI-induced CB induction and microcephaly is presented in Fig. 31.

Therapeutic Potential of MTs as a CB Antagonist. During the acute phase, MTs prevent CB formation by serving as potent free radical scavengers and antioxidants. During the chronic phase, MTs enhance charnolophagy and stabilize CS to provide neuroprotection and facilitate ICD. MTs translocate in the nucleus to initiate Zn^{2+}-induced transcriptional activation of genes involved in AgNOR activation implicated in ribosomal synthesis for the generation of new proteins (mitofusin) at the RER. MTs, as potent antioxidant, anti-apoptotic, and anti-inflammatory factors sustain ICD, in addition to regulating Zn^{2+}-induced cell growth, proliferation, migration, differentiation, and development through post-transcriptional activation of microRNAs. A pictorial diagram illustrating the therapeutic potential of MTs as CB antagonists is presented in Fig. 32.

Non-Specific Induction of CB in MDR Malignancies. Non-specific induction of CB in normal tissues can induce CB formation to cause adverse effects such as alopecia, GIT distress, myelosuppression, nephrotoxicity, cardiotoxicity, pulmonary fibrosis, and neurotoxicity depending on the genetic susceptibility and tissue-specific induction of CB formation during the treatment of MDR malignancies. Hence, drugs may be developed to prevent or inhibit particularly the cancer stem cell-specific CB formation, instead of apoptosis of normal proliferating cells involved in undesirable adverse effects. A pictorial diagram illustrating how non-specific induction of CB can cause undesirable adverse effects in MDR malignancy is presented in Fig. 33.

Quantitative Assessment of ICD. ICD can be quantitatively assessed by estimating the functional relationship between (a) CB and α-synuclein index (SI), (b) CS and SI,

Therapeutic Potential of Metallothioneins as Charnoloy Body Antagonists

Metallothioneins	
Antioxidants	Free Radical Scavenger

Charnoly Body Prevention	
Charnolophagy Induction	Charnolosome Stability

Zinc-Induced AgNOR Activation	
Anti-inflammation/ICD	Growth, Proliferation, Anti-apoptosis, Immortalization

Fig. 32: Therapeutic potential of metallothioneins as charnoly body antagonists.

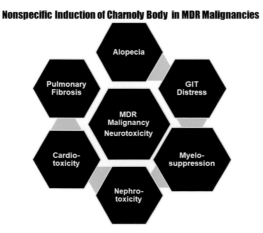

Nonspecific Induction of Charnoly Body in MDR Malignancies

Alopecia

Pulmonary Fibrosis

GIT Distress

MDR Malignancy Neurotoxicity

Cardio-toxicity

Myelo-suppression

Nephro-toxicity

Fig. 33: Nonspecific induction of charnoly body in MDR malignancies.

(c) charnolophagy and SI, and (d) CS and SI. From these analyses, we can determine the line of best fit to calculate the correlation coefficients (r-values). A positive r-value establishes a functional relationship between CB formation and SI. The SI is a ratio of the nitrative α-synuclein vs native α-synuclein and determines the oxidative and nitrative stress in a cell during DPCI. A pictorial diagram illustrating the quantitative assessment of ICD is presented in Fig. 34.

Free Radical-induced CB Molecular Pathogenesis. It is now well-established that DPCI induce PFA due to increased mitochondrial oxidative and nitrative stress. Free radicals are reactive oxygen species ($\cdot$OH, NO$\cdot$, CO$\cdot$) and induce lipid peroxidation to cause the structural and functional breakdown of PUFA. Mitochondrial membranes are highly susceptible to a free radical attack because these are highly rich in PUFA. The PFA is associated with down-regulation of $\Delta\Psi$, mega-pore formation due to TRPC delocalization and enhanced intra-mitochondrial Ca^{2+} accumulation, which induces mitochondrial hypertonicity. Consequently, a lot of water accumulates in the mitochondria to cause hypotonicity. Hence, the mitochondria become swollen during PFA. In general, PFA is reversible and can be overcome by endogenous antioxidants such as glutathione, MTs, SOD, and catalase. The mitochondria can resume their normal function as PFA can be reversed by these antioxidants. During SFA, the swollen mitochondria are disintegrated into small fragments. The fragmented mitochondrial membranes are disseminated all over the intracellular compartment. The fragmented mitochondrial membranes form pleomorphic, electron-dense, multi-lamellar stacks (also named as CB as an initial attempt of ICD). The Cyt-C in the inner mitochondrial membrane is non-covalently attached and can be easily delocalized and scatter in the entire intracytoplasmic compartment. To contain the Cyt-C and other toxic ingredients of degenerating mitochondria, CB formation occurs as an intracellular inclusion. As CB is nonfunctional, it is phagocytosed by lysosomes. Usually, CB is phagocytosed by ATP-driven lysosomal activation (also named as charnolophagy) during the secondary phase of ICD. Exogenously-administered antioxidants derived from fresh fruits and vegetables and antioxidant drugs can prevent or inhibit CB formation, augment charnolophagy and stabilize CS to prevent disease progression.

Quantitative Assessment of Intracellular Detoxification

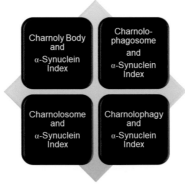

Fig. 34: Quantitative assessment of ICD.

During TFA, a CPS is transformed to CS, when the phagocytosed CB is hydrolyzed by the lysosomal enzymes. During TFA, further lipid peroxidation of the CS membranes occurs to form CS bodies. The CS bodies are pinched off from the CS and fuse with the plasma membrane to form apoptotic bodies (A-bodies) due to the release of highly toxic mitochondrial metabolites. The TFA is refractory to endogenous as well as exogenous antioxidants. Particularly during the chronic phase, CB becomes lysosome-resistant, charnolophagy is delayed and/or inhibited, and eventually the cell undergoes non-DNA-dependent apoptotic degeneration. Hence, drugs may be developed to prevent and/or inhibit CB formation and augment charnolophagy during the acute phase; and stabilize or augment CPS or CS exocytosis during the chronic phase as a basic molecular mechanism of ICD to remain healthy even during aging. A pictorial diagram illustrating the free radical-induced CS molecular pathophysiology is presented in Fig. 35.

Free Radical-induced Induction of Charnolopathies in Chronic Diseases.
Charnolopathies can occur in chronic diseases in response to DPCI. The requirement of energy (ATP) is significantly increased during these stressful situations. ATP synthesis occurs during oxidative phosphorylation in the mitochondrial electron transport chain. Free radicals are generated as a byproduct of oxidative phosphorylation. Free radicals are highly reactive oxygen species (ROS) such as ·OH and NO·. The degenerated mitochondrial membranes condense to form pleomorphic electron-dense multi-lamellar (penta or hepta) stacks as intracellular inclusions. These nonfunctional, yet toxic inclusions are identified as CB. CB is phagocytosed by lysosomes. This energy (ATP)-dependent process of CB autophagy is called as charnolophagy. A lysosome becomes significantly enlarged following charnolophagy and is recognized as an electron-dense CPS. The CPS is then transformed to CS when the phagocytosed CB is hydrolyzed by the lysosomal enzymes. The stability of CS depends on the microenvironment and inducers during DPCI. Usually, a free radical attack can be divided into three major phases: (i) PFA, (ii) SFA, and (iii) TFA. CB formed during a PFA is easily subjected to charnolophagy and efficiently exocytosed as a basic molecular mechanism of ICD. The CB formed due to a SFA is usually eliminated by endogenous

Free Radical-Induced Charnolosome Pathophysiology

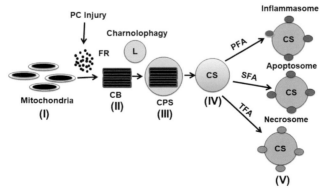

Fig. 35: Free radical-induced charnolosome pathophysiology.

antioxidants as well as by pharmacologically-synthesized antioxidant drugs. Hence, both endogenous as well as exogenous antioxidants scavenge free radicals to augment charnolophagy as well as CS stabilization and its exocytosis to maintain ICD. The TFA is most devastating, as it induces either lysosomal-resistant CB formation, and/or CS destabilization to cause membrane blebs (named as CS bodies). The incidence of CS bodies is increased due to the induction of pro-inflammatory cytokines. The CS bodies fuse with the plasma membranes and release highly toxic mitochondrial metabolites and destabilize plasma membranes to cause the formation of apoptotic bodies. The apoptotic bodies release intracellular contents and eventually induce cellular demise. The most significant toxic metabolites include: iron, Cyt-C, 8-OH, 2dG, 2,3-dihydroxy-nonenal, monoamine oxidases, ammonia, acetaldehyde, H_2O_2, caspase-3, and AIF. These toxic CS biomarkers induce proinflammatory apoptosis and eventually cellular demise to cause chronic diseases, as illustrated in Fig. 36.

MTs-induced CS Stabilization. MTs induce CS stabilization particularly during SFA and TFA of DPCI. MTs provide cytoprotection by stabilizing the CS. In a normal or MT_{trans} cell, a CS remains protected from the deleterious attack of free radicals by antioxidant MTs around it. A CS remains in a hostile microenvironment of free radicals, generated as a byproduct of oxidative phosphorylation during ATP synthesis in the electron transport chain. By donating –SH functional groups of cysteine residues, MTs scavenge free radicals to prevent CS destabilization. As CS is a structurally-unstable and functionally-labile organelle, it is exocytosed from a normal or MT_{trans} cell as a basic molecular mechanism of ICD. MTs knock out cell is devoid of MTs which serve as a defensive mechanism of CS stabilization. Usually CS remains in a hostile microenvironment of free radicals, which induce lipid peroxidation of PUFA to cause CS blebbings (also named as CS bodies). The CS bodies are ruptured to release highly toxic mitochondrial metabolites. CS sequestration releases toxic substances leading to non-nuclear DNA-dependent apoptosis. MTs-induced CS stabilization is illustrated in Fig. 37.

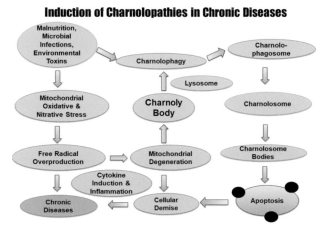

Fig. 36: Induction of charnolopathies in chronic diseases.

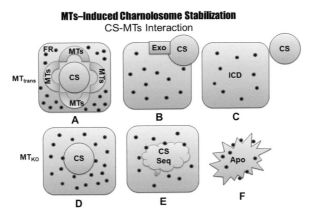

Fig. 37: MTs-induced charnolosome stabilization (CS-MTs interaction).

Conclusion

It is well-established that DPCI induce CMB due to free radical overproduction as a byproduct of oxidative phosphorylation during ATP synthesis in the electron transport chain. Depending on the severity and frequency of exposure to DPCI, free radical-induced lipid peroxidation may induce reversible or irreversible damage to mitochondrial membranes and mtDNA. The mitochondrial membranes are rich in PUFA, which render them highly susceptible to lipid peroxidation due to free radicals. Free radicals are highly reactive oxygen and nitrogen species (RONS) and induce down-regulation of the MB, implicated in ICD to remain healthy. The degenerated mitochondrial membranes condense to form CBs as an initial attempt to contain highly toxic iron, Cyt-C, ammonia, acetaldehyde, H_2O_2, lactate, membrane oxidation product, 2,3 dihydroxy nonenal, and mtDNA oxidation product, 8OH, 2dG. These toxic substances induce CS destabilization, CS permeabilization, and ultimately apoptotic degeneration. Moreover, epigenetic modification can occur more readily in the mtDNA as compared to nDNA because it is intron-less and G-C rich. Methylation occurs at the N-4 position of the cytosine residue in the mtDNA. The mtDNA is naked, and devoid of histone and protamines, which facilitates epigenetic modifications. However, the nDNA is supercoiled and possesses histones and protamines, which provide protection and control on the epigenetic modifications. The histone acetylation occurs first at the lysine residues to cause uncoiling and exposure of the cytosine residues in the nDNA. Hence, epigenetic changes are strictly regulated in the nDNA as compared to the mtDNA which remains constantly in a hostile microenvironment of free radicals, being generated as a byproduct of oxidative phosphorylation in the electron transport chain during ATP synthesis. Hence, drugs may be developed to inhibit CB formation and augment charnolophagy during the acute phase and stabilize CPS and CS to enhance their exocytosis during the chronic phase as a basic molecular mechanism of ICD for normal cellular function and homeostasis to remain healthy. Indeed! Mitochondrial bioenergetics plays a pivotal role in health and disease, particularly during aging, when their synthesis and repair is compromised due to the down-regulation of the mitochondrial genome, AgNOR, mitofusin, and depletion of endogenous antioxidants such as MTs, glutathione, SOD, and catalase. Hence, an adequate intake of antioxidants from natural as well as synthetic sources can prevent chronic diseases and promote health and well-being during aging.

References

Ebadi, M. and S.K. Sharma. 2003. Peroxynitrite and mitochondrial dysfunction in the pathogenesis of Parkinson's disease. Antioxid Redox Signal 5: 319–335.

Ebadi, M., S.K. Sharma, S. Wanpen and A. Amornpan. 2004. Coenzyme Q_{10} inhibits mitochondrial complex-1 down-regulation and nuclear factor-kappa B activation. J Cellular & Molecular Medicine 8: 231–222.

Kooncumchoo, P., S. Sharma, J. Porter, P. Govitrapong and M. Ebadi. 2006. Coenzyme Q_{10} provides neuroprotection in iron-induced apoptosis in dopaminergic neurons. Journal of Molecular Neuroscience 28: 125–141.

Sharma, S.K. and M. Ebadi. 2003. Metallothionein attenuates 3-morpholinosydnonimine (SIN-1)-induced oxidative stress in dopaminergic neurons. Antioxid Redox Signal 5: 251–264.

Sharma, S., J. Choga, V. Gupta, P. Doghor, A. Chauhan, F. Kalala, A. Foor, C. Wright, J. Renteria, K.E. Theberge and S. Mathur. 2016. Charnoly body as a novel biomarker of nutritional stress in Alzheimer's disease. Functional Foods in Health and Disease 6: 344–377.

Sharma, S. 2017a. *ZIKV* Disease, Prevention and Cure. Nova Science Publishers, New York, U.S.A.

Sharma, S. 2017b. Fetal Alcohol Spectrum Disorder. Concepts, Mechanisms, and Cure. Nova Science Publishers, New York, U.S.A.

Sharma, S. 2017c. Charnolosome-antioxidants interaction in health and disease. Conference: 22nd International Conference on Functional Foods, At Harvard Medical School, Boston, Mass, U.S.A. (Invited lecture). Sep 22, 2017.

CHAPTER-5

Antioxidants Prevent Charnoly Body Formation, Augment Charnolophagy, and Stabilize Charnolosome to Enhance Mitochondrial Bioenergetics and Intracellular Detoxification

INTRODUCTION

This chapter describes the molecular pathogenesis of CB in response to DPCI including severe malnutrition, environmental neurotoxic insult, and microbial (bacteria, virus, and fungal) infection in the most vulnerable cell such as NPCs and CPCs, derived from iPPCs. The chapter focuses primarily on the basic molecular mechanism of CB formation, intracellular pathophysiology of CB during the acute phase, intermediate phase, and chronic phase to elucidate the basic molecular mechanism of progressive neurodegeneration in chronic MDR diseases such as PD, AD, ALS, schizophrenia, MDDs, multiple drug abuse, CVDs, and MDR malignancies.

It is well-established that the mitochondrial oxidative and nitrative stress is significantly augmented during DPCI. The requirement of energy (ATP) is significantly elevated in response to DPCI. Free radicals induce lipid peroxidation associated with the structural and functional breakdown of PUFA. These changes at the molecular level cause degeneration of the mitochondrial membranes to synthesize electron-dense, multilamellar stacks (also named as CBs) as an initial and early attempt to contain highly toxic mitochondrial metabolites to maintain ICD for normal cellular function.

CB as a universal pre-apoptotic biomarker of CMB was initially discovered in the developing UN rat Purkinje neurons. It appears as a pleomorphic, electron-dense, multi-lamellar, quasi-crystalline stack of degenerated mitochondrial membranes and the down-regulation of the mitochondrial genome and its bioenergetics due to free radical overproduction in the most vulnerable cells (Sharma et al. 1985; Sharma et al. 1986; Sharma et al. 1987; Sharma 1988). CB originates by the aggregation of degenerated mitochondrial membranes, due to free radical-induced CMB. Free radicals induce lipid peroxidation by the structural and functional breakdown of PUFA. In general, free radicals induce proteases to cause proteolysis, lipases to cause lipolysis, nucleases to cause DNA fragmentation and apoptosis in the most vulnerable cells to induce charnolopathies involved in diversified embryopathies.

We divided the CB life cycle into 4 major phases: (i) origin, (ii) development, (iii) maturation, and (iv) degradation (Sharma et al. 1993) and defined CB autophagy as charnolophagy, and lysosome containing phagocytosed-CB as CPS. The CPS is transformed to CS, when the phagocytosed-CB within the CPS is hydrolyzed by the lysosomal enzymes (Sharma 2017). These neurodegenerative changes are triggered due to CMB, and can be ameliorated initially by endogenously-synthesized antioxidants such as glutathione, MTs, SOD, and catalase, and subsequently by exogenously-synthesized antioxidants including; vitamin A, D, E, CoQ_{10}, melatonin, selegiline, resveratrol, sirtuin, rutin, lycopene, and catechin to prevent CB molecular pathogenesis involved in early embryopathies and neuropathies. The antioxidants serve as free radical scavengers and augment mitochondrial synthesis as well as enhance their regeneration and bioenergetics in different body organs, particularly in the CNS and cardiovascular tissue.

This chapter describes the molecular pathogenesis of CB in response to DPCI in the most vulnerable cell such as NPCs and CPCs, derived from iPPCs. The chapter also describes the basic molecular mechanism of CB formation, the intracellular pathophysiology of CB during the acute, intermediate, and chronic phases to elucidate the basic molecular mechanism of neurodegeneration in PD, AD, ALS, schizophrenia, MDDs, multiple drug abuse, and CVDs and vice versa for the molecular pathogenesis of MDR malignancies.

We have shown that CoQ_{10}, melatonin, and MTs prevent thiol oxidation of the brain regional mitochondrial complex-1, α-synuclein, and parkin to provide neuroprotection in PD (Ebadi et al. 2001). By employing potent complex-1 inhibitors, MPP^+, rotenone, and salsolinol as experimental models of PD, we established that CoQ_{10} provides neuroprotection by inhibiting mitochondrial oxidative and nitrative stress (Ebadi et al. 2001); and a specific MAO-B inhibitor, selegiline, provides neuroprotection by MTs induction in the cultured human DA-ergic (SK-N-SH) neurons (Ebadi et al. 2002). Furthermore, we established a functional relationship between α-synuclein and MTs in PD (Ebadi and Sharma 2002) and discovered that MTs provide CoQ_{10}-mediated neuroprotection by preventing free-radical overproduction, whereas, selegiline attenuates MPP^+-induced mitochondrial degeneration and CB formation by MTs induction and inhibit apoptotic signal transduction by suppressing c-fos and c-jun proto-oncogenes in cultured SK-N-SH neurons (Sharma et al. 2003).

We determined that MTs attenuate $ONOO^-$ induced oxidative and nitrative stress in PD (Sharma and Ebadi 2003; Ebadi and Sharma 2003; Ebadi et al. 2004; Sharma et al. 2004), and wv/wv mice exhibit typical symptoms of progressive neurodegeneration and Parkinsonism due to the down-regulation of the mitochondrial complex-1 and reduction in CoQ_{10} (Ebadi et al. 2004) and established that CoQ_{10} stabilizes MTs (Ebadi et al. 2004), whereas MTs attenuate ONOO⁻-induced oxidative stress in PD (Ebadi et al. 2005; Ebadi et al. 2006). This was further confirmed in various α-synuclein and MTs gene-manipulated mouse models of PD and aging (Ebadi et al. 2005; Sharma and Ebadi 2014). CoQ_{10} inhibited mitochondrial complex-1 down-regulation and NFκβ activation in cultured SK-N-SH neurons as well as in wv/wv mice (Ebadi et al. 2004). A potent mitochondrial complex-1 inhibitor, MPP^+, inhibited TRPC-1, a calcium channel protein on the mitochondrial membranes to cause apoptosis in cultured SH-S-Y5Y neurons (Bollimuntha et al. 2005); whereas cocaine and METH-induced neurotoxicity in the SK-N-SH neurons as well as in C57BL/6J mice was attenuated by CoQ_{10}, further confirming the therapeutic potential of CoQ_{10} through mitochondrial neuroprotection (Klongpanichapak et al. 2006).

It is well-established that iron participates in the Fenton reaction to synthesize ONOO⁻ ions in the presence of ·OH and NO· radicals, generated as a byproduct of mitochondrial oxidative phosphorylation during ATP synthesis in the electron transport chain. ONOO⁻ ions not only induce oxidative but also nitrative stress in the mitochondria to trigger CB formation. In addition, iron causes the mitochondrial translocation of α-synuclein to induce oxidative and nitrative stress due to free radical overproduction (Sangchot et al. 2002). Iron-induced oxidative stress, mitochondrial aggregation, and α-synuclein translocation in SK-N-SH cells to cause progressive neurodegeneration (Sangchot et al. 2002); whereas a potent iron chelator, deforoxamine, attenuated iron-induced oxidative stress by inhibiting α-synuclein translocation in the cultured SK-N-SH cells (Sangchot et al. 2002). Pretreatment with CoQ_{10} prevented iron-induced apoptosis in cultured SK-N-SH neurons (Kooncumchoo et al. 2006). We established that the mitochondrial complex-1 activity and ¹⁸F-DOPA uptake are significantly reduced in the genetically engineered mouse model of PD; whereas CoQ_{10} provides neuroprotection in the cellular and animal models of PD (Sharma et al. 2006). Furthermore, CoQ_{10} augments brain regional ¹⁸F-DOPA and ¹⁸FdG uptake in wv/wv-MTs mice (Sharma and Ebadi 2008a) and MTs provide therapeutic potential in PD (Sharma and Ebadi 2008b). Hence, MTs can be used as early and sensitive biomarkers of redox signaling in various NDDs (Sharma and Ebadi 2011a), including nicotinism, ethanol addiction, and ZIKV charnolopathies; involved in diversified embryopathies in developing infants and Guillain Barre' Syndrome, menigoncephalitis, and sterility in adults (Sharma 2016a–e; Sharma et al. 2016a,b). In a similar study, we established that a circadian regulating hormone, melatonin, also provides neuroprotection in cultured SH-SY5Y neurons from exogenously-administered TIQs such as salsolinol and 1-benzyl TIQ (Shavali et al. 2004).

We discovered for the first time, IL-10 receptors on the rat cortical and hippocampal cultured neurons and established that IL-10 directly protects cortical neurons by activating PI-3 kinase and STAT-3-mediated signal transduction cascade (Sharma et al. 2011). Just like MTs, IL-10 provides anti-apoptotic and anti-inflammatory neuroprotection through the Zn^{2+}-mediated transcriptional regulation of genes involved in growth, proliferation, differentiation, and development. It is known that IL-10 attenuates pro-inflammatory responses following ischemic stroke primarily by acting on the microglial and endothelial cells, however there is limited information regarding the direct effects of IL-10 on the cortical neurons primarily destroyed in AIS. By employing RT-PCR and immunohistochemical methods, we confirmed that IL-10 receptors are localized on the cortical neurons. Treatment of primary cortical neurons in culture with IL-10 augmented neuronal survival following exposure to oxygen-glucose deprivation (OGD) or glutamate toxicity. IL-10 also induced phosphorylation of AKT in cortical neurons. IL-10 mediated neuroprotection against OGD and glutamate was significantly attenuated by pretreatment with the specific PI-3K inhibitor, wortmannin. In addition, STAT-3 phosphorylation was significantly induced by IL-10. Pre-treatment with IL-10 receptor antibody inhibited both STAT-3 and AKT phosphorylation as well as IL-10 mediated protection of cortical neurons, suggesting that IL-10 provides direct neuroprotection by acting through IL-10 receptor, PI3K/AKT, and STAT-3 signal transduction pathways involved in the inhibition of CB molecular pathogenesis.

The potential MB-based drugs described in this chapter include: CB antagonists, charnolophagy agonists, CPS stabilizers, CS stabilizers, and CB sequestration inhibitors to prevent and/or cure diversified charnolopathies, involved in NDDs, CVDs, and MDR malignancies. In general, mitochondrially-targeted drugs can be classified as (a) CB agonists/antagonists, (b) charnolophagy agonists/antagonists, CPS/CS stablilizers/destabilizers, and (c) CB sequestrants/desequestrants, in addition to charnolostatics, charnolocidals, and charnolomimetics.

Molecular Mechanism of CB Formation. A possible molecular mechanism of CB formation and its prevention by nutritional rehabilitation, physiological Zn^{2+}, and MTs is proposed. Pharmacological agents and nutritional rehabilitation act synergistically to prevent CB formation involved in progressive degeneration. Hence, drugs may be targeted to inhibit CB formation in NDDs and CVDs and augment cancer stem cell–specific CB formation to eliminate or minimize undesirable adverse effects of chronic diseases, including MDR malignancies.

CB Molecular Pathogenesis. There is limit beyond which lysosomes are unable to eradicate CB from the intracellular compartment. It depends on the frequency of CB formation in the most vulnerable cell in response to DPCI. CB formation also depends on the intensity and frequency of free radicals generated during DPCI as discussed earlier. The frequency and size of CB depends on the severity of DPCI. When a small-sized CB is subjected to charnolophagy, it is rapidly eliminated by the lysosomal enzymes. However, a large CB is partially eliminated due to the limited number of lysosomes in a cell. A partial elimination of CB occurs when the size of CB is abnormally increased or the frequency of its formation exceeds the normal capacity of a cell to eliminate them through energy (ATP)-driven charnolophagy. Therefore, in chronic conditions, CB is either partially eliminated or becomes resistant to lysosomal hydrolysis. These changes at the molecular level result in the formation of intracellular aggregates of degenerated proteins. The CS destabilization due to a SFA induces the formation of CS bodies. CS bodies are pinched off to fuse with the plasma membrane. The fusion of CS bodies with the plasma membrane causes PS externalization and ballooning to form apoptotic bodies, which release highly toxic substances to cause membrane perforations and release intracellular constituents, resulting in cellular demise. Hence, ICD through CB formation, charnolophagy, and CS exocytosis depends on the intensity and frequency of the free radical attack and genetic as well as epigenetic susceptibility of a cell.

Experimental Studies

To establish the novel concept of charnolopharmacotherapeutics for the prevention and cure of progressive NDDs, CVDs, MDR malignancies, and infections (including ZIKV, cytomegalovirus, and rubella virus) diseases, we performed several *in vivo*, *ex vivo, and in vitro* experiments on gene-manipulated animals and cultured SK-N-SH and SH-S-Y5Y neurons, in addition to NG-108/15 cells lines. These experiments were accomplished by conducting *in vitro* and *in vivo* studies on developing normal and protein malnourished, pyridoxine (B_6) deficient, and vitamin-D deficient developing rats, MTs and α-synuclein gene-manipulated mice, aging cultured RhO_{mgko} SK-N-SH and SH-S-Y5Y neurons, neuronal stem cells, and bone marrow-derived mononuclear cells. TEM, SEM, confocal microscopy, and digital fluorescence imaging microscopy were utilized to discover different phases of CB life cycle, charnolophagy, CPS, CS and CB sequestration in the developing UN rat cerebellar Purkinje neuron. Initially, $\Delta\Psi$ in response to toxic exposure of MPP^+, salsolinol, and rotenone was determined by digital fluorescence microscopic and confocal microscopic analyses, using JC-1 as a sensitive fluorochrome in SK-N-SH and SH-S-Y5Y neurons. Subsequently, several nuclear and mitochondrial genes, involved in growth, proliferation, differentiation, development, and apoptosis, were analyzed at the translational and transcriptional levels by immunoblotting, RT-PCR, and cDNA microarray analyses. Nuclear magnetic resonance spectroscopy (MRS) and MRI were performed to correlate and confirm the molecular imaging data derived from microPET neuroimaging. The PET RPs, ^{18}FdG and ^{18}F-DOPA were synthesized in the cyclotron and microPET imaging labs as molecular imaging biomarkers of brain regional MB and DA-ergic neurotransmission, respectively. Siemens Molecular Solutions, microPET Imaging System equipped with *micoPET Manager* for the data acquisition in List mode, and *AsiPro* for the image reconstruction in multidimensional mode was employed for acquiring *in vivo* molecular imaging data of brain regional MB and DA-ergic neurotransmission in normal control and toxins-exposed gene-manipulated mice, respectively. The detailed methodology is described in several of our earlier and recent publications and in my books by Nova Science Publishers, New York, U.S.A.

Mosquito-Borne Diseases and Cancer

It is now being realized that mosquito-borne diseases have increased the global incidence of cancer. Hence, it will be highly prudent to prevent their outbreak, spread, and transmission by a targeted, safe, and effective vector eradication program to reduce not only early morbidity and mortality but also MDR malignancies, in addition to progressive NDDs of known and unknown etiopathogenesis, as noticed in ZIKV disease. Non-specific induction of CB formation causes GIT symptoms, myelosuppression, alopecia, myocardial infarction, neurotoxicity, nephrotoxicity, hepatotoxicity, pulmonary toxicity, and infertility during the chronic treatment of MDR malignancies. Hence, drugs may be developed to induce cancer stem cell-specific CB formation, inhibit charnolophagy, and augment CPS and CS destabilization and CB sequestration in highly proliferative cancer stem cells to successfully eradicate MDR malignancies and infections such as mosquito (Aedes aegypti)–borne ZIKV disease with minimum or no adverse effects and vice versa for the personalized theranostics of NDDs and CVDs.

Clinical Significance of CB Theranostics

We reported that the accumulation of CB at the junction of the axon hillock can cause impaired axoplasmic transport of various ions, enzymes, hormones, neurotransmitters, neurotropic factors (BDNF, NFG-1, IGF-1), and mitochondria at the synaptic terminals to cause impaired synaptic transmission, synaptic atrophy, and eventually progressive degeneration due to dendritic pruning and synaptic degeneration, resulting in cognitive impairments accompanied with early morbidity and mortality (Sharma and Ebadi 2014; Sharma 2017a; Sharma 2017b). In addition, basic knowledge acquired through modern omics biotechnology, next generation sequencing (NGS), molecular genetics, epigenetics, and molecular imaging, is remarkable, which will certainly help to control any other virulent viral, bacterial, and/or fungal outbreak in future. Although charnolostatic agents will have therapeutic potential during the acute phase of ZIKV disease, charnolocidals will be needed for immediate and complete remission from ZIKV disease, FASD, and nicotinism. We need to be fully-prepared much ahead of time so that innocent victims (particularly developing infants from socioeconomically-poor countries) may not suffer from the undesirable and deleterious consequences of nicotine, ethanol, ZIKV or other viral-linked charnolopathies involving; microcephaly, embryopathies, GBS, and reproductive anomalies. In addition to classical omics (vaccinomics), next generation sequencing (NGS), and emerging molecular biological approaches, will improvise charnolosomics and charnolopharmacotherapeutics of not only nicotine, ethanol, and ZIKV disease but also several other NDDs, CVDs, and MDR malignancies.

Clinical Significance of CB Formation in Nicotine, Ethanol, ZIKV, and Other Diseases

It is now proposed that intrauterine nicotine, ethanol, and ZIKV exposure can induce organ and disease-related MOA-A or MOA-B specific CB formation, accompanied with Cyt-C, iron, TRPC, Ca^{2+}, and TSPO (18 kDa: cholesterol channel) delocalization in the NPCs or in any other highly vulnerable cell; including NPCs, OSCs, CPCs, EPCs, spermatogonia, spermatocytes, Sertoli cells, and oocytes to cause diversified embryopathies and craniofacial abnormalities. These pathophysiological events can cause selective loss of brain regional NE-ergic, 5-HT-ergic, and DA-ergic neurotransmission due to synaptic degeneration, leading to cognitive impairments and deficits in learning, intelligence, memory, and behavior, resulting in early morbidity and mortality, as noticed in FASD, MDDs, chronic drug addiction, aging, and AD. A significant impairment in sensorimotor performance has been noticed in recent victims of ZIKV microcephaly in Brazil, Colombia, and several other countries including U.S.A. and Caribbean islands. Hence, various prophylactic and therapeutic biomarkers as well as drug discovery targets have been proposed based on the systematic pathophysiological consequences of ZIKV-induced CB formation. These include but are not limited to ZIKV-induced down-regulation of MB, CB formation, triggering charnolophagy through lysosomal activation as a basic molecular mechanism of ICD, CPS formation (a waste disposal container), CS destabilization (permeabilization, sequestration, and fragmentation), CB sequestration, and apoptosis. These deleterious events at the cellular and molecular level induce microcephaly and other diversified spectrum of embryopathies in young developing infants, and infertility and GBS in adults.

Clinical Significance of CB in Personalized Nanotheranostics

It is envisaged that emerging nanotechnology will provide better, safe, effective, and economical EBPT options for MDR cancer and other drug-resistant chronic diseases including AD, PD, drug addiction, and MDDs, where conventional medical treatment has limited prospectus. Hence, future development in innovative NPs, nanomaterials, and nanodevices for the targeted drug delivery, utilizing novel chronopharmacological and charnolosomic approaches may provide better theranostics and reduce the cost of time-consuming, cumbersome, potentially-painful, and futile therapeutic interventions with serious adverse effects. Personalized medicine can design time- and cost-effective protocols for each patient while taking into consideration the genetic predisposition and individual variability to accomplish best EBPT with minimum or no adverse effects. For instance, treatment with patient-specific stem cells is a promising effort in this direction. Recently, micellar NPs for the topical and transdermal drug delivery of pharmaceuticals and personal care products have been developed (Lee et al. 2010). Particularly, specific CB and/or chronolophagy agonists and antagonists can be developed for the effective treatment of NDDs, CVDs, and MDR malignancies. In addition to possible therapeutic strategies with siRNA; the miRNAs are involved in post-transcriptional control and are de-regulated in chronic diseases and aging (Wang 2009, 2011). Recently, lactosyl gramicidine-based lipid NPs (Lac-GLN) for targeted delivery of anti-mir-155 to hepatocellular carcinoma were developed (Zhang et al. 2013). Further studies to explore the exact pathophysiological significance of dysregulated miRNAs in CMB (inducing CB formation) in chronic illnesses will expand our nanotheranostic capabilities (Hamburg et al. 2010; Sharma 2017).

FAS and ZIKV Disease

It is well-established that alcohol consumption during any phase of pregnancy is deleterious. Alcohol induces deleterious effects during the first trimester (gastrulation phase) of pregnancy, which may be further complicated with intrauterine exposure to environmental toxins and/or microbial infections including ZIKV infection. Differential diagnosis of FAS is still a significant challenge. Hippocampal somatostatin and BDNF are reduced in FAS. Particularly, hippocampal NPCs are highly susceptible to ethanol and nicotine, in addition to ZIKV. Recently, we reported CB as a biomarker as well as novel drug discovery target for the safe and effective prevention and treatment of ZIKV, nicotine, and ethanol-induced embryopathies, including microcephaly. ZIKV induces selective apoptosis of highly vulnerable NPCs, derived from iPPs through CB formation (Sharma 2016a, 2016b). CB appears due to free radical overproduction and CMB in a highly vulnerable cell (NPCs) in response to DPCI, whereas "charnolophagy" is an energy (ATP)-driven basic molecular mechanism of ICD to remain healthy (Sharma and Ebadi 2014; Sharma 2015, 2016, 2017). Recently, I proposed that antiviral drugs preventing CB formation and/or augmenting "charnolophagy" will be highly beneficial for the prevention and/or effective treatment of ZIKV disease, FASD, and nicotinism during the early acute phase, whereas, CPS stabilizers, tissue-specific charnolophagy agonists, and CB sequestration inhibitors, CS stabilizers, and CS exocytosis enhancers will have promising therapeutic potential during the chronic phase (Sharma 2016, 2017).

Clinical Significance of Autophagy vs Charnolophagy

Christian de Duve, the Nobel Laureate from Belgium, discovered lysosomes and introduced the term "Autophagy". He was awarded the shared Nobel Prize for Physiology or Medicine in 1974, along with Albert Claude and George E. Palade, for describing the structure and function of organelles (lysosomes and peroxisomes) in biological cells. Recently, the Nobel Prize in Physiology or Medicine was awarded to Prof. Yoshinori Ohsumi from Japan for discovering basic molecular mechanisms of Autophagy. I discovered CB as a pre-apoptotic biomarker of CMB in the developing UN rat cerebellar Purkinje neurons and introduced the term "charnolophagy" which occurs by lysosomal activation due to free radical overproduction during nutritional stress, toxic insult (nicotine, ethanol), and/or infection including "ZIKV Disease". CB is a universal biomarker of cell injury, whereas "charnolophagy" is a novel drug discovery target to evaluate ICD. Nicotine, ethanol, and ZIKV compromise "charnolophagy" to cause microcephaly and several diversified embryopathies involving charnolopathy.

The term autophagy can be used for eukaryotic as well as prokaryotic cells having no mitochondria and/or nuclei. However, charnolophagy is more specific and restricted term which represents especially CB phagocytosis, and is formed due to CMB by free radical overproduction in a highly vulnerable cell in response to DPCI. Thus, charnolophagy can occur only in highly sensitive and specialized (particularly in eukaryotes) cells, possessing structurally-well-defined mitochondria as well as nuclei. Both mitochondria as well as nuclear genes are involved in oxidative phosphorylation, growth, proliferation, differentiation, development, and apoptosis during DPCI.

It is important to highlight that charnolophagy is one of the most significant molecular event which occurs during conception because of primarily nuclear DNA in the head and spirally-arranged condensed mitochondria in the middle piece of a spermatocyte. The tail does not enter in the oocyte during fertilization. Almost all the mitochondrial energy is consumed to translocate male nuclear DNA near the female nuclear DNA during fertilization. The degenerated mitochondrial membranes of the middle piece are condensed to form CB, which is eliminated through energy-driven lysosomal activation in the oocytes by charnolophagy as a basic molecular mechanism of ICD for the normal growth and development of the zygote. Hence, paternal charnolophagy in the oocyte immediately after fertilization is highly crucial event for the normal and spatio-temporally-regulated growth and development of the fetus. As charnolophagy is an energy (ATP)-driven lysosomal-dependent highly intricate spatio-temporal process of ICD, Mother Nature has provided as many as 200,000 to 600,000 mitochondria in an oocyte as compared to only 22–75 mitochondria in the middle piece of the spermatocyte, involved in only specialized task of motility and conception. However, any restriction and/or inhibition in this spatio-temporally-intricate process due to DPCI can induce abortion, still birth, craniofacial abnormalities including microcephaly. Inhibition of charnolophagy during fertilization can cause either zygotic death or diversified embryopathies. Hence, the term "charnolophagy" should not be used indiscriminately and misinterpreted with general autophagy. Charnolophagy represents particularly an energy-driven CB autophagy in a highly vulnerable cell as we discovered in the developing UN Purkinje neurons and in the cultured mice hippocampal CA-3 and dentate gyrus neurons of mice exposed to intrauterine DOM during pregnancy (Sharma et al. 1985; Sharma et al. 1986; Sharma et al. 1987; Sharma et al. 1993; Dakshinamurti et al. 1991; Sharma and Dakshinamurti 1992; Dakshinamurti et al. 1993; Sharma et al. 1994; Sharma et al. 2013a; Sharma et al. 2013b; Sharma et al. 2013c; Sharma and Ebadi 2014a, 2014b; Sharma 2015, 2016a, 2016b; Sharma et al. 2016).

Usually, mitochondrial abundance in a cell depends on its metabolic activity and physiological energy (ATP) requirement. For instance, cardiomyocytes and smooth muscle cells have the maximum number of mitochondria arranged systematically and compactly as compared to nephrons, hepatocytes, and neurons. Hence, the term charnolophagy will be more specific to organs rich in mitochondria and diseases associated with organs like heart, muscle, brain, liver, and kidneys. Nevertheless, natural abundance of mitochondria and genetic and epigenetic susceptibility of the mtDNA renders any metabolically active cell highly vulnerable to CB formation during oxidative and/or nitrative stress. As described earlier, almost every cell in our body has mitochondria, except erythrocytes, hair, and nails, where we cannot expect CB formation. Nevertheless, various CS biomarkers of mitochondrial metabolism can be estimated from nail and hair samples to evaluate the overall MB and CB molecular pathogenesis of a patient requiring the targeted, safe, and effective EBPT. The reduced life span (110 days) of erythrocytes is due to the lack of mitochondria in these highly specialized cells. Hence, mitochondria are vital organelles in a living cell.

During neurotropic ZIKV infection, ATP requirement is significantly elevated and free radical synthesis is augmented, which causes extensive mitochondrial degeneration with limited regenerative potential. Free radicals induce $\Delta\Psi$ collapse and lipid peroxidation of mitochondrial membranes to cause structural and functional breakdown of PUFA. Due to the natural abundance of free radicals in the mitochondria, particularly during oxidative and nitrative stress, inner mitochondrial membrane is destroyed first, as we discovered in severely UN developing rat cerebellar Purkinje neurons. Free radicals have very short half-life (10^{-13} to 10^{-14} seconds) and their overproduction can induce mitochondrial destruction, augmenting CB formation, whereas energy (ATP)-driven charnolophagy is an efficient basic molecular mechanism of ICD and is highly significant to enjoy normal health and well-being even during aging.

Phagolysosome vs Charnolophagosome

The term phagolysosome represents a significantly enlarged lysosome containing phagocytosed subcellular components including plasma membranes (ER, mitochondria, peroxisomes, Golgi body, nuclear membranes, and several other intracellular organelle), whereas CPS represents a lysosome that has specifically phagocytosed CBs. CPS is usually localized near CB, is abnormally enlarged, electron-dense, and highly unstable structure. The incidence of CPS is increased in DPCI in a eukaryotic cell (particularly in NPCs, derived from iPPCs) in the developing embryo in response to ZIKV infection and/or toxic insult. The frequency of CPS formation is increased as a function of CB formation during nutritional stress. Thus, CPS formation represents a specific event which occurs exclusively following CB formation to enhance charnolophagy as a basic molecular mechanism of ICD for normal cellular function (Sharma et al. 1986; Sharma et al. 1987; Sharma et al. 1993). The conversion of CPS to CS facilitates exocytosis as a basic molecular mechanism of ICD for normal growth and development. Hence, conversion of CPS to CS is highly intricate spatio-temporally, transcriptionally, and translationally-regulated process which requires efficient MB. Impaired conversion of CPS to CS poses a significant challenge in ICD and can induce charnolopathies, involving diversified embryopathies.

The frequency of CB formation, charnolophagy, CPS, and CS formation was significantly increased during nutritional stress and reduced by nutritional rehabilitation of 80 days in developing UN rat cerebellar Purkinje neurons. CB formation occurred particularly in the dendrites and growth cones (possessing maximum number of mitochondria) during severe nutritional stress. How many CBs can a lysosome phagocytose, is yet to be established. However, the size of CPS was ~ 2.5X increased as compared to lysosomes in the developing UN rat cerebellar Purkinje neurons. Moreover, electron density was significantly increased, which facilitated in its identification and quantitation. A positive correlation between CB, CPS, and CS formation with a correlation coefficient of 0.8 was noticed. To quantitatively estimate the MB; a kinetic equation was developed: $\Delta E = K\Delta T$, where: ΔE is the difference in the ^{14}C-labelled glucose utilization between normal well-fed and UN neurons; ΔT is the difference in the duration of firing between normal and UN neuron. ΔE and ΔT approached to zero in 30 days UN developing rats which were nutritionally-rehabilitated subsequently for 80 days.

Clinical Significance of CB, Charnolophagy, and CS Exocytosis

As described above, charnolophagy occurs as a consequence of free radical over production, which enhances lipid peroxidation to cause structural and functional breakdown of PUFA and omega-3 fatty acids in the mitochondrial membranes and highly susceptible mtDNA. The incidence of lipid peroxidation is maximum in the brain as compared to other peripheral tissues such as heart, liver, and kidney; because > 70% of the brain is composed of only lipids. Due to natural abundance of physico-chemically-labile lipids and mitochondria, we notice CB formation more frequently in the developing malnourished or aging brain compared to other tissues. For instance, stroke occurs more frequently in the aging brain, when the brain regional MB is compromised, and lipid peroxidation is induced due to free radical generation during cerebral ischemia. The brain is highly susceptible to ischemia and/or hypoglycemia. During cerebral ischemia (induced by hemorrhage or by AIS), millions of neurons are destroyed within seconds due to the down regulation of MB, mitochondrial degeneration, and CB formation. That is why stroke either kills or renders the patient crippled for the rest of his/her life. Hence, charnolophagy becomes a highly significant event in stroke, because it is one of the most crucial and efficient basic molecular mechanism of ICD during cerebral ischemia following stroke. Charnolophagy occurs more efficiently in the young adult brain as compared to the aging brain with CMB, which triggers CB formation (involved in apoptosis and progressive neuronal demise). That is why the prognosis of stroke is better in young patients as compared to old patients; because charnolophagy as well as CPS and CS stabilization occur very efficiently in young healthy neurons as compared to mitochondrial genome knock out (RhO_{mgko}) aging neurons. Aging RhO_{mgko} neurons are highly susceptible to CB formation, charnolophagy inhibition, CB sequestration, and CPS/CS destabilization, involved in NDDs; a leading cause of morbidity and mortality in aging and in ZIKV syndrome (Sharma 2016a,b). In addition, various neuro-inflammatory cytokines play a significant role in CB pathogenesis. The pro-inflammatory cytokines IL-1β, TNF-α, IL-6, inhibit charnolophagy, whereas the anti-inflammatory cytokines, IL-4, and IL-10 induce charnolophagy to restore ICD in AIS.

Various antioxidants including glutathione, SOD, catalase, and MTs provide neuroprotection by inhibiting CB formation, as free radical scavengers and efficient charnolophagy agonists. The presence of Ca^{2+} micro-crystallization in wide-spread brain regions of the ZIKV-infected developing brain with microcephaly, further confirmed extensive degeneration of mitochondria due to free radical-induced CB formation in ZIKV embryopathies. Therefore, novel drugs inhibiting organ-specific CB formation, augmenting charnolophagy, stabilizing CPS/CS, and preventing CS sequestration will be clinically significant against ZIKV disease and other related "charnolopathies" involved in a diversified spectrum of embryopathies.

MTs Confer Mitochondrial Neuroprotection as CB Antagonists

MTs are induced in nutritional stress and during clinical seizure discharge activity to prevent free radical mediated CB formation and provide mitochondrial neuroprotection. To further confirm the therapeutic potential of MTs as CB antagonists, we discovered that although MT_{dko} mice did not exhibit any overt clinical symptoms of Parkinsonism, these genotypes are mildly obese and lethargic as compared to MT_{trans} mice which were lean, thin, and agile. The chronic administration of MPTP (10 mg/kg) i.p. for 7 days induced severe body tremors, muscular rigidity, and complete immobilization in MT_{dko} mice as compared to MT_{trans} mice, which could still walk with their stiff legs and erect tail, suggesting the neuroprotective role of MTs in PD (Sharma et al. 2004).

Various antipsychotic drugs such as chlorpromazine, chlorprazine, risperidone, domeperidone, are generally anti-DArgic, as these are D-2 receptor antagonists. These typical, first generation, antipsychotic drugs alleviate the positive symptoms of schizophrenia as compared to next generation, atypical antipsychotic drugs, as quetiapine, olanzapine, clonezapine, which alleviate the negative symptoms of schizophrenia and act on D3 and D4 receptors preferentially. The atypical antipsychotic drugs do not induce extrapyramidal symptoms as typical antipsychotic drugs, but can cause agranulocytosis; hence, periodic blood analysis is required. These drugs can also induce hepatotoxicity, hypertension, hyperglycemia, obesity, and diabetes due to the down-regulation of brain region-specific MTs and other antioxidants, CB induction, charnolophagy inhibition, and CS destabilization in the mesolimbic DArgic system.

The chronic use of antipsychotic drugs can cause Parkinsonism, associated with extrapyramidal symptoms. Although synaptic changes and adverse effects may take only hrs, these drugs require minimum 2–3 weeks to have their therapeutic effect. The chronic use of these drugs can induce reversible MOA-B specific CB formation to cause Parkinsonism (associated with extrapyramidal symptoms); whereas their discontinuation eliminates adverse symptoms due to efficient MAO-B-specific CB eradication through energy driven charnolophagy, as a basic molecular mechanism of ICD.

About 70–80% chronic drug addicts become victim to psychosis associated with schizophrenia due to excess and uncontrolled mesolimbic DA-ergic neurotransmission. Hence, anti-DA-ergic drugs alleviate the most distressing symptoms of schizophrenia to a certain extent, yet with adverse extrapyramidal symptoms including dyskinesias and dystonic reactions, tardive dyskinesia, Parkinsonism, akinesia, akathisia, and neuroleptic malignant syndrome. On the other hand, drugs which enhance the DA-ergic neurotransmission and/or DA-ergic agonists are used for the treatment of PD. The chronic use of these drugs induce hyper-sexuality and aggravate symptoms of schizophrenia in PD patients due to reversible MAO-A specific CB formation in the mesolimbic DAergic system. The symptoms of schizophrenia are alleviated when these drugs are discontinued. Hence, DSST-CBs can be used as novel discovery targets for the future development of antipsychotic, anti-Alzheimer, anti-parkinsonian, anti-epileptic, antidepressant, anti-diabetic, and anti-obesity drugs with minimum or no adverse effects. As ZIKV-victims of embryopathy may suffer from poor quality of life due to sensorimotor deficits in the later life, it will be highly prudent to develop CB targeted drugs against ZIKV embryopathies, GBS, and reproductive disorders, collectively known as "ZIKV charnolopathies". It has been identified that patients with major depression, obesity, schizophrenia, and diabetes have increased the prevalence of tobacco smoking. Some researchers believe that these patients smoke tobacco because the most addictive chemical nicotine alleviates several symptoms of these NDDs by binding with the brain regional nictotine acetylcholine (nAChRs). However, several other researchers believe that preventing cigarette smoking in these patients could improve their health. A significant clinical improvement was noticed in schizophrenia patients who quit tobacco smoking.

Therapeutic Potential of Antioxidants as CB Antagonists

In addition to MTs and glutathione, various other ROS scavenging antioxidants such as resveratrol, polyphenols, lycopenes, catechin, sirtuins, rutuins, and lysine deacetylases (LSDs) derived from natural foods, can easily pass through blood brain barrier without any serious side effects and can modulate cellular epigenetic (histone acetylation, and DNA methylation) changes and thus can be used for the prevention and/or inhibition of CB formation (involved in CMB, MAOs and TRPC down-regulation, and TSPO delocalization). These therapeutic antioxidants have also anti-apoptotic and anti-inflammatory properties to inhibit progressive neurodegeneration in PD, AD, ALS, HD, MS, chronic drug addiction, schizophrenia, diabetes, obesity, ZIKV disease, and several other diseases through IL-10 induction and IL-6 inhibition.

Although wine has resveratrol (250 µg/120 ml), it is insufficient to fulfil the daily requirement of 250 mg; which is 1000X more as compared to wine. Moreover, wine contains nitrosamines, and cigarette smoke contains tobacco-specific nitrosamines, which can cause cancer. To meet the daily requirement of resveratrol from just wine, we may have to consume ~ 300 bottles of 120 ml, which will cause hepatotoxicity and neurotoxicity much earlier as compared to conferring the beneficial effects of resveratrol, derived from the wine. Hence, resveratrol derived from natural foods or fresh grapes, instead of wine will be more beneficial, as generally publicized by the wine industries and misinterpreted by the consumers. This is highly significant for the normal growth and development of fetuses of pregnant women residing or traveling in ZIKV-prone areas.

As there is limited scope of neuron-replacement therapy, therapeutic interventions with afore-mentioned antioxidants seems practically feasible as these can enter CNS freely without inducing any deleterious adverse effects. However, their inadequate target delivery and reduced potency remains a significant therapeutic challenge. Therefore, ROS scavenging antioxidant-loaded NPs will have better CNS delivery and therapeutic potential in the effective clinical management of ZIKV-induced charnolopathies, involved in diversified embryopathies.

As $\Delta\Psi$ is an extremely sensitive parameter for assessing the MB, it can be considered as the primary event during CB formation. We discovered that CB formation occurs primarily during nutritional and/or toxic insult to a most vulnerable cell (particularly hyper proliferating starving cells) because; CB formation, charnolophagy, and/or CPS/CS formation were never observed in the normal healthy developing neurons. In fact, nutritional rehabilitation of 80 days prevented or eliminated CB formation in the developing UN Purkinje neurons. The elimination of CB through lysosomal activation (charnolophagy) is an efficient basic molecular mechanism of "ICD" particularly during conception of the oocyte. It is highly significant event in "Mother Nature" which can decide life and death of a zygote. Several toxins [including KA, DOM, acromelic acid, okadaic acid, quisqualic acid, heavy metal ions (Hg, Cd, As, Pb), polychlorobiphenyls (PCBs), dichloro diphenyl trichloroethane (DDT), ethanol, and tobacco smoke] can inhibit charnolophagy to induce CB sequestration. Intrauterine exposure to these toxins is involved in craniofacial abnormalities, as noticed in FASD. Several drugs including: anti-epileptic drugs, ACE inhibitors, anesthetic agents, and ZIKV can also induce congenital charnolopathies involved in diversified embryopathies (Sharma et al. 2014; Sharma 2016). During chronic conditions, when CB becomes lysosomal resistant, it cannot be efficiently phagocytosed. A lysosome-resistant CB formation can pose a serious problem of ICD, which occurs in progressive NDDs, CVDs, and in MDR malignancies. Moreover, CB sequestration destroys the neighboring cells during atherosclerotic plaque rupture in obesity and in diabetes due to the release of iron, Cyt-C, caspase-3, Bax, and many other toxic substances.

Nutritional rehabilitation, physiological Zn^{2+} supplementation, and/or MTs can prevent CB formation, particularly during early neuronal development and aging so that a healthy young life and aging can be enjoyed. By contrast, unhealthy lifestyle choices such as alcohol intake, cigarette smoking, a high-fat and salt-rich diet, or malnutrition (because of ignorance and poverty), may cause morbidity and early mortality due to brain region-specific CB formation. The antioxidants such as glutathione and MTs can be induced by intake of Zn^{2+}, regular diet, and moderate exercise to circumvent free radical overproduction, prevent CB formation and progressive NDDs, including chronic drug addiction. Inhibition of charnolophagy may lead to NDDs accompanied with accumulations of neuronal inclusions. MTs, as antioxidants, anti-apoptotic, and anti-inflammatory agents store, buffer, and release Zn^{2+} to dissolve amyloid plaques in AD. Hence, drugs may be developed to inhibit CB formation to prevent or treat NDDs and CVDs; and enhance cancer stem cell-specific CB formation for the clinical management of MDR malignancies.

We established that MTs, as potent free radical scavengers, prevent CB formation and serve as anti-inflammatory and apoptotic agents in polysubstance abuse (Sharma and Ebadi 2011b; Sharma 2015). We also established the clinical significance of MTs in CB prevention in nanomedicine and proposed primarily three types of NPs, based on their response to the MB. Neutral NPs have no effect of CB formation, toxic NPs enhance CB formation, whereas neuroprotective NPs inhibit CB formation and enhance charnolophagy. Hence, ROS-scavenging antioxidants-loaded NPs can be developed for the therapeutic intervention in neurotoxins-induced charnolopathies, involved in diversified embryopathies, including ZIKV, cytomegalomegalovirus, rubella virus and other drug-induced (antidepressants, antipsychotics, anesthetics, and antiepileptics) microcephaly (Sharma et al. 2013a; Sharma et al. 2013b; Sharma et al. 2013c; Sharma 2015a,b; Sharma 2016a–e).

We established the clinical significance of CB formation in KA and DOM-induced apoptosis of cultured neurons and hippocampal CA-3 and dentate gyrus neurons in the developing rat and mouse brain (Sharma et al. 2014a–c). We highlighted the clinical significance of antioxidants as promising charnolopharmacotherapeutics for the safe and effective treatment of MDR malignancies and other chronic diseases (Sharma 2014, 2015, 2016b). Intrauterine exposure of ethanol causes FAS, represented by typical craniofacial abnormalities as noticed in nicotinism and ZIKV embryopathies due to CB formation in the most susceptible NPCs in the developing embryo (Sharma et al. 2014; Chabenne et al. 2014) and CB formation occurs in the hippocampal CA-3 and dentate gyrus regions due to cerebral ischemia in vascular dementia (Jagtap et al. 2015). We emphasized that hippocampal CB formation is involved in MDDs. Hence, physiological and/or pharmacological intervention to prevent or inhibit free radical overproduction by antioxidants such as MTs and glutathione can provide neuroprotection (Sharma 2014a,b). Moreover, physicochemical injury and/or stress can induce hippocampal CB formation to cause MDD and PTSD (Sharma 2015), whereas the MAO-B inhibitor, selegiline, provides neuroprotection by preventing brain regional disease-specific CB formation through MTs induction (Sharma 2015).

Recently, I reported ZIKV-induced CB formation in the most vulnerable developing NPCs to trigger charnolopathies, involved in a diversified spectrum of embryopathies, and recommended the therapeutic potential of protein-rich-alcohol-free, well-nourished diet, B-vitamins, folate, and antioxidants such as MTs, glutathione, and melatonin in the prevention of diversified charnolopathies, because these antioxidants inhibit CB formation, involved in apoptosis, alopecia, neurodegeneration, early morbidity and mortality due to impaired synaptic transmission and loss of cognition (Sharma 2016a,b; Sharma 2017a, 2017b).

Clinical Significance of Charnolopharmacotherapeutics in Evidence-based Personalized Theranostics

Currently there is a dire need for the safe and effective EBPT of various NDDs, CVDs, cancer, and MDR bacterial, viral (including ZIKV), and fungal infections. Hence, novel MB-based CB antagonists, charnolophagy agonists, CPS/CS stablilizers, and CB sequestration-based drugs can be developed to prevent and/or cure chronic diseases. More specifically, drugs can be developed to enhance either the MB and/or prevent disease-induced CB formation in a highly vulnerable cell including: iPPCs, NPCs, CPCs, EPCs, radial glial cells, hematopoietic stem cells, osteoblasts, placental Hofbaur cells, oocytes, Sertoli cells, spermtogonia, spermatocytes, Leydig's cells, hair follicular cells, GIT cells, and numerous other cells to evaluate their prophylactic as well as therapeutic potential in chronic NDDs, CVDs, cancer, infertility, and microbial infections (including, ZIKV).

During the acute phase, the most appropriate strategy would be to develop drugs to inhibit DSST-CB formation and enhance charnolophagy as a basic molecular mechanism of ICD (also called as intracellular sanitation). Recently, frequent abortions have been reported in ZIKV infected pregnant women due to zygotic death as noticed in FASD and chronic nicotinism, depending on the extent of alcohol consumed during pregnancy due to persistence of CB formation, failure of charnolophagy, and CB sequestration. Zygotic death occurs due to inefficient elimination of CB in the zygote soon after conception due to maternal nicotine and alcohol abuse and/or ZIKV infection (Sharma et al. 2015; Sharma 2016). DSST charnolophagy is a highly crucial biological event in the etiopathogenesis of diversified embryopathies in newborn infants particularly during the first trimester (gastrulation period) of pregnancy. Hence, it will be clinically significant to prevent CPS/CS destabilization and CB sequestration (involved in toxic Cyt-C, caspase-3, AIF, and iron release), resulting in apoptosis, progressive neurodegeneration, diversified embryopathies (including microcephaly) in new born infants and GBS in adults. In addition, it will be clinically significant to develop CB sequestration inhibitors during the chronic phase to prevent and/or cure ZIKV disease by developing either an effective and safe vaccine and/or anti-viral drug. In addition, novel vaccine and/or antiviral drug(s) can be developed by targeting different phases of viral lytic cycle, specific structural proteins, nonstructural proteins (NS-1), the enzyme helicase, and noncoding RNA against ZIKV disease beyond the scope of this chapter. Ultimately, we will have both preventive as well as therapeutic options available for the successful EBPT of ZIKV disease and chronic addiction of ethanol and nicotine to prevent their deleterious consequences on the developing embryo.

The clinical significance of CB formation, charnolophagy induction, CPS/CS stabilization, and CB sequestration cannot be over-emphasized, because these basic molecular events occur due to DPCI. These deleterious events induce free radical overproduction because the energy (ATP) requirements are significantly increased during DPCI. Natural abundance of mitochondria having highly sensitive uncoiled double-stranded, intron less DNA in metabolically-active and functionally-significant vulnerable cells including, but not limited to, NPCs and CPCs, are highly susceptible to CB formation due to frequent epigenetic modifications. Moreover, the mtDNA is

GC-rich which renders it highly susceptible to oxidation at guanosine and epigenetic modification by methylation at the cytosine. Hence, charnolophagy becomes the most viable option for the cell to get rid of toxic substances and remain healthy.

Various flaviviruses have been associated with the ER in WNV infected HeLa cells. In a recent study, electron-dense virions and vesicles packets were noticed under TEM of WNV infected HeLa cells (Saiz et al. 2016). These investigators reported ER autophagy and cell signaling pathways of the UPR, autophagy, and flaviviruses, including three arms of PERK (UPR, ATF-6, IRE-1) of autophagy. Undoubtedly, ER autophagy will occur in cells rich in ER, whereas charnolophagy is the earliest and predominant event, which occurs primarily in highly vulnerable developing cells, rich in mitochondria during DPCI. Hence, ER autophagy can be distinguished from charnolophagy as described in this chapter. Other organelles including peroxysomes, Golgi bodies, and/or nuclear membranes are also phagocytosed and eliminated by autophagy during DPCI. However, charnolophagy remains the primary, most sensitive, and frequent event in the proper maintenance of MB, epigenetic modulation, and ICD in the CNS and cardiovascular system because of the natural abundance of mitochondria, their highly toxic metabolites, and their crucial involvement in maintaining the bioenergetics and ICD. Charnolophagy may also occur rarely under normal physiological conditions as a basic molecular mechanism of ICD. Nevertheless, it becomes a highly prevalent and clinically-significant intracellular event in response to DPCI. It is important to emphasize that moderate exercise may also enhance charnolophagy and CS exocytosis as a basic molecular mechanism of ICD to remain healthy even during aging.

Conclusion

DPCI including nutritional stress, nicotine, ethanol, and microbial (including ZIKV, cytomegalovirus, rubella virus) and toxoplasma infections compromise MB and enhance free radical overproduction to induce lipid peroxidation in the most vulnerable cells of our body. Lipid peroxidation causes structural and functional breakdown of PUFA to induce disintegration of the mitochondrial membranes. The mitochondrial membranes are highly susceptible to free radical-induced lipid peroxidation as they are rich in PUFA. In addition, genetic and epigenetic changes in the mtDNA occurs readily because it is GC-rich and remains in a hostile microenvironment where free radicals are generated continuously as a byproduct of oxidative phosphorylation in the electron transport chain. These deleterious events induce CB formation as an initial attempt of ICD to contain toxic mitochondrial metabolites particularly in highly vulnerable developing NPCs. Hence, CB can serve as a universal biomarker and charnolophagy and CS as novel drug discovery targets to accomplish the targeted, safe and effective EBPT of NDDs, CVDs, MDR malignancies, microbial infections, and numerous proinflammatory conditions beyond the scope of this chapter. Early therapeutic interventions to inhibit CB formation by nutritional rehabilitation, physiological Zn^{2+} supplementation, antioxidants, and healthy life-style choices (including personal and environmental hygiene), moderate exercise, reduced fat, sugar, and salt intake, and avoiding tobacco smoking and ethanol consumption will go a long way in the prevention and/or treatment of microcephaly induced due to intrauterine nicotine and alcohol abuse, toxins, and/or microbial (ZIKV) infections and other chronic diseases of aging. Eventually molecularly well-defined and genetically-sculptured practice of EBPT by developing novel ROS scavenging NPs and nano-drug delivery devices/systems preventing CB formation and augmenting charnolophagy during the acute phase, and stabilizing CPS and CS and their exocytosis, as a basic molecular mechanism of ICD during the chronic phase, will offer the targeted, safe, effective and painless EBPT of chronic MDR diseases without any adverse effects to improve the quality of our life.

References

Bollimuntha, S., B. Singh, S. Shavali, S. Sharma and M. Ebadi. 2005. TRPC-1-mediated inhibition of MPP⁺ toxicity in human SH-S-Y5Y neuroblastoma cells. Journal of Biological Chemistry 280: 2132–2140.

Chabenne, A., C. Moon, C. Ojo, A. Khogali, B. Nepal and S. Sharma. 2014. Biomarkers in fetal alcohol syndrome (Recent Update). Biomarkers and Genomic Medicine 6: 12–22.

Dakshinamurti, K., S.K. Sharma and M. Sundaram. 1991. Domoic acid induced seizure activity in normal rat. Neuroscience Letters 127: 193–197.

Dakshinamurti, K., S.K. Sharma, T. Watanabe and M. Sundaram. 1992. Hippocampal changes in postnatal mice following intrauterine exposure to domoic acid. Epilepsia Vol. Suppl (Abstract) p. 45. Proceedings of the American Epilepsy Society, Seattle, Washington, USA. Dec.

Dakshinamurti, K., S.K. Sharma, M. Sundaram and T. Watanabe. 1993. Hippocampal changes in developing postnatal mice following intra-uterine exposure to domoic acid. Journal of Neuroscience 13: 4486–4495.

Ebadi, M., P. Govitrapong, S. Sharma, D. Muralikrishnan, S. Shavali, L. Pelletm, R. Schaffer, C. Albano and J. Ekens. 2001. Ubiquinone (Coenzyme Q_{10}) and mitochondria in oxidative stress of Parkinson's disease. Biological Signals and Receptors 10. 224 253.

Ebadi, M., S.K. Sharma, S. Shavali and H.E.I. Rafaey. 2002a. Neuroprotective action of selegiline. J Neuroscience Research 67: 285–289.

Ebadi, M. and S.K. Sharma. 2002b. Mitochondrial α-synuclein-metallothionein interaction in Parkinson's disease. The FASEB Journal 16: 697.6.

Ebadi, M., S. Wanpen, S. Shavali and S. Sharma. 2004a. Coenzyme Q_{10} stabilizes metallothionein in Parkinson's disease. *In*: Hiramatsu, M., L. Packer and T. Yoshikava (eds.). Molecular Interventions and Protection in Life Style-Related Diseases. Markel Dekker, Inc. New York.

Ebadi, M., S. Sharma, S. Wanpen and A. Amornpan. 2004b. Coenzyme Q_{10} inhibits mitochondrial complex-1 downregulation and nuclear factor-kappa B activation. Journal of Cellular & Molecular Med 8: 213–222.

Ebadi, M., H. Brown-Borg, S. Garrett, B. Singh, S. Shavali and S. Sharma. 2005a. Metallothionein-mediated neuroprotection in genetically-engineered mice models of Parkinson's disease and aging. Molecular Brain Research 134: 67–75.

Ebadi, M., S. Sharma, P. Ghafourifar, H. Brown-Borg and H.E.I. Refaey. 2005b. Peroxynitrite in the pathogenesis of Parkinson's disease. Method in Enzymology 396: 276–298.

Ebadi, M. and S. Sharma. 2006. Metallothioneins 1 and 2 attenuate peroxynitrite-induced oxidative stress in Parkinson's disease. Experimental Biology and Medicine 231: 1576–1583.

Hamburg, M.A. and F.C. Collins. 2010. The path to PM. New Eng J Med 363: 301–304.

Jagtap, A., S. Gawande and S. Sharma. 2015. Biomarkers in vascular dementia (A Recent Update). 7: 43–56.

Klongpanichapak, S., P. Govitropong, S. Sharma and M. Ebadi. 2006. Attenuation of *Cocaine* and METH neurotoxicity by coenzyme Q_{10}. Neurochem Res 31: 303–311.

Kooncumchoo, P., S. Sharma, J. Porter, P. Govitrapong and M. Ebadi. 2006. Coenzyme Q_{10} provides neuroprotection in iron-induced apoptosis in DArgic neurons. Journal of Molecular Neuroscience 28: 125–141.

Lee, R.W., D.B. Shenoy and R. Sheel. 2010. Micellar nanoparticles: Applications for topical and passive transdermal drug delivery. Chapter 2: pp. 37–58. Handbook of Non-Invasive Drug Delivery

Systems (Non-Invasive and Minimally-Invasive Drug Delivery Systems for Pharmaceutical and Personal Care Products) A Volume in Personal Care & Cosmetic Technology.

Li, Z., Q. Lin, Q. Ma, C. Lu and C.M. Tzeng. 2014. Genetic predisposition to Parkinson's disease and cancer. Curr Cancer Drug Targets 14: 310–321.

Saiz, J.C., A. Ángela Vázquez-Calvo and A.B. Blázquez. 2016. *ZIKV*: the latest newcomer. Frontiers in Microbiology 7: 496.

Sangchot, P., S.K. Sharma, B. Chetsawang, P. Govitropong and M. Ebadi. 2002. Deferoxamine attenuates iron-induced oxidative stress and prevents mitochondrial aggregation and α-synuclein translocation in SK-N-SH cells in culture. Developmental Neuroscience 24: 143–153.

Sharma, S. and M. Ebadi. 2003. Metallothionein attenuates 3-morpholinosydnonimone (SIN-1)-induced oxidative and nitrative stress in DArgic neurons. Antioxidant and Redox Signaling 5: 251–264.

Sharma, S., E. Carlson and M. Ebadi. 2003. The neuroprotective actions of selegiline in inhibiting 1-methyl, 4-phenyl, pyridinium ion (MPP+)-induced apoptosis in DArgic neurons. Journal of Neurocytology 32: 329–343.

Sharma, S., M. Kheradpezhou, S. Shavali, H.E.I. Refaey, J. Eken, C. Hagen and M. Ebadi. 2004. Neuroprotective actions of coenzyme Q_{10} in Parkinson's disease. Methods in Enzymology 382: 488–509.

Sharma, S., H.E.I. Refaey and M. Ebadi. 2006. Complex-1 activity and ^{18}F-DOPA uptake in genetically engineered mouse model of Parkinson's disease and the neuroprotective role of coenzyme Q_{10}. Brain Research Bulletin 70: 22–32.

Sharma, S. and M. Ebadi. 2008a. Coenzyme Q_{10} augments brain regional ^{18}F-DOPA and 2-^{18}F-Fluoro, 2-deoxy, D-glucose uptake in metallothionein over-expressing weaver mouse. Proceedings of the World Congress of Molecular Imaging (WMIC 2008). Sep 10–13, 2008.

Sharma, S. and M. Ebadi. 2008b. Therapeutic potential of metallothioneins in Parkinson's disease. pp. 1–28. *In*: Timothy F. Hahn and Julian Werner (eds.). New Research on Parkinson's Disease. Nova Science Publishers, New York.

Sharma, S. and M. Ebadi. 2011a. Metallothioneins as early & sensitive biomarkers of redox signaling in neurodegenerative disorders. Journal of Institute of Integrative Omics & Applied Biotechnology (IIOAB Journal) 2: 98–106.

Sharma, S. and M. Ebadi. 2011b. Therapeutic potential of metallothioneins as anti-inflammatory agents in polysubstance abuse. Journal of Institute of Integrative Omics & Applied Biotechnology IIOAB Journal 2: 50–61.

Sharma, S., B. Yang, X. Xi, J. Grotta, J. Aronowski and S. Savitz. 2011. IL-10 directly protects cortical neurons by activating PI-3 kinase and STAT-3 pathways. Brain Research 1373: 189–194.

Sharma, S. 2013. *CB* as a sensitive biomarker in nanomedicine. International Translational Nanomedicine Conference. Boston, July 26–28 (Invited Speaker).

Sharma, S. and M. Ebadi. 2013. *In vivo* molecular imaging in Parkinson's disease. pp. 787–802. *In*: Pfeiffer, R.F., Z.K. Wszolek and M. Ebadi (eds.). Parkinson's Disease. IInd Edition, Chapter 58, CRC Press Taylor & Francis Group. Boca Rotan, FL, USA.

Sharma, S., A. Rais, R. Sandhu, W. Nel and M. Ebadi. 2013. Clinical significance of metallothioneins in cell therapy and nanomedicine. International Journal of Nanomedicine 8: 1477–1488.

Sharma, S., 2014a. Beyond Diet and Depression (Volume-2). Book Nova Science Publishers, New York, U.S.A.

Sharma, S. 2014b. Beyond Diet and Depression (Volume-1). Book Nova Sciences Publishers, New York, U.S.A.

Sharma, S. 2014c. Molecular pharmacology of environmental neurotoxins. pp. 1–47. *In*: Kainic Acid: Neurotoxic Properties, Biological Sources, and Clinical Applications. Nova Science Publishers, New York.

Sharma, S. 2014d. *CB* as a universal biomarker in nanomedicine. 2nd International Translational Nanomedicine Conference. Boston, July 25–27 (Invited Speaker).

Sharma, S. 2014e. Mitochondrially-targeted nanomedicines. 5th World Gene Conference. Haikou, China Nov 13–15 (Invited Speaker and Chairperson).

Sharma, S. 2014f. *CB* as a universal biomarker in drug discovery. 12th International Conference on Drug Discovery. Suzhou, China Nov 18–20 (Invited Speaker & Chair Person).

Sharma, S. 2014g. Nanotheranostics in evidence based personalized medicine. Current Drug Targets 15: 915–930.

Sharma, S. 2014h. Charnolopharmacotherapy in multi-drug resistant diseases. 5th International Conference in MediChem. Suzhou, China, Nov 18–20 (Invited Speaker).

Sharma, S. 2014i. Charnolopharmacotherapy of cancer and other diseases. 5th International Conference, Suzhou, China, Nov 18–20 (Invited Speaker).

Sharma, S and M. Ebadi. 2014a. Antioxidants as potential therapeutics in neurodegeneration. pp. 1–30. *In*: Laher, I. (ed.). System Biology of Free Radicals and Antioxidants. Springer Verlag, Heidelberg, Germany, Chapter 85.

Sharma, S. and M. Ebadi. 2014b. *CB* as a universal biomarker of cell injury. Biomarkers and Genomic Medicine 6: 89–98.

Sharma, S. and M. Ebadi. 2014c. Significance of metallothioneins in aging brain. Neurochemistry International 65: 40–48.

Sharma, S., S. Gawande, A. Jagtap, R. Abeulela and Z. Salman. 2014a. Fetal alcohol syndrome: Prevention, diagnosis, & treatment. *In*: Alcohol Abuse: Prevalence, Risk Factors. Nova Science Publishers, New York, U.S.A.

Sharma, S., B. Nepal, C.S. Moon, A. Chabenne, A. Khogali, C. Ojo, E. Hong, R. Goudet, A. Sayed-Ahmad, A. Jacob, A. Murtaba and M. Firlit. 2014b. Psychology of craving. Open Jr of Medical Psychology 3: 120–125.

Sharma, S. 2015a. Alleviating Stress of the Soldier & Civilian. Nova Science Publishers, New York, U.S.A.

Sharma, S. 2015b. Monoamine Oxidase Inhibitors: Clinical Pharmacology, Benefits, & Adverse Effects. Nova Science Publishers, New York, U.S.A.

Sharma, S. 2015c. *CB* as a Universal Biomarker in Drug Addiction. 3rd International Drug Addiction Conference. Oralando, Florida. USA Aug 2–5.

Sharma, S., J. Choga, V. Gupta et al. 2016. *CB* as a novel biomarker of nutritional stress in Alzheimer's disease. Functional Foods in Health & Disease 6: 344–377.

Sharma, S. 2016a. Personalized Medicine (Beyond PET Biomarkers). Nova Science Publishers, New York, U.S.A.

Sharma, S. 2016b. Progress in PET RPs. Nova Science Publishers, New York, U.S.A.

Sharma, S. 2016c. Disease-specific *CB formation* in neurodegenerative & other diseases. Drug Discovery & Therapy World Congress. Aug 22–25. Hynes International Convention Center. Boston Mass, U.S.A. (Invited Speaker).

Sharma, S. 2016d. *CB* as novel biomarker of nutritional stress in Alzheimer's disease. 20th International Conference of Functional Foods in Health & Disease. Josheph P. Martin Memorial Convention Center, Harvard Medical School, Boston, Mass, U.S.A. Sep 22–23 (Invited Speaker).

Sharma, S. 2016e. *CB* as a novel biomarker in *ZIKV*-induced *microcephaly*. Drug Discovery & Therapy World Congress (DDTWC-2016). Hynes Memorial Conventional Center, Boaton, Mass, U.S.A. Aug 21–25 (Invited Speaker).

Sharma, S., J. Choga, P. Doghor et al. 2016a. *CB* as a novel biomarker of nutritional stress in Alzheimer's disease. 20th International Conference on Functional Foods in Health & Disease. Joseph P. Martin International Convention Center, Harvard Medical School, Boston, Mass, U.S.A. Sep 22–23.

Sharma, S., J. Choga, V. Gupta et al. 2016b. *CB* as a novel biomarker of nutritional stress in Alzheimer's disease. Functional Foods in Health and Disease 6: 344–378.

Sharma, S.K. 1985. Mossy fiber evoked unit activity in developing normal and undernourished rat Purkinje cells. Presented and Published in the Proceedings of the 13th World Congress of Neurology at Hamburg, Germany. Sep 1–6, Vol. 232. p. 95.

Sharma, S.K., U. Nayar, M.C. Maheshwari and G. Gopinath. 1986. Ultrastructural studies of P-cell morphology in developing normal and undernourished rat cerebellar cortex. Electrophysiological Correlates Neurology India 34: 323–327.

Sharma, S.K., U. Nayar, M.C. Maheshwari and B. Singh. 1987. Effect of undernutrition on developing rat cerebellum: Some electrophysiological and neuromorphological correlates. Journal of Neurological Sciences 78: 261–272.

Sharma, S.K. 1988. Nutrition and brain development. Published in the Proceedings of the First World Congress of Clinical Nutrition. New Delhi (India) pp. 5–8.

Sharma, S.K., W. Selvamurthy and K. Dakshinamurti. 1993a. Effect of environmental neurotoxins in the developing brain. Biometeorology 2: 447–455.

Sharma, S.K., U. Nayar, M.C. Maheshwari and B. Singh. 1993b. Purkinje cell evoked unit activity in developing undernourished rats. Journal of Neurolological Sciences 116: 212–219.

Shavali, S., E.C. Carlson, J.C. Swinscoe and M. Ebadi. 2004. 1-Benzyl-1,2,3,4-tetrahydroisoquinoline, a Parkinsonism-inducing endogenous toxin, increases alpha-synuclein expression and causes nuclear damage in human dopaminergic cells. J Neurosci Res 76(4): 563–571.

Zhang, S., C. Lei and P. Liu. 2015. Association between variant amyloid deposits and motor deficits in FAD-associated presenilin-1 mutations: A systematic review. Neuroscience & Biobehavioral Reviews 56: 180–192.

Wang, J.J., Z.W. Zeng, R.Z. Xiao et al. 2011. Recent advances of chitosan nanoparticles as drug carriers. International Journal of Nanomedicine 6: 765–774.

Wang, E. 2009. microRNA regulation and its biological significance in PM and aging. Current Genomics 10: 143.

CHAPTER-6

Metallothioneins Inhibit Charnoly Body Formation and Confer Structural and Functional Stability to Charnolosome

INTRODUCTION

MTs are low molecular weight (6–7 kDa), metal-binding, cysteine-rich antioxidant, anti-inflammatory, and antiapoptotic proteins, which confer neuroprotection through Zn^{2+}-induced microRNA-mediated post-transcriptional regulation of genes involved in the DNA cell cycle, growth, proliferation, differentiation, migration, and development.

In our earlier studies, we reported that MTs prevent MPP^+-induced apoptosis in cultured SK-N-SH neurons by attenuating mtDNA oxidation and prevent the formation of 8-OH, 2dG by developing multiple fluorochrome comet assay (Sharma and Ebadi 2003; Ebadi and Sharma 2003). We also reported that MPTP-induced protein nitration is attenuated by MT overexpression in the striatal DAergic neurons of mice (Ebadi and Sharma 2003). In addition, MTs attenuate a potent $ONOO^-$ ion generator, 3-morpholinosydnonimine (SIN-1)-induced oxidative and nitrative stress in SK-N-SH and SH-SY5Y neurons, suggesting their theranostic potential in NDDs such as AIS, PD, AD, MDD, schizophrenia, and multiple drug addiction. SIN-1 induces oxidative as well as nitrative stress as noticed in diversified neurodegenerative α-synucleinopathies.

A progressive loss of DAergic neurons in the substantia nigra zona compacta and in other subcortical nuclei associated with a widespread occurrence of Lewy bodies occurs in PD. Although, the exact cause of cellular demise in PD remains poorly understood, a defect in the mitochondrial oxidative phosphorylation and enhanced oxidative stress have been proposed. We examined SIN-1-induced apoptosis in control and MTs-overexpressing DAergic neurons to determine the neuroprotective potential of MTs against $ONOO^-$-induced neurodegeneration in PD. SIN-1 induced lipid peroxidation and plasma membrane blebbing accompanied with apoptosis of cultured DA-ergic (SK-N-SH) neurons, DNA fragmentation, α-synuclein nitration, intramitochondrial accumulation of metal ions (Cu^{2+}, Fe^{3+}, Zn^{2+}, and Ca^{2+}), and enhanced the synthesis of 8-OH, 2dG (a mitochondrial DNA oxidation product) in addition to enhanced production of 2,3 dihydroxy nonenal (lipid peroxidation product of mitochondrial membranes). SIN-1 down-regulated Bcl-2 and PARP expression and up-regulated caspase-3 and Bax expression. In addition, SIN-1 induced apoptosis in aging RhO_{mgko} neurons, α-synuclein-transfected cells, MT_{dko} cells, and caspase-3-overexpressed DA-ergic neurons. SIN-1-induced deleterious changes were attenuated with a selective MAO-B inhibitor, selegiline or in MTs-transgenic mesencephalic fetal stem cells. SIN-1-induced oxidation of dopamine to dihydroxyphenylacetaldehyde (DOPAL) was attenuated in MT_{trans} fetal stem cells and in cells transfected with a mitochondrial genome encoding complex-1, and enhanced in aging RhO_{mgko} cells, in MT_{dko} cells, and caspase-3 gene-overexpressing DA-ergic neurons. Selegiline, melatonin, CoQ_{10}, and MTs inhibited SIN-1-induced down-regulation of a mitochondrial genome and up-regulation of caspase-3 as determined by the RT-PCR analysis. The synthesis of mitochondrial 8-OH, 2dG and AIF were induced by MPP^+ ions or by a potent mitochondrial (Complex-1) inhibitor, rotenone. Pretreatment with selegiline or MTs inhibited MPP^+ ion-, 6-OH-DA, and rotenone-induced increases in 8-OH, 2dG accumulation. Transfection of aging RhO_{mgko} neurons with mitochondrial genome encoding complex-1 or melanin inhibited SIN-1-induced lipid peroxidation. SIN-1 induced α-synuclein, caspase-3, and 8-OH, 2dG expression, and protein (α-synuclein) nitration. The afore-mentioned deleterious effects of SIN-1 were attenuated by MTs gene overexpression, providing evidence that NOS activation and $ONOO^-$ ion overproduction are involved in the etiopathogenesis of PD, whereas MTs induction may provide neuroprotection by preventing free radical-induced CB formation and CS destabilization (Sharma and Ebadi 2003; Sharma et al. 2013a; Sharma et al. 2013b; Sharma and Ebadi 2014; Sharma et al. 2016; Sharma 2017).

A defect in the mitochondrial oxidative phosphorylation and enhanced oxidative and nitrative stresses have been proposed in the etiopathogenesis of PD. Hence, we studied $control_{wt}$ (C57B1/6), MT_{trans}, MT_{dko}, α-synuclein knock out (alpha-syn_{ko}), α-synuclein-MTs triple knock out (α-syn-MT_{tko}), homozygous weaver mutant (wv/wv) mice, and Ames dwarf mice to evaluate the precise role of $ONOO^-$ ions in the etiopathogenesis of PD and aging (Ebadi et al. 2005). Although MT_{dko} mice were genetically susceptible to MPTP Parkinsonism, they did not exhibit any overt clinical symptoms of neurodegeneration and neuropathological changes as observed in wv/wv mice with significantly down-regulated brain regional MTs. Progressive neurodegenerative changes were associated with typical Parkinsonism in wv/wv mice. The neurodegenerative changes in wv/wv mice were observed primarily in the striatum, hippocampus, and cerebellum as noticed in multiple drug addiction due to free radical-induced CB formation, charnolophagy, and Cs destabilization. Various hallmarks of apoptosis including caspase-3, TNFα, NFkβ, MTs, and complex-1 nitration were increased; whereas glutathione, complex-1, ATP, and Ser(40)-phosphorylation of tyrosine hydroxylase, and striatal ^{18}F-DOPA uptake were significantly reduced in wv/wv mice as compared to other experimental genotypes. Striatal neurons of wv/wv mice demonstrated typical age-dependent increase in dense cored intra-neuronal inclusions as multi-lamellar CBs and destabilized CS, cellular aggregation, proto-oncogenes (c-fos, c-jun, caspase-3, and GAPDH) induction, inter-nucleosomal

DNA fragmentation, and neuro-apoptosis (Sharma and Ebadi 2008; Sharma and Ebadi 2013).

MT_{trans} and α-Syn_{ko} mice were genetically resistant to MPTP-Parkinsonism and Ames dwarf mice had increased concentrations of striatal CoQ_{10} and MTs and lived ~2.5X longer as compared to $control_{wt}$ mice. SIN-1-induced apoptosis was significantly attenuated in MT_{trans} fetal stem cells, suggesting that ONOO⁻ ions are involved in the etiopathogenesis of PD, whereas MTs-induced CoQ_{10} synthesis may provide neuroprotection in progressive neurodegencrative α-synucleinopathies (Sharma and Ebadi 2003).

To determine the genetic predisposition to MPTP-induced Parkinsonism, we utilized control, MT_{trans}, and MT_{dko} mice. These experimental genotypes were injected MPTP (10 mg/kg i.p.) for 7 days. MT_{dko} and $control_{wt}$ mice were completely immobilized and exhibited severe body tremors, muscle rigidity, and postural irregularities, whereas MT_{trans} mice could still walk with their stiff legs and erect tail (Sharma et al. 2004). However, the basic molecular mechanism of genetic resistance of MT_{trans} mice to MPTP neurotoxicity remains enigmatic. CS_{normal} and CS_{mtdko} were highly labile due to an inadequate amount or absence of intra-mitochondrial MTs, whereas MT_{trans} CS were structurally and functionally stable. In addition, Zn^{2+} provides structural and functional stability to MTs, whereas MTs provide structural and functional stability to *CSs* by serving as potent free radical scavengers and CB antagonists. In the absence of MTs, structural and functional degradation of *CS* disseminates highly toxic mitochondrial metabolites such as iron, Cyt-C, 8-OH, 2dG, 2,3 dihydroxy nonenal, ammonia, acetaldehyde, and H_2O_2, which pose a significant challenge to intranuclear, intracellular, intramitochondrial, extracellular, and systemic detoxification and trigger further degeneration as seen in PD, AD, ALS, MS, AIS, chronic drug addiction, depression, *CVDs*, and MDR malignancies (Sharma 2017a,b).

CSs can be classified based on MTs content as (i) normal CS (CS_{normal}), (ii) MTs transgenic CS ($CS_{MTtrans}$), and (iii) MTs double knock out CS (CS_{MTdko}). MTs induced *CS* stability plays a crucial role in sustaining intranuclear, intracellular, extracellular, and systemic detoxification to remain healthy even during aging. Hence, supplementing pharmacological doses of Zn^{2+} may not be useful to AD patients because it will remain free and uncontrolled due to the down-regulation of MTs in old age.

MTs provide neuroprotection as antioxidants, anti-inflammatory, and anti-apoptotic agents by serving as potent free radical scavengers and by storing, sequestering, and buffering Zn^{2+} ions. Zinc is involved in microRNA-mediated post-transcriptional regulation of genes involved in DNA cell cycle, growth, proliferation, differentiation, and development. Higher concentrations of Zn^{2+} may induce amyloid-β-42 aggregation to cause further neurodegeneration in AD by augmenting CB formation, by inhibiting charnolophagy and by CS destabilization. The structural and functional destabilization of MT_{trans} CS may induce malignant transformation due to cell immortalization and Zn^{2+}-induced transcriptional activation of genes involved in DNA cell cycle regulation, growth, proliferation, and differentiation. Hence, adequate Zn^{2+}-induced MTs stability is highly crucial during old age. Particularly, Zn^{2+} depleted MTs are readily disintegrated by the lysosomal enzymes in the CS. Although, MT_{dko} mice did not exhibit overt clinical symptoms of PD or epilepsy, these were highly vulnerable to exogenously-administered MPTP, MDMA, KA, and DOM. We, and other investigators reported that MT_{dko} mice and cultured human DAergic (SK-N-SH) neurons are highly susceptible to MPTP and MDMA-induced Parkinsonism, and KA and DOM-induced epileptogenesis (Sharma et al 2004; Xie et al. 2004).

Therapeutic Potential of MTs as CB Antagonists, Charnaolopagy Agonist, and CS Membrane Stabilizers in Neurodegenerative α-Synucleinopathies. METH is a well-known drug of abuse and neurotoxin that induces parkinsonian neuropathology in chronic abusers by targeting human NS- DA-ergic neurons. Hence, further understanding regarding the basic molecular mechanism of DA-regic neurodegeneration by METH may provide further insight regarding the exact molecular pathology of PD and its early EBPT. In earlier studies, we demonstrated that METH increases the production of ROS, decreases ATP, and reduces cell viability in the cultured SK-N-SH neurons, whereas pre-treatment with Zn^{2+} attenuates the loss of cell viability induced by METH treatment. Pre-treatment with Zn^{2+} increased MTs expression, attenuated METH-induced ROS production, and ATP depletion. MTs-mediated attenuation of METH toxicity was inhibited by chelating Zn^{2+} with CaEDTA, suggesting that Zn^{2+}-induced MTs induction confers neuroprotection by preventing ROS and augmenting ATP synthesis, and that MTs may provide mitochondrial neuroprotection by serving as a potent free radical scavenger in PD (Ajjimaporn et al. 2005). In a similar study, the recreational drug MDMA ("ecstasy") induced a selective toxicity in the DA-ergic neurons. In this study, Xie et al. (2004) employed cDNA microarray technology to evaluate changes in gene expression in murine MDMA-induced toxicity to DAergic neurons. Out of 15000 mouse cDNA fragments, MTs (MT1, MT2) appeared as candidate genes in MDMA-induced DAergic neurotoxicity which was authenticated by Northern blot analysis within 4–13 hrs of MDMA treatment. Immunoblot analysis also demonstrated a similar increase in MT protein levels, with peak times following induction in mRNA expression. MT_{dko} mice were more vulnerable to MDMA-induced toxicity to DAergic neurons as compared to control wild type mice. Stimulation of endogenous MTs with Zn^{2+} conferred full neuroprotection against MDMA-induced toxicity, whereas exogenously-administered MTs afforded partial protection, indicating that MDMA-induced toxicity to DAergic neurons is associated with increased MT1 and MT2 gene transcription and translation, as a neuroprotective mechanism. These findings further authenticated the therapeutic potential of MTs as CB antagonists, charnolophagy agonists, and CS membrane stabilizers in MPP+, MPTP, METH, and MDMA-induced molecular neuropathogenesis in DAergic neurons as noticed in PD and numerous other diseases (Xie et al. 2004; Ebadi et al. 2005; Ebadi and Sharma 2006; Sharma and Ebadi 2008; Sharma et al. 2013; Sharma and Ebadi 2014).

Clinical Significance of MTs as CB Antagonists in Aging. Recently, we reported that aging is an inevitable biological process, associated with gradual and spontaneous biochemical and physiological changes, and increases susceptibility to diseases. Chronic inflammation and oxidative stress are hallmarks of aging. MTs are low molecular weight, zinc-binding, anti-inflammatory, and antioxidant proteins that provide neuroprotection in the aging brain through Zn^{2+}-mediated transcriptional regulation of genes involved in cell growth, proliferation, and differentiation. In addition to Zn^{2+} homeostasis, antioxidant role of MTs is routed through –SH moieties on cysteine residues. MTs are induced in the aging brain as a defensive mechanism to attenuate oxidative and nitrative stress implicated in broadly classified neurodegenerative α-synucleinopathies involved in PD, AD, and aging. In addition, MTs as free radical scavengers inhibit CB formation and CS destabilization to provide mitochondrial neuroprotection in the aging brain. In general, MT-1 and MT-2 induce cell growth and differentiation, whereas MT-3 is a growth inhibitory factor, which is reduced in AD. MTs are down-regulated in wv/wv mice exhibiting progressive neurodegeneration, early aging, morbidity, and mortality as noticed in AD and aging. These neurodegenerative changes were attenuated in MTs over-expressing wv/wv mice, suggesting the neuroprotective role of MTs in PD, AD, and aging. We provided recent knowledge regarding the therapeutic potential of MTs in NDDs of aging as potent CB antagonists and CS stabilizers in one of our recent publications (Sharma and Ebadi 2014).

In this chapter, three types of CS, i.e., (i) CS_{normal}; (ii) $CS\text{-}MT_{dko}$; and (iii) $CS\text{-}MT_{trans}$ are described. The $CS\text{-}MT_{dko}$ are highly susceptible due to the absence of MTs which provide structural and functional stability to the plasma membrane as free radical scavengers. $CS\text{-}MT_{dko}$ demonstrates relatively enhanced susceptibility to MPTP-parkinsonism and KA/DOM-epileptogenesis due to the absence of MTs-mediated antioxidant defense. Moreover, depletion of Zn^{2+} from MTs renders them highly susceptible to proteolytic degradation. Zn^{2+}-depleted MTs become highly susceptible to oxidative and nitrative stress in DPCI. Although, aging MT_{dko} mice did not exhibit overt clinical symptoms of PD, AD, or seizures, these experimental genotypes were highly susceptible MPTP, MDMA, and METH-induced parkinsonism, KA, and DOM-induced seizures and sensorimotor impairments, associated with hippocampal CB formation, charnolophagy, and CS destabilization, involved in AD and other NDDs.

Therapeutic Potential of MTs as CB Antagonists. During the acute phase, MTs prevent CB formation by serving as potent free radical scavengers and antioxidants. During the chronic phase, MTs enhance charnolophagy and stabilize CS to provide neuroprotection and maintain ICD. MTs translocate in the nucleus to regulate Zn^{2+}-induced transcriptional activation of genes involved in AgNOR activation, implicated in ribosomal production for the synthesis of new proteins (i.e., mitofusin, involved in mitochondrial synthesis and repair) at the rough endoplasmic reticulum. MTs, as antioxidant, anti-apoptotic, and anti-inflammatory factors sustain ICD, in addition to facilitating cell growth, proliferation, migration, differentiation, and development by preventing not only mitochondrial oxidative stress but also ER stress.

Zinc Provides Structural and Functional Stability to MTs. It has been identified that Zn^{+2}-deficient MT is readily subjected to proteolytic degradation by the lysosomal enzymes. Zn^{2+} provides structural and functional stability to MTs, whereas MTs provide structural and functional stability to CS to sustain intranuclear, intracellular, intramitochondrial, extracellular, and systemic detoxification for normal cellular function to remain healthy. Any physicochemical disruption in CS-MTs interaction due to the dissemination of toxic substances triggers chronic CVDs and NDDs and vice versa in malignancies.

Interconversion of CS in Malignant Transformation. A CS can be transformed to apoptosome, inflammasome, nectroptsome, and metallosome depending on the inducers and microenvironment in a cell. This transformation occurs readily in response to DPCI or if a CS is derived from cancer stem cells and/or from iPPCs, which synthesize NPCs during brain development and CPCs during cardiovascular development during intrauterine life. Any physicochemical insult like drugs of abuse (nicotine, ethanol, METH, MDMA, morphine, and heroin) can induce chronic diseases like obesity, hepatoxicity, diabetes, pulmonary disease, and cancer in later life, if abused during pregnancy. Particularly, the gastrulation phase is highly sensitive to the deleterious consequences of DPCI.

CB formation occurs to restrict uncontrolled release of intra-mitochondrial toxic substances in the most vulnerable cell during DPCI; particularly, Cyt-C, acetate, H_2O_2, ammonia, Bax, Bak, AIF, iron, are highly toxic and induce extensive degenerative changes. The Cyt-C, iron, 8-OH 2dG, 2,3 dihydroxy nonenal, and 18 kDa, cholesterol channel (TSPO), and TRPCs delocalization induce further inflammation and chronic diseases by disrupting the normal epigenetic changes in the nucleus by S-adenosyl methionine (SAM)-induced histone acetylation and DNA methylation.

The mitochondria are arranged compactly in the cells involved in movements (spermatocytes, cardiomyocytes, and skeletal muscle cells). When the MB is down-regulated, CB is formed, which remains restricted to a specific region of a cell during a stressful situation to prevent the further spread of toxicity. Mitochondria are randomly distributed in metabolically-active cells like neurons, hepatocytes, nephrons, and oocytes. A neuron may have as many as 750–1000 mitochondria depending on the metabolic activity and energy (ATP) requirements. Their size varies from 1.2–10 μm. We can roughly estimate the approximate life span of a cell by counting the number of mitochondria. For instance, human RBCs are devoid of mitochondria and survive only 110 days, whereas spermatocytes can survive > 5 years if stored in 10% buffered glycerin in a freezer. Glycerin prevents ice crystal formation during thawing. However, it is important to emphasize that artificial fertilization is successful only in 40% of cases. In 60% cases, it remains unsuccessful due to CMB involving CB formation during prolonged storage. Spermatocytes remain alive and functional due to the availability of various trophic factors and glucose in the semen. However, in phosphate buffered saline, their motility and life span are significantly reduced due to CB formation.

Many victims escape from typical FASD symptoms due to efficient charnolophagy and CS exocytosis. However, circulating CS can release toxic substances at the synaptic terminals to induce cognitive impairments due to abnormal synaptic transmission, which is reflected as impaired learning, intelligence, memory, and behavior during adult life. Although, a destabilized circulating CS can induce synaptic silence, synaptic sequestration, and synaptic degeneration, these events occur very slowly because it requires the entrance of circulating CS through the blood brain barrier. However, direct release of toxic CS metabolites at the synaptic terminals due to intracellular induction of CB can induce accelerated neurodegeneration as noticed in severe malnutrition, chronic drug addiction, and acute ischemic, or hemorrhagic stroke, involving early morbidity and mortality. Although, MT_{dko} mice do not exhibit any overt clinical symptoms of progressive neurodegeneration, these are highly vulnerable to DPCI due to depletion of MTs, which, as potent free radical scavengers, prevent CB formation, augment charnolophagy and CS stability, and CS exocytosis to maintain intracellular sanitation and normal cellular function even during aging.

References

Ajjimaporn, A., J. Swinscoe, S. Shavali, P. Govitrapong and M. Ebadi. 2005. Metallothionein provides zinc-mediated protective effects against methamphetamine toxicity in SK-N-SH cells. Brain Research Bulletin 67: 466–475.

Ebadi, M. and S.K. Sharma. 2003. Peroxynitrite and mitochondrial dysfunction in the pathogenesis of Parkinson's disease. Antioxid Redox Signal 5: 319–335.

Ebadi, M., H. Brown-Borg, H.E.I. Refaey, B.B. Singh, S. Garrett, S. Shavali and S.K. Sharma. 2005. Metallothionein-mediated neuroprotection in genetically engineered mouse models of Parkinson's disease. Brain Res Mol Brain Res 134: 67–75.

Ebadi, M. and S. Sharma. 2006. Metallothioneins 1 and 2 attenuate peroxynitrite-induced oxidative stress in Parkinson's disease. Experimental Biology and Medicine 231: 1576–1583.

Sharma, S. and M. Ebadi. 2003. Metallothionein attenuates 3-morpoholinosydnonimone (SIN-1)-induced oxidative and nitrative stress in DArgic neurons. Antioxidants and Redox Signaling 5: 251–264.

Sharma, S. and M. Ebadi. 2008. Therapeutic potential of metallothioneins in Parkinson's disease. pp. 1–28. *In*: Timothy F. Hahn and Julian Werner (eds.). New Research on Parkinson's Disease. Nova Science Publishers, New York.

Sharma, S , A. Rais, R. Sandhu, W. Nel and M. Ebadi. 2013. Clinical significance of metallothioneins in cell therapy and nanomedicine. International Journal of Nanomedicine 8. 1477–1488.

Sharma, S. and M. Ebadi. 2014. Significance of metallothioneins in aging brain. Neurochem Int 65: 40–48.

Sharma, S. and W. Lippincott. 2017. Emerging biomarkers in Alzheimer's disease (Recent Update). Current Alzheimer Research.

Xie, T., L. Tong, U.D. McCann, J. Yuan, K.G. Becker, A.O. Mechan, C. Cheadle, D.M. Donovan and G.A. Ricaurte. 2004. Identification and characterization of metallothionein-1 and -2 gene expression in the context of (+/–)3, 4-methylenedioxymethamphetamine-induced toxicity to brain dopaminergic neurons. J Neurosci 24: 7043–7050.

CHAPTER-7

Clinical Significance of Charnoly Body as a Biomarker of Compromized Mitochondrial Bioenergetics in Multidrug Resistant Diseases

INTRODUCTION

Recently, we reported that the MB is significantly compromised in response to DPCI and NPs used in theranostic applications (Sharma et al. 2013a; Sharma et al. 2013b). CMB triggers CB formation in the most vulnerable cell, involved in apoptosis, NDDs, and CVDs. MTs inhibit CB formation by acting as potent free radical scavengers, charnolophagy enhancers, and CS stabilizers. We proposed basically three types of NPs, including: toxic, neutral, and protective. Toxic NPs induce CB formation, neutral NPs have no effect on the MB, whereas, protective NPs inhibit CB formation and provide neuroprotection as well as cardiovascular protection (Sharma et al. 2013a).

In this chapter, the clinical significance of CB formation in NDDs, CVDs, and MDR malignancies is highlighted. It is proposed that by inhibiting brain regional (hippocampal CA-3 and dentate gurus) CB formation, we can prevent memory impairments in AD and cure CVDs, and by augmenting cancer stem cell-specific CB formation, prevent or even cure MDR malignancies.

Environmental Neurotoxins, Drugs, and NPs Augment CB Formation. Recently, we reported that various drugs of abuse including cocaine, METH, MDMA, and Parkinsonian neurotoxins, rotenone, salsolinol, 1-benzyl,tetrahydroisoquinoline (1-benzyl-TIQ), and MPTP induce apoptosis in human DArgic (SK-N.SH) neurons by inhibiting mitochondrial complex-1, a rate-limiting enzyme involved in oxidative phosphorylation and ATP synthesis in the electron transport chain (Sharma et al.

2013c). MPP⁺-induced apoptosis in SK-N-SH neurons was attenuated by MAO-B inhibitor, selegiline, through MTs induction (Sharma et al. 2003). Since MTs inhibit CB formation, any pharmacological or physiological intervention augmenting MTs may provide neuroprotection. Furthermore, MTs inhibit progressive neurodegenerative α-synucleinopathies to prevent neurodegeneration by suppressing CB molecular pathogenesis in PD, AD, MDDs, chronic addiction, schizophrenia, and numerous other NDDs (Sharma and Ebadi 2011a,b, 2013; Sharma 2017). Various environmental neurotoxins including KA, DOM, and acromelic acid are rigid structural analogues of glutamate and induce permanent loss of memory by selectively causing neurodegeneration involving CB molecular pathogenesis in the hippocampal CA-3 and dentate gyrus neurons (Sharma et al. 1990; Dakshinamurti et al. 1993). These excito-toxic agents also induce CB formation and apoptosis when exposed to primary cortical neurons or in NG-108/15 cells in culture (Sharma et al. 1993; Dakshinamurti et al. 2003).

Classification of NPs. Recently, we proposed primarily three major types of NPs: (i) Inert, (ii) Toxic, and (ii) Protective. A toxic NP induces CB formation, a protective NP inhibits CB formation, whereas inert NP causes no change in the intracellular microenvironment and does not either induce or inhibit CB formation (Sharma et al. 2013a; Sharma et al. 2013b; Sharma et al. 2013c). Based on these findings, we can develop drugs and/or NPs for early safe and effective EBPT of various NDDs, CVDs, and cancer. Particularly, our interest needs to be focused on developing cancer stem cell-specific CB formation, which will be helpful in the safe and effective EBPT of MDR malignancies (Sharma et al. 2013a).

Intraneuronal Microinjector to Determine CB Formation. To examine the direct effect of various drugs, RPs, and NPs, an electro-micro-injector was invented for intra-neuronal study. With this simple motor-driven micro-device, we can determine whether developed NP or drug is inert, augmenting, or inhibiting CB formation at the subcellular level (Sharma 1982). We have now better microiontophoretic devices to examine the direct effect of drugs or NPs at the subcellular level. The inherent limitation of microiontophoretic devices is that the drug or NPs must have electrical charge on their surface. Although T.E.M. is required to confirm the existence of CB formation, charnolophagy, and CS exocytosis in a cell, a simple confocal microscopic examination of ΔΨ, 8-OH-2dG synthesis, and multiple fluorochrome comet assay can be performed initially by using specific fluorochromes (*JC-1, Rhodamine, Dihydrofluorescein, LysoTracker, MitoTracker, and ER tracker*). This simple, efficient, and economical approach can save lot of time, money, and energy of the drug-development organizations to discover novel NPs and/or drugs for the safe and effective personalized nanotheranostics of chronic MDR diseases.

Drug and NPs-induced CB Formation. The Nobel Laureate, St. Georgy discovered basic molecular mechanism of phosphorescence and fluorescence. Phosphorescence is a slow process of energy dissipation and is involved in longevity, whereas fluorescence accelerates CB formation, CS destabilization, apoptosis, and early neurodegeneration to reduce the life span. For example, thyroxine augments fluorescence involving fast energy dissipation as a potent un-coupler of the oxidative phosphorylation. Hence, in patients with thyrotoxicosis, oxidation remains active whereas, phosphorylation is inhibited, which causes diarrhea, dehydration, increased BMR, and weight loss due to CB formation, CS destabilization, and apoptosis, whereas phosphorescence is a slow process of energy dissipation and prolongs the life span of living organism as it protects the MB by inhibiting CB formation, charnolophagy induction, CS stabilization, and CS exocytosis as an efficient molecular mechanism of ICD for normal cellular function and homeostasis to remain healthy. A typical example of an agent which augments phosphorescence is the female hormone "estrogen", which possesses free radical scavenging antioxidant, anti-inflammatory, and antiapoptotic properties to confer mitochondrial protection in women as it inhibits free radical-induced CB formation in various cells and inhibits TSPO delocalization to provide protection and sustain intra-mitochondrial cholesterol transport for the synthesis of steroid hormones for membrane stability. This defensive mechanism is disrupted due to estrogen depletion during post-menopausal phase, which renders them highly susceptible to NDDs, CVDs, and osteoporosis.

Estrogen Prevents CB Formation. The MB remain intact in women due to the presence of estrogen, which augments anti-apoptotic protein, BCl-2. Hence, women can live longer as compared to males. However, they are also highly prone to breast cancer and ovarian cancer during their reproductive phase and osteoporosis during postmenopausal phase due to enhanced osteoclastic activity in the absence of estrogen. By augmenting BCl-2 expression, estrogen can inhibit NPs or drug-induced CB formation and may provide genetic resistance to certain malignant cancers. Estrogen augments osteoblast activity, prevents CB formation, osteoporosis, and CVDs in reproductive phase; whereas during post-menopausal period, due to the lack of estrogen, women develop osteoporosis due to enhanced osteoclast activity. Osteoblasts are rich in alkaline phosphate (localized in the mitochondria), whereas osteoclasts are rich in acid phosphatase (localized in the lysosomes). Alkaline phosphatase augments osteogencsis, whereas acid phosphatase causes osteoporosis leading to increased occurrence of bone fractures during the post-menopausal phase.

Hippocampal CB Formation Enhances Memory Impairment in AD. Excessive accumulation of CBs at the junction of the axon hillock blocks axoplasmic transport and proximo-distal flow of various ions, enzymes, neurotransmitters, hormones, neurotropic factors (BDNF, NGF-1, IGF-1), and mitochondria from the cell soma to the synaptic region to impair neurotransmission leading to progressive neurodegeneration due to synaptic atrophy in AD, PD, ALS, HD, and MS, etc. Protective NPs, drugs, or antioxidants inhibit CB formation to prevent NDDs and CVDs. Moreover, swollen or degenerated mitochondria find it difficult to flow through twisted neurotubules, which may further impair synaptic neurotransmission leading to dementia as noticed in Down's syndrome, autism, AD, and aging.

MTs Inhibit CB Formation. MTs-mediated CB prevention provides neuroprotection and cardiovascular protection, whereas its induction in MDR malignancies renders cancer treatment more difficult. Particularly, induction of MTs, HSPs, HIF-1α, and BCL-2 in cancer stem cells provides genetic resistance to conventional anticancer treatment. Hence, anti-cancer drugs should enhance cancer stem cell-specific CB formation. Furthermore, NPs or drugs may be targeted to induce cancer stem cell-specific CB formation for the safe and effective eradication of MDR malignancies.

Charnolophagy in Conception

It is logical to assume that mitochondria in the spermatocyte need to be structurally and functionally intact until its nDNA fuses with the maternal nDNA during conception. However, it remains uncertain whether mitochondria from the spermatocytes are destroyed spontaneously. Obviously, certain time is required for the nDNA to hybridize with the oocyte DNA and its penetration through maternal nuclear wall. Whether, charnolophagy occurring during fertilization, is similar to progressive NDDs such as MS, PA, PD, HD, MSA, PDD, HD, ALS, remains uncertain. In fact, the intracellular microenvironment of the oocyte is highly unsuitable for the structural and functional integrity of the spermatocyte mtDNA, so its existence within the oocyte remains only for a limited period, just sufficient to facilitate paternal nDNA hybridization with the maternal nDNA. Moreover, paternal CB is recognized as a foreign inclusion body in the oocyte during the post-zygotic period. Hence, mitochondria of the spermatocyte are immediately destroyed by CB formation and subjected to charnolophagy by the oocyte lysosomes. However, the exact nature, condition, and duration of charnolophagy in the intracytoplasmic compartment of an oocyte remains unknown. Further research is needed to establish the exact clinical significance of charnolophagy and CS exocytosis during fertilization in health and disease. It is important to emphasize that an oocyte has unlimited number of mitochondria (250,000 to 600,000), which can efficiently eliminate paternal CB and/or CS within a matter of few milli-seconds. However, intrauterine exposure to DPCI such as severe malnutrition, toxins (nicotine, ethanol, or other drugs), and microbial infections (including ZIKV, cytomegalovirus, and rubella virus) may prevent or even disrupt charnolophagy and/or CS exocytosis and may even render CS highly destabilized to release toxic mitochondrial metabolites to cause degeneration of NPCs and CPCs derived from iPPCs during embryonic life to cause microcephaly and dendritic and synaptic pruning in adult life to cause Gullain Barre' Syndrome (GBS) and meningoencephalopathy in immunocompromised adults as I have reported in my recent Books "ZIKV Disease: Prevent and Cure" and "Fetal Alcohol Spectrum Disorders: Concepts, Mechanisms and Cure".

Mitochondrially-Targeted Therapeutics in Fetal Alcohol Spectrum Disorders (FASD)

Maternal as well as paternal mitochondrial genetics and epigenetics is impaired in FAS due to fetal ethanol exposure, leading to CB formation, which can be prevented and/or eradicated by nutritional rehabilitation, physiological Zn^{2+}, and MTs or by developing specific agonists augmenting charnolophagy. Similarly, specific CB antagonists and charnolophagy agonists may be developed to prevent or treat NDDs and CVDs during early pre-zygotic phase of fetal development with minimum or no adverse effects on the craniofacial growth and development of FAS victims. Recently, we reported CB as a universal biomarker of cell injury (Sharma and Ebadi 2014). CB formation occurs due to ethanol-induced CMB and can be prevented by nutritional rehabilitation, physiological Zn^{2+}, and MTs. During severe malnutrition, CB is phagocytosed by ATP-dependent lysosomal charnolophagy. Hence, specific CB agonists and charnolophagy antagonists will have theranostic potential in preventing and eradicating carcinogenesis, whereas, specific CB antagonists and charnolophagy agonists will have theranostic potential in preventing and treating NDDs and CVDs during the early pre-zygotic phase of FAS. These specific MB-based CB-targeted drugs will have minimum or no side effects and will be useful in preventing/treating not only FAS but also impairments induced by early fetal exposure to general anesthetic agents, antiepileptic drugs, and/or environmental toxins.

Impaired Charnolophagy in FASD

Ethanol is converted to acetaldehyde by alcohol dehydrogenase. Acetaldehyde is highly toxic, causes oxidative stress, and free radical over-production. Ethanol induces CB formation by inhibiting protein synthesis in the zygote. There is now evidence to suggest that genetic and epigenetic changes in the maternal as well as paternal nuclear DNA and mtDNA can be induced by nutritional stress and/or environmental neurotoxins, which can compromise the MB to enhance CB formation and CS destabilization in the developing progenitor cells of FASD victims. CB is an electron-dense, multi-lamellar, pleomorphic, pre-apoptotic biomarker of cell injury that is formed in the most vulnerable cell due to free radical-induced CMB (Sharma and Ebadi 2014).

Recently, I introduced charnolophagy to describe the degenerated mitochondrial autophagy. (charnolophagy) which occurs in the zygote soon after the paternal nuclear DNA is hybridized with the maternal nuclear DNA during fertilization. However, mtDNA is naked intron less, labile structure, without any structural and functional support of histones and protamines, remains in a hostile microenvironment of free radicals, generated as a byproduct of mitochondrial oxidative phosphorylation in the electron transport chain, and can be readily destroyed. It is also well established that all mitochondrially-derived diseases in the developing embryo are originated from the maternal mtDNA, whereas paternal mtDNA is degenerated in the zygote soon after fertilization. There is now evidence to suggest charnolophagy as an ICD process of degenerated paternal mitochondrial membranes. If paternal charnolophagy is delayed or inhibited due to intrauterine nicotine, ethanol, anesthetic agents, and/or antiepileptic agents, it can have deleterious consequences and may even induce spontaneous death of the zygote due to release of toxic substances from the degenerating mitochondrial membranes such as heme, iron-sulfur proteins, Cyt-C, 8-OH, 2dG, 2, 3 dihydroxy nonenal, ammonia, acetaldehyde, H_2O_2, lactate, Bax, Bid, and AIF, and caspase-3. Depending on the physical and nutritional status of a woman, and the quantity and frequency of ethanol consumed during pregnancy, the deleterious effects appear in a FASD victim. The paternal charnolophagy occurs efficiently in the zygote soon after fertilization as it is highly crucial spatio-temporally-sensitive event essential for the survival and normal development of the fetus. The zygote is exposed to apoptotic factors released from the degenerating paternal mitochondria. However, ethanol and tobacco can significantly delay this naturally-occurring efficient process of CB elimination through charnolophagy in the maternal as well as paternal gametes. Absence or delayed charnolophagy may have deleterious consequences on the zygote, and ultimately, the future development of an embryo, as noticed in malnutrition, nicotine abuse, FASD, viral infection, and other victims of microcephaly and/or craniofacial anomalies.

CS Destabilization Causes Dendritic Pruning and Synaptic Degeneration in Malnutrition, Toxic Exposure, and in Microbial Infection. The incidence of CS was significantly increased in the developing rat cerebellar Purkinje neuronal dendrites. The frequency of CB formation and hence, CS, increased as a function of severity and duration of nutritional stress or toxic exposure. The dendrites exhibited immature developmental characteristics. The CS is highly labile and exhibits a pleomorphic electron-dense appearance. The CS releases highly toxic mitochondrial metabolites to inhibit protein synthesis in the dendrites. The sequestration of intranuclear CS is involved in the down-regulation of the AgNOR, that synthesizes ribosomes depending on Zn^{2+}-induced transcriptional regulation and microRNA-mediated post-transcriptional regulation of genes involved in DNA cell cycle, cell division, proliferation, migration, development, and differentiation. The inhibition of ribosomal synthesis is responsible for delayed or down-regulation of protein synthesis required for the dendritic growth, development, and synaptogenesis. Local release of toxic substances from the CS inhibits protein synthesis to cause reduced ER development and extensive dendritic pruning.

In addition to swollen and degenerated mitochondria, CB, and CS, a free ribosomal pool is observed in the UN rat Purkinje neuron dendrites. Intracellular, extracellular, and circulating CS can participate in dendritic pruning and synaptic degeneration to cause impaired or delayed sensorimotor and cognitive impairments in learning, intelligence, memory and behavior as noticed in FASD, ZIKV diseases, rubella virus infection, and cytomegalovirus infection in addition to intrauterine exposure to toxic heavy metal ions (Pb, Hg, Cd, NI), antidepressants, anti-psychotics, anti-epileptic drugs, and anesthetic agents. Several new born infants do not exhibit overt clinical symptoms of microcephaly, because of the well-built physical status, immune system, and adequate nutritional status of a western woman during pregnancy. Although, CB formation occurs in the developing NPCs of these pregnant women, it is efficiently phagocytosed by energy (ATP)-driven charnolophagy, exocytosed, and is released in the systemic circulation. The circulating CS is primarily involved in dendritic pruning, synaptic atrophy, and synaptic degeneration, which is reflected as impaired cognitive performance of new born children from nicotine and/or alcohol abusing women with or without exposure of toxins and microbial infections. These infants do not exhibit any symptoms of craniofacial abnormalities; however, they may suffer from diversified deficits represented by ADHD and cognitive impairments in sensorimotor learning, intelligence, memory, and behavior. Hence, drugs may be developed to prevent or inhibit CB formation and augment charnolophagy during acute phase and stabilize CS dynamics and its exocytosis during chronic phase of DPCI in response to nicotine, ethanol, or other toxic substances during pregnancy and immediate postnatal life of an infant. Furthermore, it will be clinically significant to stabilize CS by endogenous and/or exogenous antioxidants for the normal growth and development of the brain and other tissues to remain healthy even during aging.

Charnolophagy (CB Autophagy)

It is important to emphasize that charnolophagy should not be confused with any other type of mitochondrial elimination mechanisms in a cell. Usually, charnolophagy is used to describe elimination of degenerated mitochondria particularly during chronic diseases such as severe malnutrition, drug addiction, FASD, ZIKV disease, AD, PD, schizophrenia, MDDs, and CVDs, cancer, and aging. During fertilization, paternal mitochondria are eliminated by maternal oocyte exclusively through charnolophagy, because, there is no other intracellular organelle in the spermatocyte except the nDNA and spirally-arranged condensed mitochondria in the middle piece, whose bioenergetics is down-regulated during fertilization. CB is formed typically by down-regulation of the mitochondrial bioenergetics. Hence, compactly-packed degenerated mitochondria are named as paternal CB in the oocyte during fertilization. However, if mitochondria are destroyed, the nDNA cannot enter the oocyte. It requires energy (ATP) to reach near the nuclear membrane of the oocyte. During conception, paternal mitochondria must be functionally active till the paternal nDNA fuses with the maternal nuclear DNA. It is logical to assume that certain time is needed for the nDNA to get incorporated with the host cell DNA and its penetration through the maternal nuclear wall. Whether charnolophagy during fertilization of the oocyte is similar to NDDs such as, MS, PA, PD, HD, MSA, PDD, HD, and ALS remains unknown. However, intracellular microenvironment of the oocyte is unsuitable for the structural and functional integrity of the spermatocyte mtDNA, so it can stay inside the oocyte for a limited time just sufficient to facilitate paternal nuclear DNA entry into the maternal nucleus during fertilization. Hence, paternal CB is destroyed and is subjected to charnolophagy soon after fertilization. However, the exact nature, condition, and duration of charnolophagy in the oocyte cytoplasm remains uncertain. Further research is needed to establish the basic molecular mechanism of CB pathogenesis and difference between charnolophagy during fertilization and in general health and disease.

Mitochondrial-Targeted Therapeutic Agents in FASD. Maternal as well as paternal mitochondrial genetics and epigenetics is impaired in FAS due to fetal ethanol exposure, leading to CB formation, which can be prevented and/or eradicated by nutritional rehabilitation, physiological Zn^{2+}, and MTs or by developing specific antagonists augmenting charnolophagy. Similarly, specific CB antagonists and charnolophagy agonists may be developed to prevent or treat neurodegenerative and cardiovascular complications at an early pre-zygotic phase of fetal development with minimum or no adverse effects on the craniofacial growth and development of FAS victims. CB formation occurs due to ethanol-induced CMB and can be prevented by nutritional rehabilitation, physiological Zn^{2+}, and MTs. During severe malnutrition, CB is phagocytosed by charnolophagy. Hence, specific CB agonists and charnolophagy antagonists will have therapeutic potential in preventing and treating MDR malignancies, whereas specific CB antagonists and charnolophagy agonists will have theranostic potential in preventing and treating NDDs and CVDs during early pre-zygotic phase of FAS. These specific CB-targeted drugs will have minimum or no side effects and will be useful to prevent/treat not only FASD but also early fetal exposure to microbial (bacteria, virus, fungus) infections, general anesthetic agents, antiepileptic drugs, and environmental toxins.

Charnolophagy in FASD. Ethanol is converted to acetaldehyde by alcohol dehydrogenase. Acetaldehyde is highly toxic, causes oxidative stress, and free radical overproduction. Ethanol induces CB formation by inhibiting protein synthesis in the zygote. There is now evidence to suggest that genetic and epigenetic changes in the maternal as well as paternal nDNA and mtDNA, can be influenced by nutritional stress and/or environmental neurotoxins, which can compromise the MB to enhance CB formation in FASD and in ZIKV infection during pregnancy. CB is highly sensitive pre-apoptotic, universal biomarker of cell injury which is formed in a highly vulnerable cell due to CMB (Sharma and Ebadi 2014).

Recently, I introduced charnolophagy to describe the degenerated mitochondrial autophagy. Charnolophagy occurs in the zygote soon after paternal nDNA is hybridized with the maternal nDNA. However, mtDNA is a naked, intron less, labile structure without any structural and functional support of histones and protamines and can be easily destroyed by a free radical attack. Moreover, mtDNA is GC-rich, which renders it highly susceptible to epigenetic modification at the N-3 position of the cytosine residue. It is also well established that all mitochondrial-derived diseases in the developing embryo are originated from the maternal mtDNA, whereas paternal mtDNA is degenerated in the zygote soon after fertilization. We have now evidence to suggest charnolophagy as a basic elimination process of degenerated mitochondrial membranes. If charnolophagy is delayed and/or inhibited due to intrauterine ethanol, anesthetic agents, and/or antiepileptic agents, it can have deleterious consequences and may even induce spontaneous death of the zygote due to apoptosis and release of toxic substances from the degenerating mitochondrial membranes such as heme, iron-sulfur proteins, Cyt-C, acetaldehyde, ammonia, H_2O_2, TSPO (18 kDa), MAOs, TRPCs, Bax, Bid, and AIF. Depending on the quantity and frequency of ethanol consumed, the deleterious effects will appear in a FASD victim. Hence, paternal charnolophagy occurs very efficiently in the zygote under normal physiological conditions soon after fertilization as it is highly critical and spatio-temporally-sensitive event for the normal growth and survival of the developing fetus. Delayed and/or impaired paternal charnolophagy in response to malnutrition, toxins (ethanol, nicotine), and microbial (bacteria, virus, and fungus) infection can have deleterious consequences on the developing fetus and may induce charnolopathies involving diversified embryopathies, including: FASD and ZIKV embryopathies due to the release of highly toxic paternal mitochondrial metabolites. Hence, absence or delayed charnolophagy may have deleterious consequences on the zygote and development of the fetus to cause microcephaly, craniofacial anomalies and other neurodevelopmental deficits in sensorimotor learning in the absence of typical FASD symptomatology.

Conclusion

Detailed epidemiological studies of mitochondrial epigenetics and the exact role of teratogens in FAS, requires future investigations. Whether methylation of the mitochondrial transcription factor–A promotor is influenced by FASD, remains unknown. The exact molecular mechanism of epigenetic changes involved in ethanol-induced CB formation also remains uncertain. Moreover, it remains unknown whether ethanol can influence iron-sulfur protein-mediated mitochondrial epigenetics in FASD. It applies particularly to underage alcohol abusers which can be divided in three age-groups corresponding to childhood, early adolescence, and later adolescence ($\sim$ 0 to 10, 10 to 15, and 16 to 20). Age-group also allows parents, educators, and policymakers to focus on a single age-group and gain an understanding of the developmental processes operating within that group, subject to the caveats that children of the same age are not at the same place on a developmental dimension, nor are individual children equally far along in terms of different dimensions of human maturation. Currently limited studies are available on the MB and epigenetic changes in FASD. However, it is now well-established that hyper methylation of the promoter regions of IGF-1 and leptin genes induces gene silencing to cause diabetes and obesity. Similarly, hyper methylation of the promoter regions of BDNF gene causes MDDs. Hence, prevention and treatment of alcohol-related problems from a developmental perspective is a very important area for further investigation. Major complications of FAS and nicotinism such as craniofacial anomalies, delayed eye-blink conditioning, opthalamic complications, neurobehavioral impairments, late onset obesity, diabetes, CVDs, and cancer susceptibility can be prevented by developing tissue-specific CB and charnolophagy-targeted drugs in future. There is a growing realization that nutritional, physical, and genetic factors could play a significant role in FASD. Socioeconomic and educational status can also play a significant role in FASD. Although, the incidence of alcohol abuse is increasing in the western world, the nutritional and physical status of the pregnant woman may also have significant influence on FASD predisposition. In general, the Mediterranean or other diet consumed by young pregnant western women is rich in iron, folic acid, choline, and vitamin A, required for the normal growth and development of the fetus. These agents rejuvenate the MB which is significantly compromised in FASD. Therefore, even if the alcohol consumption rate is high, the deleterious effects of intrauterine alcohol are nullified to a certain extent. However, it depends on the spatio-temporal CB formation, charnolophagy, and CS induction and its exocytosis as a basic molecular mechanism of ICD to escape FASD, because the MB plays a crucial role in determining the life and death of a zygote. Although E.M. is required to determine CB formation in a cell as described above; simple confocal microscopic examination of $\Delta\Psi$, 8-OH-2dG, and 2, 3 dihydroxy nonenal synthesis, and multiple fluorochrome comet assay can be performed initially to confirm CB formation to save lot of time, money, and energy on drug development. Our primary goal should be to develop ROS scavenging NPs and/or novel charnolopharmacotherapeutics to prevent/inhibit CB formation in NDDs and CVDs to augment charnolophagy, stabilize, and exocytose CS from the neurons and cardiomyocytes, and vice versa to eradicate MDR malignancies. A further study is needed in this direction.

References

Aarin, M., M. Haque, L. Johal, P. Mathur, W. Nel, A. Rais, R. Sandhu and S. Sharma. 2013. Maturation of the adolescent brain. Neuropsychiatric Disease and Treatment 9: 449–461.

Bollimuntha, S., B. Singh, S. Shavali, S. Sharma and M. Ebadi. 2005. TRPC-1-mediated inhibition of MPP$^+$ toxicity in human SH-S-Y5Y neuroblastoma cells. J Biol Chem 280: 2132–2140.

Brenneman, M., S. Sharma, M. Harting, R. Strong, C.S. Cox, J. Aronowski, J.C. Grotta and S.I. Savitz. 2010. Autologous bone marrow mononuclear cells enhance recovery after AIS in young and middle-aged rats. J Cerebral Blood Flow & Metabolism 30: 140–149.

Dakshinamurti, K., S.K. Sharma, M. Sundaram and T. Watanabe. 1993. Hippocampal changes in developing postnatal mice following intra-uterine exposure to domoic acid. J Neurosci 13: 4486–4495.

Dakshinamurti, K., S.K. Sharma and J.D. Gieger. 2003. Neuroprotective actions of pyridoxine. Biochem Biophys Acta 1647: 225–229.

Ebadi, M., P. Govitrapong, S. Sharma, D. Muralikrishnan, S. Shavali, L. Pellet, R. Schaffer, C. Albano and J. Ekens. 2001. Ubiquinone (Coenzyme Q10) and mitochondria in oxidative stress of Parkinson's disease. Biological Signals and Receptors 10: 224–253.
Ebadi, M., S. Sharma, S. Wanpen and S. Shavali. 2004. Metallothionein isoforms attenuate peroxynityrite-induced oxidative stress in Parkinson's disease. *In*: Ebadi, M. and R.F. Pfeiffer (eds.). Parkinson's Disease. CRC Press, pp. 479–500.
Ebadi, M., S.K. Sharma, A. Ajjimaporn and S. Maanum. 2004. Weaver mutant mouse in progression of neurodegeneration in Parkinson's disease. *In*: Ebadi, M. and R.F. Pfeiffer (eds.). Parkinson's Disease. CRC Press.
Ebadi, M., S. Sharma, S. Wanpen and A. Amornpan. 2004. Coenzyme Q_{10} inhibits mitochondrial complex-1 downregulation and nuclear factor-kappa B activation. J Cellular & Molecular Medicine 8: 213–222.
Ebadi, M., S. Wanpen, S. Shavali and S. Sharma. 2005. Coenzyme Q_{10} stabilizes mitochondria in Parkinson's disease. pp. 127–153. *In*: Hiramatsu (ed.). Molecular Interventions in Life-Style-Related Diseases.
Ebadi, M., H. Brown-Borg, S. Garrett, B. Singh, S. Shavali and S. Sharma. 2005. Metallothionein-mediated neuroprotection in genetically-engineered mice models of Parkinson's disease and aging. Molecular Brain Research 134: 67–75.
Ebadi, M., S. Sharma, P. Ghafourifar, H. Brown-Borg and H.E.I. Refaey. 2005. Peroxynitrite in the pathogenesis of Parkinson's disease. Method in Enzymology 396: 276–298.
Ebadi, M., H. Brown-Borg, S. Sharma, S. Shavali, H.E.I. ReFaey and E.C. Carlson. 2006. Therapeutic efficacy of selegiline in *NDDs* and neurological diseases. Current Drug Targets 7: 1–17.
Ebadi, M. and S. Sharma. 2006. Metallothioneins 1 and 2 attenuate peroxynitrite-induced oxidative stress in Parkinson's disease. Exp Biol Med 231: 1576–1583.
Faisal, S., A. Patel, C. Mattison, S. Bose, R. Krishnamohan, E. Sweeney, R. Sandhu, W. Nel, A. Rais, R. Sandhu, R.N. Ngu and S. Sharma. 2013. Effect of diet on serotonergic neurotransmission in depression. Neurochemistry International 62: 324–329.
Klongpanichapak, S., P. Govitropong, S. Sharma and M. Ebadi. 2006. Attenuation of *Cocaine* and METH neurotoxicity by coenzyme Q_{10}. Neurochem Res 31: 303–311.
Malikarjunarao, K., B. Yang, S. Sharma, R. Strong, M. Brenneman, X. Xi, J.C. Grotta, J. Aronowski, V. Misra and S. Savitz. 2011. Cell based therapy for stroke. pp. 143–162. *In*: Charles S. Cox Jr (ed.). Therapy for Neurological Injury. Chapter 7, Humana Press. Springer Science.
Sangchot, P., S.K. Sharma, B. Chetsawang, P. Govitropong and M. Ebadi. 2002. Deferoxamine attenuates iron-induced oxidative stress and prevents mitochondrial aggregation and α-synuclein translocation in SK-N-SH cells in culture. Developmental Neuroscience 24: 143–153.
Sharma, S., E. Carlson and M. Ebadi. 2003. The neuroprotective actions of selegiline in inhibiting 1-methyl, 4-phenyl, pyridinium ion (MPP$^+$)-induced apoptosis in DArgic neurons. J Neurocytology 32: 329–343.
Sharma, S., M. Kheradpezhou, S. Shavali, H.E.I. Refaey, J. Eken, C. Hagen and M. Ebadi. 2004. Neuroprotective actions of coenzyme Q_{10} in Parkinson's disease. Methods in Enzymology 382: 488–509.
Sharma, S., H.E.I. Refaey and M. Ebadi. 2006. Complex-1 activity and ^{18}F-DOPA uptake in genetically engineered mouse model of Parkinson's disease and the neuroprotective role of coenzyme Q_{10}. Brain Res Bull 70: 22–32.
Sharma, S. and M. Ebadi. 2008. Therapeutic potential of metallothioneins in Parkinson's disease. pp. 1–28. *In*: Timothy F. Hahn and Julian Werner (eds.). New Research on Parkinson's Disease. Nova Science Publishers, New York.
Sharma, S., Y. Bing, M. Brenneman, Xi. Xiaopei, J. Aronowski, J.C. Grotta and S. Savitz. 2010. Bone marrow mononuclear cells protect neurons and modulate microglia in cell culture models of ischemic stroke. Journal of Neuroscience Research 88: 2869–2876.
Sharma, S. and M. Ebadi. 2011. Metallothioneins as early & sensitive biomarkers of redox signaling in neurodegenerative disorders. Journal of Institute of Integrative Omics & Applied Biotechnology (IIOAB Journal) 2: 98–106.
Sharma, S. and M. Ebadi. 2011. Therapeutic potential of metallothioneins as anti-inflammatory agents in polysubstance abuse. Journal of Institute of Integrative Omics & Applied Biotechnology IIOAB Journal 2: 50–61.

Sharma, S., B. Yang, X. Xi, J. Grotta, J. Aronowski and S.I. Savitz. 2011. IL-10 directly protects cortical neurons by activating PI-3 kinase and STAT-3 pathways. Brain Res 1373: 189–194.

Sharma, S. 2013. *Charnoly Body* as a sensitive biomarker in nanomedicine. International Translational Nanomedicine Conference. Boston, July 26–28, 2013 (Invited Speaker).

Sharma, S., C.S. Moon, A. Khogali, A. Haidous, A. Chabenne, C. Ojo, M. Jelebinkov, Y. Kurdi and M. Ebadi. 2013. Biomarkers of Parkinson's disease (Recent Update). Neurochemistry International 63: 201–229.

Sharma, S. and M. Ebadi. 2013. Antioxidant Targeting in Neurodegenerative Disorders. Ed. I. Laher, Springer Verlag. Germany. Chapter 85, pp. 1–30.

Sharma, S., B. Nepal, C.S. Moon, A. Chabenne, A. Khogali, C. Ojo, E. Hong, R. Goudet, A. Sayed-Ahmad, A. Jacob, M. Murtaba and M. Firlit. 2013. Psychology of craving. Open Jr of Medical Psychology.

Sharma, S., A. Rais, R. Sandhu, W. Nel and M. Ebadi. 2013. Clinical significance of metallothioneins in cell therapy and nanomedicine. International Journal of Nanomedicine 8: 1477–1488.

Sharma, S. and M. Ebadi. 2014. Significance of metallothioneins in aging brain. Neurochemistry International 65: 40–48.

Sharma, S.K. 1982. A simple motor-driven micro-injector for intra-neuronal study. pp. 2933–2937. *In*: Reynoud, C. (ed.). Proceedings of the Third World Congress of Nuclear Medicine and Biology, Paris, France. Pregmon Press.

Sharma, S.K., U. Nayar, M.C. Maheshwari and G. Gopinath. 1986. Ultrastructural studies of P-cell morphology in developing normal and undernourished rat cerebellar cortex. Electrophysiological Correlates Neurology India 34: 323–327.

Sharma, S.K., U. Nayar, M.C. Maheshwari and B. Singh. 1987. Effect of undernutrition on developing rat cerebellum: Some electrophysiological and neuromorphological correlates. J Neurol Sciences 78: 261–272.

Sharma, S.K., W. Selvamurthy, M.C. Maheshwari and T.P. Singh. 1990. Kainic acid induced epileptogenesis in developing normal and undernourished rats-A computerized EEG analysis. Ind Jr Med Res 92: 456–466.

Sharma, S.K., M. Behari, M.C. Maheshwari and W. Selvamurthy. 1990. Seizure susceptibility and intra-rectal sodium valproate induced recovery in developing undernourished rats. Ind J Med Res 92: 120–127.

Sharma, S.K., U. Nayar, M.C. Maheshwari and B. Singh. 1993. Purkinje cell evoked unit activity in developing undernourished rats. J Neurol Sci 116: 212–219.

Sharma, S.K. and K. Dakshinamurti. 1993. Suppression of domoic acid-induced seizures by 8-(OH)-DPAT. J Neural Transmission 93: 87–89.

Sharma, S.K., W. Selvamurthy and K. Dakshinamurti. 1993. Effect of environmental neurotoxins in the developing brain. Biometeorology 2: 447–455.

Sharma, S.K., B. Bolster and K. Dakshinamurti. 1994. Picrotoxin and pentylene tetrazole induced seizure activity in pyridoxine-deficient rats. J Neurol Sci 121: 1–9.

Sharma, S.K. and N.S. Dhalla. 2001. Domoic acid as a tool in molecular pharmacology. *In*: Gupta, S.K. (ed.). Pharmacology and Therapeutics in New Millinium. Narosa Publishing House, New Delhi (India) Chapter 12: 130–137.

Yang, B., R. Strong, S. Sharma, M. Brenneman, K. Malikarjunarao, X. Xi, J.C. Grotta, J. Aronowski and S.I. Savitz. 2010. Therapeutic time window and dose-response of autologous bone marrow mononuclear cells for ischemic stroke. J Neurosci Res 89: 833–839.

Part-II
Charnoly Body as a Drug Discovery Biomarker
Emerging Biotechnologies in Charnoly Body Research
(Personalized Theranostics)

CHAPTER-8

Development of Novel Charnolopharmacotherapeutics in Pharmaceutical Industry by Flow Cytometric Analysis

INTRODUCTION

It is now well-established that CB is formed as a universal biomarker of cell injury in response to intrauterine malnutrition, nicotine, ethanol, and/or ZIKV infection in the NPCs, EPCs, and CPCs, derived from iPPCs (Sharma and Ebadi 2014; Sharma et al. 2014; Sharma 2017a,b). Environmental neurotoxins such as KA and DOM also induce CB formation in the hippocampal CA-3 and dentate gyrus regions of the developing mice to induce dementia as noticed in AD due to CMB (Sharma et al. 1993; Sharma 2014; Sharma 2017c). We reported CB as a novel biomarker in drug addiction (Sharma 2015) and highlighted its clinical significance to evaluate the theranostic potential and toxicity of nanomedicines (Sharma et al. 2013). We also highlighted that MTs prevent CB formation by serving as potent free radical scavengers (Sharma and Ebadi 2014). Recently, we proposed that CB can be used as a novel biomarker of nutritional stress and CMB in AD and in the clinical evaluation of vascular dementia (Sharma et al. 2016; Jagtap et al. 2015). Various parkinsonian neurotoxins such as salsolinol, rotenone, MPTP, MPP$^+$, and 1 benzyl-TIQs induce CB formation in the cultured human DAergic (SK-N-SH and SH-S-Y5Y) neurons and genetic mouse models, whereas antioxidants such as glutathione and MTs prevent CB formation by scavenging free radicals involved in lipid peroxidation and mtDNA oxidation in progressive NDDs.

In this chapter, the clinical significance of flow cytometric analysis of cultured neuronal and hematopoietic cells is described to evaluate CMB and the therapeutic potential of novel charnolopharmacotherapeutics. More specifically, early CB, charnolophagy, CPS, and CS detection, quantitation, and characterization are described to emphasize their clinical significance in novel drug discovery based on

MB as a prerequisite of ICD for normal cellular function and homeostasis to remain healthy.

CB Formation and its Clinical Significance. CB is formed in the most vulnerable cell in response to DPCI due to free radical-induced CMB. The most vulnerable cells during embryonic development are NPCs, EPCs, and CPCs, derived from iPPCs. CB formation in these cells can induce diversified craniofacial abnormalities including microcephaly. Although TEM and SEM are the most suitable and sensitive approaches to determine CB formation in the vulnerable cells, these methods are difficult and cumbersome to perform on a routine basis, because of lengthy processing and analysis time required to perform these experiments. Moreover, these methods are costly. Hence, the most efficient strategy would be light microscopy. But it does not provide precise and quantitative information regarding the severity of disease at the basic molecular level. Hence, it is difficult to quantitatively assess the therapeutic potential of a drug employing light or fluorescence microscopy. Moreover, these methods provide a qualitative estimate of the disease process and/or prognosis. Flow cytometric analysis provides precise and quantitative estimate of biological (immunological, biochemical, physiological) activity in response to specific disease or treatment. Based on physical properties of the cells, we can determine whether they are alive, proliferating, undergoing apoptosis, or necrosis. The most fundamental physical properties employed in flow cytometry to determine apoptosis are the forward scatter and side scatter. Usually, forward scatter is increased when the cells are alive, growing, and proliferating, whereas the side scatter is increased when the granularity is increased. The increased granularity is an early indicator of cellular shrinkage, mtDNA down-regulation, CB formation, apoptosis, and/or necrosis. Thus, quantitative estimation of granularity, forward scatter, and side scatter can provide an overall information regarding number of cells alive or dead in response to linear or log doses of a drug.

Mitochondrial Bioenergetics. The mitochondrial bioenergetics can be determined by estimating $\Delta\Psi$, which is a highly sensitive indicator of mitochondrial function. Fluorescent dyes such as mitoTracker, dihydrofluorescein, rhodamine, and JC-1, can be utilized for the determination of $\Delta\Psi$. The down-regulation of $\Delta\Psi$ is represented by conversion of red fluorescence to green fluorescence. By employing fluorescence activated cell sorting (FACS), we can differentiate mitochondria with functionally intact $\Delta\Psi$ and those with $\Delta\Psi$ collapse. Usually, $\Delta\Psi$ collapse is an early and sensitive indicator of CMB and CB induction. Thus, $\Delta\Psi$ collapse can be considered the most sensitive and early indicator of CB molecular pathogenesis. The MB is compromised by the down-regulation of the mitochondrial genome. We prepared RhO_{mgko} cells by exposing SK-N-SH cells in Dulbecco's Modified Eagle Medium (DMEM) containing 5 ng/l of ethidium bromide in high glucose, sodium bicarbonate, and glutamate medium for 6–8 weeks. At these low concentrations of ethidium bromide, the structural and functional integrity of the nuclear DNA remains intact while the mtDNA is selectively destroyed. In addition to increased 2,3 dihydroxy nonenal and 8-OH, 2dG, the side scatter is increased in the RhO_{mgko} cells. Hence, we used RhO_{mgko} cells as an *in vitro* cellular model of PD, AD, drug addiction, and aging. The RhO_{mgko} cells exhibit increased granularity, indicating that these cells have CMB which triggers CB formation in these cellular models of chronic diseases.

Genetic Susceptibility of mtDNA in CB Formation. The nuclear DNA (nDNA) is double stranded super-helical coil with protection from histones and protamines which maintain its helicity and structural and functional integrity. Moreover, nDNA has introns (noncoding regions) and hence, remains protected from the deleterious effects of free radical attack. Usually epigenetic modification in the nDNA occur by first acetylation of the histones at the lysine residues by enzymes, histone acetylases. The acetylation of histones uncoils the nDNA and exposes the cytosine residues, where DNA methylation occurs at the N-3 position for epigenetic modifications involved in microRNA-mediated post-transcriptional regulation of genes during cell growth, proliferation, differentiation, and development. On the contrary, the mtDNA is highly sensitive, intron less nonhelical coil without any structural and functional support of histones and protamines. Moreover, the mtDNA remains in a hostile microenvironment of free radicals, generated as a byproduct of oxidative phosphorylation in the electron transport chain during ATP synthesis. The mitochondrial electron transport chain is down-regulated by primary, secondary, and tertiary free radical attack to destroy its structural and functional integrity to ultimately trigger CB formation.

DNA Cell Cycle Analysis. Another most sensitive parameter to evaluate DSST-CMB is the analysis of DNA cell cycle. There are 5 different stages of DNA cell cycle including (G0, G1, S, G-2, and M). During G0 and G-1 phase, the cell synthesizes DNA, whereas during the G2-M phase it undergoes mitosis. To execute all these stages of DNA cell cycle, MB play a crucial role. The downregulation of MB induces ATP depletion and CB formation, involved in the inhibition of DNA cell cycle. Hence, CB formation is the most sensitive early pre-apoptotic biomarker of physico-chemical injury. In a highly proliferating cell, the G-2-M peak is significantly enhanced. During apoptosis, the sub-G1 peak appears, which represents fragmented DNA. The increase or decrease in sub-G-1 peak determines the therapeutic potential of a drug under investigation. Usually, we find a linear positive correlation between sub-G-1 peak and the incidence of CB formation in a cell. The incidence of CB formation is increased in a cell population exhibiting increased sub-G-1 peak.

FACS Analysis of CB, Charnolophagy, CPS, and CS. By employing turbo sorting facility in a flow cytometer, we can isolate cells based on the charge on their surface. Usually positively charged cells are attracted towards the negatively charged electrode and the negatively charged cells are attracted towards the positively charged electrode and can be collected in different tubes. The mobility of uncharged cells is not influenced by an external electrical field and they are collected in the center in a test tube. Similarly, cells possessing increased granularity can be sorted and further characterized biochemically by extracting DNA, RNA, and proteins. Usually a free radical attack induces down-regulation of mtDNA, which is oxidized to synthesize 8-OH, 2dG. The normal and RhO$_{mgko}$ cells can be differentiated and sorted by fluorescence imaging. The number of cells exhibiting the red fluorescence and those exhibiting green fluorescence can be quantitatively estimated to determine the therapeutic potential of a drug under clinical trial. We can investigate the EBPT potential of various anticarcinogenic or anti-inflammatory drugs by employing FACS analysis. The normal and RhO$_{mgko}$ cells can be sorted and quantitatively estimated by flow cytometry. The sorted cell can be further subjected to single cell gel electrophoresis (*also named as comet assay*). We developed the multiple fluorochrome comet assay to determine the mtDNA vs nDNA damage in normal and RhO$_{mgko}$ cells. The appearance of green fluorescence comet tails represents mtDNA damage, whereas red fluorescence tails (due to ethidium bromide) represents nDNA damage. Thus, by combining flow cytometry and comet assays, we can quantitatively estimate the therapeutic index and margin of safety of a pharmaceutical agent under investigation.

Flow Cytometric Analysis of CB, Charnolophagy, CPS, and CS. As flow cytometric analysis deals with number of particles and their size in a suspension, it can be utilized for the quantitative estimation of sub-cellular organelles, including intracellular inclusions such as CB, CPS, and CS. The granularity of a cell is increased when the CB, CPS, and CS are formed in response to DPCI. Usually, CB is formed by condensation of multi-lamellar electron-dense membrane (usually penta or hepta-lamellar) stacks. These multi-lamellar electron–dense membrane stacks are phagocytosed by lysosomes to form CPS, which is subsequently transformed to CS, when the phagocytosed CB is hydrolyzed by the lysosomal enzymes. These intracellular organelles can be isolated based on their molecular weight in a sucrose density gradient by differential centrifugation and subsequently, each layer can be quantitated by flow cytometric analysis by multiple fluorochrome analysis with a specific biomarker. In addition, based on the forward scatter, side scatter, and granularity, we can determine the therapeutic potential of a drug under investigation. This unique approach facilitates identifying subcellular binding sites to evaluate the charnolopharmacotherapeutics potential of a drug to either boost or down-regulate the MB. Our primary focus is to induce down-regulation of the cancer stem cell-specific MB for successful clinical management of MDR malignancies. In addition, specific fluorescently-labeled charnolophagy agonists/antagonists may be utilized as sensitive biomarkers to analyze their theranostic potential in NDDs, CVDs, and MDR malignancies by employing flow cytometry. Hence, cellular, molecular, and genetic characterization of DSST-CB, charnolophagy, CPS, and CS employing flow cytometry with multiple fluorochromes, and sorting of different subcellular family of CB, can provide the precise EBPT potential of a drug.

Flow Cytometric and Confocal Microscopic Analysis of CS Dynamics in Health and Disease. The CS dynamics can be quantitatively determined by employing flow cytometry with a sorting facility and confocal microscopy, simultaneously. The CS can be isolated by tissue homogenization and differential centrifugation in sucrose density gradient. The CS-rich layer can be isolated and purified. CS destabilization (permeabilization, sequestration, and fragmentation) can be estimated by labeling with JC-1, Lyso-Tracker, Mito-Tracker, rhodamine, or dihydrofluorescein (DHF). A structurally and functionally stable CS appears as distinct particle in the flow cytometer, whereas destabilized CS exhibits increased granularity and side scatter due to permeabilization and sequestration. Hence, it is easy to distinguish stable vs unstable CS in a flow cytometer. By employing digital fluorescence imaging and confocal microscopy, simultaneously, we can determine SC destabilization more precisely *in vitro* in cultured cells. Initially, cells can be labeled with JC-1 and examined under confocal microscope to determine the number of mitochondria and $\Delta\Psi$. These are highly sensitive parameters of MB. Any physicochemical injury to a most vulnerable cell causes free radical overproduction to trigger $\Delta\Psi$ collapse, implicated in CB molecular pathogenesis. To determine charnolophagy, two

Table 1: Classical and potential charnolopharmacotherapeutics.

Several classical and potential charnolopharmacotherapeutics are proposed as illustrated in the list below. Major classification of DSST *charnopharmacotherapeutics* include:

(a) mtDNA-targeted CB/CPS/CS agonists/antagonists
(b) MB-targeted CB/CPS/CS agonists/antagonists
(c) Cyochrome-P-450 rejuvenators/protectants
(d) CS exocytosis agonists/antagonists
(e) CS endocytosis agonists/antagonists

1. Superoxide dismutase
2. Catalase
3. Transketolase
4. Aromatase
5. Aconitase
6. N-Acetyl Cysteine
7. Glutathione
8. Metallothioneins
9. Hypoxia Inducible Factor-1α
10. Heat Shock Proteins
11. Thioredoxine
12. Thiamine
13. TSPO (18 kDa)
14. Star (32 kDa)
15. TRPCs
16. GAPDH
17. Lactate Dehydrodeganase (LDH)
18. HMG-CO-A Reductase Inhibitors
19. Calcium Channel Antagonists
20. Cholesterol Absorption Inhibitors (Azetinib)
21. Thiamine Pyrophosphatase (TPPase)
22. Transketolase
23. Ubiquinone NADH-Oxidoreductase (Complex-1)
24. Complex-1-V
25. Melatonin
26. Mono amine Oxidase Inhibitors (MAOIs)
27. Xanthine Oxidase Inhibitors
28. Acetyl Choline Esterase Inhibitors
29. Erythropoietin
30. CB Agonists/Antagonists
31. Charnolophagy Agonists/Antagonists
32. CPS Agonists/Antagonists
33. CS Agonists/Antagonists

DSST-Charnolopharmacotherapeutics

34. Glucose Transporter-1-4
35. NOS
36. Hexokinase-1
37. 8-OH, 2dG
38. 4-Hydroxy Nonenal
39. Primary, Secondary and tertiary Free Radical Scavengers/Inhibitors
40. Orlistat
41. Sibutramine
42. Rimonabent
43. Leptins
44. Adiponectin

Table 1 contd. ...

fluorochromes are required: (a) MitoTracker can be used to determine the structural and functional integrity of mitochondria and the (b) LysoTracker can be used to determine the number of lysosomes. These fluorochromes can be merged to determine colocalization of the MitoTracker with the LysoTracker and hence, charnolophagy. Following charnolophagy, a CPS is formed, which is transformed to CS when the phagocytosed CB is hydrolyzed by the lysosomal enzymes. Hence, it exhibits a yellow fluorescence when the digital fluorescent images are merged. To further confirm co-localization, these cells are subjected to flow cytometric analysis by generating a scatterogram. The line of best fit at 45° angle authenticates co-localization. A stable CS appears as a distinct yellow fluorescent particle. CS destabilization (permeabilization, sequestration, and fragmentation) is represented by diffused or absence of fluorescence. The CS dynamics (stabilization/destabilization) can be further confirmed by SEM, TEM, atomic force microscopy, FRET, and by SPR spectroscopy as described in next chapters of this book.

References

Chabenne, A., C. Moon, C. Ojo, A. Khogali, B. Nepal and S. Sharma. 2014. Biomarkers in fetal alcohol syndrome (Recent Update). Biomarkers and Genomic Med 6: 12–22.

Jagtap, A., S. Gawande and S. Sharma. 2015. Biomarkers in vascular dementia. Biomarkers and Genomic Med 7: 43–56.

Sharma, S. 2013. Charnoly body as universal biomarker in nanomedicine. Invited Lecture. International Translational Nanomedicine Conference. Boston, July 26–28.

Sharma, S., A. Rais, R. Sandhu, W. Nel and M. Ebadi. 2013. Clinical significance of metallothioneins in cell therapy and nanomedicine. Internat Jr Nanomed 8: 1477–1488.

Sharma, S., C.S. Moon, A. Khogali, A. Haidous, A. Chabenne, C. Ojo, M. Jelebinkov, Y. Kurdi and M. Ebadi. 2013. Biomarkers of Parkinson's disease (Recent Update). Neurochemistry International 63: 201–229.

Sharma, S. and M. Ebadi. 2013. Antioxidant Targeting in Neurodegenerative Disorders. Ed. I. Laher, Springer Verlag. Germany. Chapter 85, pp. 1–30.

Sharma, S. 2014. Molecular pharmacology of environmental neurotoxins. *In*: Kainic Acid: Neurotoxic Properties, Biological Sources, and Clinical Applications. Nova Science Publishers. New York. pp. 1–47.

Sharma, S. and M. Ebadi. 2014. Charnoly body as a universal biomarker of cell injury. Biomarkers and Genomic Med 6: 89–98.

Sharma, S. 2015. Charnoly body as a novel biomarker in drug addiction invited lecture. 4th International Conference & Exhibition on Drug Addiction. Aug 3–5, Orlando, FL, U.S.A.

Sharma, S., J. Choga, P. Doghor, F.N. Kalala, A. Chauhan, V. Gupta, C. Wright, F. Alison and S. Mathur. 2016. Charnoly body as a novel biomarker of nutritional stress in Alzheimer's disease. Functional Foods in Health and Disease 6: 344–377.

Sharma, S. 2017a. *ZIKV* Disease (Prevention and Cure). Nova Science Publishers, New York, U.S.A.

Sharma, S. 2017b. Fetal Alcohol Spectrum Disorder (Concepts, Mechanisms, and Cure). Nova Science Publishers, New York, U.S.A.

Sharma, S. 2017c. Antioxidants and *mitochondrial bioenergetics*. pp. 81–102. *In*: Debasis Bagchi (ed.). Sustained Energy for Enhanced Human Function and Activity. Elsevier Inc. Chapter 5.

Sharma, S.K., W. Selvamurthy and K. Dakshinamurti. 1993. Effect of environmental neurotoxins in the developing brain. Biometeorology 2: 447–455.

CHAPTER-9

Charnoly Body as a Novel Biomarker in Nanomedicine

INTRODUCTION

Recently, nanotechnology has advanced medicine by developing environmentally-safe, biodegradable, biocompatible, targeted delivery systems/devices, and multifunctional nanocarriers for the safe and effective EBPT of MDR malignancies and other chronic diseases (Sanvicens and Marco 2008; Swami et al. 2012; Sharma 2014). Because of their unique properties, nanomaterials are currently utilized in the pharmaceutical industry. Nanotechnology has emerged as a promising approach by performing diagnosis as well as treatment simultaneously on a single platform (also known as nanotheranostics). Evidence based personalized medicine (EBPM) takes advantage of the genetic information along with phenotypic and environmental factors for healthcare designed specifically to a patient and eliminates the inherent limitations of conventional *"one size fits all"* therapeutic strategy. EBPM provides a unique opportunity to translate scientific knowledge from lab to clinic to diagnose and predict disease to improve patient-specific treatment based on the characteristic features of the disease and facilitates developing novel nanotheranostic strategies (Kim et al. 2013). Furthermore, EBPM takes advantage of chronopharmacological as well as charnolopharmacological aspects for theranostic applications (Clairambault 2009; Ohdo et al. 2010; Sharma 2017). Owing to limited studies and experimental protocols available for the risk assessment, these studies have also raised serious concerns of toxicity of some NPs and their negative impact on environment (Gajewicz et al. 2012). Above all, nanotechnology has gained considerable interest and momentum as a versatile strategy for novel drug discovery, drug delivery, clinical diagnosis, and treatment, simultaneously (nanotheranostics) to accomplish the ultimate goals of EBPT (Mura and Couvreur 2012). Nanotheranostics hold great promise because it provides excellent opportunity to monitor *in vivo* PKs for validating the prognosis. Hence, further efforts to practice nanotheranostics for EBPM will optimize treatment as it covers individual variability, early detection, economical therapeutic approach, and prognosis, allowing screening of patients who respond better to therapy. These unique properties make nanotheranostics attractive to evolve EBPM for achieving minimum discomfort, optimum safety, and maximum therapeutic benefits. Therefore, the solution of several unresolved problems of modern medicine may be accomplished by the development of nanotheranostics. A recent report provided an inventory of nanomedicines currently available to accomplish EBPT (Etheridge et al. 2013). Food and Drug Administration (FDA) has approved > 250 nanomedicines and several others are at various stages of clinical trials and approval. Therefore, innovations in nanotechnology will augment novel drug discovery and efficient drug delivery in future.

In this chapter, recently-developed drugs delivery systems including covalent conjugation of drugs with polyethylene glycol (PEGylation), block copolymers, dendrimers and aptamers, radiolabeled liposomes, chitosans and alginates, gellan/xanthan gels, drug delivery nanodevices, quantum dots (Q-Dots) for cell tracking, and siRNA, microRNA, MTs, CB, charnolophagy, CPS, and CS as novel drug discovery biomarkers and therapeutic targets are discussed to accomplish the targeted, safe, and effective EBPT. The chapter is focused primarily on the novel strategies of drug discovery and drug delivery systems for better, safe, economical, early, and effective treatment of chronic diseases by adopting nanotheranostic strategies to accomplish the ultimate-goal of EBPM by developing novel DSST charnolopharmacotherapeutics. This chapter also briefly describes CB, CPS, and CS as potential nanotheranostic biomarkers and drug discovery targets to accomplish EBPT.

Drug Delivery. Epidemiological studies have shown that out of 12 billion injections, improper drug deliveries cause > 100 million adverse reactions and > 20 million infections every year (Kwon et al. 2012). Hence, efficient drug delivery systems are extremely important in personalized medicine. Nanotechnology has enabled improvements in multi-functionality drug delivery systems to improve EBPT. A descriptive overview comprising stimulus-responsive polymers, smart polymers, their biomedical applications, and major obstacles to clinical translation is now available (Kwon et al. 2012; Hansen et al. 2013). However, the basic molecular mechanism of infusion-related adverse effects of nanomedicines is yet to be established. A considerable biological variability in adverse effects with complement activation has been noticed. Hence, further research is needed to determine the exact physiological link between immunological mechanisms and genetic predisposition to hypersensitivity (Moghimi et al. 2012). Clinically-significant genetic polymorphism in immune-responsive genes is currently being explored to expedite FDA approval and reduce the cost of healthcare system. Recently, freeze-dried lettuce cells expressing vaccine biopharmaceuticals were developed to provide protection from gastric acids in the stomach but are released in the circulatory system upon digestion of the cell wall by the intestinal microflora. This novel approach of drug delivery provides both mucosal as well as systemic immunity against harmful toxins of bacteria, viruses, and protozoa. Similarly type-1 diabetes and hemophilia can be clinically-managed by oral delivery of auto-antigens. Pro-insulin or extendin-4 can be expressed in plant cells to control blood glucose levels just like exogenous insulin administration. This approach provides an effective strategy to control infections or inherited diseases by avoiding cumbersome purification steps, refrigeration, and sterile conditions. Further innovations in this direction will facilitate development of biocompatible, biodegradable, environmentally-safe, and targeted drug delivery systems (Zhang et al. 2012). Particularly, hydrophilic molecules for transdermal drug delivery for skin care have been developed by estimating quantitative structure-permeability relationships (QSPR) and mechanistic models (Chen et al. 2013). However, QSPR models do not provide the exact estimate of skin permeability of hydrophobic solutes. Hence, further research is needed to improve skin permeability. Furthermore, linkers have shown promise as structural components of recombinant fusion proteins and stable and bioactive fusion proteins. Naturally-occurring multi-domain proteins can be used for constructing flexible, rigid, and cleavable linkers to obtain desirable PKs and controlled release of clinically-significant biomolecules *in vivo*.

It has been demonstrated that various methods used to incorporate proteins into a matrix may cause denaturation of the functional groups; however, the pro-drugs remain biologically–inactive before undergoing biotransformation *in vivo* (Vig et al. 2013). Since the pro-drug may change the bio-distribution, it is highly prudent to know its toxicity (by detecting CB formation, charnolophagy, and CS destabilization) and efficacy during preclinical development. In this respect, natural and synthetic amino acids may provide better physicochemical properties. Hence, amino acids as pro-drugs are currently being developed for improved solubility, permeability, sustained release, i.v. infusion, drug targeting, and drug stability.

PEGylation and Drug Delivery. Generally, PEG is used for the conjugation of biomolecules for pharmaceutical and nanotechnological applications. PEGylation provides 3 basic advantages: (i) nonimmunogenicity, (ii) less entrapment of NPs in the reticuloendothelial system (RES), and (iii) slow and sustained release of drugs at the target site. Hence it is now possible to design polymers for theranostic applications by PEGylation. The PEGylating procedures are now well-established. The modification of peptides and proteins can be achieved by PEGylation to protect antigenic and immunogenic peptides, receptor-mediated uptake of RES, and prevent degradation by proteolytic enzymes. Various functional groups can be incorporated by PEGylation to conjugate peptides and proteins. PEGylation also increases the size of the polypeptides to reduce fast renal clearance by changing their PKs (Roberts et al. 1997). It is known that the anticancer drug, paclilaxel (PTX), has reduced water solubility and acts as a substrate for P-glycoprotein (P-gp) and cytochrome-P450. A recent study on rats demonstrated the potential of PEGylated-NPs for oral paclitaxel delivery (Zabaleta et al. 2012). PEG 2000 (PTX-NP2), PEG 6000 (PTX-NP6), and PEG 10,000 (PTX-NP10) were used for loading PTX. The intestinal permeability of PTX increased 3–7 times in the jejunum by PEGylation compared to commercial product, taxol. The sustained therapeutic plasma levels for at least 48 hrs. A maximum oral bioavailability (70%) was achieved with PTX-NP2, suggesting bio-adhesive properties and inhibitory effects of PEGylated NPs on P-gp and cytochrome P450. We reported that nonspecific induction of CB formation, charnolophagy, and CS destabilization in highly proliferating cells induces myelosuppression (anemia, thrombocytopenia, neutropenia), GIT distress, alopecia, hepatotoxicity, pulmonary and renal fibrosis, neurotoxicity, and infertility during treatment of MDR malignancies including breast cancer, ovarian cancer, uterine cancer, prostate cancer, and lung cancer. PEGylation of anticancer drugs enhances target delivery in the cancer cells and provides better nanotheranostic potential to accomplish the targeted, safe, and effective EBPT (Sharma et al. 2013).

Recently, drug targeting was accomplished using a single NPs platform for the clinical management of cancer and AD (Droumaguet et al. 2012). Particularly, polyisoprenoyl Gemcitabine conjugates that self-assemble as NPs showed promise for cancer chemotherapy (Maksimenko et al. 2013). Furthermore, drug transport to the brain can be improved by using targeted NPs (Olivier 2005). Hence, protein linkers with characteristic property, design, and functionality were developed for the drug delivery to accomplish targeted, safe and effective EBPT (Chen et al. 2013). Further developments were made by improving the design, functionalization, and biodegradable/biocompatible polymer-based nanocarriers (Nicolas et al. 2013). A simple procedure to synthesize multi-compartment micelles based on biocompatible poly (3-hydroxyalkanoate) was developed (Babinot et al. 2013; Nicholas and Peppas 2012). Furthermore, clinically-significant hydrogels were developed to determine the extent of water absorption and permeation of solutes within the matrix as drug and cell carriers for constructing tissue engineering matrices (Hoffman 2002).

Although NPs can be used for site-specific drug delivery and medical imaging, these are localized preferentially in the RES following systemic delivery. The most significant organs of the RES are lungs, liver, and spleen, where NPs undergo phagocytosis and/or endocytosis to be eliminated from the biological system within minutes involving CB pharmacodynamics. Hence, amphiphilic di-blocks and multi-block co-polymers-conjugated NPs were developed to prevent opsonization and recognition by macrophages (Gref et al. 1995). These NPs possess a hydrophilic PEG coating and a biodegradable core to encapsulate hydrophobic drugs such as lidocaine. These NPs have significantly reduced RES accumulation, can be freeze-dried, reconstituted, and retain shelf stability. Although premature systemic clearance of NPs is reduced by modifying surfaces with PEGylation, it may also influence the normal performance of NPs as a drug carrier (Lin et al. 2010). Hence, alternative strategies including substitute polymers, conditional removal of PEG, and surface modification to overcome limitations of PEG were developed (Vorup-Jensen and Peer 2012; Amoozgar and Yeo 2012). For example, surface modified by polyethylene oxide (PEO) can avoid the physiological defense depending on the particle size, extent of systemic circulation, and selectivity for target sites in the body (Stolnik et al. 1995). The theranostic success of these NPs can be established by molecular imaging of CB, charnolophagy, and CS in normal and diseased conditions.

Chitosans and Alignates. Chitosans were discovered as novel drug delivery vehicles for theranostic applications. Chitosans NPs are suitable drug delivery vehicles because of their biocompatibility, biodegradability, non-immunogenicity, and flexibility as they can be modified and used for loading protein drugs, gene drugs, and anticancer drugs, via oral, nasal, i.v., and ocular routes, whereas alginates are bio-adhesive polymers and can be used for selective drug delivery to mucosal tissues. Wang et al. (2011) provided an excellent report on chitosan NPs, including methods of preparation, characterization, modification, *in vivo* metabolism, and clinical applications. Alginates can be synthesized from the naturally-occurring brown algae (Kelp) and can be used for trapping and/or delivery of drugs in the form of a matrix (Gombotz and Wee 2012). Alginates are composed of linear unbranched polysaccharides having 1,4-β-d-manuronic acid and L-α-glucronic acid residues which may vary in composition and sequence and are in the form of a block which can be cross-linked by the addition of divalent cations. Proteins, DNA, and cells can be incorporated into the alginate matrix while maintaining biological activity. Moreover, the pore size, degradation rate, and release kinetics can be regulated by selecting suitable alginate and coating material. Gels of different morphologies were developed with macrobeads (> 1 mm) and microbeads (< 0.2 mm). Alginates were used to prepare *in situ* gelling systems for ophthalmic applications and for protecting the wounds. These properties of alginates have directed their application as protein delivery vectors for theranostic applications. In addition, alginate/chitosan-coated nanoemulsions were developed for oral insulin delivery (Li et al. 2013). The alginate-containing dispersion was used by adding calcium chloride and chitosan based on poly-electrolyte cross-linking, suggesting the clinical potential of alginate/chitosan nanoemulsion for an oral delivery of polypeptides and proteins such as insulin. The positively charged $-NH_3^+$ of chitosan NPs and negatively-charged $-COO^-$ groups of alginates are highly suitable for developing coating materials for mucosal vaccines (Li et al. 2008). Coating onto bovine serum albumin (BSA)-loaded chitosan NPs with sodium alginate increased stability and prevented desorption of antigens in the GIT system for at least 2 hrs to meet the requirement of mucosal vaccine. Furthermore, to augment differentiation of human fetal osteoblasts, gellan/xanthan gels along with chitosan NPs were developed for the delivery of basic fibroblast growth factor (bFGF) and bone morphogenetic protein-7 (BMP-7) in a dual growth factor delivery system (Dyondi et al. 2013). The sustained release of growth factors from the NPs-loaded gels facilitated improved cell proliferation and differentiation. Significantly increased alkaline phosphatase and calcium deposition were noticed indicating that growth factors encapsulation within NPs and gels are clinically-significant for bone regeneration. The gellan/xanthan gels also demonstrated antibacterial activity against common pathogens involved in implant rejection. The detailed method and structure of gels were described to improve their permeability and bioavailability that can be incorporated into novel drug delivery systems to accomplish theranostic capability (Bhoyar et al. 2012).

Liposomal Drug Delivery. Drug delivery in the tumor can be accomplished at much higher concentrations as compared to normal tissue by encapsulation in the biocompatible and biodegradable liposomes. Moreover, liposomal-mediated passive as well as active drug delivery can minimize the adverse effects of anti-carcinogenic drugs and augments their therapeutic potential. Tumor targeting can be achieved by identifying specific receptor ligands or antibodies onto the surface of the liposome, or by developing stimulus-sensitive drug carriers such as acid or enzyme-induced drug release. In addition to tumor cells, the tumors also contain non-tumor cells such as endothelial cells, fibroblasts, pericytes, stromal cells, mesenchymal cells, innate and adaptive immune cells which can be targeted to prevent tumor cell growth. The non-tumor cells can also be targeted to prevent tumor cell proliferation. The liposomal NPs can be used to deliver anti-carcinogenic drugs to the tumor to control nonspecific uptake, interaction with blood components, and toxicity. The primary objective of liposomal encapsulation is to target anticancer drugs to the tumor endothelial neovasculature, macrophages, and pericytes within the tumor (Zhao and Rodriguez 2013). To target adhesion protein including focal adhesions and adherens junction, vinculin, a polymer-lipid nanoparticle (NPL) system was recently developed (Wang et al. 2013). The PLNs have an average size of 106 nm, positive charge, and lower encapsulation efficiency compared to poly (lactic-co-glycolic) acid (PGLA) NPs, with sustained release of BSA, while PGLA NPs exhibit an initial burst release. The anti-vinculin-conjugated PLNs could carry the drug to the cytoplasm of the fibroblasts and adhere it to the fibronectin-fibrin complex. The unconjugated PLNs demonstrated improved gene transfection efficiency. Moreover, PLNs could be modified by using different targeting ligands for studying the basic molecular mechanism of drug delivery in specific subcellular organelles such as lysosomes, peroxisomes, and CS to evaluate their structural and functional stability in health and disease.

Enhanced Permeability and Retention (EPR) Effect. There is a significant difference between passive tumor targeting and EPR effect. Passive tumor targeting (such as X-ray contrast agents) has a retention period of few minutes, whereas EPR of NPs requires days to weeks and occurs due to extravasation of macromolecules or NPs through tumor neovasculature. Recently, methods of augmenting EPR effect for efficient drug delivery in the tumor with improved therapeutic potential of drugs (including nitroglycerin, angiotensin-1 converting enzymes (ACE) inhibitors) were developed to accomplish better therapeutic effect and reduced systemic toxicity (Maeda et al. 2013). The EPR effect-based delivery of NPs is clinically-significant for tumor-targeted imaging using fluorescent or radionuclide labeling with a potential to accomplish the targeted, safe, and effective EBPT.

Chronopharmacology in EBPT. Recent advances in drug delivery methods evolved new concepts of spatiotemporal chronophamacology and DSST charnolopharmacology which involve drug delivery in a pulsatile manner. Chronotherapy is clinically-significant where sustained release of drugs is undesirable and the drugs are extremely toxic (Kim et al. 2013; Clairambault 2009). For example, certain anticancer drugs can cause serious adverse effects in conventional and sustained release protocols. The circadian pacemaker is localized in the suprachiasmatic nuclei and regulates biological processes including the sleep-wake cycle (Bisht 2011). The circadian genes regulate the sleep-wake cycle to maintain normal physiology and behavior. Hence, the biological circadian rhythm needs to be considered in designing the pulsatile drug delivery (PDD) of the hormones, neuropeptides, and cytokines that exert their physiological or pharmacological action in an oscillatory rhythm. Several FDA-approved chronopharmacological agents are now available to provide maximum therapeutic effect with minimum adverse effects because 24 hrs rhythms are observed for the pathophysiology of chronic diseases. However, DSST charnolopharmaceuticals need to be developed to accomplish targeted, safe, and effective EBPT. Hence, drug delivery microsystems may facilitate accomplishing EBPT. The efficacy and toxicity of therapeutic agents would depend on the exact dose and time of delivery which will also be affected by charnolopharmacokinetic and charnolopharmacodynamic properties of the drug. The charnolotherapeutic efficacy and toxicity of the pulsatile drug delivery systems can be authenticated by quantitatively estimating CB formation, charnolophagy, and CS stabilization/destabilization as described in the previous chapter. In addition, therapeutic effect of the charnolopharmacological agent will be under the influence of circadian rhythm which is influenced by biochemical, physiological, and behavioral mechanisms in the biological system. Hence, a novel nanotechnology for delivering drugs in a rhythmic manner is being developed employing micro pumps to minimize the chances of drug-resistance in conventional and sustained release systems. The primary objective is to determine the exact nature of the circadian rhythm, which serves as an indicator of drug release from the nanodevice. Currently, there is a dire need of suitable NPs or nanodevices which could be used on a routine basis for EBPT. These devices need to be economical, biocompatible, biodegradable, and responsive to a rhythmic biomarker such as CB and CS. Moreover, drug safety can be evaluated for personalized treatment. Recently, progress was made in the PDD systems which can treat diseases effectively such as insulin-resistant type-2 diabetes. Various therapeutic agents including proteins, hormones, analgesics, and other pharmacological agents are currently being investigated by using these nanodevices. The most important issues include biocompatibility and toxicity of polymers, response to external stimuli, ability to accomplish required serum drug levels, shelf life, and reproducibility. The basic advantage of PDD nanodevices is that the release of the therapeutic agent can be controlled as and when needed to prevent CB formation, charnolophagy, and CS destabilization, involved in molecular pathogenesis of NDDs, CVDs, and chronic MDR malignancies.

Oral Immunotherapy (OIT). The therapeutic efficacy of orally-administered drugs is reduced due to poor localization, low pH, and fast intestinal flow. Moreover, orally-administered drugs are influenced by peristalsis in the GIT system which accelerates drug elimination from the biological system. The acidic environment in the stomach can easily degrade the drug. Particularly, polypeptide drugs are degraded in the stomach. In addition, the drug experiences first pass effect while passing through the hepatic portal system to be metabolized by liver cytochrome P-450 isoenzymes (i.e., CYP-2D6, CYP-3A4, CYP-2D19). The drug may be acetylated, glucronated, or sulphated in the liver to become water soluble and excreted through the renal system. It is important to highlight that nicotine and alcohol abuse compromises the MB of various body organs including liver and brain by enhancing CB formation, charnolophagy inhibition, and by CPS and CS destabilization to ultimately cause hepatoencephalopathies, involving early morbidity and mortality. Furthermore, hippocampal atrophy occurs due to CB formation in the CA-3 and dentate gyrus regions in MDDs, AD, schizophrenia, and chronic ethanol abuse. Ethanol-induced Wernicke Korsakov's syndrome accompanied with memory impairments and confabulations are ameliorated by thamine administration, which provides neuroprotection by inhibiting free radicals-induced CB formation, charnolophagy, and CS destabilization (permeabilization, sequestration, and fragmentation) in alcohol abuse and AD.

Since various proteins, enzymes, peptide neurotransmitters, and hormones (such as growth hormone and insulin) are proteolyzed when administered orally; microneedles or micro or milli-osmotic pumps were developed for drug delivery in inflammatory diseases such as rheumatoid arthritis. By using microneedles and mini-osmotic pumps, a drug at low dose can be administered on a chronic basis. OIT seem to be well tolerated for food allergies which impact nearly 5% of the US population (Kulis and Burks 2013). To diminish the toxicity associated with oral drug delivery, novel NPs are being developed for controlled drug release, improved adhesion, increased tissue penetration, and selective intestinal targeting. Currently, adjuvants such as TLR9 agonists in combination with OIT are being developed for non-allergic herbal preparations. Several issues, such as optimal dosing, length of treatment, tolerance, and basic molecular mechanisms of protection from OIT are being explored (Chirra and Desai 2012). Particularly, amino acids are being used as pro-drugs to improve solubility, permeability, constant release, i.v. delivery, target ability, and stability of the drugs. The oral bioavailability of drugs was improved by developing enterically-coated tablets, capsules, and liposomes. Further developments are in progress for amino acid pro-drug delivery safely through the GIT system.

Although the role of drug transporters in the liver and kidney was investigated, there is limited information regarding the importance of influx and efflux transporters in the intestine (Wu and Benet 2005). Hence, drug transporters in PKs (drug absorption and bioavailability) have gained considerable interest. Various systems including *in vivo* experimental models, *in situ* organ perfusion, *in vitro* tissue slices, and cell lines in culture were developed to determine the effect of intestinal transporters on drug delivery. Recently biopharmaceutical drug disposition classification system (BDDCS) was introduced to determine the exact role of intestinal transporters and their enzymes on the oral drug PKs (Estudante et al. 2013). However, further studies are needed in this direction.

Microfabrication for Controlled Drug Delivery. Recently, microdevices for controlled drug delivery were developed using integrated circuits and nanosensors for designing automatic drug delivery systems with appropriate shape, size, flexibility, reservoir volume, and surface characteristics to improve nanotheranostics (Fernandes and Gracis 2012). Self-folded polymeric containers were developed to encapsulate molecules, polypeptides, proteins, bacteria, fungi, and cells. In addition, the oral, dermal and implantable reservoir-based drug delivery microsystems were improvised for increased drug stability and sustained release (Zhang et al. 2012). The reservoir-based systems for targeted drug delivery can accomplish zero order, pulsatile, and/or demand dosing as compared to conventional sustained drug delivery systems. Improved versions of these devices are now available for ocular applications as well (Peppas 2013).

NPs and CS Endocytosis in Nanotheranostics. Recent research was directed on elucidating the basic molecular mechanism of receptor-mediated endocytosis to determine delivery of NPs drug carriers to a specific cell *in vivo* (Xu et al. 2013). In addition, strategies to improve spatiotemporal cell-signaling to enhance tissue repair were described (Ekenseair et al. 2013). Indeed, the NPs-based drug-delivery (NDD) systems improved the efficacy of drugs for theranostic applications. Hence, the therapeutic potential of NDD systems increased with significantly reduced drug toxicity, improved bioavailability and circulation time, and controlled drug release (Probst et al. 2013).

The treatment of cancer with NDD vehicle will require improved knowledge of NPs, CS endocytosis/exocytosis, and their PKs *in vivo*. In this respect, quantum dots (Q dots) offered potential as these have suitable surface chemistry to allow incorporation in any NDD vehicle with minimal impact on the overall characteristics and excellent optical properties for real time monitoring of drug release at the cellular and systemic level. Although clinical application of Q-dots in NDD vehicles is restricted due to the former's potential toxicity as CB inducers, their core is highly suitable as organic drug carriers or inorganic contrast agents such as gold and magnetic NPs for photo-thermal therapy and magneto-transfection, respectively (Brannon-Peppas and Blanchette 2004). Further investigations are being made by avoiding the RES and utilizing the EPR effect for achieving tumor-specific targeting and nanotheranostics. In addition, antibody-targeted therapy and anti-angiogenic drugs are being developed by utilizing NPs composed of degradable as well as non-degradable polymers to accomplish the targeted, safe, and effective EBPT.

NPs in EBPT. NPs offer advantages as theranostic agents due to small size, flexibility, increased surface to volume ratio, surface modification with multivalent ligands to enhance molecular targeting of drugs. Recent reports provided detailed information regarding the interaction of NPs with biological systems to facilitate their use in diagnosis, imaging, and drug delivery for nanotheranostic applications (Vizirianakis and Fatouros 2012; Wieland and Fussenegger 2013). Currently, nanotheranostics evolved to regulate genes at the transcriptional and translational level, detect cancer cells, regulate T-cell proliferation, and maintain blood glucose levels. In addition, an implant can detect blood urea levels and can restore normal levels. Another implant was developed for artificial insemination that injects bull spermatocytes in the bovine ovary particularly during ovulation period by detecting luteinizing hormone levels. It may be possible to treat any disease at the cellular and molecular level by detecting specific metabolic parameters by improvising charnolosomic analyses.

A recent review identified nanomedicines that are being used in the treatment of cancer prior to FDA approval (Kim et al. 2012; Venditto and Szoka 2013). Anticancer treatment involving polymers, liposomes, and monoclonal antibodies as well as clinical trials were described (Liu 2013). The primary focus is on the analysis of NPs containing camptothecin derivatives, including two polymers and liposomal formulation. These nanoformulations had difficult time for FDA approval because presently-developed nanocarriers provide limited improvement in their overall performance. Irrespective of these limitations, the nanotheranostics approach to accomplish the targeted, safe, and effective EBPT seems quite promising.

Microneedles in Nanomedicine. Although microneedles were introduced as drug-delivery vehicles several years ago, their clinical significance was realized in mid-1990's with the development of nanotechnology which developed microneedles to enhance skin permeability, drug-coated and polymer microneedles to dissolve off skin and hallow microneedles for drug infusion into the skin (Ryu et al. 2012). Currently microneedles are used to deliver therapeutic agents, small molecules, and protein drugs. Hallow microneedles are used for the delivery of influenza vaccine, whereas solid microneedles for cosmetic applications and for ophthalmic treatments. The successful application of microneedles depends on their proper insertion and infusion into the skin, skin recovery after removal, drug stability, safety and efficacy, storage capacity and delivery, without any pain or discomfort (such as local or systemic irritation and infection) to the patient. Further developments in microneedle nanotechnology may improve nanotheranostics to accomplish the targeted, safe, and effective EBPT.

Nanothranostics and EBPT. Recently, nanotechnology improvised diagnostic and prognostic capability, and targeted drug delivery at the space occupying lesion for EBPT (Swant et al. 2012). Although EBPT seems impressive, the anticancer treatment compromised prognosis due to the absence of therapeutic response, drug resistance, relapse, and adverse effects of inadequate and non-targeted drug delivery. However, NPs revolutionized EBPT and enabled stem cell tracking for the future development of nanotheranostics. It is now known that epigenetic changes are involved in the molecular pathogenesis of cancer, and hence may further improve RBPT (Mura and Couvreur 2012). In addition to therapeutic potential, the theranostic NPs are capable of *in vivo* non-invasive imaging. Particularly, optical imaging with these NPs has distinct advantages such as sensitivity, safety, real time imaging for earlier screening, detection, treatment, and better prognosis which makes nanotheranostics attractive to develop EBPT for achieving maximum benefit and minimum adverse effects (Janowski et al. 2012). Recently, polymeric immunomicelles have been developed as nanocarriers with a potential to diagnosis, targeted drug therapy, imaging, and assessing the clinical response for the effective and efficient clinical management of chronic diseases. Hence, multi-modality immunomicelles were developed as novel nanocarriers for the personalized chemotherapy of cancer (Nicolini et al. 2012).

Although cell-based therapy has shown great promise, limited information regarding their exact fate *in vivo* and precise theranostic potential remain uncertain. The recent development of inorganic and organic NPs may evolve for tracking transplanted stem cells *in vivo*. Hence, nucleic acid programmable microarrays are being developed using cell-free systems to generate proteins as an alternative to fluorescence-labeled approach employing nanotechnology to analyze protein function and protein-protein interaction to accomplish the safe and effective EBPT. For instance, the limitations of fluorescence detection can be prevented by using quartz microcircuit nanogravimetry. Hence, protein microarrays using different gene proteins were developed. Similarly, liposomes which selectively localize in the tumor and transport drug as well as the imaging agent to accomplish EBPT were developed (Petersen et al. 2012). In addition, radiolabeled liposomes may be used for evaluating *in vivo* performance, and in the development of liposomal drugs. Moreover, multimodality fusion imaging may provide non-invasive PKs of liposomes in humans. Further developments in liposomal radiolabeling and fusion imaging will facilitate EBPT. Recently, theranostic NPs were utilized in chemotherapy, photodynamic and photothermal therapy, and siRNA therapy of cancer (Daka and Peer 2012). Thus, instead of conventional generic treatment, patient-centered therapies are now being developed employing nanotechonolgical approaches for targeted drug delivery combined with genomics and understanding of diseases at the molecular level. To accomplish the primary objectives of EBPT, radiolabeled liposomes for imaging and siRNA for therapeutic trials were evolved. However safe, specific, and effective strategies need to be developed. Colloidal NPs can be used to examine the tissue and cell distribution profile of anticancer agents. The primary objective is to enhance the anti-tumor efficacy and reduce the systemic side effects. NPs can also be useful for the selective delivery of oligonucleotides to tumor cells. The exact knowledge about the interactions of NPs with biological system will improve their design for diagnosis, imaging, and targeted drug delivery. Certain NPs can reverse MDR during cancer chemotherapy (Brigger et al. 2002). Hence, NPs toxicity, fabrication challenges, and regulatory and ethical issues were emphasized for the targeted, safe, and effective EBPT (Zhang et al. 2013).

Pharmaceutical Nanocarriers. In general, liposomes, micelles, nonoemulsions, NPs, chitosans and alginates, gellan/xanthan gels, and dendrimers and aptamers are utilized to enhance systemic drug stability for selective localization at the SOLs with compromised vasculature. Specific targeting with increased intracellular penetration with cell-penetrating molecules as peptides and contrast properties for direct visualization *in vivo* was achieved by stimulus-sensitive drug release employing immune-liposomes (Torchilin 2006). Multifunctional nanocarriers can enhance the theranostic potential whereas amphiphilic copolymers serve as micellar drug carriers (Rosler et al. 2001). Hence, chemical modification of the amphiphilic copolymer building blocks-based drug delivery system were developed to enhance stability of micellar drug carriers or block copolymer containing specific ligands that allow targeted drug delivery or by improving micellar drug carriers by addition of auxiliary agents. The spatiotemporal control over drug release could be accomplished by improving the channel kinetics of metal NPs (Kim et al. 2013). Block copolymer micelles having polyethylene oxide can be used as hydrophilic blocks, whereas poly L-amino acid micelles can be used as hydrophobic blocks. Hydrophobic drugs including doxorubicin into block copolymer micelles with prolonged systemic circulation times. The block copolymers accumulate slowly at the solid tumors and have therapeutic potential in cancer treatment just like long-circulating liposomes. Basic knowledge regarding *in vivo* degradation and cellular and tissue responses which determines the compatibility of these biodegradable microspheres is extremely important for theranostic applications. Hence, PLA and PGLA microspheres carrying bone morphogenetic protein (BPM) and leuprlin acetate and their interactions in the eye, CNS, and lymphoid tissue for vaccine development and controlled drug release were developed (Shive and Anderson 1997).

Miniaturized Drug Delivery Systems. It is important to have economical microdevices for transdermal and subcutaneous drug delivery (Ochoa et al. 2012). Miniaturized drug delivery systems were developed by employing osmotic principles of pumping. These devices can be simple microneedles arrays to complex systems equipped with micro-pumps, micro-reservoirs, sensors, and electronic circuits for remote-controlled nano-drug delivery (Stevenson et al. 2012). However, osmotic micro-pumps do not require electrical power, provide zero order drug release kinetics, and can be used for a wide range of applications for a prolonged period and are not influenced by first pass effects and GIT transit time (Herrlich et al. 2012). These mico-pumps have 3 components: osmotic agent, solvent, and drug. Water from the body fluids serves as a solvent and drug as an osmotic agent in a single compartment system. The two compartment system employs a separate osmotic agent and the multi-compartment system utilizes the solvent, drug, and osmotic agent, separately. Further innovative improvements are needed for agents used during gene therapy or agents which cannot be administered orally, topically, or i.v. (Meng and Hoang 2012). These noninvasive approaches bypass physiological barriers, release appropriate dose, and ensure bioavailability of drug for the required duration to accomplish maximum efficacy. Recently, micro-electromechanical systems (MEMS) was developed for radiolabeling, nanomedicine delivery for cancer treatment, and sustained ocular drug delivery (Li et al. 2012). Further improvements of MEMS actuators, valves, and other microstructures for on-demand dosing may provide better performance. Therefore, a regulated valve was developed for the intra-thecal delivery of insulin and other drugs using MEMS (Li et al. 2012).

In addition to bolus and the continuous flow delivery systems, a piezoelectronically-controlled silicon valve, equipped with pressure sensors was developed for controlled drug release from a mechanically-pressurized reservoir. These micro-devices have clinical significance in sensorineural hearing loss accompanied with equilibrium disorders and tinnitus by employing regenerative therapeutic approaches for the targeted and sustained drug delivery (Pararas et al. 2012). These micro-devices will repair and regenerate hearing and CNS disorders of aging patients for which there is currently no better treatment.

Recent Studies with Q-Dot NPs. To determine the PKs and theranostic potential of bone marrow-derived mononuclear stem cells (MNCs) in an experimental model of AIS, we labeled these cells with Cd/Se quantum dots (Q-Dots) NPs (Brenneman et al. 2010). Digital fluorescence imaging and confocal microscopic analyses provided evidence that MNCs exhibit preferential chemotaxis in the peri-infarct region and are exponentially-eliminated as a function of time, suggesting a therapeutic window of MNCs-mediated neuronal recovery (Yang et al. 2011). Subsequently, we provided a detailed description of cell-based therapy in AIS and discovered that MNCs provide neuroprotection by modulating microglia in a cell culture model of AIS (oxygen and glucose deprivation) and elucidated the basic molecular mechanism of MNCs-mediated neuroprotection (Sharma et al. 2010; Mishra et al. 2011). Treatment of MNCs in AIS rats increased brain regional IL-10, which led us to propose that cerebral cortex neurons are protected through MNCs-mediated paracrine release of an anti-inflammatory cytokine, IL-10, by binding to its specific receptor. Furthermore, IL-10 provides anti-inflammatory action by activating upstream PI-3 kinase and downstream STAT3-mediated signaling (Sharma et al. 2011). We discovered for the first time the presence of IL-10 receptors on the murine cortical cultured neurons. These findings were confirmed by examining the effect of transcather injection of MNCs on the viability and cytokine release of MNCs. We determined that MNCs are highly primitive and can readily release anti-inflammatory cytokines such as IL-10 and other neurotrophic factors to provide therapeutic benefit in AIS and other NDDs (Khoury et al. 2010).

Several other molecular mechanism(s) of MNCs-mediated neuroprotection remain unexplored. *In vivo* molecular imaging with ^{18}FdG and ^{18}F-DOPA as PET imaging biomarkers, strongly supported MTs as CB antagonists in stem cells as potential antioxidant neuroprotective Zn^{2+}-binding proteins in progressive NDDs (Sharma and Ebadi 2012). Hence, MTs induction in stem cells can enhance their therapeutic benefit in chronic NDDs (Sharma and Ebadi 2011a). Based on these novel findings, we investigated the pharmacological properties of NPs employing MTs and CB as universal biomarkers of neuroprotection/neurodegeneration (Sharma and Ebadi 2011b). We reported that MTs provide neuroprotection as potent CB antagonists by serving as potent free radical scavengers (Sharma et al. 2013). Further studies in this direction will not only promote nanotheranostics but also provide the precise safety and toxicity profile of NPs for successful EBPT.

α-Synuclein Index (SI) and Charnolophagy Index as Biomarkers of Novel Drug Discovery. We discovered SI and charnolophagy index as early and sensitive biomarkers of neurodegenerative α-synucleinopathies (Sharma et al. 2003; Sharma 2017). MTs inhibit α-synucleinopathies by inhibiting CB formation, α-synuclein index, charnolophagy index (a ratio of charnolophagy vs autophagy), by acting as free radical scavengers, and as anti-inflammatory agents. Hence in addition to CB; MTs, charnolophagy index, and SI may be used as novel drug discovery biomarkers for theranostic applications. Furthermore, CS destabilization was correlated with the SI. There was a linear positive correlation between CS destabilization and SI with a correlation coefficient of 0.92. CS destabilization was increased as a function of increase in SI and charnolophagy index. These molecular changes induce the release of toxic substances from the destabilized CPS and CS through permeabilization, sequestration, and fragmentation to trigger neurodegenerative apoptosis. MTs induction reduces SI as well as CPS and CS destabilization and charnolophagy index to provide neuroprotection. There was a positive linear correlation between:

(i)   CS destabilization and SI
(ii) CB formation and SI
(iii) CPS destabilization and SI
(iv) Charnolophagy and SI
(v)   Charnolophagy Index and SI

SI is a ratio of the nitrative α-synuclein and native α-synuclein as follows:

SI = Nitrative α-Syn/Native α-Syn
Charnolophagy Index = Charnolophagy/Autophagy

Parkinsonian neurotoxins: MPTP, 6-OH-DA, rotenone, salsolinol, and 1b-TIQ all induced SI as well as charnolophagy index in the cultured SK-N-SH and SH-SY5Y cells. Pre-treatment with a specific MOA-B inhibitor, selegiline, melatonin, and CoQ_{10} attenuated MPTP-induced increase in the SI as well as charnolophagy index by inducing MTs. MTs also provide neuroprotection as potent free radical scavengers to prevent CB formation, augment charnolophagy, and stabilize CPS and CS for ICD as boosters of the MB and ICD for normal cellular function and homeostasis to remain healthy.

CB, Charnolophagy, CPS, and CS as Novel Biomarkers of Drug Discovery. Depending on the extent of acute or chronic exposure to toxic NPs, free radical-mediated mitochondrial degeneration results in lysosomal-sensitive or lysosomal-resistant CB formation. Lysosomal-sensitive CB can be readily subjected to charnolophagy, resulting in neuroprotection; whereas lysosomal-resistant CB may inhibit charnolophagy, resulting in the formation of intra-neuronal inclusions and apoptosis due to the release of toxic substances from the degenerating mitochondria, resulting in progressive NDDs and CVDs. Hence, CB antagonists and charnolophagy agonists can be developed as novel charnolopharmacotherapeutics for the treatment of progressive NDDs and CVDs, and CB agonists and charnolophagy antagonist for the clinical management of MDR malignancies with minimum or no adverse effects. Furthermore, we proposed primarily 3 types of NPs, which could be developed for CB, charnolophagy, and CS targeting including: (a) inert or neutral; without any influence on CB formation; (b) toxic; augmenting CB formation; and (c) protective; ROS scavengers-loaded NPs having therapeutic potential as CB inhibitors, charnolophagy enhancers, and CS stabilizers in NDDs and CVDs as described earlier. Hence, CB formation or its elimination at the subcellular level may be used as a universal biomarker of novel drug discovery in addition to structural and functional characterization of NPs and/or drugs for theranostic applications as described in our recent publications (Chabenne et al. 2014; Sharma 2014; Sharma et al. 2013; Sharma and Ebadi 2014; Sharma et al. 2014; Sharma and Ebadi 2014; Sharma 2015; Sharma 2017a,b).

Charnolophagy as a Sensitive Biomarker of Novel Drug Discovery and Personalized Theranostics. In my recently-published books "ZIKV Disease: Prevention and Cure" and Fetal Alcohol Spectrum Disorder (FASD): Concepts, Mechanisms, and Clinical

Management' I described basic differences between charnolophagy and autophagy and their specific biomarkers to distinguish these basic molecular events of ICD. In general, fluorescently-labeled LC-1, LC-2, and LC-3 antibodies are employed to evaluate autophagy in a healthy or diseased cell. Charnolophagy can be determined by fluorescently or quantum dots (NPs)-labeled CB specific biomarkers such as Cyt-C, complex-1, TSPO (18 kDa), MAOs, 8-OH, 2dG (mtDNA oxidation product), 2,3 dihydroxy nonenal (membrane oxidation product), TRPCs (calcium channel protein), BCl_2, Bax, BOK, AIF, SOD, catalase, glutathione, MTs, HSPs, heat shock factor (HSF-1α), caspase-3, and mitofusin antibodies alone or in combination for co-localization experiments for further confirmation. Initially, ΔΨ collapse can be determined by mitotracker, dihydrofluorescein, rhodamine, or JC-1, and free radical production can be determined by digital fluorescence imaging, confocal microscopy, and multiple fluorochrome flow cytometric analysis. As CB formation is triggered by free radical overproduction and ΔΨ collapse, we can use these two parameters to initially assess CB molecular pathogenesis. Charnolophagy can be estimated by multiple fluorochrome flow cytometry with a sorting facility. We can quantitatively estimate structurally intact mitochondria, CBs, charnolophagy, and CS by utilizing two specific fluorochromes such as mitotracker and lysotracker (Invitrogen). In addition, ER and peroxisome stress can be estimated by the ER-tracker and peroxisome-tracker. Under normal physiological conditions, these fluorochromes exhibit distinct fluorescence representing a total population of structurally intact mitochondria and CBs. These subcellular organelles can also be distinguished by determining the side scatter and forward scatter depending on their size and micro-distribution in a normal and DPCI cell. Colocalization experiments can also be performed by merging mitotracker and lysotracker fluorescent images to assess charnolophagy and CS pharmacodynamics. After determining charnolophagy (which represents exclusively CB autophagy) and autophagy (which represents CB autophagy as well as autophagy of other intracellular organelles such as ER membranes, peroxisomes, microbodies, and Golgi bodies, in addition to CB), we can estimate the ratio of charnolophagy and autophagy which is represented by the charnolophagy index. Later, charnolophagy index can be utilized as a sensitive biomarker for novel drug discovery and early EBPT of chronic MDR diseases.

Charnolophagy Index = Charnolophagy/Autophagy

It is important to highlight that charnolophagy index represents exclusively CMB of a cell during DPCI. However, it may not fully represent ER membrane stress, which can be determined by a similar experimental approach, employing different fluorescent biomarkers such as ER-tracker and fluorescently-labeled AgNOR antibody.

SiRNA-mediated Gene Silencing with Fusion Proteins in EBPM. In the recent past, Winkler (2011) described the use of fusion proteins for the targeted therapy using siRNA which can be accomplished if the basic problems of pharmaceutical development are addressed such as specific arginine-rich peptides for siRNA loading capacity, stability, toxicity, and immunogenicity. In addition to liposomal and polymeric NPs, fusion proteins may be used for the targeted delivery to a certain tissue or organ and release of siRNA after cellular uptake. The fusion consists of a protein binder and an oligonucleotide including polymers and dendrimers, respectively. Recently, FDA approved 20 antibodies for therapy. Hence, researchers are now using antibody derivatives as the targeting component of fusion proteins for the siRNA delivery. For EBPT, individual gene targets can be used with the same delivery agent without purification (Watkins et al. 2010). Protamine-fusion protein was first used for specific siRNA delivery (Caravella and Lugovskoy 2010; Chen et al. 1997). In addition, the heavy chain Fab fragment of an HIV-1 envelope antibody was fused to a truncated protamine for complexation of nucleic acids and a plasmid encoding the bacterial toxin ETA was transported into HIV-infected cells. A fusion protein consisting of a single-chain antibody specific for the tumor surface protein ErbB2 and a truncated protamine fusion protein was used to deliver a luciferase plasmid into antigen-positive cells for siRNA complexation (Li et al. 2001; Song et al. 2005). The fusion protein can transport siRNA to the tumor tissue *in vitro* and in an animal xenograft, resulting in the down-regulation of the targeted mRNA, suppressing immune activation and inflammatory processes. Similarly, the scFv–Cκ–protamine construct inhibited hepatitis B protein expression in an animal model. A 65aa double-stranded RNA binding domain was fused to *Tat* protein for binding and enhancing cellular uptake of siRNA (Peer et al. 2007). In addition, gene targets were knocked down after treating mice intra-nasally. High target down-regulation and low toxicity were reported, however without any significant selectivity. Furthermore, conjugates of *Tat*-peptides with poly-amidoamine (PAMAM) dendrimers were generated to enhance oligonucleotide uptake, but this approach could not increase the uptake of siRNA and gene-silencing (Wen et al. 2007).

It is known that the tripeptide Arg-Gly-Asp (RGD) binds to αvβ3 integrin, which is expressed on endothelial cells during angiogenesis. Tethering the RGD peptide increased binding to integrin-positive cells, and intracellular accumulation of imaging agents (Kumar et al. 2008). There was no enhancement of the RGD-targeted dendrimer in cell-culture model due to enhanced membrane permeation mediated by the cationic surface groups. However, tissue penetration was increased by the RGD conjugation in a 3D cell-culture model and a larger portion of the siRNA was delivered to the tumor (Eguchi et al. 2009). Hence, dendrimers may be developed for targeted siRNA delivery provided specific uptake and gene-silencing is determined and cytotoxicity issues are resolved. For both polymeric as well as for dendrimeric carriers, the distinction between fusion proteins and NPs is diffuse, as aggregation to multi-molecular structures is noticed (Kang et al. 2005). Packaging siRNAs in poly-lysine prevented Toll-like receptor activation, and similar effects were possible for the fusion proteins (Shukla et al. 2005).

Recently, protamine-derived peptides or oligo-arginines were used due to the ease of preparation and availability. It was realized that complexation strategies such as dendrimeric structures may improve loading capacity but may also increase the particle size. In addition, unspecific cellular uptake and toxic effects may arise when using charged complexing agents, hence, optimal size and structure need to be elucidated for the safe and effective EBPT. Further research is needed to determine advantages over competing approaches, such as structurally more complex lipid- or polymer-based NPs. In addition, it is highly prudent to select carefully the siRNA structure and sequence. Usually partially 2′-O-modified oligonucleotides and LNAs (*locked nucleic acids*) are used in siRNA technology, however antisense oligonucleotides demonstrated that optimization is crucial for the success of nucleic acid-based therapeutics (Waite et al. 2009; Kunath et al. 2003; Sioud 2010). Hence, comprehensive testing of chemical modifications pertinent to efficiency, target selectivity, and charnolosomal and endosomal escape is extremely important before developing specific structures and sequences for clinical applications. For cancer chemotherapy, NPs may be designed with distinct tumor characteristics for both cell-surface antigen as well as siRNA-mediated target gene silencing (Vester and Wengel 2004; Leachman et al. 2010).

microRNA in EBPT. Recent advances in molecular biology emphasized the clinical significance of microRNA in NDDs, CVDs, and MDR malignancies. There is a significant correlation between personalized medicine and miRNAs. microRNAs are single-stranded 19–24 nucleotides non-coding RNAs, involved in the post-transcriptional regulation of genes, and have a key role in various cell processes including mRNA and protein expression. microRNAs were implicated in disease progression and regression, hence, can be used as sensitive biomarkers for the EBPT. In addition, polymorphisms in miRNA encoding their targets and factors involved in maturation can be used as novel pharmacogenomic biomarkers in cancer (Shukla et al. 2010). Dysregulated miRNAs expression is involved in MDR malignancies. Hence, miRNAs can be used as molecular targets of CB induction/inhibition, charnolophagy inducers/inhibitors, and as CS stabilizers/destabilizers to evaluate drug response in EBPT. Pharmacogenomic investigations highlighted genes that contribute to the individual patient's drug sensitivity, resistance, and toxicity genes, including the role of microRNA, DNA methylation, copy number variations, and single nucleotide polymorphisms (Aveci and Baran 2013). MiRNAs influence apoptosis, cell cycle, differentiation, and cytoskeletal organization at the post-transcriptional level through MTs-mediated Zn^{2+}-induced transcriptional regulation of target genes by binding at the coding region or by inhibiting the translation at the 3'-untranslational regions. MiRNAs in the body fluids can be used for the diagnosis, prognosis, clinical outcome, and response to treatment in various clinical conditions (Dreussi et al. 2012). Particularly, miRNAs have a crucial role in cancer etiology and in the post-transcriptional regulation of genes involved in neurodegeneration. Hence, miRNA-mimics and miRNA silencing molecules may be developed to modulate miRNA expression and CB induction in tumors as therapeutic agents (Fabbri 2013). Furthermore, the aging model of *C. alegans* indicated that 73 out of 139 miRNAs have sequence homology to human miRNAs (Ibáñez-Ventoso and Driscoll 2009). miRNAs control neuronal cell fate during development and alter gene expression of the non-coding RNA during progressive NDDs and can be detected in the peripheral mononuclear cells (Maes et al. 2010). Several disorders of aging in women after menopause can be attributed to functional decline in estrogen and CB induction in the osteoblasts to cause osteoporosis. Abnormal microRNA expression was associated with estrogen-responsive breast cancer and the target genes involved in the aging process (Klinge 2009).

Epigenetic Changes and microRNA. Recent evidence supports that epigenetic changes are involved in chromatin remodeling and can contribute to fetal metabolic programming by methylation of DNA at the cytosine residues and acetylation of histones. These epigenetic changes can be modulated by miRNAs to influence gene expression during undernutrition, environmental neurotoxicity, or fetal alcohol exposure. Maternal undernutrition during conception may also increase the risk of developing insulin resistance during adulthood (Lie et al. 2014). In singleton fetuses, exposure to prenatal undernutrition resulted in reduced expression of PIK3CB, PRKCZ, and pPRKCZ (Thr410) genes in the skeletal muscle. In PIUN singletons, there was increased expression of IRS1, PDPK1, and SLC2A4 genes. In twins, PCUN caused increased expression of IRS1, AKT2, PDK1 and PRKZ, PRKCZ, while PIUN also induced increased expression of IRS1 and PRKCZ and SLC2A4 SLC2A4 genes in fetal muscle. There were specific changes in the expression of 22 microRNAs in skeletal muscle, providing evidence that maternal undernutrition during conception induces changes in the microRNAs, which may alter the insulin-signaling in the skeletal muscle suggesting association between prenatal undernutrition and insulin resistance in adult life. In addition, stem cell pluripotency and differentiation are governed by methylation at cytosine residues and modulated by histone acetylation-deacetylation. Hence, impaired nutrition and environmental stress may induce drastic changes in the developing fetus by induction of miRNA-mediated CB formation, impaired charnolophagy, and CS destabilization involved in chronic MDR diseases. In addition, miRNA can influence the epigenetic changes leading to future risk of metabolic syndromes, fatty liver, and insulin resistant diabetes (Sookoian et al. 2013).

Regulation of Mitochondrial Function by miRNAs. It is known that the maintenance of cellular energy and homeostasis depends on the normal function of mitochondria which plays a crucial role in the apoptotic pathway and their dysfunction is associated with chronic diseases. Recently, the role of miRNAs in the regulation of the MB, and in modulating metabolic pathways in tumor suppression and their theranostic application was summarized (Tomasetti et al. 2014). Exactly, how miRNAs are involved in mitochondrial degeneration, CB induction/inhibition, charnolophagy induction/inhibition, and CPS/CS stabilization/destabilization is yet to be established. Hence, reprogramming of the energy metabolism is proposed as an emerging feature of cancer diagnosis and prognosis. microRNAs, localized in the mitochondria, emerged as key regulators of metabolism and can be affected by modulating mitochondrial proteins encoded by nuclear genes. The miRNAs regulate signaling pathways in mitochondria and may be de-regulated in various diseases including cancer. Hence, modulation of miRNAs levels may provide novel theranostic strategies for the treatment of mitochondria-related pathologies including CB, charnolophagy, and CPS/CS stabilization/destabilization in health and disease. Indeed! Elucidation of the role of miRNAs in the regulation of MB involving diversified charnolopathies will determine unknown molecular mechanisms involved in the genesis and progression of cancer. Eventually, this knowledge may promote the development of innovative theranostic approaches as discussed in this chapter.

In a study, pulmonary arterial endothelial cells were used as cell types and the iron-sulfur cluster assembly proteins (ISCU1/2) as targets for down-regulation by hypoxia-induced miRNA 210 (miR-210) (Chan et al. 2009). ISCU1/2 induced assembly of iron-sulfur clusters (involved in electron transport and redox reactions). By up-regulating miR-210 and down-regulating ISCU1/2, the structural integrity of iron sulfur clusters was impaired. Down-regulation of ISCU1/2 during hypoxia was associated with induction of miR-210, which decreased the activity of iron-sulfur proteins involved in regulating mitochondrial metabolism, including complex-1 and acotinase activities. These molecular events resulted in the down-regulation of oxidative phosphorylation and hence, MB and other functions, suggesting clinically-significant association of miRNA, iron-sulfur cluster proteins, hypoxia, and mitochondrial functions in cellular metabolism and adaptation to stress involving CB formation, charnolophagy, and CPS/CS destabilization. Further investigations are needed to improve various clinically-significant aspects of nanotheranostics relevant to DSST-MB-based charnolopharmacotherapeutics to accomplish the targeted safe, and effective EBPT of NDDs, CVDs, and MDR malignancies.

CB Pathogenesis in Response to Acute and Chronic Exposure of Toxic Drugs or NPs. Depending on the amount of acute or chronic exposure of toxic drugs or NPs, free radical-mediated mitochondrial degeneration results in lysosomal-sensitive or resistant CB formation. Lysosomal-sensitive CB can be subjected to charnolophagy, resulting in cellular recovery due to ICD; whereas lysosomal-resistant CB inhibits charnolophagy, resulting in the formation of intra-neuronal inclusions and apoptosis, causing progressive NDDs and CVDs. Hence, CB antagonists and charnolophagy agonists may be developed for the clinical management of progressive NDDs and CVDs, and DSST-CB agonists and charnolophagy antagonist for the targeted, safe, and effective EBPT of MDR malignancies with minimum or no adverse effects.

CB as a Universal Biomarker in Nanotheranostics. Genetic and epigenetic changes may induce CB formation. Nutritional stress, environmental toxins, NPs, chronic diseases, drug addiction, and aging augment CB formation due to the down-regulation of nuclear DNA, mtDNA, and microRNA, which participate in cell injury, apoptosis, and repair in progressive NDDs, CVDs, and cancer. Nutritional rehabilitation, physiological Zn^{2+}, and MTs prevent CB formation as free radical scavengers and eliminate CBs by energy (ATP)-driven "charnolophagy". During the acute phase, charnolophagy occurs to prevent further release of toxic substances such as Cyt-C, iron sulfur proteins, Bax, BID, and AIF from the degenerating mitochondria to provide cytoprotection, whereas during the chronic phase, lysosomal-resistant CB formation causes accumulation of precipitated proteins as intracellular inclusions in progressive NDDs and CVDs. Hence miRNA and CB may be used as novel biomarkers for theranostic applications. Furthermore, CB and CS-specific antagonists and charnolophagy agonists may be developed to provide neuroprotection and cardioprotection and vice versa for the eradication of MDR malignancies.

Potential Toxicity of NPs. Despite the wide use of nanoscale materials in several industrial applications as well as in biology and medicine, very little research has been carried out on the potential toxicity of NPs. Papis et al. (2007a,b) obtained 10 differentially expressed mRNAs in BALB3T3 fibroblasts exposed to different forms of cobalt, that is, microparticles, NPs, and ions. Those genes represented candidate biomarkers for indicating specific cellular effects after cobalt NPs exposure. These investigators further evaluated the expression of those genes by real-time RT-PCR after exposure to different forms of cobalt. They also tested some genes associated with cobalt toxicity, such as VEGF, HIF-1α, and Bnip3 and identified biomarkers that were sensitive to cobalt ions. These data were consistent with the possibility that cobalt NPs, due to their large surface area, once inside the cell dissolve and act as ions.

Recently, Joo et al. (2013) screened various blood biomarkers to monitor NPs neurotoxicity by analyzing bound proteins on their surface. These investigators reported that NPs are artificial or natural particles with diameters of 100 nm or less. Unique and hidden physical, chemical, electrical, and optical properties of NPs have been observed as their use has expanded in electronic, chemical, and biological applications. Due to their high surface-to-volume ratio, NPs may be toxic to cells and tissues through endocytosis, in which cells engulf a NP as if it were a protein or similar molecule. NP accumulation in the body may cause pulmonary and CVDs, spleen injury, liver DNA cleavage, and the other problems. Newly developed NPs may require risk assessment involving determination of CB molecular pathogenesis and standardized protocols and guidelines for control and regulation by performing DSST charnolosomic analysis with correlative and combinatorial bioinformatics.

NPs can enter the body through inhalation, injection, dermal penetration, or ingestion. Inhaled NPs may enter the circulatory system and spread to various organs by traveling deep into alveoli in the lungs, causing inflammation, or in the bloodstream by crossing the air-blood barrier. Can we locate the NPs in the brain? If so, what would be the mechanisms of their translocation across the BBB? Even though the mechanisms and pathways of NP penetration into the brain are uncertain, direct disruption or interactions with various blood proteins may enable them to cross the BBB. To answer this question, many studies use protein corona analysis to examine the bound proteins on the surface of NPs. Bound proteins are released from NPs and analyzed via gel electrophoresis and LC-MS. Visualization of the protein analysis network reveals potential mechanisms of NP toxicity. Adsorbed proteins on NPs may undergo conformational changes, causing rearrangement of critical domains or exposure epitopes. Consequently, the fate of NPs could be determined through interactions with associating proteins. For example, Apo-E is one of the major components of the protein corona and may act as a carrier protein for crossing the BBB (Drobne 2007; Burch 2002; Sharma 2007; Chakraborty et al. 2011; Wagner et al. 2012; Chen et al. 2012).

It is now well established that oxidative stress is an important neurotoxic mechanism. ROS could be generated through free-radical activity on the surface of NPs, using lysosome-associated and toll-like receptor-induced signaling pathways (Chen et al. 2012; Bae et al. 2009). NP interaction with toll-like receptors may activate nicotinamide adenine dinucleotide phosphate (NADP) oxidase cascades, leading to ROS generation and inflammation. After BBB penetration through interactions with carrier proteins, NPs could damage adjacent tissues through oxidative stress, leading to the expression of proinflammatory cytokines, chemokines, and-related genes involving CB molecular pathogenesis (Shimizu et al. 2009; Sharma 2017). ROS might also play a crucial role in NF-κB-dependent inflammation, and the activated NF-κB may initiate the transcription of inflammation-promoting genes such as TNF-α and IL-8. Neuroinflammation from NPs could activate glial cells and astrocytes, chronically perturbing neuronal hemostasis and eventually leading to apoptosis or necrosis (Zhang et al. 2011).

A NP-associated neurodegeneration study reported neuroinflammation and damage in the hippocampus (Win et al. 2006). Another study reported that nanosized carbon caused increased inflammation-related proteins, such as monocyte chemoattractant protein-1, IL-6, and C-reactive protein (CRP) (Niwa 2008). Moreover, mice exposed to silica NPs revealed increased haptoglobin, CRP, and serum amyloid-A, supporting neurodegeneration through chronic inflammation (Higashisaka et al. 2012). These researchers investigated the role of NPs in various NDDs, including AD, transmissible spongiform encephalopathies, PD, and ALS, by monitoring inflammation biomarkers. NDDs share a common similarity of misfolded proteins: β-amyloid, prion protein, α-synuclein, and SOD, respectively (Ross and Poirier 2004). Since oligomers of these proteins may cause neurotoxicity through ROS induction, oligomers could be an important biomarker for potential EBPT. Oligomer-based techniques, such as oligomer detection of β-amyloid and α-synuclein, chemical techniques using thioflavin, real-time quaking-induced conversion assay, protein misfolding cyclic amplification, and multimer detection systems along with imaging analysis, could be effective tools to accomplish targeted, safe, and effective EBPT (Hyeon et al. 2012). Neuroinflammatory states were noticed in transgenic animal models of AD. In these models, there was slow but significant disease progression in later stages. In transmissible spongiform encephalopathies, activated microglia and astrocytes were observed on transmission of infectious prion *in vivo*, including increased proinflammatory innate cytokines, such as TNF-α, IL-1β, and IL-6, suggesting chronic neuroinflammation as the root cause of *NDDs*. Therefore, NP-induced chronic inflammation and related neurodegeneration cannot be neglected in the risk assessment of NPs (Solito and Sastre 2012). These investigators are currently conducting neuro-nanotoxicity studies of ZnO and SiO-NPs in 20 and 100 nm sizes with both positive and negative charges by oral administration in rats and verifying blood biomarkers, in parallel with other imaging techniques such as MRI and PET to accomplish the targeted, safe, and effective EBPT of various NDDs.

Due to diverse interactions between NPs and proteins, the mechanisms of neurotoxicity remain controversial, especially in long-term exposure. Since the neurotoxicity and neurodegeneration of NPs may progress slowly, the steady loss of neurons may not present any pre-symptom until extensive neuronal damage has occurred. Hence, early detection of CB molecular pathogenesis involving charnolophagy, CS destabilization, and CS exocytosis as basic molecular mechanisms of CMB and intracellular toxicity will be highly useful to accomplish the safe and effective EBPT of chronic MDR diseases.

Conclusion

EBPT can design time- and cost-effective therapeutic protocols for each patient while identifying his/her genetic predisposition and individual variability to accomplish best theranostic options with minimum or no adverse effects. For instance, treatment with patient-specific stem cells is an effort in this direction. Recently, micellar NPs for the topical and transdermal drug delivery of pharmaceutical and personal care products were developed (Lee et al. 2010). Nanotechnology provides better, safe, effective, and economical EBPT options for cancer and other chronic MDR diseases where conventional treatment has limited success. Hence, future development in innovative NPs, nanomaterials, and nanodevices for targeted drug delivery utilizing DSST chronopharmacological and charnolopharmacological approaches may provide the safe and effective EBPT and reduce the cost of time-consuming, cumbersome, and potentially-painful conventional therapeutic options with serious adverse effects. Particularly, specific CB, charnolophagy, and CPS/CS agonists/antagonists may be developed for the targeted, safe, and effective treatment of NDDs, CVDs, and MDR malignancies. In addition to possible theranostic strategies with siRNA, the miRNAs are involved in post-transcriptional control and may be de-regulated in chronic diseases and aging (Wang 2009). Recently lactosyl Gramicidine-based lipid NPs (Lac-GLN) were developed for the targeted delivery of anti-mir-155 to hepatocellular carcinoma (Zhang et al. 2013). Hence, further studies to explore the exact pathophysiological significance of dysregulated miRNAs in CMB causing CB formation, charnolophagy induction/inhibition, and/or CPS/CS stabilization/destabilization in chronic illnesses will expand our capability in nanotheranostics to accomplish the targeted, safe, and effective EBPT of NDDs, CVDs, and MDR malignancies (Hamburg and Collins 2010; Sharma 2016, 2017). Eventually, the molecularly well-defined and genetically-sculptured practice of EBPM developing novel NPs and nano-drug delivery devices/systems will provide painless theranostics which will improve the quality of our life. Hence, the future of nanotheranostics to accomplish EBPT employing CB, charnolophagy, and CPS/CS-targeted charnolopharmacotherapeutics seems promising.

References

Amoozgar, Z. and Y. Yeo. 2012. Recent advances in stealth coating of nanoparticle drug delivery systems. Wiley Interdisciplinary Reviews: Nanomed & Nanobiotech 4: 219–233.

An, S.S., K. Limb, H. Ohb, B. Leeb, E. Zukicc, Y. Jud, T. Yokoyamae, S. Kimf and E. Welkerc. 2010. Differentiating blood samples from scrapie infected and non-infected hamsters by detecting disease-associated prion proteins using multimer detection system. Biochem Biophys Res Commun 392: 505–509.

Avci, C.B. and Y. Baran. 2013. Use of microRNA in personalized medicine. pp. 311–326. *In*: Yousef, M. and J. Allmer (eds.). miRNomics: microRNSA Biology and Computational Analysis. Methods in Molecular Biology. Vol. 1107; Springer ScimiRNA Pharmacogenomics: The New Frontier for Personalized Medicine in Cancer.

Babinot, J., E. Renard and B.Le. Droumaguet. 2013. Facile synthesis of multicompartment micelles based on biocompatible poly(3-hydroxyalkanoate). Macromol Rapid Commun 34: 362–368.

Bae, Y.S., J.H. Lee, S.H. Choi, S. Kim, F. Almazan, J.L. Witztum and Y.I. Miller. 2009. Macrophages generate reactive oxygen species in response to minimally oxidized low-density lipoprotein: toll-like receptor 4- and spleen tyrosine kinase-dependent activation of NADPH oxidase 2. Circ Res 104: 210–218.

Bhoyar, N., T.K. Giri, D.K. Tripathi, A. Alexander and Ajazuddin. 2012. Recent advances in novel drug delivery system through gels: Review. J Pharm & Allied Health Sci 2: 21–39.

Bisht, R. 2011. Chronomodulated drug delivery system: A comprehensive review on the recent advances in a new sub-discipline of 'chronopharmaceutics'. Asian J Pharm 5: 1–8.

Brannon-Peppas, L. and J.O. Blanchette. 2004. Nanoparticle and targeted systems for cancer therapy. Adv Drug Deliv Rev 56: 1649–1659.

Brenneman, M., S. Sharma, M. Harting et al. 2010. Autologous bone marrow mononuclear cells enhance recovery after AIS in young and middle-aged rats. J Cerebral Blood Flow & Metabolism 30: 140–149.

Brigger, I., C. Dubernet and P. Couvreur. 2002. Nanoparticles in cancer therapy and diagnosis. Adv Drug Deliv Rev 54: 631–651.

Burch, W.M. 2002. Passage of inhaled particles into the blood circulation in humans. Circulation 106: e141–142.

Caravella, J. and A. Lugovskoy. 2010. Design of next-generation protein therapeutics. Curr Opin Chem Biol 14: 520–528.

Chabenne, A., C. Moon, C. Ojo, A. Khogali, B. Nepal and S. Sharma. 2014. Biomarkers in fetal alcohol syndrome (Recent Update). Biomarkers & Genomic Med 6: 12–22.

Chakraborty, S., P. Joshi, V. Shanker, Z.A. Ansari, S.P. Singh and P. Chakrabarti. 2011. Contrasting effect of gold nanoparticles and nanorods with different surface modifications on the structure and activity of bovine serum albumin. Langmuir 27: 7722–7731.

Chan, S.Y., Y.Y. Zhang, C. Hemann, C.E. Mahoney, J.L. Zweier and J. Loscalzo. 2009. microRNA-210 controls mitochondrial metabolism during hypoxia by repressing the iron-sulfur cluster assembly proteins ISCU1/2. Cell Metab 10: 273–284.

Chen, G., Z. Ke, M. Xu, M. Liao, X. Wang, Y. Qi, T. Zhang, J.A. Frank, K.A. Bower, X. Shi and J. Luo. 2012. Autophagy is a protective response to ethanol neurotoxicity. Autophagy 8: 1577–1589.

Chen, L., L. Han and G. Lian. 2013. Recent advances in predicting skin permeability of hydrophilic solutes. Adv Drug Deliv Rev 65: 295–305.

Chen, S.Y., C. Zani, Y. Khouri and W.A. Marasco. 1995. Design of a genetic immunotoxin to eliminate toxin immunogenicity. Gene Ther 2: 116–123.

Chen, X., J.L. Zaro and W.C. Shen. 2013. Fusion protein linkers: Property, design and functionality. Adv Drug Deliv Rev 65: 1357–1369.

Chirra, H.D. and T.A. Desai. 2012. Emerging microtechnologies for the development of oral drug delivery devices. Adv Drug Deliv Rev 64: 1569–78.

Clairambault, J. 2009. Modelling physiological and pharmacological control on cell proliferation to optimise cancer treatments. Mathematical Modelling of Natural Phenomena 4. 12–67.

Daka, A. and D. Peer. 2012. RNAi-based nanomedicines for targeted personalized therapy. Adv Drug Deliv Rev 64: 1508–1521.

Dreussi, E., P. Biason, G. Toffoli and E. Cecchin. 2012. miRNA pharmacogenomics: the new frontier for personalized medicine in cancer. Pharmacogenomics 13: 1635–1650.

Drobne, D. 2007. Nanotoxicology for safe and sustainable nanotechnology. Arh Hig Rada Toksikol 58: 471–478.

Droumaguet, B. Le, J. Nicolas, D. Brambilla et al. 2012. Versatile and efficient targeting using a single nanoparticulate platform: application to cancer and Alzheimer's disease. ACS Nano 6: 5866–5879.

Dyondi, D., T.J. Webster and R. Banerjee. 2013. A nanoparticulate injectable hydrogel as a tissue engineering scaffold for multiple growth factor delivery for bone regeneration. Int J Nanomed 8: 47–59.

Eguchi, A., B.R. Meade, Y.C. Chang et al. 2009. Efficient siRNA delivery into primary cells by a peptide transduction domain-dsRNA binding domain fusion protein. Nat Biotechnol 27: 567–571.

Ekenseair, A.K., F.K. Kasper and A.G. Mikos. 2013. Perspectives on the interface of drug delivery and tissue engineering. Adv Drug Deliv Rev 65: 89–92.

Estudante, M., J.G. Morais, G. Soverala and L.Z. Benet. 2013. Intestinal drug transporters: An overview. Adv Drug Deliv Rev 65: 1340–1356.

Etheridge, M.L., S.A. Campbell, A.G. Erdman, C.L. Haynes, S.M. Wolf and J. McCullough. 2013. The big picture on nanomedicine: the state of investigational and approved nanomedicine products. Nanomedicine: Nanotech, Biol & Med 9: 1–14.

Fabbri, M. 2013. microRNAs and cancer: towards a personalized medicine. Curr Mol Med 3: 751–756.

Fernandes, R. and D.H. Gracias. 2012. Self-folding polymeric containers for encapsulation and delivery of drugs. Adv Drug Deliv Rev 64: 1579–1589.

Gajewicz, A., B. Rasulev, T.C. Dinadayalane et al. 2012. Advancing risk assessment of engineered nanomaterials: Application of computational approaches. Adv Drug Deliv Rev 64: 1663–1693.

Gombotz, W.R. and S.F. Wee. 2012. Protein release from alginate matrices. Adv Drug Deliv Rev 64: 194–205.

Gref, R., A. Domb, P. Quellec, T. Blunk, R.H. Müller, J.M. Verbavatz and R. Langer. 1995. The controlled intravenous delivery of drugs using PEG-coated sterically stabilized nanospheres. Adv Drug Deliv Rev 16: 215–33.

Hamburg, M.A. and F.C. Collins. 2010. The path to personalized medicine. New Eng J Med 363: 301–304.

Hansen, S., C.M. Claus-Michael Lehr and U.F. Schaefer. 2013. Modeling the human skin barrier— Towards a better understanding of dermal absorption. Adv Drug Deliv Rev 65: 149–151.

Herrlich, S., S. Spieth, S. Messner and S.R. Zengerle. 2012. Osmotic micropumps for drug delivery. Adv Drug Deliv Rev 64: 1617–1627.

Higashisaka, K., Y. Yoshioka, K. Yamashita, Y. Morishita, M. Fujimura, H.K. Nabeshi and K. Nagano. 2011. Acute phase proteins as biomarkers for predicting the exposure and toxicity of nanomaterials. Biomaterials 32: 3–9.

Hoffman, A.S. 2002. Hydrogels for biomedical applications. Adv Drug Deliv Rev 54: 3–12.

Hyeon, J.W., S. Kim, J. Park, B. Choi, S. Lee, Y. Ju S. and C. Kim. 2012. The association between prion proteins and Abeta (1)(-)(4)(2) oligomers in cytotoxicity and apoptosis. Biochem Biophys Res Commun 424: 214–220.

Ibanez-Ventoso, C. and M. Driscoll. 2009. microRNAs in C. elegans aging: Molecular insurance for robustness? Current Genomics 10: 144–153.

Janowski, M., J.W. Bulte and P. Walczak. 2012. Personalized nanomedicine advancements for stem cell tracking. Adv Drug Deliv Rev 64: 1488–1507.

Joo, J.Y., M.A. Lee, S.O. Bae and S. Soo. 2013. Blood biomarkers: from nanotoxicity to neurodegeneration. 12 Feb.

Kang, H., R. Delong, M.H. Fisher and R.L. Juliano. 2005. TAT-conjugated PAMAM dendrimers as delivery agents for antisense and siRNA oligonucleotides. Pharm Res 22: 2099–2106.

Khoury, R.E.l., V. Misra, S. Sharma et al. 2010. The effect of trans-catheter injections on viability and cytokine release of mononuclear cells. Am J Neurorad 31: 1488–1492.

Kim, T.H., S. Lee and X. Chen. 2013. Nanotheranostics for personalized medicine. Expert Rev Mol Diagn 13: 257–269.

Kim, Y.C., J.H. Park and M.R. Prausnitz. 2012. Microneedles for drug and vaccine delivery. Adv Drug Deliv Rev 64: 1547–1568.

Klinge, C.M. 2013. Estrogen regulation of microRNA expression. Curr Genomics 10: 169–183.

Kulis, M. and W.A. Burks. 2013. Oral immunotherapy for food allergy: Clinical and preclinical studies. Adv Drug Deliv Rev 65: 774–781.

Kumar, P., H.S. Ban, S.S. Kim et al. 2008. T cell-specific siRNA delivery suppresses HIV-1 infection in humanized mice. Cell 134: 577–586.

Kunath, K., T. Merdan, O. Hegener, H. Haberlein and T. Kissel. 2003. Integrin targeting using RGD-PEI conjugates for *in vitro* gene transfer. J Gene Med 5: 588–599.

Kwon, K.C., R. Nityanandam, J. Stewart and D. Henry. 2013. Oral delivery of bioencapsulated exendin-4 expressed in chloroplasts lowers blood glucose level in mice and stimulates insulin secretion in beta-TC6 cells. Plant Biotechnol J 11: 77–86.

Kwon, G.S. and K. Kataoka. 2012. Block copolymer micelles as long-circulating drug vehicles. Adv Drug Deliv 64: 237–245.

Leachman, S.A., R.P. Hickerson, M.E. Schwartz et al. 2010. First-in-human mutation-targeted siRNA phase Ib trial of an inherited skin disorder. Mol Ther 18: 442–446.

Lee, R.W., D.B. Shenoy and R. Sheel. 2013. Micellar nanoparticles: Applications for topical and passive transdermal drug delivery. Chapter 2. pp. 37–58. Handbook of Non-Invasive Drug Delivery Systems. (Non-Invasive and Minimally-Invasive Drug Delivery Systems for Pharmaceutical and Personal Care Products.) A Volume in Personal Care & Cosmetic Technology. Deliv Rev 28: 25–42.

Li, G.H., P.P. Yang, S.S. Gao and Y.Q. Zu. 2012. Synthesis and micellar behavior of poly (acrylic acid-b-styrene) block copolymers. Coll Polymer Sci 290: 1825–1831.

Li, T., A.T. Evans, S. Chiravuri, R.Y. Gianchandani and Y.B. Gianchandani. 2012. Compact, power-efficient architectures using microvalves and microsensors, for intrathecal, insulin, and other drug delivery systems. Adv Drug Deliv Rev 64: 1639–1649.

Li, X., P. Stuckert, I. Bosch, J.D. Marks and W.A. Marasco. 2001. Single-chain antibody-mediated gene delivery into erbb2-positive human breast cancer cells. Cancer Gene Ther 8: 555–565.

Li, X., J. Qi, Y. Xie, X. Zhang, S. Hu, Y. Xu, Y. Lu and W. Wu. 2013. Nanoemulsions coated with alginate/chitosan as oral insulin delivery systems: preparation, characterization, and hypoglycemic effect in rats. Int J Nanomed 8: 23–32.

Li, X.Y., X.Y. Kong, S. Shi et al. 2008. Preparation of alginate coated chitosan microparticles for vaccine delivery. BMC Biotech 8: 89–100.

Lie, S., J.L. Morrison, Q. Williams-Wyss, C.M. Suter, D.T. Humphreys, S.E. Ozanne, S.S.M. Maclaughlin, D.O. Kleemann, S.K. Walker, C.T. Roberts and I.C. McMillen. 2014.

Periconceptional undernutrition programs changes in insulin-signaling molecules and microRNAs in skeletal muscle in singleton and twin fetal sheep. Biol Reprod 9: 90(1): 5.

Lin, W.J., L.W. Juang, C.L. Wang, Y.C. Chen, C.C. Lin and K.L. Chang. 2010. Pegylated polyester polymeric micelles as a nano-carrier: Synthesis, characterization, degradation, and biodistribution. J Expt & Clin Med 2: 4–10.

Liu, S. 2013. Epigenetics advancing personalized nanomedicine in cancer therapy. Adv Drug Deliv Rev 64: 1532–1543.

Maeda, H., H. Nakamura and J. Fang. 2013. The EPR effect for macromolecular drug delivery to solid tumors: Improvement of tumor uptake, lowering of systemic toxicity, and distinct tumor imaging *in vivo*. Adv Drug Deliv Rev 65: 1375–1385.

Maes, O.C., H.M. Chertkow, E. Wang and H.M. Schipper. 2010. microRNA: Implications for Alzheimer's disease and other human CNS disorders. Curr Genomics 10: 154–168.

Maksimenko, A., J. Mougin, S. Mura et al. 2013. Polyisoprenoyl gemcitabine conjugates self-assemble as nanoparticles, useful for cancer therapy. Cancer Lett 334: 346–353.

Meng, E. and T. Hoang. 2012. MEMS-enabled implantable drug infusion pumps for laboratory animal research, preclinical, and clinical applications. Adv Drug Deliv Rev 64: 1628–1638.

Misra, V., B. Yang, S. Sharma and S. Savitz. 2011. Cell based therapy for stroke. pp. 143–162. *In*: Charles S. Cox Jr (ed.). Therapy for Neurological Injury. Chapter 7, Humana Press. Springer Science.

Moghimi, S.M., P.P. Wibroe, S.Y. Helvig, S.Z. Farhangrazi and A.C. Hunter. 2012. Genomic perspectives in inter-individual adverse responses following nanomedicine administration: The way forward. Adv Drug Deliv Rev 64: 1385–1393.

Mura, S. and P. Couvreur. 2012. Nanotheranostics for personalized medicine. Adv Drug Deliv Rev 64: 1394–1416.

Nicholas, A. and N.A. Peppas. 2012. An introduction to the most cited papers in the history of advanced drug delivery reviews (1987–2012). Adv Drug Deliv Rev 48: 139–157.

Nicolas, J., S. Mura, D. Brambilla, N. Mackiewicz and P. Couvreur. 2013. Design, functionalization strategies and biomedical applications of targeted biodegradable/biocompatible polymer-based nanocarriers for drug delivery. Chem Soc Rev 42: 1147–1235.

Nicolini, C., N. Bragazzi and E. Pechkova. 2012. Nanoproteomics enabling personalized nanomedicine. Adv Drug Deliv Rev 64: 1522–1531.

Niwa, Y., Y. Hiura, H. Sawamura and N. Iwai. 2008. Inhalation exposure to carbon black induces inflammatory response in rats. Circ J 72: 144–149.

Ochoa, M., C. Mousoulis and B. Ziaie. 2012. Polymeric microdevices for transdermal and subcutaneous drug delivery. Adv Drug Deliv Rev 64: 1603–1616.

Ohdo, S., S. Koyanagi and N. Matsunga. 2010. Chronopharmacological strategies: Intra- and inter-individual variability of molecular clock. Advanced Drug Delivery Reviews 62: 885–897.

Olivier, J.C. 2005. Drug transport to brain with targeted nanoparticles. NeuroRx 2: 108–119.

Pararas, E.L., D.A. Borkholder and J.T. Borenstein. 2012. Microsystems technologies for drug delivery to the inner ear. Adv Drug Deliv Rev 64: 1650–1660.

Papis, E., R. Gornati, M. Prati, J. Ponti, E. Sabbioni and G. Bernardini. 2007a. Gene expression in nanotoxicology research: analysis by differential display in BALB3T3 fibroblasts exposed to cobalt particles and ions. Toxicol Lett 170: 185–192.

Papis, E., R. Gornati, J. Ponti, M. Prati, E. Sabbioni and G. Bernardini. 2007b. Gene expression in nanotoxicology: a search for biomarkers of exposure to cobalt particles and ions. Nanotoxicology 1: 198–203.

Peer, D., P. Zhu, C.V. Carman, J. Lieberman and M. Shimaoka. 2007. Selective gene silencing in activated leukocytes by targeting siRNAs to the integrin lymphocyte function-associated antigen-1. Proc Natl Acad Sci USA 104: 4095–4100.

Peppas, N.A. 2013. Historical perspective on advanced drug delivery: How engineering design and mathematical modeling helped the field mature. Adv Drug Deliv Rev 65: 5–9.

Petersen, A.L., A.E. Hansen, A. Gabizon and T.L. Andresen. 2012. Liposome imaging agents in personalized medicine. Adv Drug Deliv Rev 64: 1417–1435.

Probst, C.E., P. Zrazhevsky, V. Bagalkot and X. Gao. 2013. Quantum dots as a platform for nanoparticle drug delivery vehicle design. Adv Drug Deliv Rev 65: 703–719.

Roberts, M.J., M.D. Bentley and J.M. Harris. 2002. Chemistry for peptide and protein PEGylation. Adv Drug Deliv Rev 54: 459–76.

Rosler, A.A., G.W.M. Vandermeulen and H.A. Klok. 2001. Advanced drug delivery devices via self-assembly of amphiphilic block copolymers. Advanced Drug Delivery Reviews 53: 95–108.

Ross, C.A. and M.A. Poirier. 2004. Protein aggregation and neurodegenerative disease. Nat Med 10 Suppl: S10–17.

Ryu, J.H., H. Koo, I.C. Sun et al. 2012. Tumor-targeting multi-functional nanoparticles for theragnosis: new paradigm for cancer therapy. Adv Drug Deliv Rev 64: 1447–1458.

Sanvicens, N. and M.P. Marco. 2008. Multifunctional nanoparticles—Properties and prospectus for their use in human medicine. p 425, Elsevier Publishers.

Sawant, R.R., A.M. Jhaveri and V.P. Torchilin. 2012. Immunomicelles for advancing personalized therapy. Adv Drug Deliv Rev 64: 436–446.

Shaikh, S., S. Nazim, T. Khan, A. Shaikh, M. Zameeruddin and A. Quazi. 2010. Recent advances in pulmonary drug delivery system: A review. International J Appl Pharm 2: 27–31.

Sharma, H.S. and A. Sharma. 2007. Nanoparticles aggravate heat stress induced cognitive deficits, blood-brain barrier disruption, edema formation, and brain pathology. Prog Brain Res 162: 245–273.

Sharma, S., Y. Bing, M. Brenneman et al. 2010. Bone marrow mononuclear cells protect neurons and modulate microglia in cell culture models of ischemic stroke. J Neurosci Res 88: 2869–2876.

Sharma, S. and M. Ebadi. 2011. Therapeutic potential of metallothioneins as anti-inflammatory agents in polysubstance abuse. Inst Integ Omics Appl Biotech J 2: 50–61.

Sharma, S. and M. Ebadi. 2011. Metallothioneins as early and sensitive biomarkers of redox signaling in neurodegenerative disorders. Inst Integ Omics Appl Biotech 2: 98–106.

Sharma, S., B. Yang, X. Xi, J. Grotta, J. Aronowski and S. Savitz. 2011. IL-10 directly protects cortical neurons by activating PI-3 kinase and STAT-3 pathways. Brain Res 1373: 189–194.

Sharma, S. and M. Ebadi. 2012. *In vivo* molecular imaging in Parkinson's disease. pp. 787–802. *In*: Ebadi, M. and R. Pfieffer (eds.). Parkinson's Disease. CRC Press, Chapter 58.

Sharma, S., A. Rais, R. Sandhu, W. Nel and M. Ebadi. 2013. Clinical significance of metallothioneins in cell therapy and nanomedicine. Int J Nanomed 8: 1477–1488.

Sharma, S., C.S. Moon, A. Khogali, A. Haidous, A. Chabenne, C. Ojo, M. Jelebinkov, Y. Kurdi and M. Ebadi. 2013. Biomarkers of Parkinson's disease (Recent Update). Neurochem Int 63: 201–229.

Sharma, S. 2013. charnoly body as a sensitive biomarker in nanomedicine. International Translational Nanomedicine Conference, Boston, MASS, July 25–27.

Sharma, S., B. Nepal, C.S. Moon, A. Chabenne, A. Khogali, C. Ojo, E. Hong, R. Goudet, A. Sayed-Ahmad, A. Jacob, A. Murtaba and M. Firlit. 2014. Psychology of craving. Open Jr of Med Psych 3: 120–125.

Sharma, S. and M. Ebadi. 2014. Significance of metallothioneins in aging brain. Neurochem Int 65: 40–48.

Sharma, S. and M. Ebadi. 2014. CB as universal biomarker of cell injury. Biomarkers & Genomic Med 6: 89–98.

Sharma, S. 2014. Molecular pharmacology of environmental neurotoxins. *In*: Kainic Acid: Neurotoxic Properties, Biological Sources, and Clinical Applications. Nova Science Publishers. New York. 301, Chapter 85.

Shimizu, M., H. Tainaka, T. Oba, K. Mizuo, M. Umezawa and K. Takeda. 2009. Maternal exposure to nanoparticulate titanium dioxide during the prenatal period alters gene expression related to brain development in the mouse. Particle Fibre Toxicol 6: 20.

Shive, M.S. and J.M. Anderson. 1997. Biodegradation and biocompatibility of PLA and PLGA microspheres. Adv Drug Deliv Rev 28: 5–24.

Shukla, R., T.P. Thomas, J. Peters, A. Kotlyar, A. Myc and J.R. Baker. 2005. Tumor angiogenic vasculature targeting with pamam dendrimer–RGD conjugates. Chem Commun 46: 5739–5741.

Shukla, S., C.S. Sumaria and P.I. Pradeepkumar. 2010. Exploring chemical modifications for siRNA therapeutics: A structural and functional outlook. ChemMedChem 5: 328–349.

Sioud, M. 2010. Recent advances in small interfering RNA sensing by the immune system. Nat Biotechnol 27: 236–242.

Solito, E. and M. Sastre. 2012. Microglia function in Alzheimer's disease. Front Pharmacol 3: 14.

Song, E., P. Zhu, S.K. Lee et al. 2005. Antibody mediated *in vivo* delivery of small interfering RNAs via cell-surface receptors. Nat Biotechnol 23: 709–717.

Sookoian, S., T.F. Gianotti, A.L. Burgueño and C.J. Pirola. 2013. Fetal metabolic programming and epigenetic modifications: a systems biology approach. Pediat Res 73: 531–542.

Stevenson, C.L., J.T. Jr. Santini and R. Langer. 2012. Reservoir-based drug delivery systems utilizing microtechnology. Adv Drug Deliv Rev 64: 1590–1602.

Stolnik, L., L. Illum and S.S. Davis. 1995. Long circulating microparticulate drug carriers. Adv Drug Deliv Rev 16: 195–14.

Swami, A., J. Shi, S. Gadde, A.R. Votruba, N. Kolishetti and O.C. Farokhzad. 2012. Nanoparticles for targeted and temporally-controlled drug delivery. Chapter 2. pp. 9–29. *In*: Svenson, S. and R.K. Prud; home (eds.). Multifunctional Nanoparticles for Drug Delivery Applications: Imaging, Targetting, and Delivery. Nanostructure Science and Technology. Springer Verlag Publishers.

Tomasetti, M., J. Neuzil and L. Dong. 2014. microRNAs as regulators of mitochondrial function: role in cancer suppression. Biochim Biophys Acta 1840: 1441–1453.

Torchilin, V.P. 2013. Multifunctional nanocarriers. Adv Drug Deliv Rev 58: 1532–1555.

Venditto, V.J. and F.C. Jr Szoka. 2013. Cancer nanomedicines: So many papers and so few drugs! Adv Drug Deliv Rev 65: 80–88.

Vester, B. and J. Wengel. 2004. LNA (locked nucleic acid): high-affinity targeting of complementary RNA and DNA. Biochemistry 43: 13233–13241.

Vig, B.S., K.M. Huttunen, K. Laine and J. Rautio. 2013. Amino acids as promoieties in prodrug design and development. Adv Drug Deliv Rev 65: 1375–1385.

Vizirianakis, I.S. and D.G. Fatouros. 2012. Personalized nanomedicine: paving the way to the practical clinical utility of genomics and nanotechnology advancements. Adv Drug Deliv Rev 64: 1359–1362.

Vorup-Jensen, T. and D. Peer. 2012. Nanotoxicity and the importance of being earnest. Adv Drug Deliv Rev 64: 1661–1662.

Wagner, S., A. Zensi, S.L. Wien, S.E. Tschickardt, W. Maier, T. Vogel, F. Worek, C.U. Pietrzik and J.K.H. von Briesen. 2012. Uptake mechanism of ApoE-modified nanoparticles on brain capillary endothelial cells as a blood-brain barrier model. PloS One 7: e32568.

Waite, C.L. and C.M. Roth. 2009. Pamam-RGD conjugates enhance siRNA delivery through a multicellular spheroid model of malignant glioma. Bioconjug Chem 20: 1908–1916.

Wang, J., C. Örnek-Ballanco, J. Xu, W. Yang and X. Yu. 2013. Preparation and characterization of vinculin-targeted polymer–lipid nanoparticle as intracellular delivery vehicle. Int J Nanomed 8: 39–46.

Wang, J.J., Z.W. Zeng, R.Z. Xiao et al. 2011. Recent advances of chitosan nanoparticles as drug carriers. Int J Nanomed 6: 765–774.

Wang, E. 2009. microRNA regulation and its biological significance in personalized medicine and aging. Current Genomics 10: 143.

Watkins, J., A. Marsh, P.C. Taylor and D.R. Singer. 2010. Personalized medicine: The impact on chemistry. Therapeutic Delivery 1: 651–665.

Wen, W.H., J.Y. Liu, W.J. Qin et al. 2007. Targeted inhibition of hbv gene expression by single-chain antibody mediated small interfering RNA delivery. Hepatol 46: 84–94.

Wieland, M. and M. Fussenegger. 2013. Reprogrammed cell delivery for personalized medicine. Adv Drug Deliv Rev 64: 1477–1487.

Win, S.T., S. Yamamoto, S. Ahmed, M. Kakeyama, T. Kobayashi and H. Fujimaki. 2006. Brain cytokine and chemokine mRNA expression in mice induced by intranasal instillation with ultrafine carbon black. Toxicol Lett 163: 153–160.

Winkler, J. 2011. Nanomedicines based on recombinant fusion proteins for targeting therapeutic siRNA oligonucleotide. Ther Deliv 2: 891–905.

Wu, C.Y. and L.Z. Benet. 2005. Predicting drug disposition via application of BCS: transport/absorption/elimination interplay and development of a biopharmaceutics drug disposition classification system. Pharm Res 22: 11–23.

Xu, S., B.Z. Olenyuk, C.T. Okamoto and S.F. Hamm-Alvarez. 2013. Targeting receptor-mediated endocytotic pathways with nanoparticles: Rationale and advances. Adv Drug Deliv Rev 65: 121–138.

Yang, B., R. Strong, S. Sharma et al. 2011. Therapeutic time window and dose-response of autologous bone marrow mononuclear cells for ischemic stroke. J Neurosci Res 89: 833–839.

Zabaleta, V., G. Ponchel, H. Salman, M. Agüeros, C. Vauthier and J.M. Irache. 2012. Oral administration of paclitaxel with pegylated poly(anhydride) nanoparticles: permeability and pharmacokinetic study. Eur J Pharm Biopharm 81: 514–523.

Zhang, X.Q., X. Xu, N. Bertrand, E. Pridgen, A. Swami and O.C. Farokhzad. 2012. Interactions of nanomaterials and biological systems: Implications to personalized nanomedicine. Adv Drug Deliv Rev 64: 1363–1384.

Zhang, Q.L., M. Li, J.W. Ji, F.P. Gao, R. Bai, C.Y. Chen, Z.W. Wang, C. Zhang and Q. Niu. 2011. *In vivo* toxicity of nano-alumina on mice neurobehavioral profiles and the potential mechanisms. Int'l J Immunopathol Pharmacol 24: 23S–29S.

Zhang, L.Y., J. Mena, J. Sun et al. 2012. Electrospray of multifunctional microparticles for image-guided drug delivery. Proc. SPIE 8233, Reporters, Markers, Dyes, Nanoparticles, and Molecular Probes for Biomedical Applications IV, 823303.

Zhang, M., X. Zhou, B. Wang, B.C. Yung, L.J. Lee, K. Ghoshal and R.J. Lee. 2013. Lactosylated gramicidin-based lipid nanoparticles (Lac-GLN) for targeted delivery of anti-miR-155 to hepatocellular carcinoma. J Control Release 168: 251–261.

Zhang, Y., H.F. Chan and K.W. Leong. 2013. Advanced materials and processing for drug delivery: The past and the future. Advanced Drug Delivery Reviews 65: 104–120.

Zhao, G. and B.L. Rodriguez. 2013. Molecular targeting of liposomal nanoparticles to tumor microenvironment. Int J Nanomed 8: 61–71.

CHAPTER-10

Clinical Significance of Mitochondrial Bioenergetic and Charnoly Body in Evidence Based Personalized Nanotheranostics

INTRODUCTION

The application of nanotechnology in the biomedical field (known as nanomedicine), has gained significant interest in recent years, as a unique strategy for selective drug delivery and diagnostic applications. This emerging discipline is recognized as nanotheranostics, which involves simultaneous diagnosis as well as treatment employing NPs as efficient and targeted drug delivery vehicles. This emerging trend of EBPM promises to deliver the right drug to a right patient at the right time as it considers genetic predisposition and chronopharmacological aspects of a disease to accomplish theranostic capabilities. Currently, nanotechnology that develops novel materials at size of 100 nm or less is one of the most promising areas of clinical investigation. Because of their intrinsic properties, nanomaterials are used in electronics, photovoltaic, catalysis, environmental and space engineering, the cosmetic industry, and now in the medicine and pharmaceutical industry.

Nanotechnology is evolving promising opportunities for the progress of modern medicine by developing environmentally safe, biodegradable, biocompatible, targeted delivery systems/devices, and multifunctional nanocarriers with longevity and targetability, intracellular penetration and contrast loading. However, recent studies raised concerns of toxicity of some NPs to living organisms and their negative impact on environmental ecosystems. Thus, lack of available data and low adequacy of experimental protocols prevent risk assessment in nanomedicine (Gajewicz et al. 2012). Irrespective of these inherent limitations, application of nanotechnology in nanomedicine has gained considerable interest and momentum, as a versatile strategy for selective drug delivery and diagnostic purposes (Mura and Couvreur 2012). The encouraging results obtained with multifunctional nanomedicines have directed the efforts towards the creation of theranostic nanomedicine (nanotheranostics) which combines imaging and therapeutic functions in a single platform. Thus, nanotheranostics hold great promises because these unique drug delivery systems integrate simultaneous non-invasive diagnosis as well as treatment with an excellent opportunity to monitor in real time drug release and distribution in a biological system, thus predicting and validating the disease prognosis. Due to these unique characteristics, nanotheranostics are becoming attractive strategies for optimizing the treatment of cancer and other chronic MDR diseases. Hence, attempts to use nanotheranostics for personalized medicine will consolidate optimized treatment for each patient, while taking into consideration the individual variability. Furthermore, clinical application of nanotheranostics would enable earlier detection, economical treatment, and assessment of response, thus allowing proper screening of patients, which will respond to therapy and will have favorable prognosis. This concept makes nanotheranostics extremely attractive to elaborate the targeted, safe, and effective EBPT protocols. There is no doubt that the solution of many unresolved problems of conventional medicine will be furnished by the development of nanomedicine. A recent report provided a comprehensive inventory of nanomedicines to accomplish this clinically-significant goal (Etheridge et al. 2013). A detailed information regarding FDA classification, approval status, nanoscale size, treated conditions, nanostructure, and nanomedicine products already in use in humans and several others in pipeline is now available.

This chapter focuses primarily on the most recent evolution of EBPM and novel strategies to discover better, safe, economical, early, and effective treatment of chronic diseases such as NDDs, CVDs, and MDR malignancies for a better quality of life by improvising the nanotheranostic approach which has shown promising results and potential of translation to safe and effective clinical applications. The chapter also highlights the emerging concepts and mechanisms of MB-based CB, charnolophagy, and CS exocytosis/endocytosis-targeted nanomedicines for the safe and effective clinical management of malignancies and other chronic MDR diseases.

Drug Delivery. Recent innovations in nanotechnology have augmented the advancement of drug delivery. Indeed! Nanotechnology has enabled control over size, shape, and multi-functionality of drug delivery systems. It has shaped the past and may influence the future of drug delivery and EBPM. Over the past 25 years, many interesting biomedical applications have been proposed for stimuli-responsive polymers, including diagnostics, drug delivery, regenerative medicine, and cell culture. A brief overview comprising stimuli-responsive polymers, smart polymers, their biomedical applications, and major barriers to clinical translation is available in a recent report (Hansen et al. 2012). However, the underlying mechanism of i.v. infusion-related adverse reactions inherent to regulatory-approved nanomedicines remains elusive. There are inter-individual differences in adverse reactions, including cardiovascular, bronchopulmonary, mucocutaneous, psychosomatic, and autonomic manifestations. Although nanomedicine-mediated triggering of complement activation was suggested as a contributing factor to these adverse events, complement activation may persist in non-responders as well (Moghimi et al. 2012).

Whether these reactions share similar immunological mechanisms and genetic factors with hypersensitivity syndrome is yet to be established. Hence, genetic studies could be a powerful tool to delineate causative factors and molecular pathways that induce infusion related adverse reactions. Further investigations in this direction may lead to the better design of *in vitro* tests for risk assessment and treatment decisions, thereby revolutionizing clinical medicine with novel CB-based nanopharmaceuticals. Such innovative procedures may also improve regulatory approval processes for nanomedicines currently in the pipeline and decrease the overall cost of health care. Hence, clinically-significant immunity genes and their polymorphisms in relation to nanomedicine infusion-mediated responses are being explored these days.

In an emerging new concept, freeze-dried plant cells (lettuce) expressing vaccine antigens/biopharmaceuticals are protected in the stomach from acids/enzymes but are released to the immune or blood circulatory system when the cell wall is digested by microbes that colonize the gut. Vaccine antigens encapsulated in plant cells upon oral delivery after priming provides both mucosal and systemic immunity and protection against bacterial, viral, or protozoan pathogens, or toxin challenge. Similarly, the oral delivery of autoantigens has been effective against type-1 diabetes and hemophilia. Indeed! Oral delivery of proinsulin or exendin-4, expressed in plant cells regulates blood glucose levels similar to injections. Therefore, this novel strategy offers a cost-effective alternative to deliver therapeutic proteins to combat infectious or inherited diseases by eliminating inactivated pathogens, expensive purification protocols, cold storage/transportation, and sterile injections. Furthermore, innovation in material chemistry has allowed the generation of biodegradable, biocompatible, environment-responsive, and targeted delivery systems (Zhang et al. 2012). Particularly, understanding the permeation of hydrophilic molecules is of relevance to many applications including transdermal drug delivery, skin care, and risk assessment of occupational, environmental, or consumer exposure.

Recently advances in modeling skin permeability of hydrophilic solutes, including quantitative structure–permeability relationships (QSPR) and mechanistic models have been highlighted (Chen et al. 2012). A dataset of human skin permeability of hydrophilic and low hydrophobic solutes has been compiled. Generally, statistically derived QSPR models under-estimate skin permeability of hydrophilic solutes. Hence, including an additional aqueous pathway is necessary to improve the prediction of skin permeability of hydrophilic solutes. However, it remains to be established as to how the aqueous pathway should be modeled. Nevertheless, it has been demonstrated that the contribution of aqueous pathway can constitute up to > 95% of the overall skin permeability. Furthermore, linkers have shown promise as components of recombinant fusion proteins and in the construction of stable, bioactive fusion proteins. Hence, general properties of linkers derived from naturally-occurring multi-domain proteins may be considered as the foundation in their design. Empirical linkers can be classified into 3 categories: (a) flexible linkers, (b) rigid linkers, and (c) *in vivo* cleavable linkers. Besides the basic role in linking the functional domains together (as in flexible and rigid linkers) or releasing the free functional domain *in vivo* linkers may be utilized for the synthesis of fusion proteins, improving biological activity, increasing expression yield, and achieving desirable PKs. A variety of both natural and synthetic polymeric systems have been investigated for the controlled release of proteins. Many of the procedures used to incorporate proteins into a polymeric matrix can be harsh and often cause denaturation of the functional groups. However, prodrugs are biologically inactive that upon biotransformation *in vivo* result in active drug molecules (Vig et al. 2012).

Since prodrugs might alter the tissue distribution, efficacy, and the toxicity of their design should be considered at the early stages of preclinical development. In this regard, natural and synthetic amino acids may offer significant structural diversity and physicochemical properties. Hence, amino acid as prodrugs have been developed to improve poor solubility, poor permeability, sustained release, i.v. delivery, drug targeting, and metabolic stability of the parent drug. Furthermore, pulmonary drug delivery has served as an excellent route of drug administration and remains the preferred route for various drugs. A recent report summarized the rationale of pulmonary drug delivery system, technologies, devices, formulation, and applications of pulmonary drug delivery system (Shaikh et al. 2010). Pulmonary drug delivery is an important area of investigation which may impact the treatment of several diseases including asthma, COPD, and other diseases, as inhalation provides the most direct access to drug target. Moreover, pulmonary delivery is a needle-free treatment, avoids first pass effect, and can minimize systemic side effects in the treatment of COPD, provide rapid response, and minimize the required dose since the drug is delivered directly to the conducting zone of the lungs. Recently, inhaler, aerosol, pulmonary drug delivery devices, dry powder inhaler, meter dose inhaler, nebulizer, and fine particle fraction have been developed to improve the quality of pulmonary drug delivery systems.

PEGylation and Drug Delivery. PEG is a highly investigated polymer for the covalent conjugation of biological macromolecules and surfaces for many pharmaceutical and biotechnological applications. The PEG chemistry and methods of preparation with new (*second-generation*) PEG derivatives, reversible conjugation, and PEG structures are now well established. Pegylation provides three basic advantages: nonimmunogenicity, less entrapment of NPs in the RES, and the slow and sustained release of drug(s) at the target site. These unique properties prevent nonspecific induction of *CB formation* in normal proliferating cells during the treatment of MDR malignancies involving undesirable adverse effects including GIT distress, myelosuppression, alopecia, hepatotoxicity, pulmonary fibrosis, nephrotoxicity, neurotoxicity, and infertility.

Peptides and proteins are extremely important in the modification of biological macromolecules. Thus, PEGylating of peptides and proteins include shielding of antigenic and immunogenic epitopes, shielding of receptor-mediated uptake by the RES, and preventing recognition and degradation by proteolytic enzymes. Furthermore, PEG conjugation increases the size of the polypeptide, thus reducing the renal filtration and altering the PKs of drugs (Roberts et al. 1997). An important aspect of PEGylation is the incorporation of various functional groups that can be used to attach the peptide or protein. A recent study on rats demonstrated the potential of PEGylated NPs as carriers for the oral delivery of Paclitaxel (PTX), an anticancer drug, characterized by its low aqueous solubility and to act as a substrate of the P-glycoprotein (P-gp) and cytochrome P450. For the PEGylating of NPs, 3 different PEGs were used: PEG 2000 (PTX-NP2), PEG 6000 (PTX-NP6), and PEG 10,000 (PTX-NP10). The loading of PTX in PEGylated NPs increased 3 to 7 times the intestinal permeability of paclitaxel through the jejunum compared with the commercial formulation, taxol.

The permeability of PTX was significantly higher for PTX-NP2 and PTX-NP6 than for PTX-NP10, and sustained and therapeutic plasma levels of paclitaxel for at least 48 hrs. The oral bioavailability was 70% for PTX-NP2, 40% for PTX-NP6, and 16% in case of PTX-NP10 suggesting bio-adhesive properties of PEGylated NPs and the inhibitory effect of PEG on the activity of P-gp as well as cytochrome P450 (Zabaleta et al. 2012).

Recently, versatile and efficient targeting has been accomplished using a single NPs platform for the clinical management of cancer and AD (Droumaguet et al. 2012). Particularly, polyisoprenoyl gemcitabine conjugates that self-assemble as NPs have shown promise for cancer therapy (Maksimenko et al. 2012). Furthermore, drug transport to the brain can be improved by targeted NPs (Olivier 2005). Hence, fusion protein linkers with characteristic property, design, and functionality have been developed for targeted drug delivery (Chen et al. 2012). Further developments have been made in improvising the design, functionalization strategies, and biomedical applications of biodegradable/biocompatible polymer-based nanocarriers for targeted drug delivery (Nicolas et al. 2012). A simple procedure to synthesize multicompartment micelles based on biocompatible poly(3-hydroxyalkanoate) has been developed (Babinot et al. 2012) and most cited papers of advanced drug delivery reviews are now available in a recent report (Nicolas and Peppas 2012). Furthermore, the composition and synthesis of hydrogels, the character of absorbed water, and permeation of solutes within swollen matrices have been explored. The important properties of hydrogels relevant to their biomedical applications have been identified as drug and cell carriers, and as tissue engineering matrices (Hoffman 2002).

Although NPs have significant therapeutic application in site-specific drug delivery or medical imaging, these are generally eliminated by the RES within minutes after systemic administration and accumulate in the lung, liver, and spleen. To obtain a coating that might prevent opsonization and subsequent recognition by the macrophages, sterically stabilized nanospheres have been developed using amphiphilic diblock or multiblock copolymers (Gref et al. 1995). These nanospheres are composed of a hydrophilic PEG coating and a biodegradable core in which various drugs can be encapsulated. Hydrophobic drugs, such as lidocaine could be entrapped up to 45 wt % and its release kinetics are governed by the physicochemical characteristics of the polymer. Plasma protein adsorption was significantly reduced on PEG-coated particles and protein concentrations were time-dependent. The nanospheres exhibited increased systemic circulation times and reduced liver accumulation, depending on the coating, PEG molecular weight, and surface density. The pegylated NPs could be freeze-dried, redispersed in aqueous solutions and retained shelf stability. Hence, it is possible to design optimal polymers for a given therapeutic application.

It is well known that to exert its activity a drug must reach its pharmacological site(s) of action(s) within the body. One of the current approaches to achieve site-specific drug delivery utilizes the use of a carrier. Although modifying surfaces of NPs with pegylation is commonly used for reducing premature clearance of NPs from the circulation, pegylation may negatively impact the performance of NPs as a drug carrier (Lin et al. 2010). Hence, alternative surface modification strategies, including substitute polymers, conditional removal of PEG, and surface modification, may provide solutions to prevent limitations of PEG (Vorup-Jensen and Peer 2012; Amoozgar and Yeo 2012). Surface modified by polyethylene oxide (PEO) can bypass the normal physiological defense processes depending on its particle size and layer properties, remain for a prolonged period in the systemic circulation, and have selectivity for target sites within the body (Stolnik et al. 1995).

Chitosans and Alignates. Recently nanotechnology has evolved to discover chitosans as novel drug delivery systems. Chitosan NPs are better drug carriers because of their biocompatibility, biodegradability, and flexibility as they can be easily modified. The chitosans have attracted attention for their applications in loading protein drugs, gene drugs, and anticancer drugs via various routes of administration including oral, nasal, i.v., and ocular. Wang et al. (2011) furnished a report on chitosan NPs, including their methods of preparation, characteristics, modification, *in vivo* metabolic processes, and clinical applications. Similarly, Alginate, a naturally occurring biopolymer extracted from brown algae (kelp), has several unique properties that could be used as a matrix for the entrapment and/or delivery of biological agents (Gombotz and Wee 2012). Alginates are bio-adhesive polymers and can be used for the site-specific delivery to mucosal tissues. Alginate is a family of linear unbranched polysaccharides which contain varying amounts of 1, 4′-linked β-D-mannuronic acid and α-L-guluronic acid residues. The residues may vary in composition and sequence and are arranged in blocks along the chain. Alginates can be cross-linked by the addition of divalent cations in aqueous solution. The relatively mild gelation process enables not only proteins, but also cells and DNA which can be incorporated into alginate matrices with retention of full biological activity. By selection of the type of alginate and coating agent, the pore size, degradation rate, and release kinetics can be controlled. Gels of different morphologies can be prepared including large block matrices, large beads (> 1 mm in diameter), and microbeads (< 0.2 mm in diameter). *In situ* gelling systems have also been developed by the application of alginate to the cornea or on the surfaces of wounds. All these extraordinary properties, in addition to the non-immunogenicity, have led to an increased use of alignates as protein delivery vehicles.

Recently, nanoemulsions coated with alginate/chitosan for oral insulin delivery have been developed (Li et al. 2013). Coating of the nanoemulsion was achieved based on polyelectrolyte cross-linking, with sequential addition of calcium chloride and chitosan to the bulk nanoemulsion dispersion that contained alginate. The particle size of the nanoemulsion was about 488 nm, and the insulin entrapment ratio was 47.3%. Circular dichroism spectroscopy confirmed conformational stability of insulin and *in vitro* leakage study indicated well-preserved integrity of the nanoemulsion in simulated gastric juices. Hypoglycemic effects were noticed in both normal and diabetic rats. The pharmacological bioavailability of the coated nanoemulsion with 25 and 50 IU/kg insulin were 8.42% and 5.72% in normal rats and 8.19% and 7.84% in diabetic rats, respectively. Moreover, there were prolonged hypoglycemic effects after the oral administration of the coated nanoemulsion compared to s.c. insulin suggesting that the nanoemulsion coated with alginate/chitosan is a potential delivery system for oral delivery of polypeptides and proteins. Due to the electrostatic interaction between the positively charged $-NH_3^+$ of chitosan microparticles and negatively charged $-COO^-$ of alginate, absorption of antigens onto chitosan microparticles via electrostatic interaction is relatively mild process suitable for mucosal vaccine (Li et al. 2008).

To increase the stability of antigens and prevent an immediate desorption of antigens from chitosan carriers in GIT, coating onto BSA-loaded chitosan microparticles with sodium alginate was performed by layer-by-layer technology to meet the requirement of mucosal vaccine. The prepared alginate coated chitosan microparticles, with mean diameter of about 1 μm, was suitable for the oral mucosal vaccine. Moreover, alginate coating onto the surface of chitosan microparticles could modulate the release behavior of BSA from alginate coated chitosan microparticles and could effectively protect model protein (BSA) from degradation in acidic medium *in vitro* for at least 2 hrs, indicating that alginate coated chitosan microparticles might be an effective vehicle for oral administration of antigens. Usually gels are transparent or translucent semisolid formulations containing a high ratio of solvent/gelling agent. When dispersed in an appropriate solvent, the gelling agent merges to form a 3D colloid network structure, which limits fluid flow by entrapment and immobilization of the solvent molecules. The network is also responsible for gel resistance to deformation and hence, its viscoelastic properties. Topical gel formulation provides a suitable delivery system for drugs because they are less greasy and can be easily removed from the skin. Hence, gel formulation provides better property and suitability in comparison to cream and ointments.

In a recent study, gellan/xanthan gels along with chitosan NPs of 297 ± 61 nm diameter, basic fibroblast growth factor (bFGF), and bone morphogenetic protein 7 (BMP7) in a dual growth factor delivery system were developed to promote the differentiation of human fetal osteoblasts for bone regeneration (Dyondi et al. 2013). The NPs loaded gels exhibited improved cell proliferation and differentiation due to the sustained release of growth factors. Dual growth factor loaded gels exhibited a higher alkaline phosphatase and calcium deposition compared to single growth factor loaded gels suggesting that encapsulation and stabilization of growth factors within NPs and gels are promising strategies for bone regeneration. Gellan/xanthan gels also exhibited an antibacterial effect against Pseudomonas aeruginosa, Staphylococcus aureus, and Staphylococcus epidermidis, the common pathogens in implant rejection.

Recently, the method and structure of gels have been discussed in detail to improve their permeability and bioavailability that can be incorporated into a novel drug delivery system like solid dispersion into gel, emulgel, hydrogel, *in situ* gel, and solid lipid NPs into gel and microemulsion gels (Bhoyar et al. 2012). The gels are semisolid transparent or translucent, 3D polymeric matrices comprising small quantity of solid dispersed in relatively large quantity of liquid yet possessing solid-like characteristics. They form a high degree of physical reticulation. The gels are composed of long disordered chains those are reversibly-connected at certain points and form a colloidal dispersion system. They exhibit mechanical properties as solid state. Both the dispersed component and the dispersion medium extend continuously throughout the entire gelling system. The gels contain a high ratio of solvent/gelling agents. When dispersed in an appropriate solvent, gelling agent merge to form a 3D colloidal network, which restricts fluid flow by entrapment and immobilization of the solvent molecules.

Similarly, liposomes are biodegradable and can be used to deliver drugs at a much higher concentration in tumor tissues than in normal tissues. Both passive and active drug delivery by liposomal NPs can reduce the toxic side effects of anticancer drugs and enhance the therapeutic efficacy. Active liposomal targeting of tumors can be achieved by recognizing specific tumor receptors through tumor-specific ligands or antibodies coupled onto the surface of the liposomes, or by stimulus-sensitive drug carriers such as acid-triggered or enzyme-triggered drug release.

It is known that tumors are often composed of tumor cells and nontumor cells, which include endothelial cells, pericytes, fibroblasts, stromal, mesenchymal cells, innate, and adaptive immune cells. The nontumor cells form the tumor microenvironment, which could be targeted and modified so that it is unfavorable for tumor cells to grow. Recently, liposomal NPs have been used to deliver anticancer drugs to the tumor microenvironment and to overcome nonspecific uptake, interaction with components in blood, and toxicity with an emphasis on the liposomal targeting of anticancer drugs to the endothelium of tumor neovasculature, tumor associated macrophages, fibroblasts, and pericytes within the tumor microenvironment (Zhao and Rodriguez 2013). I have proposed CSscs as a novel drug discovery target for the safe and effective EBPT of MDR malignancies.

Furthermore, a polymer–lipid nanoparticle (PLN) system has been developed for targeting vinculin, a focal adhesion protein associated with cellular adhesive structures, such as focal adhesions and adherens junctions (Wang et al. 2013). The PLNs possessed an average size of 106 nm and had a positively charged surface. With a lower encapsulation efficiency of 32% compared with poly (lactic-co-glycolic) acid (PLGA) NPs (46%), the PLNs exhibited a sustained release of BSA, while PLGA NPs demonstrated an initial burst-release. Cell-uptake experiments using mouse embryonic fibroblasts cultured in fibrin–fibronectin gels established that the anti-vinculin conjugated PLNs could ship the cargo to the cytoplasm of fibroblasts and adhered to fibronectin–fibrin. Thus, unconjugated PLNs have demonstrated high gene transfection efficiency. Furthermore, PLNs can be manipulated via a different type of targeting ligands and could be used for studying molecular mechanisms by delivering drugs to specific cellular organelles.

Effective Treatment with EPR. There is a major difference between passive tumor targeting and the enhanced permeability and retention (EPR) effect. Particularly in relation to drug retention, passive targeting of low-molecular-weight X-ray contrast agents involves a retention period of less than a few minutes, whereas the EPR effect of NPs involves a prolonged retention time (usually days to weeks) in tumors. The EPR effect results from the extravasation of macromolecules or NPs through tumor blood vessels. Detailed information on the EPR effect, including its features, vascular mediators in both cancer and inflamed tissue is now available in a recent report (Maeda et al. 2012). In this chapter, various methods of augmentation of the EPR effect have been described, that result in better tumor delivery and improved therapeutic effect, where nitroglycerin, angiotensin I-converting enzyme (ACE) inhibitor, or angiotensin II-induced hypertension are used to accomplish better therapeutic effect and reduced systemic toxicity. The EPR effect-based delivery of NPs is also clinically-useful for tumor-selective imaging using fluorescent or radionuclide labeling.

Chronopharmacology in EBPM. With the advancement in chronobiology, modern drug delivery approaches have evolved to a new concept of chronopharmacology, that is, the ability to deliver the therapeutic agent to a patient in a staggered profile. Chronotherapy is particularly applicable where sustained action is not required, and the drugs are extremely toxic. For instance, some anticancer drugs are extremely toxic and can cause serious side effects in conventional and sustained release therapies. The mammalian circadian pacemaker resides in the suprachiasmatic nuclei and influences several biological processes, including the sleep-wake rhythm (Bisht 2011). The clock genes control the circadian rhythms in physiology and behavior. 24 hrs rhythms are observed for the pathophysiology of diseases. Hence, the efficacy and toxicity of several drugs vary depending on the dosing time. Such chronopharmacological phenomena are influenced by pharmacokinetic and pharmacodynamic properties of the medicine. The underlying mechanisms are associated with the 24-hrs rhythms of biochemical, physiological, and behavioral processes under the control of the circadian clock. Hence, a new nanotechnology for delivering medications precisely in a time-modulated fashion, by bedside or ambulatory pumps, is being developed for the clinical management of human diseases. As a result, the chances of development of drug resistance, as seen in conventional and sustained release formulations, can be minimized. A key point in the development of this formulation is to determine the circadian rhythm, which is a suitable indicator to trigger the release of the drug from the nanodevice. Indeed! There is a dire need of suitable rhythmic biomaterials or nanodevices which should be biodegradable, biocompatible, and reversibly responsive to specific biomarkers in a rhythmic fashion. At present, pulsatile drug delivery is gaining popularity. The major advantage in this system is that the drug can be released as and when required. The application of a biological rhythm to pharmacotherapy may be accomplished by the appropriate timing of conventionally formulated tablets and capsules, and a special drug delivery system, to synchronize the drug concentrations with the rhythms in the disease activity. Moreover, the dose and time-dependent alterations in the therapeutic outcome and safety of the drug can be evaluated. Several FDA-approved chronopharmacological agents are now available to provide maximum therapeutic effect with minimum undesirable side effects. A significant progress has been made in pulsatile drug delivery systems that can effectively treat diseases with intermittent dosing therapies, such as, diabetes. The drugs that are currently under development are for the delivery of proteins, hormones, pain medications and other pharmaceutical agents. The major considerations in the design of polymer-based pulsatile systems are the biocompatibility and toxicity of the polymers, response to external stimuli, ability to maintain the desired serum drug levels, shelf life, and reproducibility. Besides, the body's biological circadian rhythm needs to be considered in the designing of the pulsatile drug delivery systems for neuropeptides, hormones, cytokines, or other agents that exert their physiological or pharmacological action in an oscillatory manner. These considerations, along with the potential therapeutic benefits of pulsatile drug delivery microsystems may increase the quality of life.

Oral Immunotherapy and Drug Delivery. Orally-administered drugs suffer from poor localization and reduced therapeutic efficacy due to physiological conditions such as low pH, and high intestinal fluid flow. Moreover, orally administered drugs are influenced by peristalsis in the GIT system which accelerates drug elimination from the biological system. Furthermore, the acidic environment in the stomach can structurally degrade the drug. Particularly, polypeptide drugs are difficult to administer as they can be easily degraded by the acidic environment in the stomach. In addition, the drug experiences first pass effect while passing through the hepatic portal system to be metabolized by liver cytochrome P-450 isoenzymes. The drug may be acetylated, glucronated, or sulphated in the liver to become water soluble and excreted through the renal system. Since various proteins, enzymes, peptide neurotransmitters, and hormones (such as growth hormone and insulin) can be easily proteolyzed when administered orally, microneedles or micro or miliosmotic pumps are preferred for chronic administrations of drugs particularly in inflammatory conditions such as rheumatoid arthritis. By using microneedles and micro-osmotic pumps, we can administer a drug at a low dose on a chronic basis. In recent years, oral immunotherapy (OIT) has been tested in clinical trials for food allergies. Food allergies (peanut, milk, and egg allergies in young children) affect ~ 5% of the U.S. population and have increased in the last decade. OIT seems to be fairly well tolerated and leads to desensitization with increased threshold of allergen to induce reactions (Kulis and Burks 2012). Novel platforms combining controlled release, improved adhesion, tissue penetration, and selective intestinal targeting may overcome these issues and potentially diminish the toxicity and high frequency of administration practiced with conventional oral delivery. Further investigations in mouse models indicate the potential of using adjuvants, such as TLR9 agonists in combination with OIT, peptide OIT, and non-allergen applications such as herbal formulations. Several questions, including the optimal dosing and length of treatment, whether tolerance can be developed, and the cellular mechanisms resulting in protection following OIT are being investigated now. In addition, amino acids are used as prodrugs to improve poor solubility, poor permeability, sustained release, i.v. delivery, drug targeting, and metabolic stability of the parent drug. A variety of delivery systems such as enterically coated tablets, capsules, particles, and liposomes have been developed to improve the oral bioavailability of drugs. Particularly, challenges associated with the development of amino acid prodrugs are now being addressed. Further developments of oral drug delivery platforms for administering drugs in a safe and effective manner across the GIT epithelium have been made (Chirra and Desai 2012).

While much research has been focused on the role of drug transporters in the liver and kidney, less is known about the importance of uptake and efflux transporters in the intestine. Recently the importance of drug transporters as one of the determinants of PKs has become increasingly important. Over the past years the effects of intestinal transporters have been studied using *in vivo* models, *in situ* organ perfusions, *in vitro* tissue preparations, and in cell lines (Wu and Benet 2005). Recently, the biopharmaceutics drug disposition classification system (BDDCS) that allows the prediction of transporter effects on the disposition of orally administered drugs has been proposed. Furthermore, BDDCS predictions have been discussed with respect to the role of intestinal transporters and transporter-metabolizing enzyme on the oral drug PKs (Estudante et al. 2012). However, the importance of these transporters on drug absorption and bioavailability requires further investigations.

Microfabrication for Controlled Drug Delivery. Microfabrication along with appropriate surface chemistry, provide a means to fabricate platforms with flexibility in tailoring the shape, size, reservoir volume, and surface characteristics of microdevices. The same technology can be used to integrate circuits and sensors for designing sophisticated autonomous drug delivery devices that may improve diagnostic as well as therapeutic applications. A recent review sheds light on some of the fabrication techniques and addresses microdevices that can be effectively used for controlled oral drug delivery (Fernandes and Gracias 2012).

Self-folding refers to self-assembly processes where thin films or interconnected planar templates curve, roll-up, or fold into 3D structures such as cylindrical tubes, spirals, corrugated sheets, or polyhedrals. This process has been demonstrated in metallic, semiconducting and polymeric films and has been used to generate nanotubes with diameters as small as 2 nm and fold polyhedra as small as 100 nm, with a surface resolution of 15 nm. Self-folding methods are important for drug delivery since they provide a means to construct 3D, biocompatible, polymeric containers with well-tailored composition, size, shape, wall thickness, porosity, surface patterns, and chemistry. Self-folding is also a parallel process, and it can encapsulate or self-load therapeutic cargo during assembly. A variety of therapeutic cargos including small molecules, peptides, proteins, bacteria, fungi, and mammalian cells have been encapsulated in self-folded polymeric containers. Self-folding of all-polymeric containers has been demonstrated along with the mechanisms involving differential stresses or surface tension forces, and the applications of self-folding polymers in drug delivery. A reservoir-based drug delivery system that incorporates microtechnology has also been developed with emphasis on oral, dermal, and implantable systems. Important features such as working principles, fabrication methods, dimensional constraints, and performance criteria have been discussed. Reservoir-based systems include a subset of microfabricated drug delivery systems and provide unique advantages. Furthermore, reservoirs, whether external to the body or implanted, provide a well-controlled environment for a drug formulation, allowing increased drug stability and prolonged delivery durations (Zhang et al. 2012).

Reservoir systems have the flexibility to accommodate various delivery schemes, including zero order, pulsatile, or on demand dosing, as opposed to sustained release profile. The development of reservoir-based systems for targeted delivery for difficult to treat applications (ocular) has resulted in platforms for patient therapy. The fundamental aspects of microtechnology and how it augmented the collaboration of pharmaceutical scientists, chemists, biologists, engineers, and medical scientists towards the development of advanced drug delivery systems have been recently highlighted with an emphasis on the advances of biomaterials and on the use of design equations and mathematical modeling to achieve a wide range of successful treatments (Peppas 2012).

Targeting of drugs and their carrier systems by using receptor-mediated endocytotic pathways had been in its nascent stages 25 years ago. The recent explosion of knowledge has focused on the design and synthesis of NPs delivery systems as well as elucidation of the cellular complexity of what was previously termed receptor-mediated endocytosis to design and test the feasibility of delivery of highly specific NPs drug carriers to specific cells and tissue. The mechanisms governing the major modes of receptor-mediated endocytosis used in drug delivery, and approaches using these targets for *in vivo* drug delivery of NPs have been explored. Some of the inherent complexities associated with the simple shift from a ligand–drug conjugate versus a ligand–NPs conjugate, in terms of ligand valency and its relationship to the mode of receptor-mediated internalization have been reported (Xu et al. 2012). Hence, the controlled drug delivery of bioactive molecules is an essential component of engineering strategies for tissue repair. Recently challenges to regenerate complex tissues utilizing drug delivery and the development of translational tissue engineering therapies which promote spatiotemporal cell-signaling cascades to maximize the rate and quality of repair have been discussed (Ekenseair and Kasper 2012). Thus, NPs-based drug delivery (NDD) has emerged as a promising approach to improve the efficacy of existing drugs and enable the development of new therapies. Therefore, the therapeutic potential of NDD systems to simultaneously achieve reduced drug toxicity, improve bio-availability, increase circulation times, controlled drug release, and targeting is remarkable (Probst et al. 2012).

However, the clinical translation of NDD vehicles with a primary goal of treating challenging diseases, such as cancer, will require a thorough knowledge of how NPs influence their fate in biological systems, especially *in vivo*. Consequently, a model system for systematic evaluation of all stages of NDD with high sensitivity, high resolution, and low cost is required. In theory, this system should maintain the properties and behavior of the original NDD vehicle, while providing mechanisms for monitoring intracellular and systemic nanocarrier distribution, degradation, drug release, and clearance. For such a model system, Q-Dots have offered great potential. Q-Dots possess small size and versatile surface chemistry, allowing their incorporation within any NDD vehicle with minimal effect on overall characteristics, and superb optical properties for real-time monitoring of NDD vehicle transport and drug release at both cellular and systemic levels. Although the direct use of Q-Dots for drug delivery remains questionable due to their toxicity as potential CB enhancers and CS destabilizers, the Q-Dot core can be easily replaced with organic drug carriers or biocompatible inorganic contrast agents (such as gold and magnetic NPs) by their similar size and surface properties, facilitating translation of well-characterized NDD vehicles to the clinic, maintaining NDD imaging capabilities, and providing additional therapeutic functionalities such as photothermal therapy and magneto-transfection. Unique features that make Q-Dots an ideal platform for nanocarrier design and how this model can be applied to study NDD vehicle behavior for diverse drug delivery applications have been described in detail (Brannon-Peppas and Blanchette 2004). Further studies have been directed towards more targeted treatment of cancer, through more specific anti-cancer agents or through methods including delivery by avoiding the RES, utilizing the EPR effect, and tumor-specific targeting. In addition, treatment using antibody-targeted therapies the ability to treat cancer by targeting delivery through angiogenesis, antiangiogenic drugs in clinical trials, and delivery methods that utilize NPs composed of degradable as well as nondegradable polymers have been discussed.

NPs in Personalized Medicine. NPs offer distinct advantages as theranostic agents due to their flexibility, small sizes, large surface-to-volume ratio, and ease of surface modification with multivalent ligands to increase avidity for target molecules. The application of nanotechnology to personalized medicine provides an excellent opportunity to improve the treatment of many chronic and degenerative diseases. NPs can be engineered to interact with specific biological components, allowing them to benefit from personalized medicine strategies. To improve these interactions, a comprehensive knowledge of how NPs interact with biological systems is extremely important. How the interactions of NPs with biological systems can guide their design for diagnostic, imaging and drug-delivery purposes have been discussed in a recent report (Vizirianakis and Fatouros 2012). An overview of NPs has been provided with an emphasis on systems that have reached clinical trials. Furthermore, considerations for the development of personalized nanomedicines such as the potential toxicity due to CB induction and CS destabilization, scientific and technical challenges of fabrication, and regulatory and ethical issues have been discussed. In most therapeutic approaches, personalized medicine requires time- and cost-effective characterization of an individual's genetic background to achieve the best-adapted therapy. For this purpose, cell-based drug delivery offers a promising alternative. A recent review has highlighted the progress made in synthetic biology-based cell engineering toward advanced drug delivery (Wieland and Fussenegger 2012).

Starting from basic one-input responsive transcriptional or post-transcriptional gene control systems, the field has reached a level on which cells can be engineered to detect cancer cells, to obtain control over T-cell proliferation, and to restore blood glucose homeostasis upon blue light illumination. In addition, a cellular implant can detect blood urate level disorders and restore homeostasis while another cellular implant has been fabricated as an artificial insemination device that releases bull sperm into bovine ovary only during ovulation time by recording endogenous luteinizing hormone levels. It is envisaged that this field may reach a stage at which cells can be reprogrammed to detect multiple metabolic parameters and treat any disorder connected to them. A recent review has identified a timeline for nanomedicine anticancer drug approval using the business model of inventors, innovators, and imitators. By evaluating the publication record of nanomedicine cancer therapeutics, the investigators have identified a trend of few publications prior to FDA approval (Venditto and Szoka 2012; Kim et al. 2012).

The publications related to cancer involving polymers, liposomes, or monoclonal antibodies and the number of citations as well as clinical trials have been described (Liu et al. 2012). The investigators have focused on the analysis of nanomedicines containing camptothecin derivatives, including two polymers as innovations and liposomal formulation. The conclusion that may be drawn from the analysis of the camptothecins is that approved drugs reformulated in polymeric and liposomal cancer nanomedicines have a more difficult time navigating through the approval process because reformulating currently approved drugs in a nanocarrier provides a small increase in performance. Moreover, the drug carriers have a more difficult path through the clinic than monoclonal antibodies. The added complexity of nanocarriers also deters their use to deliver new molecular entities.

Microneedles in Nanomedicine. Microneedles were first conceptualized for drug delivery many decades ago, but only became the subject of significant interest in the mid-1990's when microfabrication technology enabled their manufacture as (i) solid microneedles for skin pretreatment to increase skin permeability, (ii) microneedles coated with drug that dissolves off in the skin, (iii) polymer microneedles that encapsulate drug and fully dissolve in the skin, and (iv) hollow microneedles for drug infusion into the skin. Microneedles have been used to deliver low molecular weight drugs, biotherapeutics, and vaccines, including human studies with a number of small-molecule and protein drugs and vaccines (Ryu et al. 2012). Influenza vaccination using a hollow microneedle is now in clinical use and solid microneedle products are being used for cosmetic purposes. In addition to applications in the skin, microneedles have also been adapted for delivery of therapeutic agents into the eye and into cells. Indeed! Successful application of microneedles depends on the function of the device that facilitates their insertion and infusion into skin, skin recovery after removal, drug stability during manufacturing, storage and delivery, and on patient outcomes, including lack of pain, skin irritation, and skin infection, drug efficacy, and safety. Hence, building a technology base and demonstrations of successful drug delivery, microneedles may enable better pharmaceutical therapies, vaccination, and other applications.

CB in Nanothransotics and EBPM. The diversity of NPs has revolutionized EBPM and enabled individualized tailoring of stem cell labeling materials for the specific needs of each patient. Thus, the successful implementation of stem cell tracking will contribute to the further development of nanotheranostics. While selective personalized therapies are impressive, majority of cancer therapies have a compromised outcome. Such therapeutic failure could result from no response, drug resistance, disease relapse, or adverse side effect from improper drug delivery. Nanomedicine has a potential to advance the identification of diagnostic and prognostic biomarkers and the delivery of right drug to disease sites. Personalized medicine promises to offer unique opportunities to integrate new technologies and concepts to disease prognosis, diagnosis, and therapeutics (Sawant et al. 2012). This report has dissected the interface of personalized medicine with nanomedicine and epigenetics and outlined the progress and challenging areas that can be explored to perfect personalized health care. It is known that epigenetic aberrations contribute to cancer pathogenesis. Given the individualized traits of epigenetic biomarkers, epigenetic considerations would significantly refine personalized nanomedicine. Thus, nanotheranostics seeks to afford tailored therapeutic regimens for individual patients and is emerging as a new paradigm in the diagnosis and treatment of diseases (Mura and Couvreur 2012). For diagnostic function, theranostic NPs require the inclusion of noninvasive imaging modalities as well. Among them, optical imaging has several advantages including sensitivity, real-time and convenient use, and non-ionization safety, which make it the leading approach for theranostic applications (Janowski et al. 2012). Furthermore, clinical application of nanotheranostics would enable earlier detection and treatment of diseases and assessment of the response, thus allowing screening of patients which would potentially respond to therapy and have higher possibilities of a favorable outcome. This concept makes nanotheranostics attractive to elaborate EBPM protocols for achieving maximal benefit along with a high safety profile. This chapter has focused on the nanotheranostics which illustrates the potential of translation to clinical applications and may transform into practice EBPM. Polymeric immunomicelles as a class of nanocarriers have the potential to combine diagnosis, targeted drug therapy, as well as imaging and monitoring of therapeutic response, to render EBPM for the effective and efficient clinical management of diseases. Hence, smart multi-functional immunomicelles, as the next generation of nanocarriers, are poised for facilitating personalized cancer treatment. Indeed! Nanotechnology developments have facilitated the generation of data on the anatomical, physiological, and molecular level for individual patients to accomplish EBPT. The encouraging results obtained with monofunctional nanomedicines have directed the efforts towards the creation of "nanotheranostics" which integrate imaging and therapeutic capabilities in a single platform (Nicolini et al. 2012).

This attempt for performing a real personalized medicine will tailor optimized treatment to each patient, considering the individual variability. For instance, generation of patient-specific stem cells exemplifies the efforts toward this new approach. Cell-based therapy is a highly promising treatment paradigm; however, due to the lack of consistent and unbiased data about the fate of stem cells *in vivo*, interpretation of therapeutic effects remains challenging. Thus, the advent of nanotechnology with development of inorganic and organic NPs may expand methods for tracking transplanted stem cells *in vivo*. Recent emphasis has been focused to explore the role of cell tracking using currently-available NPs. Nucleic acid programmable protein arrays utilize a complex mammalian cell free expression system to produce proteins *in situ*. As an alternative to fluorescent-labeled approaches, a new label free method, emerging from the combined utilization of 3 independent and complementary nanotechnological approaches, seems capable to analyze protein function and protein–protein interaction studies required to accomplish EBPM. Quartz micro circuit nanogravimetry, based on frequency and dissipation factor, mass spectrometry, and anodic porous alumina overcomes the limitations of fluorescence detection. This could be further optimized by a well-defined bacterial cell free expression system to quantify the regulatory protein networks in humans. Hence, implications for personalized medicine of the protein array using different genes proteins have been reported. Furthermore, the importance of molecular and diagnostic imaging has increased significantly in the therapeutic strategies of many diseases, particularly in cancer therapy. Engineered liposomes that selectively localize in tumor tissue can transport both drugs and imaging agents, which allows for a theranostic approach with potential in EBPM (Petersen et al. 2012).

For example, radiolabeling of liposomes used in preclinical studies for evaluating *in vivo* performance and has been an important tool in the development of liposomal drugs. However, advanced multimodality imaging systems may provide new possibilities for non-invasive monitoring of liposome bio-distribution in humans. Advances in imaging and developments in liposome radiolabeling techniques permit to enter a new arena where we consider how to use imaging for patient selection and treatment monitoring. Thus, nanocarrier imaging agents could have interesting properties for disease diagnostics and staging.

Recently, theranostic NPs have been applied to chemotherapy, photodynamic therapy, siRNA therapy, and photothermal therapy (Daka and Peer 2012). Thus, the idea of casting aside generic treatments in favor of patient-centric therapies has become feasible owing to advances in nanotechnology and drug delivery coupled with the knowledge of genomics and an understanding of disease at the molecular level. The major advances in the development of radiolabeled liposomes for imaging as a tool in EBPM have been recently proposed. Particularly RNA interference (RNAi) has just made it through the pipeline to clinical trials. However, for RNAi as an ideal personalized therapeutic and to be clinically approved, safe, specific, and potent strategies must be devised for efficient delivery of RNAi payloads to specific cell types, which remains a challenge. Through evaluating the recent studies in this field, the progress in designing targeted nano-scaled strategies that are anticipated to overcome the delivery drawbacks and along with the exciting "omics" discipline to personalize RNAi-based therapeutics have been reported. Numerous investigations have shown that both tissue and cell distribution profiles of anticancer drugs can be controlled by their entrapment in colloidal NPs. The rationale behind this approach is to increase antitumor efficacy, while reducing systemic side-effects. NPs are also beneficial for the selective delivery of oligonucleotides to tumor cells. Moreover, certain types of NPs exhibit capabilities to reverse MDR, which is a major problem in chemotherapy. The experiments, aiming to decorate NPs with molecular ligand for 'active' targeting of cancerous cells, have also been addressed with a focus on the imaging for cancer diagnosis. Thus, the application of nanotechnology to EBPM will provide unique opportunity to improve the treatment of many diseases. In this regard NPs offer several advantages as therapeutic and diagnostic tools due to design flexibility, small sizes, large surface-to-volume ratio, and ease of surface modification with multivalent ligands to increase avidity for target molecules (Brigger et al. 2002). Furthermore, NPs can be engineered to interact with specific biological components, allowing them to benefit from the insights provided by EBPM technology. To consolidate these interactions, a comprehensive knowledge of how NPs interact with biological systems is critical. The interactions of NPs with biological systems can guide their design for diagnostic, imaging, and drug delivery purposes. Finally, basic considerations for the development of EBPM have been summarized including potential toxicity, scientific, and technical challenges in fabrication, and regulatory and ethical issues by utilizing NPs (Zhang et al. 2012).

Pharmaceutical Nanocarriers. Currently used pharmaceutical nanocarriers, such as liposomes, micelles, nanoemulsions, polymeric NPs, chitosans, alginates, and many others furnish numerous properties, such as longevity in the blood allowing for their accumulation in pathological areas with compromised vasculature, specific targeting to certain disease sites due to ligands attached to the surface, enhanced intracellular penetration with the help of surface-attached cell-penetrating molecules, contrast properties due to the carrier loading with various contrast materials allowing for direct visualization *in vivo*, and stimuli-sensitivity allowing for drug release from the carriers under certain physiological conditions (Torchilin 2006).

Some of the pharmaceutical carriers are on their way into clinic, while others are still under preclinical development. Immunoliposomes capable of prolonged residence in the blood and specific target recognition represent one of few examples of this kind. Simultaneously, multifunctional pharmaceutical nanocarriers combining several useful properties of one particle can significantly enhance the efficacy of many therapeutic and diagnostic protocols. Current status, and future directions in the emerging area of multifunctional nanocarriers with primary attention on the combination of such properties as longevity, targetability, intracellular penetration, and contrast loading has been highlighted. Amphiphilic copolymers serve as building blocks for the preparation of micellar drug carriers. Over the past decade, the effectiveness of such self-assembled drug delivery devices has been demonstrated (Rösler et al. 2001).

Two approaches can be used to improve the effectiveness of amphiphilic block copolymer-based drug delivery systems. The first approach involves the chemical modification of the block copolymer building blocks. Several examples have been discussed of amphiphilic block copolymers modified with cross-linkable groups to increase the stability of the micellar drug carriers, or of block copolymers containing specific ligands that could allow targeted drug delivery. The second approach to improve the performance of micellar drug carriers is the addition of auxiliary agents. The feasibility of channel proteins and metal NPs to improve temporal control over the drug release process has been addressed. Furthermore, the development of block copolymer micelles as long-circulating drug vehicles has been described as well as a recent fundamental study of block copolymer micelles, where much insight into their structures and properties is summarized to shed light on their properties *in vivo*. There is emphasis on block copolymer micelles having poly (ethylene oxide) as the hydrophilic and poly (L-amino acid) as the hydrophobic block, with emphasis on the molecular properties of poly (ethylene oxide) (Kwon et al. 2012). Hydrophobic drugs, such as doxorubicin, distribute into block copolymer micelles and evidence of the long circulation times of block copolymer micelles has been presented. Like long-circulating liposomes, block copolymers that form micelles, accumulate passively at solid tumors and thus have potential for anti-cancer drug delivery. Hence, basic understanding of the *in vivo* biodegradation as well as cellular and tissue responses which determine the biocompatibility of biodegradable PLA and PLGA microspheres are important in the design and development of biodegradable microspheres containing bioactive agents for theranostic application (Shive and Anderson 1997). A review of biodegradation, biocompatibility, and tissue/material interactions, and selected examples of PLA and PLGA microsphere-controlled release systems have been provided. Selected examples include microspheres incorporating bone morphogenetic protein (BMP) and leuprorelin acetate as well as interactions with the eye, CNS, and lymphoid tissue and their relevance to vaccine development. A subsection of NPs and nanospheres has been also provided with an emphasis on their biodegradation and biocompatibility in this chapter.

Miniturized Drug Delivery Systems. Low cost manufacturing of microdevices for transdermal and subcutaneous drug delivery will have a major impact on next generation devices for administration of biopharmaceuticals and other emerging formulations (Ochoa et al. 2012).

These devices range in complexity from simple microneedle arrays to more complicated systems incorporating micro-pumps, micro-reservoirs, on-board sensors, and electronic intelligence (Stevenson and Santini 2012). Miniaturized drug delivery systems have been developed by applying osmotic principles for pumping. Osmotic micropumps require no electrical energy and enable drug delivery of smallest size for a wide range of new applications. These pumps provide constant (zero-order) drug release rates (Herrlich et al. 2012). This facilitates systems for long term use not limited by GIT transit time and first-pass effect. Osmotic pumps consist of 3 building blocks: osmotic agent, solvent, and drug. This is used to categorize pumps into (i) single compartment systems using water from body fluids as solvent and the drug itself as the osmotic agent, (ii) two compartment systems employing a separate osmotic agent, and (iii) multi-compartment employing solvent, drug, and osmotic agent, separately. In parallel to the micropumps, relevant applications and therapies have been discussed. Further innovation in implantable drug delivery devices is needed for novel pharmaceuticals such as certain biological agents, gene therapy, and other small molecules that are unsuitable for administration by oral, topical, or i.v. routes (Meng and Hoang 2012).

This invasive dosing scheme seeks to directly bypass physiological barriers presented by the human body, release the appropriate drug amount at the site of treatment, and maintain the drug bioavailability for the required duration of administration to achieve drug efficacy. Advances in novel micro electromechanical systems (MEMS) enabled implantable drug infusion pumps with unique performance. The micropumps for lab animal research and preclinical studies include acute rapid radiolabeling, short-term delivery of nanomedicine for cancer treatment, and chronic ocular drug dosing. Thus, further investigation of MEMS actuators, valves, and other microstructures for on-demand dosing control may enable next generation implantable pumps with high performance within a miniaturized form for clinical applications.

Recently a valve-regulated architecture, for intrathecal, insulin, and other drug delivery systems has been developed that offers high performance and volume efficiency by MEMS components (Li et al. 2012; Li et al. 2012). A piezoelectrically-actuated silicon microvalve with embedded pressure sensors is being used to regulate dosing by throttling flow from a mechanically-pressurized reservoir. A preliminary prototype system has been developed with two reservoirs, pressure sensors, and a control circuit board within a 130 cm^3 metal casing. Different control modes of the programmable system have been evaluated to mimic clinical applications. In addition, bolus and continuous flow deliveries have been demonstrated.

Recently, the prevalence of sensorineural hearing loss and other auditory diseases, along with balance disorders and tinnitus, has augmented efforts to develop therapeutic compounds and regenerative approaches to treat these conditions, necessitating advances in MEMS capable of targeted and sustained drug delivery (Pararas et al. 2012). The delicate nature of hearing structures and relative inaccessibility of the cochlea by means of conventional delivery routes necessitate advancements in both the precision and miniaturization of delivery systems, and the nature of the molecular and cellular targets. Moreover, multiple compounds may need to be delivered in a time-sequenced fashion over an extended time-period. Various approaches are now being developed for inner ear drug delivery, including micropump-based devices, reciprocating systems, and cochlear prosthesis-mediated delivery systems suitable for clinical use. These developments represent exciting advances that have the potential to repair and regenerate hearing structures in millions of patients for whom no currently available medical treatments exist, a situation that requires them to function with electronic hearing augmentation devices or to live with severely impaired auditory function particularly in aging patients. These advances will have the potential for clinical applications that share similar requirements and challenges with drug delivery to the CNS.

Assessment of Mitochondrial Bioenergetics by Q-Dots-Labelled Charnolosomes. Recently, we used Cd/Se (Q-Dots) NPs-labeled bone marrow derived mononuclear stem cells (MNCs) to determine their bio-distribution, PKs, and therapeutic potential in experimental model of AIS (Brenneman et al. 2010). By digital fluorescence microscopy and confocal microscopic analysis, we discovered that MNCs exhibit preferential chemotaxis and are exponentially eliminated from the peri-infarct region as a function of time. These findings led us to determine the therapeutic window of MNCs-mediated recovery following AIS (Yang et al. 2011). We also provided a detailed description of cell-based therapy in AIS (Misra et al. 2011). Furthermore, we discovered for the first time that MNCs protect cortical neurons by modulating microglia in cell culture models of AIS and elucidated the basic molecular mechanism of MNCs-mediated neuroprotection (Sharma et al. 2010). Treatment of MNCs in AIS rats significantly increased brain regional IL-10, hence we proposed that cortical neurons are protected directly by MNC-s-mediated paracrine release of IL-10. Indeed, IL-10 can directly bind to its specific IL-10 receptor to execute anti-inflammatory response by activating upstream PI-3 kinase and downstream STAT-3-mediated signal transduction cascade (Sharma et al. 2011). That cortical neurons possess IL-10 receptors, was our original discovery. To further confirm these findings, we examined the effect of trans-catheter injections on the viability and cytokine release of mononuclear cells, which indicated that MNCs are highly primitive, fragile, and can release anti-inflammatory cytokines such as IL-10 and other neurotrophic factors to exert their therapeutic effect in AIS and other NDDs (Khoury et al. 2010). There could be several other molecular mechanisms of MNCs-mediated neuroprotection which remain unexplored yet. However, *in vivo* molecular imaging studies from our labs employing ^{18}FdG and ^{18}F-DOPA as PET biomarkers strongly support *MTs* as potent antioxidant neuroprotective factors in the *NDDs* such as PD, AD, and drug addiction (Sharma and Ebadi 2012). Recently, we reported that MTs induction in stem cell can enhance their therapeutic potential in *NDDs* (Sharma and Ebadi 2011a). Based on these findings, we proposed to further investigate detailed pharmacological properties of NPs using *MTs* and CB formation as sensitive biomarkers of neuroprotection/neurodegeneration (Sharma and Ebadi 2011b). Moreover, MTs as potent free radical scavengers, provide neuroprotection by inhibiting CB formation, by augmenting charnolophagy, and by stabilizing CS in the most vulnerable cells including NPCs derived from iPPCs. Further studies in this direction will not only promote practice of EBPT but also the safety measure of NPs for future biomedical applications.

Conclusion

Nanotechnology promises to provide better, safe, effective, and economical EBPT strategies for cancer and other drug-resistant chronic diseases whereas conventional medical treatment has a currently limited prospectus. Future development in innovative NPs and nanomaterials along with nanodevices for the targeted drug-delivery utilizing chronopharmacological, charnolopharmacological, and charnolosomic approaches may provide better theranostic opportunities and reduce the cost of time-consuming, cumbersome, and painful therapeutic options. It is envisaged that molecularly well-understood and genetically-chiseled practice of EBPM employing novel nano drug delivery devices/systems will provide painless and effective theranostic strategies which may improve prolongevity as well as quality of life. In addition, development of novel ROS scavenging antioxidant drug-loaded NPs will have improved theranostic potential to serve as potent disease-specific CB agonists/antagonists, charnolophagy agonists/antagonists, and CS stabilizers/destabilizers for the safe and effective clinical management of chronic diseases including MDR malignancies.

References

Amoozgar, Z. and Y. Yeo. 2012. Recent advances in stealth coating of nanoparticle drug delivery systems. Wiley Interdisciplinary Reviews: Nanomedicine and Nanobiotechnology 4: 219–233.

Babinot, J., E. Renard, B. Le Droumaguet, J.M. Guigner, S. Mura, J. Nicolas, P. Couvreur and V. Langlois. 2013. Facile synthesis of multicompartment micelles based on biocompatible poly(3-hydroxyalkanoate). Macromol Rapid Commun 34: 362–368.

Bhoyar, N., T.K. Giri, D.K. Tripathi and A. Alexander. 2012. Recent advances in novel drug delivery system through gels: Review. Journal of Pharmacy & Allied Health Sciences 2: 21–39.

Bisht, R. 2011. Chronomodulated drug delivery system: A comprehensive review on the recent advances in a new sub-discipline of 'chronopharmaceutics'. Asian J Pharm 5: 1–8.

Brannon-Peppas, L. and J.O. Blanchette. 2004. Nanoparticle and targeted systems for cancer therapy. Adv Drug Deliv Rev 56: 1649–1659.

Brenneman, M., S. Sharma, S.M. Harting, R. Strong, C.S. Cox, J. Aronowski, J.C. Grotta and S.I. Savitz. 2010. Autologous bone marrow mononuclear cells enhance recovery after AIS in young and middle-aged rats. J Cerebral Blood Flow & Metabolism 30: 140–149.

Brigger, I., C. Dubernet and P. Couvreur. 2002. Nanoparticles in cancer therapy and diagnosis. Adv Drug Deliv Rev 54: 631–651.

Chen, L., L. Han and G. Lian. 2012. Recent advances in predicting skin permeability of hydrophilic solutes. Advanced Drug Delivery Reviews 65: 295–305.

Chen, X., J.L. Zaro and W.C. Shen. 2013. Fusion protein linkers: Property, design and functionality. Adv Drug Deliv Rev 65: 1357–1369.

Chirra, H.D. and T.A. Desai. 2012. Emerging microtechnologies for the development of oral drug delivery devices. Adv Drug Deliv Rev 64: 1569–1578.

Daka, A. and D. Peer. 2012. RNAi-based nanomedicines for targeted personalized therapy. Adv Drug Deliv Rev 64: 1508–1521.

Dyondi, D., T.J. Webster and R. Banerjee. 2013. A nanoparticulate injectable hydrogel as a tissue engineering scaffold for multiple growth factor delivery for bone regeneration. International Journal of Nanomedicine 8: 47–59.

Ekenseair, A.K., F.K. Kasper and A.G. Mikos. 2013. Perspectives on the interface of drug delivery and tissue engineering. Adv Drug Deliv Rev 65: 89–92.

Estudante, M., J.G. Morais, G. Soveral and L.Z. Benet. 2012. Intestinal drug transporters: An overview. Adv Drug Deliv Rev 64: 95–109.

Etheridge, M.L., S.A. Campbell, A.G. Erdman, C.L. Haynes, S.M. Wolf and J. McCullough. 2013. The big picture on nanomedicine: the state of investigational and approved nanomedicine products. Nanomedicine: Nanotechnology, Biology and Medicine 9: 1–14.

Fernandes, R. and D.H. Gracias. 2012. Self-folding polymeric containers for encapsulation and delivery of drugs. Adv Drug Deliv Rev 64: 1579–1589.

Gajewicz, A., B. Rasulev, T.C. Dinadayalane, P. Urbaszek, T. Puzyn, D. Leszczynska and J. Leszczynski. 2012. Advancing risk assessment of engineered nanomaterials: Application of computational approaches. Advances in Drug Delivery Reviews 64: 1663–1693.

Gombotz, W.R. and S.F. Wee. 2012. Protein release from alginate matrices. Advanced Drug Delivery Reviews 64: 194–205.

Gref, R., A. Domb, P. Quellec, T. Blunk, R.H. Müller, J.M. Verbavatz and R. Langer. 1995. The controlled intravenous delivery of drugs using PEG-coated sterically stabilized nanospheres. Advanced Drug Delivery Reviews 16: 215–233.

Hansen, S., S.M. Claus-Michael Lehr and U.F. Schaefer. 2012. Modeling the human skin barrier towards a better understanding of dermal absorption. Advanced Drug Delivery Reviews 65: 251–264.

Herrlich, S., S. Spieth, S. Messner and R. Zengerle. 2012. Osmotic micropumps for drug delivery. Adv Drug Deliv Rev 64: 1617–1627.

Hoffman, A.S. 2002. Hydrogels for biomedical applications. Adv Drug Deliv Rev 54: 3–12.

Janowski, M., J.W. Bulte and P. Walczak. 2012. Personalized nanomedicine advancements for stem cell tracking. Adv Drug Deliv Rev 64: 1488–1507.

Khoury, R.E.I., V. Misra, S. Sharma, C. Cox, P. Walker, J.C. Grotta, J.C. Gee, A. Suzuki and S.I. Savitz. 2010. The effect of trans-catheter injections on viability and cytokine release of mononuclear cells. American J Neuroradiology 31: 1488–1492.

Kim, Y.C., J.H. Park and M.R. Prausnitz. 2012. Microneedles for drug and vaccine delivery. Adv Drug Deliv Rev 64: 1547–1568.

Kulis, M. and W.A. Burks. 2012. Oral immunotherapy for food allergy: Clinical and preclinical studies. Adv Drug Deliv Rev 65: 774–781.

Kwon, G.S. and K. Kataoka. 1995. Block copolymer micelles as long-circulating drug vehicles. Adv Drug Deliv Rev 16(2-3): 295–309.

Kwon, K.C., D. Verma, N.D. Singh, R. Herzog and H. Daniell. 2013. Oral delivery of human biopharmaceuticals, autoantigens and vaccine antigens bioencapsulated in plant cells. Advanced Drug Delivery Reviews 65: 782–799.

Le Droumaguet, B., J. Nicolas, D. Brambilla, S. Mura, A. Maksimenko, L. De Kimpe, E. Salvati, C. Zona, C. Airoldi, M. Canovi, M. Gobbi, N. Magali, B. La Ferla, F. Nicotra, W. Scheper, O. Flores, M. Masserini, K. Andrieux and P. Couvreur. 2012. Versatile and efficient targeting using a single nanoparticulate platform: application to cancer and Alzheimer's disease. ACS Nano 6: 5866–5879.

Li, G.H., P.P. Yang, S.S. Gao and Y.Q. Zu. 2012. Synthesis and micellar behavior of poly (acrylic acid-b-styrene) block copolymers. Coll Polymer Sci 290: 1825–1831.

Li, T., A.T. Evans, S. Chiravuri, R.Y. Gianchandani and Y.B. Gianchandani. 2012. Compact, power-efficient architectures using microvalves and microsensors, for intrathecal, insulin, and other drug delivery systems. Adv Drug Deliv Rev 64: 1639–1649.

Li, X., J. Qi, Y. Xie, X. Zhang, S. Hu, Y. Xu, Y. Lu and W. Wu. 2013. Nanoemulsions coated with alginate/chitosan as oral insulin delivery systems: preparation, characterization, and hypoglycemic effect in rats. International Journal of Nanomedicine 8: 23–32.

Li, X.Y., X.Y. Kong, S. Shi, X. Zheng, G. Guo, Y. Wei and Z.Y. Qian. 2008. Preparation of alginate coated chitosan microparticles for vaccine delivery. BMC Biotechnology 8: 89–100.

Lin, W.J., L.W. Juang, C.L. Wang, Y.C. Chen, C.C. Lin and K.L. Chang. 2010. Pegylated polyester polymeric micelles as a nano-carrier: Synthesis, characterization, degradation, and biodistribution. Journal of Experimental & Clinical Medicine 2: 4–10.

Liu, S. 2012. Epigenetics advancing personalized nanomedicine in cancer therapy. Adv Drug Deliv Rev 64: 1532–1543.

Maeda, H., H. Nakamura and J. Fang. 2013. The EPR effect for macromolecular drug delivery to solid tumors: Improvement of tumor uptake, lowering of systemic toxicity, and distinct tumor imaging *in vivo*. Adv Drug Deliv Rev 88: 53–71.

Maksimenko, A., J. Mougin, S. Mura, E. Sliwinski, E. Lepeltier, C. Bourgaux, S. Lepêtre, F. Zouhiri, D. Desmaële and P. Couvreur. 2013. Polyisoprenoyl gemcitabine conjugates self-assemble as nanoparticles, useful for cancer therapy. Cancer Lett 334: 346–353.

Meng, E. and T. Hoang. 2012. MEMS-enabled implantable drug infusion pumps for laboratory animal research, preclinical, and clinical applications. Adv Drug Deliv Rev 64: 1628–1638.

Misra, V., B. Yang, S. Sharma and S.I. Savitz. 2011. Cell based therapy for stroke. pp. 143–162. *In*: Charles S. Cox Jr (ed.). Therapy for Neurological Injury. Chapter 7, Humana Press. Springer Science.

Moghimi, S.M., P.P. Wibroe, S.Y. Helvig, S.Z. Farhangrazi and A.C. Hunter. 2012. Genomic perspectives in inter-individual adverse responses following nanomedicine administration: The way forward. Advanced Drug Delivery Reviews 64: 1385–1393.

Mura, S. and P. Couvreur. 2012. Nanotheranostics for personalized medicine. Adv Drug Delivery Rev 64: 1394–1416.

Nicholas, A. and N.A. Peppas. 2013. An introduction to the most cited papers in the history of advanced drug delivery reviews (1987–2012). Adv Drug Deliv Rev 48: 139–157.

Nicolas, J., S. Mura, D. Brambilla, N. Mackiewicz and P. Couvreur. 2013. Design, functionalization strategies and biomedical applications of targeted biodegradable/biocompatible polymer-based nanocarriers for drug delivery. Chem Soc Rev 42: 1147–1235.

Nicolini, C., N. Bragazzi and E. Pechkova. 2012. Nanoproteomics enabling personalized nanomedicine. Adv Drug Deliv Rev 64: 1522–1531.

Ochoa, M., C. Mousoulis and B. Ziaie. 2012. Polymeric microdevices for transdermal and subcutaneous drug delivery. Adv Drug Deliv Rev 64: 1603–1616.

Olivier, J.C. 2005. Drug transport to brain with targeted nanoparticles. NeuroRx 2: 108–119.

Pararas, E.E.L., D.A. Borkholder and J.T. Borenstein. 2012. Microsystems technologies for drug delivery to the inner ear. Adv Drug Deliv Rev 64: 1650–1660.

Peppas, N.A. 2013. Historical perspective on advanced drug delivery: How engineering design and mathematical modeling helped the field mature. Adv Drug Deliv Rev 65: 5–9.

Petersen, A.L., A.E. Hansen, A. Gabizon and T.L. Andresen. 2012. Liposome imaging agents in personalized medicine. Adv Drug Deliv Rev 64: 1417–1435.

Probst, C.E., P. Zrazhevsky, V. Bagalkot and X. Gao. 2013. Quantum dots as a platform for nanoparticle drug delivery vehicle design. Adv Drug Deliv Rev 65: 703–718.

Roberts, M.J., M.D. Bentley and J.M. Harris. 1997. Chemistry for peptide and protein PEGylation. Adv Drug Deliv Rev 28: 25–42.

Rösler, A.A., G.W.M. Vandermeulen and H.A. Klok. 2001. Advanced drug delivery devices via self-assembly of amphiphilic block copolymers. Advanced Drug Delivery Reviews 53: 95–108.

Ryu, J.H., H. Koo, I.C. Sun, S.H. Yuk, K. Choi, K. Kim and I.C. Kwon. 2012. Tumor-targeting multi-functional nanoparticles for theragnosis: new paradigm for cancer therapy. Adv Drug Deliv Rev 64: 1447–1458.

Sawant, R.R., A.M. Jhaveri and V.P. Torchilin. 2012. Immunomicelles for advancing personalized therapy. Adv Drug Deliv Rev 64: 1436–1446.

Shaikh, S., S. Nazim, T. Khan, A. Shaikh, M.A. Zameeruddin and A. Quazi. 2010. Recent advances in pulmonary drug delivery system: A review. International Journal of Applied Pharmaceutics 2: 27–31.

Sharma, S., Y. Bing, M. Brenneman, X. Xi, J. Aronowski, J. Grotta and S.I. Savitz. 2010. Bone marrow mononuclear cells protect neurons and modulate microglia in cell culture models of ischemic stroke. Journal of Neuroscience Research 88: 2869–2876.

Sharma, S., B. Yang, X. Xi, J.C. Grotta, J. Aronowski and S.I. Savitz. 2011. IL-10 directly protects cortical neurons by activating PI-3 kinase and STAT-3 pathways. Brain Res 1373: 189–194.

Sharma, S. and M. Ebadi. 2011a. Therapeutic potential of metallothioneins as antiinflammatory agents in polysubstance abuse. Institute of Integrative Omics and Applied Biotechnology Journal 2: 50–61.

Sharma, S. and M. Ebadi. 2011b. Metallothioneins as early and sensitive biomarkers of redox signaling in neurodegenerative disorders. Institute of Integrative Omics and Applied Biotechnology Journal 2: 98–106.

Sharma, S. and M. Ebadi. 2012. *In vivo* molecular imaging in Parkinson's disease. pp. 787–802. *In*: Ebadi, M. and R. Pfieffer (eds.). Parkinson's Disease. CRC Press, Published Oct 18, Chapter 58.

Shive, M.S. and J.M. Anderson. 1997. Biodegradation and biocompatibility of PLA and PLGA microspheres. Adv Drug Deliv Rev 28: 5–24.

Stevenson, C.L., J.T. Santini Jr and R. Langer. 2012. Reservoir-based drug delivery systems utilizing microtechnology. Advanced Drug Delivery Reviews 64: 1590–1602.

Stolnik, L., L. Illum and S.S. Davis. 1995. Long circulating microparticulate drug carriers. Advanced Drug Delivery Reviews 16: 195–214.

Torchilin, V.P. 2006. Multifunctional nanocarriers. Adv Drug Deliv Rev 58: 1532–1555.

Venditto, V.J., Jr and F.C. Szoka. 2013. Cancer nanomedicines: So many papers and so few drugs! Adv Drug Deliv Rev 65: 80–88.

Vig, B.S., K.M. Huttunen, K. Laine and J. Rautio. 2013. Amino acids as promoieties in prodrug design and development. Adv Drug Deliv Rev 65: 1370–1385.

Vizirianakis, I.S. and D.G. Fatouros. 2012. Personalized nanomedicine: paving the way to the practical clinical utility of genomics and nanotechnology advancements. Adv Drug Deliv Rev 64: 1359–1362.

Vorup-Jensen, T. and D. Peer. 2012. Nanotoxicity and the importance of being earnest. Advanced Drug Delivery Reviews 64: 1661–1662.

Wang, J., C. Örnek-Ballanco, J. Xu, W. Yang and X. Yu. 2013. Preparation and characterization of vinculin-targeted polymer–lipid nanoparticle as intracellular delivery vehicle. International Journal of Nanomedicine 8: 39–46.

Wang, J.J., Z.W. Zeng, R.Z. Xiao, T. Xie, G.L. Zhou, X.R. Zhan and S.L. Wang. 2011. Recent advances of chitosan nanoparticles as drug carriers. International J Nanomedicine 6: 765–774.

Wieland, M. and M. Fussenegger. 2012. Reprogrammed cell delivery for personalized medicine. Adv Drug Deliv Rev 64: 1477–1487.

Wu, C.Y. and L.Z. Benet. 2005. Predicting drug disposition via application of BCS: transport/absorption/elimination interplay and development of a biopharmaceutics drug disposition classification system. Pharm Res 22: 11–23.

Xu, S., B.Z. Olenyuk, C.T. Okamoto and S.F. Hamm-Alvarez. 2013. Targeting receptor-mediated endocytotic pathways with nanoparticles: Rationale and advances. Adv Drug Deliv Rev 65: 121–138.

Yang, B., R. Strong, S. Sharma, M. Brenneman, K. Malikarjunarao, X. Xi, J.C. Grotta, J. Aronowski and S.I. Savitz. 2011. Therapeutic time window and dose-response of autologous bone marrow mononuclear cells for ischemic stroke. J Neurosci Res 89: 833–839.

Zabaleta, V., G. Ponchel, H. Salman, M. Agüeros, C. Vauthier and J.M. Irache. 2012. Oral administration of paclitaxel with pegylated poly(anhydride) nanoparticles: permeability and pharmacokinetic study. Eur J Pharm Biopharm 81: 514–523.

Zhang, X.O., X. Xu, N. Bertrand, E. Pridgen, A. Swami and O.C. Farokhzad. 2012. Interactions of nanomaterials and biological systems: Implications to personalized nanomedicine. Adv Drug Deliv Rev 64: 1363–1384.

Zhang, L.Y., J. Mena, J. Sun, A. Letson et al. 2012. Electrospray of multifunctional microparticles for image-guided drug delivery. Proc. SPIE 8233, Reporters, Markers, Dyes, Nanoparticles, and Molecular Probes for Biomedical Applications IV, 823303.

Zhang, Y., H.F. Chan and K.W. Leong. 2013. Advanced materials and processing for drug delivery: The past and the future. Advanced Drug Delivery Reviews 65: 104–120.

Zhao, G. and B.L. Rodriguez. 2013. Molecular targeting of liposomal nanoparticles to tumor microenvironment. International J Nanomedicine 8: 61–71.

CHAPTER-11

Translational Multimodality Neuroimaging of Charnoly Body, Charnolophagy, and Charnolosome for Personalized Theranostics of Chronic Multidrug Resistant Diseases

INTRODUCTION

Recently, high-resolution, noninvasive, multimodality *in vivo* molecular imaging with PET, SPECT, CT, and MRI, employing fusion algorithms has revolutionized EBPT of NDDs, CVDs, and MDR malignancies. However, specific RPs for the accurate diagnosis and effective clinical treatment of AD, PD, drug addiction, and other cognitive impairments remains a significant challenge. Currently, multimodality fusion neuroimaging is utilized for the determination of PKs and pre-clinical development of RPs, *in vivo* monitoring of stem cell transplantation therapy, nicotinic acetylcholine receptors (nAChRs) investigations, regional cerebral blood flow, and glucose utilization studies in cognitively-impaired subjects employing noninvasive microPET and nano-SPECT imaging. Furthermore, multimodality imaging is performed to detect CNS infections using ^{99m}Tc-HMPAO SPECT and ^{18}F-FDG PET/CT.

In this chapter, recent knowledge regarding multimodality fusion imaging is provided with a primary emphasis on nanoSPECT/CT, PET-CT, and PET-MRI to evaluate the PKs and PDs of CB and associated molecular events of ICD. Furthermore, limitations of individual imaging system are highlighted to emphasize the importance of complementary multimodality imaging employing Q-dots or radiolabeled diseases-specific CBs, CPS, and CS biomarkers for cell tracking and exploring the intracellular micro-distribution of these ultrastructural organelles to accomplish the targeted, safe and effective EBPT of chronic MDR diseases.

Future developments in specific RPs to localize DSST-CB, charnolophagy, and CS will facilitate early differential diagnosis, prevent, slowdown and/or cure NDDs, CVDs, and cancer. Eventually, conventional and functional neuroimaging, combined with clinical, laboratory, and -omics analyses will facilitate theranostic evaluation of intracellular MB of chronic diseases.

The incidence of NDDs (such as AD, PD, and drug addiction) CVDs, diabetes, obesity, and MDR malignancies is increasing alarmingly due to global increase in the life span and growing number of aging population (Rocca et al. 2011; Qui et al. 2009). AD is the most common cause of dementia in aging subjects. It is characterized by the presence of amyloid-β plaques, neurofibrillary tangles, reactive gliosis, and synaptic loss (Shulman et al. 2011; Serrano-Pozo et al. 2011; Lacor 2007; Lemere and Masliah 2010; Danysz and Parsons 2012; Mokhtar et al. 2013; Nasrallah and Wolk 2012). Currently, AD and other NDDs such as MS are diagnosed by neuropsychological tests, clinical examination, and by multimodality *in vivo* molecular neuroimaging (Harvey 2012; Brenner 2011; Chang et al. 2010; Liu et al. 2015; Albert et al. 2015; Eshaghia et al. 2015).

In earlier studies, Schillaci et al. (2009) summarized the results of radionuclide imaging and MRI in AD and recommended PET, CT, and MRI for the routine clinical evaluation of dementias. Molecular imaging employing, PET, SPECT, MRI, and MR spectroscopy has the potential to discover novel biomarkers to detect AD during the asymptomatic and prodromal dementia stage. Recent developments in specific molecular imaging agents and MRI have shown promise in the early differential diagnosis and evaluating theranostic efficacy in AD. *In vivo* molecular imaging including PET, SPECT, CT, fMRI, and MRS in combination with *in vitro* detection of serum and CSF biomarkers such as amyloid-β-42, total tau, and phosphorylated tau facilitates early differential diagnosis of AD and its possible prognosis. Currently, novel therapeutic agents for AD are being developed to reduce amyloid-β-42 burden in the CNS. Hence, there is a quest for the novel discovery of PET and SPECT-RPs, and MRI contrast agents to quantitatively determine its level noninvasively at an earlier stage of diseases progression.

In this chapter, recent information on multimodality imaging is described with a primary emphasis on PET-CT, SPECT-CT, and PET-MRI to quantitatively analyze DSST-CB formation, charnolophagy, CPS, and CS micro-distribution and its exocytosis by specific biomarkers of MB to quantitatively assess ICD. The complementary role of multimodality molecular imaging and technical limitations of individual imaging system are also described with a primary objective to accomplish the targeted, safe, and effective EBPT of chronic MDR diseases.

In Vitro and *In Vivo* CS Imaging in Health and Disease

A CS can be detected *in vitro* employing cells in culture. The cultured cells may be subjected to serum and glucose deprivation to enhance free radical overproduction, induce CB formation, and trigger charnolophagy, which is an ATP-driven lysosomal-dependent process. A lysosome containing phagocytosed CB is named as CPS, which is transformed to CS when the phagocytosed CB is hydrolyzed by the lysosomal enzymes. A CS is almost 1.5–2.5 times larger than the size of a lysosome

(0.25–1.25 μm). The size of CS varies from 2.5–3.5 μm and it is more electron dense as compared to a lysosome.

A CS is a single layered, short-lived (usually 3 hrs) organelle. However, its half life depends on the concentration of antioxidants (glutathione, MTs, BCl_2, HSP-70, P^{53}, and GAPDH) in a cell. The stability of a CS is enhanced with the induction and expression of endogenously-synthesized antioxidants and/or by exogenously administered antioxidant drugs.

A CS contains all toxic mitochondrial metabolites. The most important molecules which are localized in the CS are: Cyt-C, MAO-A or MAO-B, cholesterol, TSPO (18 kDa): a cholesterol transporter channel protein, and TRPCs (calcium regulating protein). These molecules can be used as biomarkers for its proper identification by specific antibodies with immunoprecipitation, immunoblotting, ELISA, and by RT-PCR by using specific primers. A Ca^{2+} channel protein, TRPC and two important molecules, 8-OH, 2dG (as mt-DNA oxidation product) and 2, 3, dihydroxy nonenal (as membrane oxidation product), can be determined by specific fluorescently-labelled antibodies and digital fluorescence imaging. A confocal or digital fluorescence microscopy can be utilized to authenticate their presence in a typical CS. In addition, oxidation products of MAOs (acetaldehyde, ammonia, and H_2O_2) can be determined to assess the toxicity of CS. A short list of molecular probes can be further investigated for the precise identification and characterization of CS biomarkers by performing DSST-CS analysis as follows:

Table 2: Molecular probes for identification and characterization of disease-specific spatiotemporal charnolosome (DSST-CS) biomarkers.

Charnolosome Biomarker	Probe
Mitochondrial ΔΨ	Rhodamine, JC-1, Dihydrofluorescein
TSPO (18 kDa) Cholesterol Channel Protein	PK-11129 to evaluate inflammation
Monoamine Oxidase-B	Selegiline, Rasagiline, Moclobemide, Safinamide
Complex-1	^{11}C or ^{18}F-labeleld Rotenone or MPTP 1-Benzyl, tetrahydroisoquinoline (1-Benzyl TIQ)
Ca^{2+}	Fura-2
All other ions (Fe^{3+}, Na^+, Heavy Metals: Pb, Pb, Ni, Co, Cd)	X-Ray microprobe analysis and Inductively- coupled plasma mass spectrophotometry (ICP-MS)
Real Time Free Radicals (Half Life: 10^{-13}–10^{-14} Sec)	Electron spin resonance spectroscopy
8-OH, 2dG 2,3 Dihydroxy Nonenal	Fluorescence or Q-Dot-labeled antibodies
TRPC	Fluorescence, Q-Dot, or radiolabeled (^{11}C, ^{18}F-TRPC) for *in vivo* molecular imaging of *CS*

A typical DSST-CS can be isolated from highly susceptible severely-malnourished neuron or cell or following exposure to heavy metal ion toxicity, or in response to microbial (bacteria, virus, fungal) infections for the targeted, safe, and effective EBPT of a patient.

CS Isolation

A CS can be isolated from the cultured cells or in an intact tissue by differential ultracentrifugation in a sucrose-density gradient. We obtain different layers depending on the molecular mass of each intracellular organelle. The dense nuclear fraction settles at the bottom of the centrifuge tube, followed by CS, mitochondria, lysosomes, and ribosomes in the supernatant. The number of CS depends on the severity of DPCI. The nuclear fraction settles down at the bottom because it is highly dense. It is followed by CS fraction, mitochondrial fraction, lysosome/peroxisome fraction, and the ribosomal fraction, which remains predominantly in the supernatant because these are very light. The CS (as a byproduct of CB) fraction can be identified by TEM and biochemically characterized by using specific CS biomarkers as described above.

Biochemical Characterization of CS. A CS can be characterized biochemically by specific biomarkers. We can have multimodality molecular imaging of CS by MRI, employing Fe^{3+} as a probe. A routine biochemical method and NMR spectroscopy can be utilized to determine the N-acetyl aspartic acid (NAA) in the CS as a quantitative estimate of neurodegeneration. Multimodality molecular imaging of the CS can be performed by fusion imaging with PET/MRI/MRS. In addition, MRS analysis can provide information about lactate, PCr/Cr ratio, and NAA as biomarkers of CMB to detect CB formation and CS induction *in vivo*. *In vivo* analyses of complex-1 can be conducted by utilizing ^{18}F-rotenone or ^{18}F-MPTP as specific radiolabeled PET neuroimaging probes.

In Vitro Analyses of CS. In a cell free system, ^{45}Ca uptake can be studied by employing β-scintillation counting and autoradiography. By estimating the metals from the CS fraction (particularly Fe^{3+}, Cu^{2+}, Zn^{2+}, and Ca^{2+}), we can quantitatively determine environmental toxicity of heavy metal ions.

CS Interconversion

The CS interconversion to inflammasome, apoptosome, necrosome, necro-apoptosome, and metallosome can be quantitatively estimated biochemically by determining the levels of specific biomarkers as well as by utilizing DSST-PET imaging biomarkers of CS. An inflammosome has increased concentrations of pro-inflammatory cytokines such as IL-1β, IL-6, TNFα, and NFκβ, and can be evaluated *in vivo* by employing ^{11}C-PK-11129 as a PET imaging RP to assess inflammation. This PET imaging probe determines TSPO (18 kDa) delocalization (a cholesterol transporter protein) as a biomarker of inflammation. An apoptosome can be determined by estimating AIF, caspase-3 activation, and PARP cleavage, BCl-2/Bax, Bak, HSP-72, P53, MTs, and gluathione by developing multiple antibody microarrays or by developing pathways-specific RT-PCR micro-arrays. Metallosome can be evaluated by atomic absorption spectrophotometer (AAS) or ICP-MS. Although, AAS is quite sensitive and specific, and it can estimate a single metal ion at any given time, for multiple estimations of metal ions, we need to have multiple lamps. During their replacement, the alignment changes, which can significantly influence the detection sensitivity and introduce variation in the sensitivity of detection. This method allows to determine the concentration of metal ions as low as parts per million to parts per billion from a biological sample including metallosome. The most suitable equipment to quantitatively estimate various metal ions from the CS or metallosome is the ICP-MS. This sophisticated equipment can estimate as many as 32 metal ions in 20 minutes in a detection range of parts per billion to part per zillion. The entire procedure is simple, does not require difficult extraction, and is matrix-independent. The Argon plasma torch burns at 5000–8000°C in vacuum, which can induce pyrolysis, atomation, and ionization within a fraction of second to facilitate fast, simple, and accurate determination of metal ion concentration from the CS isolated from chronic NDDs, CVDs, and MDR malignant patients to clinically evaluate meta ion toxicity. Thus, based on the nature of metal ion and chemical abundance in the CS, their classification may change to inflammasome, apoptosome, necrosome, necro-apoptosome, or metallosome. These sophisticated investigations in combination with LC-MS, capillary electrophoresis, flow cytometry, cDNA microarrays, and next generation DNA sequencing can objectively analyze the exact pathophysiological significance of CS in the clinical prognosis of a patient.

Clinical Diagnosis of AD. Currently, neurophysiological and neurobiological tests, anatomical and functional neuroimaging, and clinical evaluation are performed for the differential diagnosis of AD. Gueguen et al. (1997) emphasized that recognizing memory disorders in AD involves an early diagnostic strategy to identify the primary cause. Although significant effort has been made in recent years to discover specific diagnostic biomarkers based on quantitative EEG (Q-EEG), there is no consensus on which items are most relevant, and whether the patient is awake or asleep. In addition, cognitive potentials are used to distinguish between different types of dementias. Exaggerated pupil dilation in response to a mydriatric drug has been proposed as a diagnostic biomarker of AD with controversial results. Although studies on the proteins tau and P-97 are promising, currently, there is no specific biomarker that could be utilized routinely for the differential diagnosis of AD. Molecular genetics studies have identified chromosomal abnormalities in certain families. Apart from chromosome 19 and APO-3, these biomarkers have no definite theranostic significance. However, Allele sigma 4 is now considered as a risk factor for AD. In addition, APO-E phenotyping might have some diagnostic value, yet it is not better than neuropsychological evaluation and *in vivo* molecular neuroimaging. It is difficult to develop an accurate diagnostic strategy without multimodality neuroimaging as highlighted in this chapter. In fact, the value of morphological imaging (with CT/MRI) and diagnosis of dementias (with PET/SPECT) becomes highly crucial in these patients. In addition, volumetric measurements of certain brain structures can be beneficial for the early detection of neurodegeneration in AD. Hence *in vivo*, non-invasive neuroimaging with CT, MRI, PET, and SPECT has a pivotal role for the early differential diagnosis of degenerative dementias.

PET/SPECT Neuroimaging. We reported that high-resolution microPET imaging can be utilized non-invasively to perform translational studies. However, its limited resolution restricts a detailed morphological analysis (Sharma and Ebadi 2008). The SPECT imaging system can be utilized to overcome these limitations. The nanoSPECT/CT imaging system has better resolution to confirm microPET imaging data and establish a detailed functional anatomy of the NDDs in experimental animals. This noninvasive imaging modality significantly reduces the cost and number of particularly gene-manipulated murine models of neurodegeneration and can be used to study PKs of newly-developed drugs such as charnolopharmacotherapeutics. Moreover, it is a unique and most attractive approach to obtain basic information of the NDDs at the cellular, molecular, and genetic level to accomplish the targeted, safe, and effective EBPT. However, very limited studies are available in this direction.

Further improvements in the spatio-temporal resolution will enhance the quality of *in vivo* multimodality translational neuroimaging of CB, charnolophagy, CPS, and CS employing specific NPs or radionuclides. This unique molecular imaging strategy will be very promising for drug development and accomplish personalized nanotheranostics.

Non-Invasive Monitoring of Transplanted Cells. Recently, noninvasive monitoring of transplanted cells by baculovirus-mediated sodium iodide symporter gene delivery to monitor functional viability of islet transplants using fluorescence imaging and ^{125}I-NanoSPECT/CT imaging was developed (Liu et al. 2013). The GFP expression of Bac-GFP-infected rat islets was detected *in vitro* by fluorescence microscopy. Iodine uptake and its inhibition by $NaClO_4$ in Bac-NIS-infected islets were monitored *in vivo* by ^{125}I-NanoSPECT/CT imaging. Bac-GFP- or Bac-NIS-infected islets were implanted into the axillary cavity of NOD-SCID mice, and fluorescence imaging and ^{125}I NanoSPECT/CT imaging were performed. Bac-GFP infected islets, and GFP expression remained for ~ 2 weeks and $NaClO_4$ could inhibit iodine uptake in Bac-NIS-infected islets. The fluorescence intensity of the transplanted sites in Bac-GFP-infected groups was increased and the grafts could be differentiated by ^{125}I NanoSPECT/CT imaging for up to 8 hrs, suggesting that baculovirus may be used as a NIS gene delivery vector for non-invasive monitoring of transplanted islets *in vivo*.

It has been shown that TGF-β activation by the αvβ6 integrin is implicated in pulmonary fibrosis as its expression is enhanced in pulmonary fibrosis; hence, it could be used as a theranostic target (John et al. 2013). Currently, the immuno-histochemical analysis of lung biopsy is performed to detect αvβ6 integrin and evaluate the therapeutic response, which is invasive and clinically-challenging for certain patients with pulmonary fibrosis. These investigators used Bleomycin to induce murine lung fibrosis. NanoSPECT/CT imaging was performed by ^{111m}In-αvβ6-specific (diethylenetriamine pentaacctate-tetra [DTPA]-A20FMDV2) or control (DTPA-A20FMDVran) peptide. Hydroxyproline, αvβ6 protein, and itgb6 messenger RNA were estimated to assess lung fibrosis. ^{111}In-labeled A20FMDV2 peptide was bound to αvβ6 integrins within one hr after i.v. administration. Bleomyin-treated mice exhibited enhanced integrin binding compared to saline-treated controls. Pretreatment with αvβ6-blocking antibody reduced integrin binding. A positive correlation between ^{111m}In-A20FMDV2 peptide and hydroxy proline, αvβ6 protein, and itgb6 mRNA, suggested that this novel approach is highly sensitive, quantifiable, and noninvasive for estimating αvβ6 integrin and may be used for monitoring the therapeutic response in patients with pulmonary fibrosis. Furthermore, it was demonstrated that injured but functionally intact spleen can be saved by surgical interventions (Furka et al. 2013). These investigators developed a partial spleen resection by embracing suture lines and spleen auto-transplants by implantation of spleen chips between the sheets of the omentum, by the "spleen-apron" procedure. Functional and structural follow-up, including lab tests (hematological, hemorheological, enzymological, chemical, and immunological), imaging procedures (abdominal US, scintigraphy, SPECT, nanoSPECT/CT), morphological (histological, immunohistochemical, and E.M.) analyses, and the investigation of the hematopoietic stem cells confirmed the viability of auto-transplants. The implanted spleen chips could restore the functions following remodellation and recolonization after neovascularization; an aspect that was highly significant in the prevention of post-splenectomy infection and DIC. In addition, Skaliczki et al. (2012) developed a rat model of compromised bone healing. These investigators performed nanoSPECT to evaluate osteoblast activity, and μCT and histology to evaluate bone formation, and demonstrated that bone regeneration can be detected 4 weeks after the spacer removal, establishing the reproducibility of this experimental model to evaluate bone regeneration.

Non-Invasive Tracking of Transplanted Stem Cells. Recent studies have shown that the transplanted stem cells can be tracked *in vivo* by radionuclide-labeled reported gene imaging. The radionuclide imaging was performed to monitor stem cell therapy by using recombinant baculovirus carrying the sodium channel-inducible (NIS) gene (Pan et al. 2013). Induced pluripotent stem cells (hiPSCs), embryonic stem cells (hESCs), and umbilical cord blood mesenchymal stem cells (hUCB-MSCs) were used to infect with recombinant baculovirus carrying NIS and GFP reported genes. Flow cytometry was employed to determine transfection efficiency, fluorescence intensity, and duration of gene expression. CCK-8 assays were performed to assess proliferative/cytotoxicity effects of baculovirus on hUCB-MSCs and Bac-NIS-infected hUCB-MSCs were used to determine ^{125}I uptake and perchlorate inhibition. NanoSPECT/CT imaging was performed on mice transplanted with Bac-NIS-infected hUCB-MSCs. The infection efficiency of these cells increased as a function of increase in MOIs. The cell proliferation was negligibly-influenced and no cytotoxicity was observed by transfection. GFP expression could be detected even after 8 days post-infection. The NIS gene products accumulated the radioiodide within 30 minutes, which correlated with hUCB-MSCs cell number, and was inhibited by perchlorate, suggesting that recombinant baculovirus carrying the NIS gene can be used for stem cell monitoring *in vivo*, employing nanoSPECT/CT imaging in NDDs and other chronic illnesses.

NPs-Conjugated Radioligands for Fusion Imaging. Recently, Polyák et al. (2013) developed ^{99m}Tc-labeled 75–200 nm folate-poly-glutamate chitosan NPs for SPECT or SPECT/CT imaging. These self-assembled NPs are biodegradable, biocompatible, and are internalized by folate receptor-overexpressing rat hepatocellular carcinoma cells. Their specificity and targeting efficiency was assessed by *in vivo* SPECT and nanoSPECT/CT imaging. The bio-distribution studies revealed maximum localization in the kidney tumors, and minimum in the lungs and thyroid gland, confirming their utility for translational studies.

Radiation-induced Apoptosis In Vivo. Recently, Lin et al. (2012) used N-terminal extension of six histidine residues to radiolabel recombinant annexin A5 with ^{99m}Tc, with a radiochemical yield of > 95%, for imaging apoptosis in the internal organs of γ-irradiated mouse. This probe was tested in 20 Gy-irradiated Jurkat T cells which demonstrated 20-fold higher uptake than the sham-irradiated cells. The translational capability of ^{99m}Tc (I)-his (6)-annexin A5 probe was assessed by bio-distribution studies employing nanoSPECT/CT imaging in 10 Gy γ-irradiated C57BL/6J mice, which exhibited 3–5-fold higher splenic uptake than those of the sham-irradiated mice. The immunohistochemical staining of the spleen and intestine for activated caspase-3 confirmed that ^{99m}Tc (I)-his(6)-annexin A5 can be used effectively as a translational imaging probe for detecting radiation-induced apoptosis in animal models of NDDs. These novel *in vivo* probes can also be utilized to quantitatively assess CS-dependent and CS-independent apoptosis *in vivo* in real time as a function of disease progression/ regression.

Comparison of SPECT vs PET Imaging. Recently ^{99m}Tc-glucarate, a radiolabeled glucose analogue, was proposed as a SPECT alternative to ^{18}F-FdG-PET for non-invasive detection of certain tumors. So far there have been few studies on ^{99m}Tc-glucarate for tumor imaging and for comparing ^{99m}Tc-glucarate with ^{18}F-FdG-PET. For ^{99m}Tc-glucarate as a possible substitute for ^{18}F-FdG-PET, mice bearing xenografts of 4 tumor types were imaged (Cheng et al. 2011). *In vivo* imaging with ^{18}F-FdG-PET, provides basic information regarding the CMB and indirectly CB pathogenesis in a diseased organ. ^{99m}Tc-glucarate imaging will be a simple and economical substitute to quantitatively assess brain regional CMB to assess CB pathogenesis and determine the clinical benefits of charnolopharmacotherapeutics.

Two mice bearing SUM-190 breast cancer xenografts received 1 mCi of ^{99m}Tc-glucarate and were imaged on a nanoSPECT/CT. One day later, the same animals received 1 mCi of ^{18}F-FdG and were imaged on animal Mosaic-HP PET. ^{99m}Tc-Glucarate (0.5–1 mCi) was administered to mice bearing xenografts induced by BxPC3 pancreatic cancer cells, HEK-293 renal cell carcinomas cells, or HCT-116 colorectal tumor cells. NanoSPECT/CT imaging was performed to evaluate tumor localization. In the SUM190 xenografted mice, the average tumor localization was 1.4% for ^{99m}Tc-glucarate and 2.1% for ^{18}F-FdG. While slightly higher than ^{99m}Tc-glucarate, the tumor accumulation of ^{18}F-FdG was accompanied by higher bone marrow and muscle accumulations, which could interfere with the imaging depending upon the location. The whole-body clearance of ^{99m}Tc-glucarate was faster than ^{18}F-FdG. The accumulation of ^{99m}Tc-glucarate varied among tumor types but was readily visible in all images. SPECT images obtained with ^{99m}Tcglucarate compared favorably with PET images obtained with ^{18}F-FdG. Tumor images with ^{99m}Tc-glucarate were also positive in 3 additional tumor models, suggesting that it could be used as a convenient and economical alternative to ^{18}F-FdG for animal studies on tumorigenesis. However, limited studies are currently available for human applications to quantitatively assess the DSST-CMB, charnolophagy, and CS stabilization/destabilization.

Although, PET imaging with ^{18}F-FdG provides direct estimate of tissue-specific CMB involving CB, charnolophagy, and CS dynamics, it remains uncertain whether ^{99m}Tc-glucarate could be used as more convenient and economical approach to determine DSST-CMB and CB pharmacodynamics (PDs) to quantitatively assess the potential benefit of novel charnolopharmacotherapeutics.

Although anatomical referencing of PET and SPECT images in experimental animals is based on CT, it requires a high radiation dose which may cause DNA damage (Kersemans et al. 2011). These researchers investigated whether CT can be utilized without compromising radiotherapy by determining radiation dose, biological damage, and image quality. NanoSPECT/CT imaging was performed to generate CT dose index and compared with the EBT2 film. Two mice strains, differing in radiation sensitivity were used to determine the effect of microCT. DNA damage was assessed in the leukocytes, liver, and jejunum by analyzing γH2AX foci, and jejunum damage by hematoxylin and eosin staining. The image quality was evaluated by estimating signal-to-noise ratio (SNR), contrast-to-noise ratio (CNR), and scanner linearity (SL). This study revealed that nanoSPECT/CT underestimates the absorbed dose because γH2AX formation in leukocytes, liver, and jejunum was significantly increased within

40 min. The radiosensitive strain demonstrated more DNA damage in the jejunum after 3 days. However, SNR, CNR, and SL permitted anatomical referencing which could be acquired without DNA damage and/or compromising image quality by using reduced radiographic voltage, flux, and duration for PET and SPECT imaging.

Noninvasive Imaging to Determine PKs and PDs of DSST-CS. In general, bio-distribution and PKs of newly-developed RPs is performed by the time-consuming and invasive approach of sacrificing animals and counting radioactivity from each organ. This conventional approach can increase the radiation exposure particularly when several RPs are evaluated for their translational utility. Currently, these studies can be performed efficiently and safely by *in vivo* non-invasive PET or SPECT imaging. However, recent studies revealed a mismatch in the bio-distribution of ^{111}In-labeled antibodies in the liver and kidneys when the *in vivo* imaging data was compared with *ex vivo* counting (Cheng et al. 2010). These researchers explored whether this mismatch could be reduced by selecting the proper ROI, adequate color thresholds, and correcting for the circulating radioactivity. Vials of known radioactivity of [111m]In were used as phantoms and [111m]In-DTPA-IgG antibody was administered by i.v. for imaging employing Bioscan NanoSPECT/CT in rats. The animals were sacrificed after imaging for *ex vivo* counting of radioactivity in each organ. However, higher values were obtained in *in vivo* imaging due to circulating radioactivity, which was resolved by correcting for blood pool radioactivity. These experiments confirmed that the counting accuracy depends on the proper setting of color thresholds and ROIs.

MicroPET vs Micro-SPECT Imaging. Recently, performance of microPET and microSPECT imaging systems was compared by using ^{18}F and ^{99m}Tc-labeled anti-Her2 NPs in Her2-positive tumor bearing mice, respectively (Cheng et al. 2010). Initially, phantoms and then tumor bearing mice injected with ^{99m}Tc-NPs were used for Bioscan NanoSPECT/CT imaging and ^{18}F-NPs injected mice for Philips Mosaic HP PET imaging. Although phantom imaging revealed that the resolution of SPECT was better, the detection sensitivity remained 15X lower. However, chelation of NPs with ^{99m}Tc was easier and safer compared to covalent radiolabeling with [18]F. The quantitation of radioactivity was accurate in both imaging systems. To develop multimodality imaging agents, Liang et al. (2010) synthesized streptavidin-conjugated NPs for both fluorescence and nuclear imaging in a tumor mouse model. These investigators attached 4 functions to the NPs without compromising the bio-distribution and PKs, including biotinylated anti-Her2 antibody for tumor targeting, [111m]In-labeled DOTA chelator for SPECT imaging, Cy5.5 to NPs for fluorescence imaging. Multimodality imaging with improved T/NT ratio was accomplished by IVIS fluorescence camera and a nanoSPECT/CT imaging in SUM190 (Her2+) tumor bearing mice. These data confirmed the significance of multimodality imaging for translational research.

It is now well-recognized that the patients suffering from bone metastasis are subjected to radionuclide therapy (RNT). [177]Lu is promising due to its long half-life (t1/2 = 6.73 days) and relatively low β energies, suitable for theranostic applications. The bio-distribution and toxicity of ^{177}Lu-EDTMP were studied in mice and rabbits by performing nanoSPECT/CT imaging and autoradiography, and dogs were used for imaging with γ-camera before initiating the human clinical trials (Mathe et al. 2010). The radioactive uptake of ^{177}Lu-EDTMP was observed in remodeling bone with negligible renal retention. However, the platelet count was depleted in dogs receiving the highest radioactivity. Radiolabeling of ^{177}Lu did not alter the biological behavior of EDTMP as a bone-localizing radiotracer, as determined by effective half lives in the animals, however, in PKs, differences were noticed. Furthermore, the dogs did not exhibit any adverse effect, suggesting that ^{177}Lu-EDTMP may be used as a bone-localizing agent for clinical applications.

In earlier studies, ^{99m}Tc-radiolabeled, HYNIC-derivatized minigastrin analogs have been synthesized for the molecular imaging of gastrin (von Guggenberg et al. 2009). NanoSPECT/CT was performed on tumor bearing nude mice to determine radiolabeling efficiency, stability, cell internalization, and binding on the CCK-2 receptor expressing AR4J2 cells. Radio-HPLC employed to estimate metabolites in liver, kidneys, and urine indicated rapid enzymatic degradation *in vivo*. These RPs demonstrated high stability and receptor mediated uptake in AR42J cells with increased renal clearance and target to non-target ratios in mouse models of tumor, suggesting their translational utility.

NanoSPECT/CT for Pre-Clinical Development of RPs. Nuclear imaging has been proposed for the novel discovery of novel RPs for translational imaging and drug delivery (Garrood et al. 2009). ^{99m}Tc-labeled anti-selectin antibody was used in human synovial tissue-transplanted SCID mice for nanoSPECT/CT imaging. The tissue vasculature was stimulated by injecting TNF-α in the grafts, 5 hrs prior to imaging at different time intervals. A significantly-increased target to non-target ratios confirmed that nanoSPECT/CT imaging in the SCID mouse model can be used to develop RPs for localizing human synovial tissue *in vivo*.

Focal Brain Lesions in HIV/AIDs. It is difficult to diagnose the exact etiology of focal brain lesions (BL) in HIV patients. These lesions could be due to infections such as tuberculosis, toxoplasmosis, or due to lymphoma. Serological, molecular biological, and *in vivo* molecular imaging is performed to determine the exact etiopathogenesis, which differ in their sensitivity and specificity. When therapy remains unsuccessful, stereotaxic biopsy (STB) of lesions is performed. Recently, histopathological diagnosis derived by STB or autopsy in HIV-1 type C seropositive patients was compared with diagnostic neuroimaging with CT, MRI, and ^{201}Th/^{99m}Tc SECT imaging with reference to toxoplasmosis (Shyam babu et al. 2013). The most common cause of FBL was toxoplasmosis, followed by tuberculoma, progressive multifocal leukoencephalopathy (PML), primary CNS lymphoma (PCNSL), and measles inclusion body encephalitis (MIBE). Histopathological confirmation could be accomplished in 14/21, CT, and MRI demonstrated comparable specificities (75%), whereas, MRI had slightly better sensitivity in detecting multiple lesions. The positive predictive value of both CT and MRI suggested that CT could be more suitable for evaluating FBL. Although ^{99m}Tc SPECT imaging could diagnose 75% inflammatory lesions accurately, it could not differentiate PCNSL from toxoplasmosis.

Nicotinic ACh Receptors Study with SPECT Imaging. It is now realized that patients with MDDs may be treated by modulating the β2 subunit containing nicotinic acetylcholine receptors. SPECT imaging was performed with ^{123}I-5-I-A-85380 to examine β2-subunit-containing nAChRs (β2*-nAChRs) in depressed patients (Saricicek et al. 2012). These investigators also examined β2*-nAChR binding in the postmortem brain samples of MDD patients. ^{123}I-5 -I-A-85380 SPECT and MRI were performed in 23 drug-free, non-smokers with depression.

Acutely ill and recovered patients exhibited reduced β2*-nAChR compared to controls. The receptor occupancy reduced in acutely ill patients compared to those who recovered and correlated with the frequency of depressive episodes, anxiety scores, and trauma scores. These data were analogous to DAergic PET ligands and DA receptors for the differences between β2*-nAChR *in vivo* and in post-mortem analysis. Reduced receptor occupancy for the SPECT ligand was attributed to increased acetylcholine in the CNS.

Fusion Imaging in CNS Infections. Although the incidence of CNS opportunistic infections (OIs) has been significantly reduced following highly active antiretroviral therapy (HAART); the likelihood of OIs such as toxoplasmosis, cryptococcosis, tuberculosis, and progressive multifocal leukoencephalopathy (PML) has not changed (Manzardo et al. 2005). Moreover, the differential diagnosis should include primary lymphoma in all cases with FBL. Differential diagnosis can be accomplished by performing multimodality neuroimaging with SPECT, PET, MRI, and/or CT, and molecular analysis of CSF and serum, and by evaluating the therapeutic response. Stereotaxic biopsy should be reserved for those patients with atypical lesions or those who remain resistant to conventional therapy. To prevent the recurrence of OIs, life-long treatment has been recommended. Certain HIV/AIDs patients on HART therapy develop worsening of OIs, characterized by immune reconstitution inflammatory syndrome (IRIS) and low CD4+ T-cell counts. Patients with CNS cryptococcosis, tuberculosis, or PML may present symptoms of IRIS, whereas HAART-induced immune reconstitution may improve the prognosis of PML and may allow maintenance therapy to be discontinued in patients with high CD4+ T-cell response.

Multimodality Neuroimaging in AD. It is now known that AD is associated with deterioration in cognition and behavior. With the availability of newly-developed drugs for symptoms relief, there is need of an early diagnosis and the development of novel sensitive imaging modalities and biomarkers, to identify and/or monitor early cerebral changes, suggestive for AD (Gualdi et al. 2004). Multimodality CT and MRI are recommended for the clinical evaluation, to exclude treatable cases of dementia and to evaluate the extent of cerebral atrophy and the presence of parenchymal signal abnormalities. Functional neuroimaging, including PET, SPECT, and fMRI, can be used to investigate cerebral function, such as blood perfusion, metabolism, activation, molecular composition, water diffusion; and have the potential to detect subtle pathological changes earlier during the disease. MRI can provide both morphological as well as functional evaluation. Further studies are needed to determine the exact role of various fMRI procedures. Disease-Specific PET radionuclides (^{18}F, ^{11}C)-labeled CB, charnolophagy, and CS biomarkers will confer excellent *in vivo* molecular imaging strategy for early differential diagnosis, prognosis, and treatment of AD. A comprehensive evaluation of AD will include conventional and functional imaging, combined with clinical, laboratory, omics (particularly charnolosomics), and genetic analyses.

Brain Regional Perfusion and Glucose Metabolism. In a study, ^{99m}Tc-HMPAO SPECT and ^{18}F-FDG PET/CT imaging was used to estimate brain regional blood flow and glucose metabolism respectively (Banzo et al. 2011). Twenty-two patients with cognitive impairment were studied: four subjective memory complaints (SMC), 8 amnestic mild cognitive impairment (MCI), 5 prodromic AD and 5 AD. Fifteen patients demonstrated brain regional hypoperfusion and 19 demonstrated hypometabolism. Similar abnormalities in brain regional perfusion as well as hypometabolism were observed in 9 patients. These were 2 SMC, 2 amnestic MCI, 3 prodromic AD, and 3 AD patients. In six patients (1 amnestic MCI, 2 prodromic AD, and 3 AD), hypometabolism was more evident than the cerebral hypoperfusion. Four patients (1SMC, 3 amnestic MCI) demonstrated abnormal ^{18}F-FdG-PET/CT and normal ^{99m}Tc-HMPAO SPECT imaging. There were 3 patients (1 SMC 2, amnestic MCI) with normal ^{99m}Tc-HMPAO SPECT and ^{18}F-FdG-PET/CT scans. Patients with cognitive impairment as well as SMC demonstrated reduced brain regional perfusion as well as hypometabolism. In some patients with a normal cerebral blood flow, cerebral hypometabolism was detected and vice versa. However, it remains to be established whether ^{99m}Tc-HMPAO SPECT and ^{18}F-FDG PET/CT imaging could be reliably utilized to quantitatively assess DSST mitochondrial bioenergetics and CB pharmacodynamics involving charnolophagy induction/inhibition and CS stabilization/de-stabilization as a function of disease progression/regression.

Ethanol-mediated Comorbidity in Drug Addiction. We performed a study on C57Bl/6J mice to determine the deleterious consequences of ethanol on cocaine and METH-induced neurotoxicity in C57Bl/6J mice employing longitudinal microPET neuroimaging (Sharma and Ebadi 2008). Chronic treatment of cocaine and METH induced a dose and time-dependent reduction in the striatal ^{18}F-DOPA and ^{18}FdG uptake, which was further reduced when cocaine and METH were co-administered along with ethanol, indicating that ethanol enhances cocaine and METH neurotoxicity by compromising brain regional DAergic neurotransmission and MB, respectively. An active metabolite, coca-ethylene is formed by co-administration of cocaine along with ethanol, which is more potent and induces severe neurotoxicity particularly in FAS victims due to CB formation, charnolophagy inhibition, and CS destabilization in the developing NPCs derived from iPPC to induce diversified embryopathies including microcephaly and other craniofacial abnormalities (Chabenne et al. 2014; Sharma et al. 2014; Sharma 2017).

Therapeutic Potential of MTs as CB Antagonists. It is well established that CBs are pre-apoptotic, multi-lamellar electron-dense membrane stacks of degenerated mitochondria, which are formed due to free radical overproduction during DPCI. The CB was discovered as a pre-apoptotic biomarker of cell injury in developing UN rat cerebellar Purkinje neurons and in the mice hippocampal neurons in response to intrauterine DOM exposure (Sharma 2014; Sharma and Ebadi 2014). Recently, we reported the clinical significance of CB as a universal biomarker of cell injury to further confirm our original hypothesis: "MTs provide ubiquinone (CoQ_{10})-mediated neuroprotection by inhibiting CB formation, augmenting charnolophagy, CS stabilization, and by serving as potent free radical scavengers." We reported that MTs are down-regulated in the aging brain, particularly in AD patients (Sharma and Ebadi 2014); hence, could be used as early and sensitive biomarkers for the clinical diagnosis of PD, AD, and drug addiction in addition to SI and charnolophagy index (Sharma et al. 2013a; Sharma 2017, 2018). MTs inhibit CB formation, augment charnolophagy, and stabilize CS by serving as potent antioxidants and free radical scavengers. Furthermore, we highlighted the clinical significance of MTs in cell therapy and nanomedicine (Sharma et al. 2013b).

The distribution kinetics of ^{18}F-DOPA was significantly impaired in *wv/wv* mice and these genotypes exhibited progressive neurodegeneration in the striatum, hippocampus, and cerebellum as observed in patients suffering from multiple drug addiction (Sharma and Ebadi 2005). The *wv/wv* mice exhibited age-dependent reduction in the striatal ^{18}D-DOPA as well as ^{18}FdG uptake as determined by high-resolution microPET imaging employing *MicroPET Manager* for the data acquisition and *AsiPro* for the 3D image reconstruction (Sharma et al. 2006; Sharma and Ebadi 2006).

These original findings further confirmed free radical-induced molecular mechanism of neurodegeneration and the therapeutic potential of MTs as CB antagonists, charnolophagy agonists, and CS stabilizers. In addition to significant reduction in the striatal ^{18}F-DOPA, wv/wv mice exhibited progressive reduction in the brain regional MB as determined by molecular imaging with ^{18}FdG (Sharma and Ebadi 2013). To further establish the therapeutic potential of MTs in progressive NDDs, we raised genetically-modified mouse models including: (i) MT_{trans} mice, MT_{dko} mice, α-Syn-MT_{tko} mice, wv/wv, and wv/wv-MTs mice (Sharma and Ebadi 2014). These experimental genotypes further confirmed our original hypothesis that progressive neurodegeneration occurs due to CMB, whereas MTs provide neuroprotection as free radical scavengers and CB antagonists, charnolophagy agonists, and CS stabilizers. The brain region-specific ^{18}FdG was significantly reduced in wv/wv mice, whereas it was improved in wv/wv-MTs mice, suggesting the therapeutic potential of MTs in NDDs through their boosting action on MB. Hence, MTs can be used as novel theranostic biomarkers for the early detection of NDDs such as PD, AD, and drug addiction.

Early Detection of Suicidality by Neuroimaging. It is well-known that suicidal tendencies are most common among patients suffering from MDDs and is a universal challenge. Every year > 750,000 victims try to commit suicide in the U.S.A. Out of which 30,000 become successful in taking away their lives. The majority of these suicide victims are > 85 years old living alone with limited resources. There are subtle differences in the cognitive performance of suicidal patients; however, currently, the knowledge of underlying molecular neuropharmacology is limited. Multi-modality molecular imaging with theranostic capabilities may confer unique opportunity to determine the exact spatio-temporal psychopharmacology of the brain in these patients. Recently, multimodality neuroimaging was performed to determine alternations in the neurotransmitters, transporters, and receptors to explain the possible molecular mechanism of suicidal behavior (Desmyter et al. 2011). These investigators reviewed neuroimaging articles comprising structural imaging with CT, and functional imaging with SPECT and fMRI. CT as well as structural MRI could not differentiate between the normal and suicidal brain. fMRI in subjects with a history of suicide attempt provided reduced volumes of the frontal and temporal lobe, with a trend towards reduced grey matter volume in the frontal lobe among white populations. Functional neuroimaging revealed reduced perfusion and perfusion defect in the prefrontal cortex during cognitive action in suicidal patients. The mitochondrial metabolism of prefrontal cortex was inversely correlated with the lethality of previous suicide attempters following the fenfluramine challenge. There was also no significant difference in the binding potential of the serotonin transporter. However, these victims exhibited a negative correlation between impulsivity and SERT binding. Recent suicide attempters exhibited reduced 5-HT$_{2A}$ receptor binding. The 5-HT$_{2A}$ receptor binding index was lower in the deliberate self-injury patients compared to self-poisoning patients. No significant difference in the DAT activity between suicide victims and controls was observed. However, suicide attempters demonstrated a negative correlation between DAT binding potential and mental energy. Although there is no systematic study on the binding potential of NE and GABA transporters or their receptor in these patients, impaired GABA-ergic neurotransmission has been reported in MDDs. In addition, depletion in IGF-1 and BDNF in the hippocampal pyramidal neurons involving CB formation, charnolophagy inhibition, and CS destabilization are implicated in MDDs and schizophrenia (Sharma 2015).

Several studies have linked stress to the development of MDD and suicidal behavior. Recent preclinical studies demonstrated that in rodents, chronic stress and the stress hormone cortisol causes oxidative damage to mitochondrial function and membrane lipids in the brain (Du et al. 2016). Mitochondria play a pivotal role in synaptic neurotransmitter signaling by providing ATP, mediating lipid and protein synthesis, buffering $[Ca^{2+}]_i$, and regulating apoptotic signal transduction. Membrane lipids are essential to CNS function because cholesterol, PUFA, and sphingolipids form a lipid raft region on the membrane that mediates neurotransmitter signaling through G-protein-coupled receptors and ion channels. Low serum cholesterol levels, low antioxidant capacity, and abnormal early morning cortisol levels are potential biomarkers of depression and suicidal behavior. A recent review summarized the basic molecular mechanism by which nutrients protect against oxidative damage to mitochondria and lipids in the brain regional neurocircuitry associated with cognitive and affective disorders. These nutrients include ω3 fatty acids, antioxidants (vitamin C and Zn^{2+}), members of the vitamin B family (Vitamin B^{12} and folic acid), and magnesium. There is currently evidence to suggest that these nutrients can enhance cognitive performance and may have therapeutic benefit for depression and suicidal behavior. Hence, regular intake of these nutrients may prevent the onset of mood disorders and suicidal behavior in vulnerable individuals or may augment the therapeutic benefit of antidepressants. These findings are clinically-significant for the health and well-being of both military as well as civilian population. Furthermore, it has been shown that short telomere length (TL) occurs in individuals under psychological stress, and with various psychiatric diseases. Recent studies reported mtDNA copy number (mtDNAcn) alterations in several psychiatric diseases. Hence, Otsuka et al. (2017) analyzed TL and mtDNAcn in post-mortem samples from 528 suicide completers without severe physical illness (508 peripheral bloods; 20 brains) and 560 samples from control subjects (peripheral bloods from 535 healthy individuals; 25 post-mortem brains) by qPCR analysis. Suicide completers had significantly shorter TL and higher mtDNAcn of peripheral bloods with sex/age-dependent differences (shorter TL was more remarkable in female/young suicides, whereas, higher mtDNAcn was more so in male/elderly suicides). The normal age-related decline of TL and mtDNAcn were altered in suicide completers. Shorter TL and lower mtDNAcn of post-mortem prefrontal cortex were seen in suicide completers compared to controls, indicating the association of aberrant telomeres and mtDNA content with suicide completion. Hence, further research on telomere shortening and mitochondrial dysfunction involving CB induction, charnolophagy, and CS destabilization may elucidate the basic molecular mechanism of suicide-related pathophysiology.

Recent preclinical data suggest that chronic stress may cause cellular damage and mitochondrial dysfunction involving CB molecular pathogenesis, leading to the release of mtDNA into the bloodstream. MDDs were associated with an increased mtDNA in leukocytes from blood and saliva samples. Therefore, Lindquist et al. (2016) quantified free circulating mtDNA in plasma samples from 37 suicide attempters, who had undergone a dexamethasone suppression test (DST), and 37 healthy controls. They hypothesized that free circulating mtDNA would be elevated in the suicide attempters and would be associated with hypothalamic–pituitary–adrenal (HPA)-axis hyperactivity involving elevated plasma cortisol levels. Suicide attempters had significantly higher plasma levels of free-circulating mtDNA compared with healthy controls, which was related to impaired HPA-axis negative feedback. Pre-DST plasma levels of mtDNA were correlated with post-DST cortisol levels. The peripheral cortisol index was consistent with an increased mitochondrial or cellular damage. Recently, we reported that stress-induced elevated circulating and salivary cortisol is involved in microglial activation and hippocampal atrophy through CB formation in progressive NDDs including PD, AD, schizophrenia, MDDs, and suicide attempters (Sharma 2016; Sharma et al. 2016). It is now known that suicide and related behaviors are complex phenomena associated with different risk factors.

Although most individuals who display suicidal behavior do not have a history of early-life adversity, a significant minority does. Recent experimental and clinical evidence suggest that early-life adversity leads to epigenetic changes of genes involved in stress-response systems. In a review, Ernst et al. (2012) suggested that early-life adversity increases risk of suicide in susceptible individuals by influencing the development of emotional, behavioral and cognitive phenotypes that result from the epigenetic regulation of the HPA axis and other systems in responses to stress. Hence, future studies are needed to better understand the relevance of increased free-circulating cortisol and mtDNA in relation to the pathophysiology underlying suicidal behavior and depression through CB formation, charnolophagy, and CS destabilization implicated in apoptotic neurodegeneration and suicidal ideation.

Neuroimaging in Schizophrenia. PET and SPECT neuroimaging have significantly enhanced our knowledge regarding schizophrenia and its clinical management (Erritzoe et al. 2003). During episodes of illness, the striatal presynaptic DArgic activity is enhanced and is associated with positive symptoms and better therapeutic response. However, the exact role of the prefrontal DA-ergic system remains enigmatic. The major limitations in these studies were: (i) a limited number of patients, (ii) lack of proper controls, and (iii) the cost of investigation. Moreover, it was difficult to find drug-free patients with schizophrenia. These investigators recommended that development of novel ^{18}F-labeled PET RPs may provide precise pharmacological mechanisms and effective treatment of EBPT of schizophrenia in future.

Differential Diagnosis of PD. A basic understanding of the imaging setup, post-processing procedures, and neuro-anatomy of SPECT for the differential diagnosis of PD is now well established (Morano and Seibyl 2003; Seibyl 2008). Guilford Pharmaceuticals company developed a sensitive and specific tropane derivative (Iometopane [123]I β-CIT, GPI 200, RTI 55) as a SPECT imaging agent for the differential diagnosis of PD and supranuclear palsy patients, as it binds specifically to the striatal (caudate and putamen) DA transporter (Anonymous 2003). The severity of both disease traits could be determined as a function of DAergic degeneration as this agent demonstrated reduced striatal localization in PD patients. It was envisaged that DOPA-scan will be beneficial to distinguish PD from other types of tremors to avoid inappropriate psychotropic medications and unnecessary investment in CT and MRI.

Differential Diagnosis of AD. There is no doubt that a NDDs such as AD is a devastating dementing illness with serious morbidity and mortality (Silverman et al. 1999). Early and accurate diagnosis of AD makes it possible to treat and prevent the disease progression. Neuroimaging with ^{18}FdG-PET has provided the brain regional metabolic pattern to help in this direction. The diagnostic accuracy of ^{18}FdG-PET in distinguishing AD from other cognitive impairments at an earlier stage is far better than CT, MRI, and SPECT and exceeds the clinical diagnosis based on history, physical examination, cognitive testing, and blood and CSF analyses as it provides a sensitive measure of brain regional CMB, involving CB formation, charnolophagy, and CS destabilization, implicated in AD pathogenesis.

SPECT Imaging with ^{99m}***TC-labeled RBCs.*** In earlier studies, we determined the sites of ^{99m}Tc binding on the RBCs for blood pool scanning (Rehani and Sharma 1980). ^{99m}Tc-RBC imaging is highly specific, noninvasive, and easy to perform; it provides an accurate diagnosis for the management of orbital hemangioma and avoids invasive imaging or biopsy (Burroni et al. 2012). SPECT imaging with ^{99m}Tc-labeled RBCs supplemented CT, MRI, and US findings, especially when performed along with multimodality fusion imaging (SPECT/MRI, SPECT/CT) in suspected cases of orbital hemangiomas (Pilecki et al. 2008).

MicroPET Neuroimaging of Drug Abused Mice. We studied the effect of multiple drug abuse in C57/BJ6 mice. Chronic intoxication of cocaine and METH reduced the striatal ^{18}F-DOPA uptake. By microPET neuroimaging, we established that the co-intoxication of cocaine and METH along with ethanol further reduces ^{18}F-DOPA uptake, suggesting that alcohol may serve as a gateway to multiple drug abuse (Sharma and Ebadi 2008). In a recent study, we reported that MTs provide neuroprotection by binding, donating, and buffering Zn^{2+} and are down-regulated in the hippocampal region of AD patients. The exact pathophysiological significance and therapeutic potential of MTs remains unknown. It is known that by donating Zn^{2+}, MTs are involved in the transcriptional activation of genes involved in growth, development, and differentiation in the CNS and other organs. Hence, MTs may have therapeutic potential in cell therapy and nanomedicine (Sharma et al. 2013). Similar molecular approaches may be developed in future for the safe and effective EBPT of AD as highlighted in our recent report (Sharma 2014). Moreover, MTs provide neuroprotection by preventing CB formation during the acute phase and by inhibiting CB formation, augmenting charnolophagy, and by stabilizing CS during the chronic phase as potent free radical scavengers to provide neuroprotection in chronic MDR diseases (Sharma 2016, 2017, 2018).

Molecular Imaging in Translational Research. Indeed, high-resolution molecular imaging can provide an *in vivo*, noninvasive, quantitative, and real time estimate of the basic biological process in a living system (Villemagne et al. 2006). In addition, the biological variability can be minimized by molecular imaging under physiological conditions, reducing the number and cost of animals for the longitudinal analysis.

Future developments in target selection, RPs development, and imaging technology to quantitatively assess tissue and DSST-CB formation, charnolophagy induction, and CS stabilization employing novel NPs or radiotracers may provide in-depth knowledge regarding the disease process which will be highly significant in translational research to successfully accomplish EBPT of NDDs, CVDs, and chronic MDR malignancies. This unique approach may revolutionize the existing concept(s) of the healthcare system (Massoud and Gambhir 2007; Eckelman et al. 2008). Hence, novel NPs and PET-RPs may be developed to target receptor, transport protein, proliferation, angiogenesis, and inflammation, in addition to CMB-based CB, CPS, and CS evaluation to accomplish the targeted, safe, and effective personalized-theranostics of NDDs, CVDs, and MDR malignancies. However, for accurate drug development and PKs and PDs analyses, the number of control patients need to be small for molecular imaging.

PET imaging with targeted RPs facilitates noninvasive molecular characterization of biological changes, leading to earlier detection of disease, monitoring of therapies, and better prognostication. Recently, Li et al. (2014) provided the current knowledge of PET RPs in CVDs. In addition, gene-manipulated animal models of diseases have contributed significantly in translational research for molecular theranostics to solve challenging healthcare problems (Cunha et al. 2014). In fact, this unique approach provides novel *replacement, reduction, and refinement* strategies to accomplish EBPT. Molecular imaging for small animals include: microPET and nanoSPECT, optical imaging, CT, MRI, MRSI, and ultrasound with distinct merits and limitations. To overcome inherent limitations of individual imaging system, multimodality imaging systems are being developed. The combination of high-resolution micro-CT/micro-MRI, micro-PET/micro-SPECT, and micro-PET/micro-SPECT/CT has improved translational research in neurology, cardiology, and oncology. Furthermore, this unique and promising approach has improved our basic understanding of disease process and novel theranostic strategies. Indeed, multimodality imaging employing novel NPs and RPs targeting organ and disease-specific CMB, CB, charnolophagy, and CS stabilization will be highly beneficial to the pharmaceutical industries and research organizations for novel drug discovery.

Personalized Cancer Therapy. Although gene-manipulated murine models of human diseases (*particularly cancer*) is gaining popularity in translational research, these models lack tumor heterogeneity and genetic diversity of human cancers. Recently, Malaney et al. (2014) introduced two mouse models called *"Mouse Avatars" and Co-Clinical Trials* to accomplish EBPT. To determine drug efficacy, tumor cells are implanted in *"Mouse Avatars"*, which allows individual patient to have his/her own tumor growth for personalized treatment and eliminates the cost and toxicity of the conventional non-targeted chemotherapeutic approach. This novel strategy allows real-time integration and interpretation of the murine and human tumor data simultaneously to quantitatively assess the therapeutic response. It is envisaged that the combination of molecular profiling with omics technology ("Mouse Avatar" and Co-Clinical Trials), along with MB, CB, charnolophagy, and CS-targeted charnolopharmacotherapeutics may revolutionize the drug development industry to accomplish the targeted, safe, and effective EBPT of NDDs, CVDs, and chronic MDR malignancies.

Treatment of Malignant Gliomas. It is known that majority of malignant gliomas relapse after surgery and standard radio-chemotherapy (Keunen et al. 2014). Therefore, novel cellular and molecular therapies are being developed to target tumor growth. Although histopathology remains the gold standard for tumor classification, neuroimaging has taken a pivotal role in detecting and localizing space occupying lesions (SOLs), define the target area for biopsies, plan surgical and radiation interventions, and assess tumor progression and treatment, in addition to safe and effective theranostics of brain tumors. The development of anti-angiogenic agents that affect the tumor vasculature, has improved the quality of brain tumor imaging. To accurately evaluate the therapeutic decision, multi-modality neuroimaging, with novel contrast agents, radiotracers, and technological advances in the data analysis and interpretation may help in the discovery of relevant biomarkers. The clinical management of patients may be improved by utilizing DSST charnolopharmacotherapeutics involving CB prevention/inhibition, charnolophagy induction, CS stabilization, and CS-exocytosis/endocytosis as basic molecular mechanisms of MB and ICD for normal cellular function and homeostasis to remains healthy.

PET/MR Fusion Imaging. Recently, the diagnostic potential of integrated PET/MRI system was summarized (Czernin and Herrmann 2014). PET/MRI provides improved clinical assessments of cancers that may not be characterized with MRI and CT. Functional capabilities of MRI along with the molecular PET, provide new knowledge regarding the disease process and reduces the radiation exposure to vulnerable populations such as children and women of child-bearing age.

Iron Oxide NPs for Personalized Medicine. Iron oxide nanoparticles (IONPs), with theranostic potential, can be used in personalized medicine as these are inexpensive, non-toxic, and biodegradable. However, progress in their use has been limited due to inefficient drug loading and delivery. Recently, DA has been used to modify the surface of IONPs that could be encapsulated into human serum albumin (HSA) as a drug carrier (Xie et al. 2010). The HSA coated IONPs (HSA-IONPs) were labeled with ^{64}Cu-DOTA and Cy5.5, for testing in a U87MG xenograft mouse model. The *in vivo* multimodality PET, MRI, near-infrared fluorescence (NIRF), and *ex vivo* histological imaging were performed to explore the *in vivo* behavior of these NPs. HSA-IONPs demonstrated prolonged circulation half-life and specific tumor localization, extravasation rate, and reduced uptake by macrophages.

Dopamine-D$_3$ Receptor Imaging. D$_3$ receptors are a subtype of D$_2$ receptors, and currently their exact functional role is difficult to differentiate. There is considerable interest in developing selective D$_3$ receptor ligands for PD, schizophrenia, anxiety, depression, and drug addiction (Le Foll et al. 2014). Recently, [^{11}C]-(+)-PHNO was developed as a selective and sensitive D$_3$ receptors imaging agent with increased T/NT ratio in the ROI. [^{11}C]-(+)-PHNO was superior to ^{11}C-raclopride, which is unable to differentiate between D$_2$ and D$_3$ receptors to provide precise information regarding the functional significance of D$_3$ receptors in drug addiction and schizophrenia.

Biomarker Imaging in AD. Recently, significant interest was developed to discover surrogate biomarkers for the diagnosis of AD during the asymptomatic stage. Currently, putative disease-modifying agents are being tested in clinical trials. However, treatment need to be initiated before molecular changes progress to an early prodromal dementia phase or an irreversible stage of irreversible metabolic, functional, and morphological impairment (Malaney et al. 2014; Keunen et al. 2014; Czernin and Herrmann 2014;

Xie et al. 2010; Le Foll et al. 2014). It is now emphasized that the primary objective of any CNS drug development is to elucidate the molecular mechanism rather than molecule to advance further research on clinical trials (Hargreaves and Rabiner 2014). Indeed, PET imaging biomarkers provide confirmation of targeted drug delivery for neuropsychiatric drug development, facilitate exploring the neuropharmacological basis of psychiatric diseases, and the optimization of drug therapy. Since, CB formation, charnolophagy, and CS have been discovered as early, pre-apoptotic biomarkers of CMB in progressive NDDs, CVDs, and chronic MDR malignancies which can be detected at much earlier and initial stages of disease progression, these novel biomarkers may be utilized to define the preclinical stages of these chronic diseases (Sharma 2016, 2017, 2018).

Gd-Enhanced MRI for Brain Tumors. Gd-enhanced MRI plays a significant role in the clinical assessment of brain tumors. Although canine brain tumors are utilized as a translational model for evaluating human brain tumors, there is no standardized neuroimaging response assessment criteria in veterinary trials. Moreover, the assessment of solid tumors is complicated by pathophysiologic features inherent to brain tumors and the surrounding brain tissue (Rossmeis et al. 2014). In this respect, multimodality perfusion imaging, PET, and MRSI has shown great promise in differentiating tumor progression from treatment-induced necrosis.

^{89}Zr-Labeled Antibody (immuno-PET) Imaging. Recently, ^{89}Zr has been introduced as a diagnostic probe with excellent physical and chemical properties for immuno-PET imaging to characterize tumor lesions. It can be used to identify patients who may benefit from a specific therapy and monitor prognosis for personalized treatment (van de Watering et al. 2014). However, further research is needed to develop better conjugation methods and improved chelators to minimize Zr^{4+} released from the antibodies to validate their translational utility. It is expected that the development of new ^{89}Zr-labeled antibodies directed against novel tumor targets may enhance clinical applications of ^{89}Zr-labeled immuno-PET for translational imaging in future.

PET and MRI to Study Epigenetic Changes. It is now believed that abnormal gene regulation due to impaired epigenetic mechanisms may be involved in the initiation and persistence of human diseases including NDDs, CVDs, and chronic MDR malignancies. However, the association of epigenetic dysfunction with disease and the development of therapeutic agents for the treatment are still lacking. Future developments to visualize chromatin-modifying enzymes in the human brain employing recently-improved molecular imaging will help in the early and differential diagnosis of CNS and other disorders and novel drug discovery. Recently, invasive and noninvasive methods have been developed for estimating histone deacetylase (HDAC) enzymes in the CNS (Wang et al. 2014). The majority of these methods are invasive and difficult to translate to the human brain. However, molecular imaging may provide novel and noninvasive strategies to visualize epigenetic changes in the human brain. To identify and validate the proper CNS radiotracer for imaging HDACs and other histone-modifying enzymes implicated in epigenetic mechanisms involving CB induction/inhibition, charnolophagy induction/inhibition, CS stabilization/destabilization, and CS exocytosis/endocytosis agonists will be a significant future challenge. Eventually translational neuroimaging with PET and MRI will be a valuable addition to *ex vivo* methods to evaluate CNS and other diseases and understand epigenetic changes in health and disease. Moreover, it remains unknown whether epigenetic changes in the mtDNA can modify CB, charnolophagy, and CS pharmacodynamics in chronic diseases. Further study is required in this direction.

EEG and Fusion Neuroimaging. Recently, the clinical significance of the simultaneous acquisition of EEG and fMRI has been highlighted (Neuner et al. 2014). As MRI advances towards using ultra-high magnetic fields to enhance T/NT ratio, combined EEG-fMRI can be feasible at 7T or higher magnetic field strengths. These authors also discussed the challenges of MRI-EEG and reviewed the proposed solutions. Further developments in multimodality neuroimaging employing MRI, PET, and EEG in the same subject will lead to successful translational research to accomplish safe and effective EBPT.

Translational PET/MRI Neuroimaging in Drug Addiction. Translational neuroimaging with PET and MRI can elucidate neurobehavioral impairments in drug addiction (Jupp and Dalley 2014). These noninvasive neuroimaging modalities have further elucidated the etiology of drug seeking behavior and the influence of environment and neuronal impairments in chronic drug abuse. Mostly these studies were performed in rats, monkey, and humans to discover specific biomarkers of impaired DA-ergic neurotransmission. The neuroimaging studies were correlated and confirmed with neurobehavioral analyses to understand the basic molecular mechanism of drug-seeking impulsive behavior. Recently, the importance of environmental variables on cocaine self-administration in nonhuman primate models of drug addiction was reported employing noninvasive translational PET. These studies demonstrated that environmental stimuli can influence brain function and drug self-administration. Furthermore, non-drug alternatives (e.g., food reinforcement and social variables (e.g., social rank, social stress)) can influence drug-seeking behavior, suggesting individual variability in pharmacological response to drug abuse treatment. It is known that cocaine-related cognitive deficits cause increased rates of relapse in nonhuman primate models. Recently, the utility of PET imaging to study the neurobiological vulnerability to cocaine addiction and subsequent adaptations following chronic self-administration and long-term consequences were highlighted (Nader and Banks 2014). These authors emphasized the involvement of environmental (e.g., social rank) and gender-specific influences on DAergic function and sensitivity to the reinforcing effects of cocaine. PET neuroimaging and behavioral analyses facilitated the designing of personalized pharmacological and behavioral treatment strategies in patients with drug seeking behavior. Moreover, recent advances in radiochemistry of novel PET ligands and multimodality neuroimaging can further enhance our understanding regarding drug addiction and its early safe and effective EBPT (Gould et al. 2014).

In Vivo Brodmann Mapping. Recently "*In vivo* Brodmann mapping" or non-invasive cortical parcellation employing MRI, has become an important research topic. Hence, Glasser et al. (2014) reviewed *in vivo* myelin mapping studies and methods for estimating myelin content. They discussed strategies to improve myelin maps surface registration for comparisons, and neurobiological aspects of myelination. Myelin content was inversely correlated with cortical circuit complexity. By using PET imaging data and functional network analyses, these investigators examined metabolic differences in the myelinated cortical networks. Lightly myelinated cognitive networks had higher aerobic glycolysis than heavily myelinated motor cortex, reflecting greater anabolic processes involving MB, confirming that cortical myelination stabilizes circuits and inhibits synaptic plasticity.

Conclusion

In this chapter, the clinical significance of *in vitro* and *in vivo* molecular imaging of MB, CB, charnolophagy, and CS-labelled NPs and radiotracers to assess ICD and to discover novel DSST charnolophamacotherapeutics for the targeted, safe, and effective EBPT of NDDs, CVDs, and chronic MDR malignancies is highlighted. Although the analyses of functional genomics through *in vivo* molecular imaging involves relatively costly equipment and state of the art computer-controlled RPs synthesis modules, the acquisition of high-resolution, non-invasive dynamic functional images provides detailed, valuable, and precise information regarding the disease process on a longitudinal basis under physiological conditions. Hence, the future of multimodality *in vivo* fusion imaging seems promising as well as challenging to combat these chronic diseases with currently limited therapeutic success. The most significant challenge is to develop novel PET RPs and NPs for the differential diagnosis of progressive NDDs of unknown etiopathogenesis (such as PD, AD, ALS, HD, MS, MDD, schizophrenia, and drug addiction), CVDs, and MDR malignancies. An early stage detection of these chronic diseases will facilitate safe and effective EBPT. Hence, DSST radiolabeled or fluorescently labeled CB biomarkers, charnolophagy agonists/antagonists, CPS agnonists/antagonists, CS agonists/antagonists, and CS endocytosis/endocytosis agonists/antagonists will provide early and more sensitive measures of MB and ICD for the targeted, safe, and effective EBPT of chronic intractable diseases.

References

Albert, M., C. DeCarli, S. DeKosky, M.D. Leon, N.L. Foster, N. Fox. R. Frank, R. Frackowiak et al. 2015. The Use of MRI and PET for Clinical Diagnosis of Dementia and Investigation of Cognitive Impairment: A Consensus Report Prepared by the Neuroimaging Work Group1 of the Alzheimer's Association. pp. 1–15.

Anonmous. 2003. Iometopane: (123)I beta-CIT, dopascan injection, GPI 200, RTI 55. Drugs R *D* 4: 320–22.

Banzo, I., R. Quirce, I. Martínez-Rodríguez, J. Jiménez-Bonilla, H. Portilla-Quattrociocchi, P. Medina-Quiroz, F. Ortega, E. Rodríguez, I. Mateo, J.L. Vázquez-Higuera, M. de Arcocha and J.M. Carril. 2011. Molecular neuroimaging in the study of cognitive impairment: contribution of the cerebral blood flow SPECT with ^{99m}Tc-HMPAO and ^{18}F-FDG PET/CT scan. Rev Esp Med Nucl 30: 301–306.

Brenner, LA. 2011. Neuropsychological and neuroimaging findings in traumatic brain injury and post-traumatic stress disorder. Dialogues in Clin Neurosci 13: 311–323.

Burroni, L., G. Borsari, P. Pichierri, E. Polito, O. Toscano, G. Grassetto, A. Al-Nahhas, D. Rubello and A.G. Vattimo. 2012. Preoperative diagnosis of orbital cavernous hemangioma: a ^{99m}Tc-RBC SPECT study. Clin Nucl Med 37: 1041–1046.

Chabenne, A., C. Moon, C. Ojo, A. Khogali, B. Nepal and S. Sharma. 2014. Biomarkers in fetal alcohol syndrome (Recent Update). Biomarkers and Genomic Medicine 6: 12–22.

Chang, C.C., C.C. Lui, J.J. Wang, S.H. Huang, C.H. Lu, C. Chen, C.F. Chen, M.C. Tu, C. Huang and W.N. Chang. 2010. Multi-parametric neuroimaging evaluation of cerebrotendinous xanthomatosis and its correlation with neuropsychological presentations. BMC Neurology 10: 1–8.

Cheng, D., Y. Wang, X. Liu, P.H. Pretorius, M. Liang, M. Rusckowski and D.J. Hnatowich. 2010. Comparison of ^{18}F PET and 99mTc SPECT imaging in phantoms and in tumored mice. Bioconjug Chem 21: 1565–1570.

Cheng, D., M. Rusckowski, Y. Wang, Y. Liu, G. Liu, X. Liu and D. Hnatowich. 2011. A brief evaluation of tumor imaging in mice with ^{99m}Tc-glucarate including a comparison with ^{18}F-FDG. Curr Radiopharm 4: 5–9.

Cheng, D., M. Rusckowski, P.H. Pretorius, L. Chen, N. Xiao, Y. Liu, G. Liu, M. Liang, X. Liu, S. Dou and D.J. Hnatowich. 2011. Improving the quantitation accuracy in noninvasive small animal single photon emission computed tomography imaging. Nucl Med Biol 38: 843–848.

Cunha, L., I. Horvath, S. Ferreira, J. Lemos, P. Costa, D. Vieira, D.S. Veres, K. Szigeti, T. Summavielle, D. Máthé and L.F. Metello. 2014. Preclinical imaging: an essential ally in modern biosciences. Mol Diagn Ther 18: 153–173.

Czernin, J., L. Ta and K. Herrmann. 2014. Does PET/MR Imaging Improve Cancer Assessments? Literature evidence from more than 900 patients. J Nucl Med 55: 59S–62S.

Danysz, W. and C.G. Parsons. 2012. Alzheimer's disease, b-amyloid, glutamate, NMDA receptors and memantine—searching for the connections. British Journal of Pharmacology 167: 324–352.

Desmyter, S., C. van Heeringen and K. Audenaert. 2011. Structural and functional neuroimaging studies of the suicidal brain. Prog Neuropsychopharmacol Biol Psychiatry 35: 796–808.

Du, J., M. Zhu, H. Bao, B. Li, Y. Dong, C. Xiao, G.Y. Zhang, I. Henter, M. Rudorfer and B. Vitiello. 2016. The role of nutrients in protecting mitochondrial function and neurotransmitter signaling: Implications for the treatment of depression, PTSD, and suicidal behaviors. Crit Rev Food Sci Nutr 56: 2560–2578.

Ebadi, M. and S. Sharma. 2006. Metallothioneins 1 and 2 attenuate peroxynitrite-induced oxidative stress in Parkinson's disease. Exp Biol Med 231: 1576–1583.

Eckelman, W.C., R.C. Reba and G.I. Kelloff. 2008. Targeted imaging: an important biomarker for understanding disease progression in the era of personalized medicine. Drug Discovery Today 13: 748–759.

Erritzoe, D., P. Talbot, W.G. Frankle and A. Abi-Dargham. 2003. Positron emission tomography and single photon emission CT molecular imaging in schizophrenia. Neuroimaging Clin N Am 13: 817–832.

Ernst, C., F. Jollant, B. Labonte and N. Mechawar. 2012. The neurodevelopmental origins of suicidal behavior. Trends in Neuroscience 35: 14–23.

Eshaghia, A., S. Riyahi-Alama, R. Saeedia, T. Roostaeia, A. Nazeria et al. 2015. Classification algorithms with multi-modal data fusion could accurately distinguish neuromyelitis optica from multiple sclerosis. NeuroImage Clinical 7: 306–314.

Furka, I., N. Németh and I. Mikó. 2013. The spleen in experimental surgery. Magy Seb 66: 156–160.

Garrood, T., M. Blades, D.O. Haskard, S. Mather and C.A. Pitzalis. 2009. A novel model for the pre-clinical imaging of inflamed human synovial vasculature. von Guggenberg. Rheumatology (Oxford) 48: 926–931.

Glasser, M.F., M.S. Goyal, T.M. Preuss, M.E. Raichle and D.C. Van Essen. 2014. Trends and properties of human cerebral cortex: correlations with cortical myelin content. Neuroimage 93: 165–175.

Gould, R.W., A.N. Duke and M.A. Nader. 2014. PET studies in nonhuman primate models of *Cocaine* abuse: translational research related to vulnerability and neuroadaptations. Neuropharmacology 84: 138–151.

Gualdi, G.F., M.C. Colaiacomo, L. Bertini, A. Melone, M. Rojas and C. Di Biasi. 2004. Neuroimaging of Alzheimer disease: current role and future potential. Clin Ter 155: 429–438.

Gueguen, B., J. Touchon and D. Campion. 1997. Memory disorders in the elderly: complementary examinations—for whom? Therapie 52: 499–502.

Hampel, H., S. Lista, S.J. Teipel, F. Garaci, R. Nisticò, K. Blennow, H. Zetterberg, L. Bertram, C. Duyckaerts, H. Bakardjian, A. Drzezga, O. Colliot, S. Epelbaum, K. Broich, S. Lehéricy, A. Brice, Z.S. Khachaturian, P.S. Aisen and B. Dubois. 2014. Perspective on future role of biological markers in clinical therapy trials of Alzheimer's disease: a long-range point of view beyond 2020. Biochem Pharmacol 88: 426–449.

Hargreaves, R.J. and E.A. Rabiner. 2014. Translational PET imaging research. Neurobiol Dis 61: 32–38.

Harvey, P.D. 2012. Clinical applications of neuropsychological assessment. Dialogues in Clinical Neuroscience 14: 91–99.

John, A.E., J.C. Luckett, A.L. Tatler, R.O. Awais, A. Desai, A. Habgood, S. Ludbrook, A.D. Blanchard, A.C. Perkins, R.G. Jenkins and J.F. Marshall. 2013. Preclinical SPECT/CT imaging of αvβ6 integrins for molecular stratification of idiopathic pulmonary fibrosis. J Nucl Med 54: 2146–52.

Jupp, B. and J.W. Dalley. 2014. Behavioral endophenotypes of drug addiction: Etiological insights from neuroimaging studies. Neuropharmacology 76: 487–497.

Kersemans, V., J. Thompson, B. Cornelissen, M. Woodcock, P.D. Allen, N. Buls, R.J. Muschel, M.A. Hill and S.C. Smart. 2011. Micro-CT for anatomic referencing in PET and SPECT: radiation dose, biologic damage, and image quality. J Nucl Med 52: 1827–1833.

Keunen, O., T. Taxt, R. Grüner, M. Lund-Johansen, J.C. Tonn, T. Pavlin, R. Bjerkvig, S.P. Niclou and F. Thorsen. 2014. Multimodal imaging of gliomas in the context of evolving cellular and molecular therapies. Adv Drug Deliv Rev 76: 98–115.

Lacor, P.N. 2007. Advances on the understanding of the origins of synaptic pathology in AD. Current Genomics 8: 486–508.

Le Foll, B., A.A. Wilson, A. Graff, I. Boileau and P. Di Ciano. 2014. Recent methods for measuring DA D3 receptor occupancy *in vivo*: importance for drug development. Front Pharmacol 5: 161.

Lemere, C.A. and E. Masliah. 2010. Can Alzheimer disease be prevented by amyloid-β immunotherapy? Nat Rev Neurol 6: 108–119.

Li, Y., W. Zhang, H. Wu and G. Liu. 2014. Advanced tracers in PET imaging of cardiovascular disease. Biomed Res Int 2014: 504532.

Liang, M., X. Liu, D. Cheng, G. Liu, S. Dou, Y. Wang, M. Rusckowski and D.J. Hnatowich. 2010. Multimodality nuclear and fluorescence tumor imaging in mice using a streptavidin nanoparticle. Bioconjug Chem 21: 1385–1388.

Lin, K.J., C.C. Wu, Y.H. Pan, F.H. Chen, S.Y. Fu, C.S. Chiang, J.H. Hong and J.M. Lo. 2012. *In vivo* imaging of radiation-induced tissue apoptosis by (99m)Tc(I)-his (6)-annexin A5. Ann Nucl Med 26: 272–280.

Lindqvist, D., J. Fernström, C. Grudet, L. Ljunggren, L. Träskman-Bendz, L. Ohlsson and A. Westrin. 2016. Increased plasma levels of circulating cell-free mitochondrial DNA in suicide attempters: associations with HPA-axis hyperactivity. Translational Psychiatry 6: 971.

Liu, S., Y. Pan, J. Lv, H. Wu, J. Tian and Y. Zhang. 2014. Feasibility of baculovirus-mediated reporter gene delivery for efficient monitoring of islet transplantation *in vivo*. Nucl Med Biol 41: 171–178.

Liu, S., W. Cai, S. Liu, F. Zhang, M. Fulham, D. Feng, S. Pujol and R. Kikinis. 2015. Multimodal neuroimaging computing: a review of the applications in neuropsychiatric disorders. Brain Informatics 2: 167–180.

Malaney, P., S.V. Nicosia and V. Davé. 2014. One mouse, one patient paradigm: New avatars of personalized cancer therapy. Cancer Lett 344: 1–12.

Manzardo, C., M. Del Mar Ortega, O. Sued, F. García, A. Moreno and J.M. Miró. 2005. Central nervous system opportunistic infections in developed countries in the highly active antiretroviral therapy era. J Neurovirol Suppl 3: 72–82.

Massoud, T.F. and S.S. Gambhir. 2007. Integrating noninvasive molecular imaging into molecular medicine: an evolving paradigm. Trends in Molecular Medicine 13: 183–191.

Mathe, D.A., B.R. Polyak, D. Keraly, J. Pawlak, M. Zakunun, M. Pillai and G.A. Janoki. 2010. Multispecies animal investigation on biodistribution, pharmacokinetics and toxicity of 177Lu-EDTMP, a potential bone pain palliation agent. Nucl Med Biol 37: 215–26.

Mokhtar, S.H., M.M. Bakhuraysah, D.S. Cram and S. Petratos. 2013. The beta-amyloid protein of Alzheimer's disease: Communication breakdown by modifying the neuronal cytoskeleton. International Journal of Alzheimer's Disease. Article ID 910502, 15 pages.

Morano, G.N. and J.P. Seibyl. 2003. Technical overview of brain SPECT imaging: improving acquisition and processing of data. J Nucl Med Technol 31: 191–95.

Nader, M.A. and M.L. Banks. 2014. Environmental modulation of drug taking: Nonhuman primate models of *Cocaine* abuse and PET neuroimaging. Neuropharmacology 76: 510–517.

Nasrallah, I.M. and D.A. Wolk. 2014. Multimodality imaging of Alzheimer disease and other neurodegenerative dementias. J Nucl Med 55: 2003–2011.

Neuner, I., J. Arrubla, J. Felder and N.J. Shah. 2014. Simultaneous EEG-fMRI acquisition at low, high and ultra-high magnetic fields up to 9.4T: Perspectives and challenges. Neuroimage 102P1: 71–79.

Otsuka, I., T. Izumi, S. Boku, A. Kimura, Y. Zhang, K. Mouri, S. Okazaki, K. Shiroiwa, M. Takahashi, Y. Ueno, O. Shirakawa, I. Sora and A. Hashimoto. 2017. Aberrant telomere length and mitochondrial DNA copy number in suicide completers. Sci Rep 7: 3176.

Pan, Y., S. Liu, H. Wu, J. Lv, X. Xu and Y. Zhang. 2013. Baculovirus as an ideal radionuclide reporter gene vector: a new strategy for monitoring the fate of human stem cells *in vivo*. PLoS One 8: e61305.

Pilecki, S., M. Gierach, J. Gierach, Z. Serafin, N. Sulima, A. Grzela, E. Olejarz, S. Wałek, W. Lasek, J. Kałużny and R. Junik. 2008. Single photon emission computed tomography (SPECT) in the diagnosis of orbital cavernous hemangioma. Pol J Radiol 73: 59–62.

Polyák, A., I. Hajdu, M. Bodnár, G. Trencsényi, Z. Pöstényi, V. Haász, G. Jánoki, G.A. Jánoki, L. Balogh and J. Borbély. 2013. (^{99m})Tc-labelled nanosystem as tumour imaging agent for SPECT and SPECT/CT modalities. Int J Pharm 449: 10–17.

Qiu, C., M. Kivipelto and E.V. Strauss. 2009. Epidemiology of Alzheimer's disease: occurrence, determinants, and strategies toward intervention. Dialogues Clin Neurosci 11: 111–128.

Rehani, M.M. and S.K. Sharma. 1980. Site of Tc-99m binding to the red blood cells. J Nuclear Medicine 22: 676–78.

Roccaa, W.A., R.C. Petersen, D.S. Knopmanb, L.E. Hebert, D.A. Evans, K.S. Hallf, S. Gaog, F.W. Unverzagtf, K.M. Langah, E.B. Larsonk and L.R. White. 2011. Trends in the incidence and prevalence of Alzheimer's disease, dementia, and cognitive impairment in the United States. Alzheimers Dement 7: 80–93.

Rossmeisl, J.H. Jr, P.A. Garcia, G.B. Daniel, J.D. Bourland, W. Debinski, N. Dervisis and S. Klahn. 2014. Neuroimaging response assessment criteria for brain tumors in veterinary patients. Vet Radiol Ultrasound 55: 115–132.

Saricicek, A., I. Esterlis, K.H. Maloney, Y.S. Mineur, B.M. Ruf, A. Muralidharan, J.I. Chen, K.P. Cosgrove, R. Kerestes, S. Ghose, C.A. Tamminga, B. Pittman, F. Bois, G. Tamagnan, J. Seibyl, M.R. Picciotto, J.K. Staley and Z. Bhagwagar. 2012. Persistent β2*-nicotinic acetylcholinergic receptor dysfunction in major depressive disorder. Am J Psychiatry 169: 851–59.

Schillaci, O., L. Travascio, C. Bruni, G. Bazzocchi, A. Testa, F.G. Garaci, M. Melis, R. Floris and G. Simonetti. 2009. Molecular imaging and magnetic resonance imaging in early diagnosis of Alzheimer's disease. A literature review. Neuroradiol J 21: 755–71.

Seibyl, J.P. 2008. Single-photon emission computed tomography and positron emission tomography evaluations of patients with central motor disorders. Semin Nucl Med 38: 274–286.

Serrano-Pozo, A., M.P. Frosch, E. Masliah and B.T. Hyman. 2011. Neuropathological alterations in Alzheimer disease. *In*: Selkoe, D.J., D.M. Holtzman and E. Mandelkow (eds.). Cold Spring Harb Perspect Med 1: 1–23.

Sharma, S. and M. Ebadi. 2005. Distribution kinetics of ^{18}F-DOPA in weaver mutant mice. Molecular Brain Research 139: 23–30.

Sharma, S., H.El. Refaey and M. Ebadi. 2006. Complex-1 activity and ^{18}F-DOPA uptake in genetically engineered mouse model of Parkinson's disease and the neuroprotective role of coenzyme Q_{10}. Brain Res Bull 70: 22–32.

Sharma, S. and M. Ebadi. 2008. SPECT neuroimaging in translational research of CNS disorders. Neurochem Internat 52: 352–362.

Sharma, S., A. Rais, R. Sandhu, W. Nel and M. Ebadi. 2013. Clinical significance of metallothioneins in cell therapy and nanomedicine. International Journal of Nanomedicine 8: 1477–1488.

Sharma, S. and M. Ebadi. 2013. *In vivo* molecular imaging in Parkinson's disease. pp. 787–802. *In*: Pfeiffer, R.F., Z.K. Wszolek and M. Ebadi (eds.). Parkinson's Disease. IInd Edition, Chapter 58, CRC Press Taylor & Francis Group. Boca Rotan, FL, USA.

Sharma, S., C.S. Moon, A. Khogali, A. Haidous, A. Chabenne, C. Ojo, M. Jelebinkov, Y. Kurdi and M. Ebadi. 2013a. Biomarkers of Parkinson's disease (Recent Update). Neurochemistry International 63: 201–229.

Sharma, S., A. Rais, R. Sandhu, W. Nel and M. Ebadi. 2013b. Clinical significance of metallothioneins in cell therapy and nanomedicine. International Journal of Nanomedicine 8: 1477–1488.

Sharma, S. 2014. Nanotheranostics in evidence based personalized medicine. Curr Drug Targets 15: 915–930.

Sharma, S., S. Gawande, A. Jagtap, R. Abeulela and Z. Salman. 2014. Fetal alcohol syndrome: Prevention, diagnosis, & treatment. pp. 39–94. *In*: Jeffrey Raines (ed.). Alcohol Abuse: Prevalence, Risk Factors. Nova Science Publishers, New York, U.S.A. Chapter 3.

Sharma, S. and M. Ebadi. 2014. Significance of metallothioneins in aging brain. Neurochemistry International 65: 40–48.

Sharma, S. and M. Ebadi. 2014. Antioxidant Targeting in Neurodegenerative Disorders. Ed. I. Laher, Springer Verlag. Germany. Chapter 85, pp. 1–30.

Sharma, S. and M. Ebadi. 2014. *Charnoly body* as a universal biomarker of cell injury. Biomarkers and Genomic Medicine 6: 89–98.

Sharma, S. 2014. Molecular pharmacology of environmental neurotoxins. *In*: Kainic Acid: Neurotoxic Properties, Biological Sources, and Clinical Applications. Nova Science Publishers. New York. pp. 1–47.

Sharma, S. 2014. Nanotheranostics in evidence based personalized medicine. Current Drug Targets 15: 915–930.

Sharma, S. 2015. Alleviating Stress of the Soldier and Cvilian. Nova Science Publishers. New York, U.S.A.

Sharma, S. 2015. Beyond Diet and Depression: Disease-Specific Depression and Biomarkers (Nutrition and Diet Research Progress). Nova Science Publishers, New York, U.S.A.

Sharma, S. 2015. Beyond Diet and Depression: Basic Knowledge, Clinical Symptoms and Treatment of Depression (Nutrition and Diet Research Progress). Nova Science Publishers, New York, U.S.A.

Sharma, S. 2015. Monoamine Oxidase Inhibitors: Clinical Pharmacology, Benefits, and Potential Health Risks. Nova Science Publishers, New York. U.S.A.

Sharma, S. 2016. Progress in PET RPs. Quality Control and Theranostics. Nova Science Publishers, New York, U.S.A.

Sharma, S. 2016. PET RPs for personalized medicine. Curr Drug Targets 17(16): 1894–1907.

Sharma, S., J. Choga, V. Gupta, P. Doghor, A. Chauhan, F. Kalala, A. Foor, C. Wright, J. Renteria, K.E. Theberge and M. Mathur. 2016. Charnoly body as a novel biomarker of nutritional stress in Alzheimer's disease. Functional Foods in Health and Disease 3: 344–378.

Sharma, S. 2016. Disease-specific charnoly body formation in neurodegenerative and other diseases. Conference: Drug Discovery and Therapy World Congress: Wyne Memorial Convention Center, Boston, Mass, U.S.A. Aug 23–25 (Invited lecture).

Sharma, S. and W. Lipincott. 2017. Biomarkers in Alzheimer's disease—Recent update. Curr Alzheimer Res Feb 20.

Sharma, S. 2017. Fetal Alcohol Spectrum Disorder (Concepts, Mechanisms, and Cure). Nova Science Publishers, New York, U.S.A.

Sharma, S. 2017. *ZIKV* Disease. Prevention and Cure. Nova Science Publishers, New York, U.S.A.

Shulman, J.M., P.L. De Jager and M.B. Feany. 2011. Parkinson's disease: genetics and pathogenesis. Annual Review of Pathology 6: 193–222.

Shyam babu, C., P. Satishchandra, A. Mahadevan, V. Pillai Shibu, S. Ravishankar, N. Sidappa, R. Udaykumar, V. Ravi and S.K. Shankar. 2013. Usefulness of stereotactic biopsy and neuroimaging in management of HIV-1 Clade C associated focal brain lesions with special focus on cerebral toxoplasmosis. Clin Neurol Neurosurg 115: 995–1002.

Silverman, D.H., G.W. Small and M.E. Phelps. 1999. Clinical value of neuroimaging in the diagnosis of dementia. sensitivity and specificity of regional cerebral metabolic and other parameters for early identification of Alzheimer's disease. Clin Positron Imaging 2: 119–130.

Skaliczki, G., M. Weszl, K. Schandl, T. Major, M. Kovács, J. Skaliczki, H. Redl, M. Szendrői, K. Szigeti, D. Máté, C. Dobó-Nagy and Z. Lacza. 2012. Compromised bone healing following spacer removal in a rat femoral defect model. Acta Physiol Hung 99: 223–32.

van de Watering, F.C., M. Rijpkema, L. Perk, U. Brinkmann, W.J. Oyen and O.C. Boerman. 2014. Zirconium-89 labeled antibodies: a new tool for molecular imaging in cancer patients. Biomed Res Int 2014: 203601.

von Guggenberg, E., W. Sallegger, A. Helbok, M. Ocak, R. King, S.J. Mather and C. Decristoforo. 2009. Cyclic minigastrin analogues for gastrin receptor scintigraphy with technetium-99m: preclinical evaluation. J Med Chem 52(15): 4786–4793.

Villemagne, V.L., S. Ng, R. Cappai, K.J. Barnham, M.T. Fodero-Tavoletti, C. Rowe and C.L. Masters. 2006. La lunga attesa: Towards a molecular approach to neuroimaging and therapeutics in Alzheimer's disease. Neuroradiol J 19: 453–474.

Von Sallegger, W., A. Helbok, M. Ocak, R. King, S.J. Mather and C. Decristoforo. 2009. Cyclic Minigastrin analogs for gastrin receptor scintigraphy with Technetium-99m: preclinical evaluation. J Med Chem 52: 4786–4793.

Wang, C., F.A. Schroeder and J.M. Hooker. 2014. Visualizing epigenetics: current advances and advantages in HDAC PET imaging techniques. Neuroscience 264: 186–197.

Xie, J., K. Chen, J. Huang, S. Lee, J. Wang, J. Gao, X. Li and X. Chen. 2010. PET/NIRF/MRI triple functional iron oxide nanoparticles. Biomaterials 31: 3016–3022.

CHAPTER-12

PET Radiopharmaceuticals and Surface Plasmon Resonance Spectroscopy for Charnoly Body and micro-RNA Based Personalized Theranostics

INTRODUCTION

The development of new PET-RPs for imaging and their theranostic application is increasing globally for chronic diseases as it provides clinically-significant *in vivo*, non-invasive, multimodality, 5D-spatiotemporal information of the SOL at the cellular, molecular, and genetic level to accomplish the targeted, safe, and effective EBPT of chronic MDR diseases. Although currently available remote-controlled GMP-compliant automated synthesis modules and self-shielded cyclotrons for radionuclide synthesis facilitate PET-RPs synthesis and enable multicenter trials for regulatory approval, the development of new RPs requires proper identification of the target, lead compound, well-defined synthesis steps, chemical characterization, preclinical, and clinical evaluation, and the therapeutic benefit to accomplish EBPT.

PET is a promising, noninvasive, *in vivo*, multi-modality imaging system which provides basic information regarding the spatio-temporal physiology and biochemistry of living organism. It is an excellent approach for quantifying pathophysiological events in the human body and has been used successfully in novel drug discovery, staging cancer and other chronic diseases, evaluating prognosis, and accomplishing EBPT (Hendrikse et al. 2014). PET imaging takes advantage of the conventional imaging technologies as well as positron-emitting RPs to discover specific biomarkers at different stages of disease progression/regression. More specifically, PET imaging utilizes coincident annihilated γ-photons to acquire spatiotemporal information of organs to reconstruct 5D images for the longitudinal analyses and quantitative estimation of dynamic functional studies. It is analogous to *ex vivo* autoradiography and permits non-invasive evaluation of the diseases in a live human body. This sophisticated biotechnology provides basic information regarding receptor/enzyme interactions and cellular metabolism by utilizing efficiently-synthesized RPs. Unlike MRI and CT, which provide primarily anatomical information, PET imaging can quantitatively estimate real time biochemical changes in CMB involving CB molecular pathogenesis even before morphological symptoms become evident during prodromal stages of disease progression. This imaging technology provides a clinically-significant relationship between molecular mechanisms of disease progression/regression and effective theranostic interventions. Moreover, it can provide efficient and cost-effective strategies to prevent failures in drug development and screen novel drugs for EBPT. Hence, future developments in PET radiochemistry employing DSST-CB, charnolophagy, and CS-labeled novel RPs or fluorochrome-labeled antibodies for *in vivo* targeted imaging will minimize time-consuming and cumbersome futile therapeutic attempts for the clinical management of chronic MDR diseases as described in this chapter.

The growth of PET imaging relies primarily on the development in the synthesis of new ^{18}F and ^{11}C-labeled RPs. Recently, novel strategies have been developed for radiolabeling clinically-significant molecules with ^{18}F, including ^{18}F radiochemistry, late stage fluorination reactions, as well as microfluidics and solid-phase radiochemistry for efficient production of PET-RPs (Cole et al. 2014). In addition, novel strategies to synthesize ^{11}C-labeled PET-RPs have been developed with specific examples of how these compounds have unique properties to determine intricate molecular events in a biological system and the applications of ^{13}N and ^{15}O in PET imaging (Langstrom et al. 2013). Labeled endogenous compounds are particularly important to elucidate real-time biochemical, physiological, and pharmacological events occurring in the body in health and disease to accomplish EBPT. The information provided in this chapter is by no means exhaustive as several investigators have already contributed remarkably in this highly specialized discipline. Particularly, the synthesis of (a) cyclotron and (b) generator-based PET-RPs, radiolabeled with ^{18}F, ^{11}C, ^{13}N, ^{15}O, ^{68}Ga, ^{64}Cu, ^{82}Ru, ^{89}Zr, ^{110}Lu, and ^{124}I radionuclides for current applications and future developments in PET is discussed. The detailed synthesis steps for specific PET-RPs are now available in other publications (Li and Conti 2010; Coenen et al. 2010; Miller et al. 2008; Antoni and Langsgtrom 2008; Iwata 2004; Okarvi 2001).

This chapter presents emerging knowledge regarding the synthesis of most commonly-used clinically-significant PET-RPs as well as novel radioligands to motivate young investigators, researchers, nuclear medicine technologists, and clinicians interested in improving the accuracy of EBPT employing DSST-CB-based ^{18}F and ^{11}C-labelled RPs. A systematic knowledge of emerging PET-RPs for the personalized theranostics of NDDs, CVDs, cancer, and other diseases is provided. More specifically, ^{18}F and ^{11}C-labelled CB, charnolophagy, and CS agonists/antagonists, CS exocytosis agonists/antagonists, and microRNA agonists/antagonists may be utilized as novel biomarkers to quantitatively assess real-time MB *in vivo* in health and disease. Similarly, charnolophagy and CS exocytosis biomarkers may be labelled with PET radionuclides to determine precise DSST-MB and ICD in normal and diseased organs to assess the clinical prognosis and therapeutic outcome in a patient. Particularly, this chapter describes CB and microRNA-based EBPT employing novel PET-RPs and SPR spectroscopy.

Mitochondrial Bioenergetics and microRNAs in CS Stability and Disease-Specific Spatio-Temporal Charnolopathies

Recent studies emphasized the roles of mitochondria in cellular functions including immune defense, epigenetics, and stem cell (SC) development for the prevention and treatment of diseases (Swai et al. 2016). It is recognized that the nuclear-mitochondrial interaction is disrupted in response to DPCI in the most vulnerable cell. Mitochondria play a pivotal role in the immune system by detecting foreign invaders through signaling pathways (e.g., inflammasomes) and generating immune responses. Hence, modulation of this role might confer new therapeutic potential. Methylation by DNA methyltransferases contributes to the epigenetic modification of mtDNA and nDNA. Dysregulation of the mitochondrial epigenome is implicated in various diseases. Mitochondria participate in tissue regeneration and integrity; maintained by stem cell renewal and differentiation. Stem cells present promising EBPT potential in regenerative medicine. Hence, understanding DSST-MB and CB dynamics in stem cells is highly crucial. New therapeutic interventions are emerging with scientific knowledge linking mitochondria to immunity, epigenetics, and stem cell biology. Recently, I emphasized the clinical significance of DSST-charnolopathies in progressive NDDs, CVDs, and chronic MDR malignancies (Sharma 2016, 2017). This chapter highlights the pivotal role of nuclear and mitochondrial microRNAs in CB molecular pathogenesis and CS destabilization in NDDs (including PD, AD, and stroke), CVDs, and MDR malignancies.

microRNAs and Mitochondrial Bioenergetics. The miRNAs are small, single-stranded, non-coding molecules that serve as post-transcriptional gene regulators. In addition to nucleocytoplasmic compartments, they are also localized in the mitochondria and can inhibit target protein-coding genes, by repressing mRNA translation or promoting their degradation. Initially, miRNAs were observed to be originated from nuclear genome and exported to cytosol, where they exert most of their actions. Recently, Durate et al. (2014) reported that miRNAs are also present in the mitochondria (even originated from mtDNA), regulating genes coding for mitochondrial proteins, and mitochondrial function. Since miRNAs are involved in numerous biological processes, they are now considered highly crucial to better understand, explain, and prevent/cure not only the pathogenesis of diseases but also mitochondrial dysfunction and associated diseases. Certain microRNAs can even serve as regulators of mitochondrial function to prevent malignant transformation (Tomasetti et al. 2014). Mitochondria maintain cellular homeostasis, are highly crucial to the intrinsic apoptotic pathway, and their dysfunction is associated with numerous diseases. miRNAs regulate signaling pathways in mitochondria and many of them are deregulated in various diseases including cancers. miRNAs are implicated in the regulation of the MB and in modulating metabolic pathways resulting in tumor suppression and their therapeutic applications. They are the key regulators of metabolism and can affect mitochondria by modulating mitochondrial proteins coded by nuclear genes.

It has been postulated that reprogramming of the mitochondrial energy metabolism is a characteristic feature of cancer. Hence, modulation of miRNAs levels may provide novel therapeutic strategies for the treatment of mitochondria-related pathologies, including malignancies. The elucidation of the role of miRNAs in the regulation of MB will enhance our understanding regarding the basic molecular mechanism of cell biology associated with the genesis and progression of neoplastic diseases, which will promote the development of innovative pharmacological interventions, including CB and CS-based charnolopharmacotherapeutics as proposed in this book. Although, therapies targeting epigenetic changes for cancer treatment are in Phase I/II trials, all these target only nuclear DNA. Emerging evidence suggests the presence of methylation markers on mtDNA, but their contribution to cancer and other diseases is yet to be established. It is currently known that expression of genes encoded on mtDNA are altered in cancer cells, along with increased glycolytic flux. The glycolytic flux and elevated ROS are supported by increased antioxidants: glutathione and MTs. Particularly, microRNA-34a translocates to mitochondria, mediates downstream apoptotic effects of tumor suppressor P^{53}, and inhibits the antioxidant response element Nrf-2, resulting in glutathione depletion. Recently, Trivedi et al. (2017) encapsulated microRNA-34a in the hyaluronic-Acid NPs and delivered to cisplatin-sensitive and cisplatin-resistant A549-lung adenocarcinoma cells. The uptake of these NPs in cells resulted in altered ATP levels, decreased glycolytic flux, Nrf-2 and glutathione levels, resulting in caspase-3 activation and apoptosis. Concomitant molecular changes in epigenetic status of D-loop on the mtDNA and transcription of mtDNA-encoded genes were also observed. These investigators provided a novel therapeutic approach of altered MB and redox signaling in cancer cells with underlying changes in epigenetic status of mtDNA that resulted in induction of cancer cell apoptosis.

microRNAs and Mitochondrial Dysfunction in CVDs. It is now well established that mitochondria are semiautonomous cellular organelles with their own genome, which not only supply energy but also participate in cell death pathways. MiRNAs are small non-coding RNAs, which inhibit the stability and/or translation of mRNA and play a pivotal role in NDDs, CVDs, and cancer. microRNAs are usually 19 to 25 nt long, involved in post-transcriptional gene regulation by binding to the 3'-untranslated regions of the target mRNA, which impact diverse cellular processes. To determine if nuclear miRNAs translocate into the mitochondria and regulate their function with pathophysiological implications in cardiac myocytes, Das et al. (2012) conducted a study to discover that miR-181c is encoded in the nucleus, assembled in the cytoplasm, and eventually translocated into the mitochondria of cardiac myocytes. Immunoprecipitation of *Argonaute 2* from the mitochondrial fraction indicated binding of cytochrome c oxidase subunit 1 (mt-COX1) mRNA from the mitochondrial genome with miR-181c. Also, a luciferase reporter construct showed that mi-181c binds to the 3'UTR of mt-COX1. To study whether miR-181c regulates mt-COX1, these investigators overexpressed precursor miR-181c (or a scrambled sequence) in primary cultures of neonatal rat ventricular myocytes. Overexpression of miR-181c did not change mt-COX1 mRNA but decreased mt-COX1 protein, suggesting that miR-181c is primarily a translational regulator of mt-COX1. In addition to altering mt-COX1, overexpression of miR-181c increased mt-COX2 mRNA and protein content, with an increase in both mitochondrial respiration and ROS in neonatal rat ventricular myocytes, indicating that miR-181c can enter and target the mitochondrial genome, inducing electron transport chain complex IV remodeling, and mitochondrial dysfunction. The nuclear miR-181c translocated into the mitochondria and regulated mitochondrial genome expression. These observations may augment our understanding of MB and the role of miRNA in mitochondrial dysfunction. These investigators reported miRNA-mediated regulation of mitochondria and the involvement of rat mitomiR miR-181c in electron chain complex IV remodeling in cardiomyocytes. Similar to other reports on mitomiRs, rat cardiomyocyte mitochondria harbored a unique miRNA expression pattern, with miR-181c enriched 2-fold in the mitochondrial fraction with respect to the whole heart because of its translocation into the other organelles. The immunoprecipitation assay of Argonaute 2—the catalytic component found in the protein complex of which miRNAs are part—revealed that miR-181c and Cyt-c oxidase subunit 1 (COX1) mRNA co-immuno-precipitated from the mitochondrial pellet. COX1 mRNA was identified as a target for miR-181c with luciferase assay. Overexpression of miR-181c caused a decrease in COX1 protein content but not in the amount of its mRNA, suggesting reduced translation rather than mRNA degradation. In addition, there was an increased rate of O_2 consumption by complex IV, induced by increased generation of ROS. Intriguingly, the mRNAs of COX2 and COX3—two other complex IV subunits that are transcribed in a polycistronic unit from mtDNA along with COX1—were upregulated. Based on these findings, these investigators hypothesized that this remodeling of complex IV might be due to miR-181c-activated feedback loop that increases transcription of mtDNA, but because miR-181c binds only to COX1 mRNA, inhibiting its translation, COX1 protein levels decrease while the other subunits become more abundant. In a further study, Das et al. (2014) reported that miR-181c regulates the mitochondrial genome, MB, and propensity for heart failure *in vivo*. However, the *in vivo* influence of miR-181c remains unknown. These investigators reported an *in vivo* method for the administration of miR-181c in rats, which results in reduced exercise capacity and signs of heart failure, by targeting the 3′-end of mt-COX1 (Cyt-c oxidase subunit 1). They cloned miR-181c and encapsulated it in lipid-based NPs for systemic delivery. The plasmid DNA complexed nanovector revealed no overt toxicity. The mRNA levels of mitochondrial complex IV genes in the heart, but not any other mitochondrial genes, were significantly altered with miR-181c overexpression, suggesting selective mitochondrial complex IV remodeling due to miR-181c targeting mt-COX1. Isolated heart mitochondrial studies showed altered O_2-consumption, ROS production, matrix Ca^{2+}, and $\Delta\Psi$ in miR-181c-treated animals, suggesting that miRNA delivered to the heart *in vivo* can lead to cardiac dysfunction by regulating mitochondrial genes.

microRNAs and Mitochondrial Dysfunction in PD. Parkinson's disease (PD) is a complex neurological disorder of the elderly population with a selective loss of DAergic neurons in the substantia nigra pars compacta (SNpc). Although, the exact molecular mechanism of DAergic neuronal demise remains poorly understood, TNF-α, a pro-inflammatory cytokine is elevated in the blood, CSF, and striatal region of the brain in PD patients. The elevated levels of TNF-α and its role in the pathogenesis of PD are yet to be established. Hence, Prajapati et al. (2015) investigated the role of TNF-α in the regulation of cell death and miRNA mediated mitochondrial functions employing, DAergic (SH-SY5Y) cell line. The cells were treated with low dose of TNF-α for prolonged period induced cell death which was rescued in the presence of zVAD. fmk, a caspase inhibitor and N-acetyl-cysteine (NAC), an antioxidant. It has been identified that TNF-α alters complex-I activity, decreases ATP levels, and increases ROS levels and mitochondrial turnover through autophagy (more precisely through charnolophagy). In addition, TNF-α regulates miRNA expression involved in PD pathogenesis. Bioinformatic analysis demonstrated that the putative targets of altered miRNA included both pro/anti apoptotic genes and subunits of the mitochondrial complex. The cells treated with TNF-α exhibited decreased level of nuclear encoded transcript of mitochondrial complexes, the target of miRNA, indicating that TNF-α is a regulator of miRNAs which may impact mitochondrial functions and neuronal demise via CB molecular pathogenesis having an important implication for PD progression as we have reported (Sharma et al. 2013a; Sharma et al. 2013b). We reported that CoQ_{10} serves as an antiapoptotic, antioxidant, and anti-inflammatory agent in the wv/wv mouse model of PD, AD, and drug addiction. CoQ_{10} rejuvinated complex-1, a rate-limiting enzyme for oxidative phosphorylation, and inhibited TNF-α-induced NFκβ activation to provide neuroprotection in these genotypes (Ebadi et al. 2004). Furthermore, MTs provided ubiquinone (CoQ_{10})-mediated neuroprotection in chronic NDDs by serving as potent free radical scavengers, CB antagonists, and CS stabilizers (Sharma et al. 2004; Sharma et al. 2014; Sharma and Ebadi 2014; Sharma 2017).

microRNAs and Mitochondrial Dysfunction in Stroke. Recently, Ouyang et al. (2014) reported that stroke is one of the leading causes of death and disability worldwide. Because stroke is a multifactorial disease with a short therapeutic window, many clinical stroke trials have failed, and the only currently approved therapy is thrombolysis. microRNAs are endogenously expressed noncoding short single-stranded RNAs that regulate gene expression at the post-transcriptional level, via degradation or translational inhibition of their target mRNAs. Recent studies revealed a significant role of miRNAs in ischemic diseases. miRNAs are especially important candidates for stroke therapeutics because of their ability to simultaneously regulate many target genes and since targeting single genes for therapeutic intervention has not yet succeeded in the clinic. Although there are already reports about miRNA in ischemic heart disease, much less is currently known about miRNAs in cerebral ischemia. These investigators summarized current knowledge about miRNAs and cerebral ischemia, focusing on the role of miRNAs in ischemia (both changes in expression and identification of potential targets), as well as miRNAs as biomarkers and therapeutic targets in cerebral ischemia. However, the precise role of microRNAs in CB molecular pathogenesis involving charnolophagy, CS stabilization/destabilization, and CS exocytosis/endocytosis leading to CVDs, AIS, and other diseases is yet to be established.

microRNAs Regulate Mitochondrial Function in Cerebral Ischemia-Reperfusion Injury. Cerebral ischemia-reperfusion injury involves numerous fatal terminal pathways in the mitochondria, including ROS generation caused by changes in $\Delta\Psi$ and $[Ca^{2+}]_i$ overload, resulting in apoptosis via Cyt-c release and eventually, induction of CB molecular pathogenesis. In addition, numerous microRNAs are associated with the overall process. Hu et al. (2015) summarized the mitochondrial changes in cerebral ischemia-reperfusion and described the molecular mechanism of miRNA-regulated mitochondrial function, which included oxidative stress and energy metabolism, as well as apoptosis. They concluded that studies of microRNAs that regulate mitochondrial function inhibiting molecular pathogenesis will expedite the development of treatments for cerebral ischemia-reperfusion injury and other associated CVDs.

Astrocyte-Targeted Approaches for Stroke Therapy: Role of Mitochondria and microRNAs. Astrocytes are known as critical regulators of neuronal function and an effective target for stroke therapy in animal models. Identifying individual targets with the potential for simultaneous activation of multiple downstream pathways that regulate astrocyte homeostasis may be necessary for successful clinical translation. Stary et al. (2015) suggested that mitochondria and microRNAs represent individual targets with multi-modal therapeutic potential. Mitochondria regulate metabolism and apoptosis, while microRNAs bind and inhibit numerous mRNAs to inhibit CB formation and promote CS stabilization. Hence, by combining strategies targeted at maintaining astrocyte function during and following cerebral ischemia, a synergistic therapeutic effect may be achieved.

Glial-Mitochondrial Function for Protection from Cerebral Ischemia: The Role of microRNAs. It has been identified that astrocytes and microglia play crucial roles in response to cerebral ischemia and are effective targets for stroke therapy in animal models. microRNAs are important post-transcriptional regulators of gene expression that function by inhibiting the translation of specific target genes. Li et al. (2016) recently reported that in astrocytes, miR expression patterns regulate mitochondrial function in response to oxidative stress via targeting BCl_2 and HSP-70 family members. Mitochondria play a crucial role in microglial activation, and miRs regulate the neuroinflammatory response. As endogenous miR expression patterns can be altered with exogenous mimics and inhibitors, miR-targeted therapies represent a unique intervention to optimize glial mitochondrial function and improve the therapeutic outcome following cerebral ischemia by inhibiting CB molecular pathogenesis. These investigators highlighted that astrocytes and microglia play a crucial role in neuronal function and fate following ischemic stress, discussed the relevance of mitochondria in the glial response to injury, and presented evidence implicating miRs as potential regulators in the glial mitochondrial response to cerebral ischemia.

Therapeutic Potential of microRNAs to Modulate Redox and Immune Response in Stroke. Cerebral ischemia is a major cause of death and disability throughout the world, yet therapeutic options remain limited. The interplay between the cellular redox state and the immune response plays a critical role in determining the extent of neural cell injury after ischemia and reperfusion. Excessive amounts of ROS generated by mitochondria and other sources act both as triggers and effectors of inflammation. Ouyang et al. (2015) focused on the interplay between these two mechanisms. It is currently known that miRNAs are important post-transcriptional regulators that interact with multiple target mRNAs regulating target genes, including those involved in controlling mitochondrial function, redox state, inflammatory pathways, and the induction of DSST charnolopathies. These investigators focused on the regulation of mitochondria, ROS, and inflammation by miRNAs in deleterious intra- and intercellular events involving CB formation and CS destabilization that lead to brain cell death after cerebral ischemia. Although pretreatment using miRNAs was effective in cerebral ischemia in rodents, testing treatment after the onset of ischemia is highly essential in the development of acute stroke treatment. In addition, miRNA formulation and delivery into the CNS remain a significant challenge in the translation of miRNA therapy. Hence, future research should focus on post-treatment and potential clinical use of miRNAs. microRNAs and mitochondrial dysfunction involving DSST charnolopathies for other diseases such as AD, MS, depression, and FASD are described in the next chapters.

Cyclotron-based PET-RPs for Charnoly Body and microRNA-based Personalized Theranostics

Quality Control and Radiation Safety. It is extremely important to emphasize that the theranostic potential of PET imaging depends primarily on the wise and far-sighted site planning and proper design of the cyclotron and radiochemistry lab, well-qualified staff to ensure quality control and discovery of novel RPs, and state of the art computer-based (remote-controlled) technologies (Jacobson et al. 2002). Currently, there are limited number of trained and certified radiopharmaceutical scientists, health physicists, and nuclear medicine physicians all over the world. Unlike conventional chemical synthesis where parameters such as time, temperature, pH, ionic concentrations, and radiation safety measures may not be of critical significance, all these physicochemical conditions must be maintained in a perfect order and preferably performed in remote (computer)-controlled synthesis modules, because radiation safety and quality control measures are extremely important at each and every step during the automated, semi-automated, or manual synthesis of PET-RPs. Improper design and operation of the cyclotron, hot cells, and/or radiochemistry synthesis modules may not only reduce the efficiency of the production runs but also provide unnecessary radiation burden to the personnel and premises. Particularly, the radiation worker should avoid leakage of delivery lines, spillage of reagents, and unnecessary radiation exposure during PET-RPs synthesis. We published basic guidelines of quality control and radiation safety during ^{18}FDG and ^{18}F-DOPA synthesis in the PET-RPs lab (Sharma et al. 2006; Sharma et al. 2007).

Although time, distance, shielding, and ALARA principles of radiation safety are strictly followed and PET-RPs synthesis is generally performed in remote-controlled synthesis modules in properly-designed video-monitored hot cells for theranostic applications; a typical research and development unit may not require specially-designed hot cells where the requirements of newly-synthesized RPs might be limited. However, for research and development of novel PET-RPs, we would not only require efficient and cost-effective synthesis modules such as microfluidic systems with computer-controlled graphics user interface (GUI) but also strict quality control (QC) including: radiation safety measures during radionuclide production, radiochemical synthesis, purification, and eventually accurate formulation for theranostic applications.

Quality Control of Short-Lived PET-RPs. Generally, cyclotron-based radionuclides used for the PET-RPs synthesis have short half-lives ($t_{1/2}$) (^{13}N: 10 Min; ^{82}Rb: 75 Sec, ^{15}O: 120 Sec, ^{62}Cu: 9.7 Min, ^{68}Ga: 68 Min, ^{18}F- 110 Min). Hence it is difficult to perform all necessary QC experiments before injection to the patient as per United States Pharmacopoeia (USP) and Food and Drug Administration (FDA) guidelines. Testing sterility and pyrogenicity are time-consuming and are generally performed after administration of PET-RPs to a patient. Although pyrogenicity can be checked within 20 min using Charles River device, the Limulus Amoebocyte Lysate (LAL) test requires at least 1 hr. Moreover, a sterility test to detect slow-growing bacteria such as Mycobacterium tuberculi may require several days. Since short-lived PET-RPs are synthesized in well-designed modules under strict criteria of regulatory agencies; standard operating procedures (SOPs) including isotonicity, radiochemical, radionuclidic, chemical purity, and pH are integrated to the production process by remote-controlled radionuclide production, purification, and formulation steps, so that all crucial QC measures could be strictly followed before theranostic applications.

Detection of Trace Elements in PET-RPs. Usually, minute quantities of radioisotopes are synthesized due to radioactivation of metal targets during proton bombardment in the cyclotron. Hence, the metallic impurities must be checked soon after the target material, target body, or target window rebuild during system maintenance. It is highly prudent to bombard protons only after loading the target body with [^{18}O] H$_2$O water and by accurately centering and focusing the proton beam on the target, rather than on the target body. Proton bombardment without the target will produce silver NPs as a major contaminant in the subsequent runs for ^{18}F$^-$ production. Similarly, aluminum (Al) could be a possible contaminant if the vacuum window bursts during the production run particularly in Siemens RDS-111 Eclipse cyclotrons. However, this limitation has been rectified by improvising a copper grid in recently–designed cyclotrons. We used the Varian atomic absorption spectrophotometer (AAS) equipped with Win-Lab software for the estimation of metal ion impurities (Ag, Co, Ni, Mn, Al, and Cu) in the ^{18}F$^-$ water. In addition to γ-ray spectrometry, these metal ion impurities were analyzed employing Fisher-Thermo-Scientific ICP-MS. Although sensitivity of both ICP-MS as well as AAS was similar, the latter is time-consuming and cumbersome. At any given time, we change the lamp for the detection of an element; the alignment of the instrument is disturbed, which reduces the sensitivity; whereas ICP-MS can analyze > 32 elements in just 20 min in a 10 μl sample. Moreover, detection of radio-metal impurities employing ICP-MS does not require specialized preparation protocols as it is matrix-independent. The argon plasma torch burns at 5000–8000°C under vacuum, where dissociation, atomization, and ionization occur within fraction of a second, which facilitates detection of elements up to parts per zillion. With a conventional AAS, we can estimate as low as parts per billion using 20 μl samples. In addition, it requires cumbersome sample processing procedures, lamps of specific wavelength, and their proper alignment. However, ICP-MS is 10X costly as compared to AAS.

Requirements of PET-RPs Radiolabeling. There are some extremely important basic requirements of radiolabeling molecules with ^{18}F or other radionuclides. For instance, it should have: easy and simple synthesis steps; sufficient chemical reactivity; extremely low concentrations (< 10^{-4} M); negligible steric hindrance of target molecule following incorporation of radionuclide; high specific activity, sufficient radiochemical yield, minimum purification steps, and should be free from side products.

Commonly used PET Radionuclides. A brief list of commonly used short-lived PET radionuclides with their production mode and nuclear reactions is provided below:
^{11}C, [^{11}C]CO$_2$, [^{11}C]CH$_4$ (t$_{1/2}$ = 20 min; NR: ^{14}N(p, a); TP: ^{11}C N$_2$(+O$_2$); DP: N$_2$(+H$_2$); ^{11}B, ^{13}N, [^{13}N]NOx (t$_{1/2}$ = 9.97 min; NR: ^{16}O(p, a); TP: ^{13}N H$_2$O; DP: H$_2$O+EtOH; [^{13}N] NH$_3$: NR ^{13}C; ^{15}O (t$_{1/2}$ = 2.04 min; NR: ^{15}N(d,n)^{15}O; TP; N$_2$(+O$_2$) [^{15}O]O$_2$; DP: ^{15}N; ^{18}F, [^{18}F]F$_2$, ^{18}F-, (t$_{1/2}$ = 110 min; NR: ^{20}Ne(d, a)^{18}F; ^{18}O(p, n)^{18}F; TP: [^{18}O]H$_2$O; Ne(+F$_2$), ^{18}O [Abbreviations: NR: Nuclear Reaction; TP: Target Product: DP: Decay Product].

These radionuclides can be utilized for labeling various biomarkers of CB molecular pathogenesis as described in this book.

Commonly-used PET-RPs. Many PET-RPs used in clinical diagnosis are radiolabeled versions of molecules in the body, such as: ^{13}N-ammonia, ^{15}O-water, ^{11}C-acetate, ^{11}C-methionine, and ^{18}F-fluoride. ^{15}O water is synthesized by bombarding cyclotron-generated (8–10 MeV) deuteron or protons on enriched ^{14}N target by d-n reaction [^{14}N (d-n) ^{15}O]. ^{18}F is preferred because of its ideal physicochemical and nuclear properties (635 KeV positron energy; 97% positron decay ratio; 2.3 mm maximum range), required for satisfactory imaging resolution and dosimetry. Moreover, the radius of ^{18}F (1.34A) and hydrogen (1.25A) nuclei is almost similar, which facilitates substitution reactions. ^{15}O water vapors react with carrier ^{16}O to produce ^{15}O$_2^-$ over Pd-Al alloy. The ^{15}O water vapors are trapped in saline solution by bubbling N$_2$ as a carrier under sterilized conditions. Due to natural abundance of C, N, O in biomolecules such as; DNA, RNA, proteins, neurotransmitters, hormones, enzymes, and phospholipids; ^{11}C, ^{13}N, ^{15}O-labeled RPs have shown great promise for future developments in CB-based theranostics. However, ^{13}N and ^{15}O-labeled RPs are currently of limited use because of their relatively reduced half-lives for routine clinical applications. Moreover, it requires onsite cyclotron, imaging system, and patient's bed, where these could be delivered directly to the patient. Similarly, transportation of ^{11}C-labeled RPs poses a significant challenge owing to their reduced half-lives.

Although ^{18}F is currently utilized for radiolabeling PET RPs due to its highly suitable physical properties to perform molecular imaging, further improvements in computer technology and efficient radio synthesis modules will facilitate labeling specific CB, charnolophagy, and CS biomarkers with short-lived radionuclides such as ^{11}C, ^{13}N, and ^{15}O for the DSST analysis of mitochondrial bioenergetics and ICD in health and disease. In my recently-published books "ZIKV Disease (Prevention and Cure) and Fetal Alcohol Spectrum Disorders (Concepts, Mechanisms, and Cure)" I have described potential CB and CS biomarkers for PET radiolabeling to quantitatively assess the MB and ICD in health and disease.

Potential CB, Charnolophagy, CS, and microRNA Biomarkers. Recently, I proposed several biomarkers of CB, charnolophagy, and CS including, but not limited to Cyt-C, lactate, inorganic phosphate, iron, Cr/PCr, NAA, acetate, acetaldehyde, acetone, ammonia, H$_2$O$_2$, MAOs, manoldialdehyde (MDA), LDH, SOD, catalase, phosphatidyl serine, ATP, MTs, glutathione, CoQ$_{10}$, NADH oxidase, TSPO (18 kDa), cholesterol, S-adenosyl methionine, homocysteine, dihydroepindiasterone, thioredoxine, caspase-3/PARP, p^{53}, BCl$_2$, Bax, Bak, BCl-X, GAPDH, aromatase, aconitase, mitochondrial complexes (I-V), 8OH, 2dG, 2,3 dihydroxy nonenal, APO-E, cholesterol, HSP-70, HSF, TRPCs, Ca^{2+}, caspase-3, and AIF. These CB, charnolophagy, and CPS/CS biomarkers can be quantitively estimated by Luminex multiplex ELISA, antibody microarray, cDNA microarray, microRNA microarrays, RT-PCR, immunoblotting, and by SPR spectroscopic analysis, in addition to radiolabeling with specific PET radionuclides for *in vivo* molecular imaging of DSST-MB and ICD.

Radiolabeling of CB, Charnolophagy, CS, and microRNA Biomarkers with [^{18}F]. Although [^{18}F]F$^-$ is not a natural agent for radiolabeling, as it may even alter chemical properties of the compound and may not even behave as naturally as ^{11}C-labeled molecules in a biological system, it is currently the most acceptable and suitable strategy for molecular imaging particularly where the cyclotron facility is unavailable at the PET imaging center. Moreover, we can produce a high specific activity [^{18}F]F⁻. This radionuclide has relatively low energy and provides a low radiation dose. Moreover, its practically-reasonable half-life allows synthesis and imaging for the *in vivo* non-invasive dynamic function studies. Relatively longer half-life allows distribution of ^{18}F-labeled PET-RPs to neighboring PET imaging centers without onsite cyclotron and PET radiochemistry facility. These distinct advantages of ^{18}F over ^{11}C, ^{13}N, and ^{15}O radionuclides, allow onsite as well as remote production of PET-RPs for basic as well as clinical studies. It can also be used for radiolabeling macromolecules such as proteins, peptides, and antibody fragments with slow PKs. Hence, currently it will be more appropriate to radiolabel afore-mentioned CB, charnolophagy, and CPS/CS biomarkers with ^{18}F⁻. The information derived from studies employing ^{18}F-labeled CB, charnolophagy, and CPS/CS biomarkers can be extended to ^{11}C-labelled PET RPs subsequently for the precise DSST assessment of MB and ICD as an excellent theranostics criteria of health and well-being.

Usually ^{18}F is prepared in two chemical forms; (a) [^{18}F]F$_2$ from ^{20}Ne (d,α) ^{18}F nuclear reaction. The cold ^{19}F$_2$ gas is added as a carrier which reduces the specific activity of [^{18}F]F$_2$ whereas the reaction, ^{18}O (p, n) ^{18}F is used for the synthesis of nucleophilic [^{18}F]fluoride. (b) ^{18}F⁻ in aqueous phase is not sufficiently nucleophilic, hence, water is evaporated by aziotropic distillation using krytopfix (K-222) in acetonitrile as an ion trapping agent, which renders the fluorine (F$_2^-$) ion naked and highly reactive for nucleophilic substitution to replace the hydrogen atom with ^{18}F. The inherent limitations of [^{18}F]F$_2$ is that it is not a natural agent for radiolabeling, may alter the chemical properties of the compound, and may not even behave as naturally as ^{11}C-labeled molecules. Nevertheless, it is presently the most suitable and acceptable radionuclide for molecular imaging particularly where the cyclotron facility is unavailable. Hence, only ^{18}F-labeled RPs with practically feasible half-life (110 min) and moderate energy have shown great promise in routine clinical practice.

Radiolabeling with ^{75}Br. Although ^{75}Br ($t_{1/2}$ = 97 min) can be produced at higher specific activities, as ^{18}F and can be used for PET imaging, its higher positron emission energy (1.74 MeV) prevents replacement for ^{18}F unless labeling of a specific compound with ^{18}F is difficult. Other halogens including; ^{76}Br ($t_{1/2}$: 16 hrs) and ^{124}I ($t_{1/2}$: 4.15 days) are also clinically less significant due to the reduced positron emission rate and high energy, whereas high-resolution imaging can be achieved with ^{18}F as it allows quantitative analysis of metabolites and improved statistics to perform longitudinal analyses.

Radiolabeling with ^{11}C and other Radionuclides. While developing novel PET-RPs, detailed PKs data is required using experimental animals for translational research. In general, the synthesis and transportation time of a PET-RPs should not exceed > 3 physical half-lives. Hence, any PET-RPs synthesis requiring > 3 physical half-lives could pose a challenge in its radiochemical synthesis, clinical utility, and may even provide an unnecessary radiation burden. Although specific activity of a radionuclide may be high, the final product may be insufficient to perform PET imaging even for a single patient. Hence, time-consuming and cumbersome procedures may not be clinically-significant for short-lived radionuclides such as ^{11}C, ^{13}N, and [15]O. However, in research and development units where experimental animals such as mice and rats are used, and the radioactivity requirement is of the order of couple of hundred μCi, lengthy yet innovative and clinically-significant procedures for the novel discovery of PET-RPs are worth exploring. Hence, in addition to ^{18}F-labeled compounds, ^{11}C, ^{13}N, and ^{15}O-labeled compounds are now being developed in PET imaging centers for basic and clinical applications. Particularly, it will be highly promising to develop specific CB, charnolophagy, and CS-targeted PET- RPs which can be labeled with afore-mentioned radionuclides for *in vivo* assessment of DSST-CMB in real time and its amelioration with noval drug development, which will facilitate accomplishing the targeted, safe, and effective EBPT of chronic MDR diseases. In fact, several clinically-significant ^{18}F-labeled RPs were developed initially from painstaking and cumbersome procedures with ^{3}H, ^{14}C, and ^{11}C radionuclides. Hence, a considerable effort is being made to acquire molecular imaging data using efficient computer-based algorithms and associated technology using these short-lived radionuclides to accomplish EBPT of chronic intractable diseases. Future developments in this direction seem very promising for a successful EBPT of currently challenging NDDs, CVDs, and chronic MDR malignancies.

Routine Synthesis of PET-RPs. ([18]FdG and ^{18}F-DOPA) Recently ^{18}F-labeled RPs were utilized for *in vivo*, non-invasive PET imaging in the healthcare, personalized medicine, and drug discovery to accomplish EBPT. In general, two procedures are utilized for the synthesis of PET-RPs: (a) nucleophilic substitution and (b) electrophilic substitution. A versatile PET-RP, [18]FDG is synthesized by bombarding protons on the oxygen-enriched $H_2^{18}O$ water target through a p-n reaction followed by a (SN-2) nucleophilic substitution reaction. Although initially hydrolysis step was performed using 1N HCl, it was banned by FDA because the pH of the final product is ~ 4.5, which produces pain in some patients. Hence, alkaline hydrolysis with 1N NaOH is recommended. However, the radiochemical impurities exist in both synthesis procedures (Hung 2002; Yu 2006). With acid hydrolysis, 2 chloro, 2-deoxy, D mannose, and with basic hydrolysis, 2-fluoro, 2-deoxy-D mannose is detected as potential impurity. For QC assurance, the final product must be > 95% pure before administration to the patient (Sharma and Ebadi 2014).

Generally, [18]FdG is utilized to determine hypometablic brain regions in AD, employing PET neuroimaging. Thus, *in vivo* PET imaging employing [18]FdG is an excellent imaging biomarker to assess MB and hence, CB molecular dynamics of an organ in health and disease. PET neuroimaging with [18]FdG supersedes all other presently-available molecular imaging modalities such as SPECT, CT, and MRI for the differential diagnosis of AD, because it provides real-time estimate of brain regional MB and hence, precise information regarding the molecular pathology of CB and associated events such as: charnolophagy and CPS/CS dynamics. [18]FdG is also utilized in the diagnosis and prognosis of at least 70 other clinical conditions as a robust PET imaging biomarker of MB. Its uptake is significantly enhanced in inflamed tissues and in malignant cancers, indicating that MB is significantly enhanced, which induces hyerproliferation and MDR malignant transformations in cancer cells. Glucose metabolism is also significantly enhanced in vascular smooth muscle cells in neointimal hyperplasia, restenosis, resulting in plaque rupture due to uncontrolled CB sequestration and/or CS destabilization (involving permeabilization, sequestration, and fragmentation). Usually, ^{18}F-DOPA is utilized to determine brain regional nigrostriatal DA-ergic neurotransmission in PD patients. ^{18}F-DOPA uptake is also significantly enhanced in neuroendocrine tumors. We synthesized ^{18}F-DOPA and ^{18}FdG employing the regio-selective electrophilic substitution method and nucleophilic method, respectively, as sensitive biomarkers of brain regional DA-ergic neurotransmission, and MB, respectively, with a primary objective to investigate basic molecular mechanism of PD, AD, and drug addiction in α-synuclein and MTs gene manipulated mice. We have described detailed methods to synthesize ^{18}D-DOPA and ^{18}FdG in our publications (Sharma and Ebadi 2005; Ebadi et al. 2005; Klongpanichapak et al. 2006; Sharma et al. 2006; Ebadi and Sharma 2006; Sharma and Ebadi 2008a; Sharma and Ebadi 2008b). ^{18}F-DOPA synthesis required 45 min and the yield was 30–35%. The electrophilic substitution required cold F_2 gas to passivate the delivery lines. Since a considerable amount of fluorine gas is adsorbed on the internal wall of the steel delivery lines, fluorinated polyethylene tubing was recommended, which avoids repeated passivation and increases the radiochemical yield. As fluorine is used as a carrier gas during proton bombardment, the radiochemical yield is always poor. Moreover, fluorine is inflammable, caustic, foul smelling, and can produce blisters in the lungs; hence, its leakage can be disastrous in the radiochemistry lab. Generally, electrophilic substitution reaction is used to synthesize ^{18}F-DOPA, with relatively reduced specific activity (Adam et al. 1988; Namavari et al. 1992; de Vries et al. 1999). However, recent improvements provided better production of quality-controlled ^{18}F-DOPA for clinical applications. Initially, [^{18}F]-DOPA was synthesized to determine the brain regional distribution of DA by PET neuroimaging (Loane and Politis 2011). Now it is also used for early detection of neuroendocrine tumors (NETs) and pancreatic cancer (Minn et al. 2009).

PET neuroimaging with [^{18}F]-DOPA for imaging somatostatin receptors is better than SPECT imaging for the early detection of NETs. However, ^{68}Ga-DOTA-TATE demonstrated superior results compared to ^{18}F-DOPA. As ^{18}F-DOPA is relatively less sensitive in detecting non-secreting NETs, it may be used along with receptor imaging for the clinical managements of NETs. However, the carcinoid crisis directed the importance of the nucleophilic labeling method for ^{18}F-DOPA (Koopmans et al. 2005). For environmental safety, non-carrier added nucleophilic substitution reaction using $^{18}F_2^-$ ion in the form of fluorinated water is used to synthesize ^{18}F-DOPA. A four-step procedure was developed for the synthesis of ^{18}F-DOPA by nucleophilic substitution reaction. This involves the nucleophilic fluorination followed by iodination. Then glycine is coupled with the ^{18}F-labeled benzyl iodide and hydrolysis is performed to eliminate amino as well as hydroxyl groups with a yield of 20 ± 4%. However, nucleophilic substitution method requires multiple synthesis steps. Hence ^{18}F-DOPA is generally synthesized by regio-selective electrophilic substitution by destannylation of its precursor as described above. Although, ^{18}F-DOPA can be synthesized using radiofluorinated water and is environmentally-friendly; the entire procedure is time-consuming (105 min), costly, and requires extensive cleaning due to cumbersome multiple synthesis steps (Haug et al. 2009; Shen et al. 2009).

Recently, general procedures to synthesize ^{18}F-labeled RPs by nucleophilic radiofluorination for the synthesis of several PET-RPs with their merits and limitations were described. In addition, Lodi et al. (2008) described major steps for ^{11}C-labeled RPs synthesis which require production of either $^{11}CO_2$ under oxidizing conditions or $^{11}CH_4$ under reducing conditions. Several ^{11}C-labeled PET-RPs were synthesized using $^{11}CO_2$ or $^{11}CH_4$ and Grignard's (Methyl-Mg-Bromide) reagent. The carboxy-acetyl moiety prepared by Grignard's reagent can be reacted with serotonin to obtain ^{11}C-acetyl serotonin (^{11}C-melatonin) to image brain melatonin-binding sites. Ren Iwata from Tohku PET Imaging Center (Japan) published a comprehensive list of ^{11}C-labeled PET-RPs which can be utilized to acquire information for the synthesis of a specific PET-RP (Iwata 2004). These methods can also be utilized to radiolabel specific CB, charnolophagy, and CS biomarkers as described in this chapter.

Experimental Studies with ^{18}FDG and ^{18}F-DOPA. We synthesized ^{18}FDG by nucleophilic substitution reaction and ^{18}F-DOPA by regio-selective electrophilic substitution reaction using Siemens 11 MeV negative ion RDS Eclipse Cyclotron, $^{18}F_2$ gas and fluostannalyl DOPA as a precursor, F_2 gas as carrier, and HBr and ammonia for the hydrolysis employing RayBioteck GINA Star synthesis module for experimental studies on PD and drug addiction in MTs gene-manipulated mice, α-Syn$_{ko}$ mice, α-SynMT$_{tko}$ mice, wv/wv mice, and wv/wv/MTs mice to evaluate brain regional MB in PD, AD, and drug addiction (Ebadi et al. 2005; Sharma and Ebadi 2005; Ebadi and Sharma 2006; Sharma et al. 2006; Klongpanichapak et al. 2006; Sharma and Ebadi 2008; Sharma and Ebadi 2008b).

Metal-Catalyzed Cross-Coupling. Recently cross coupling reactions for radiolabeling evolved the PET imaging as a promising technology for theranostics (Pretze et al. 2011). Advances in ^{11}C and ^{18}F-labeled RPs using metal mediated carbon-carbon, carbon-heterocarbon atom cross coupling (using Stille, Suzuki, and Songashira cross-coupling), click chemistry, and microfludic systems are highly significant for future development of PET-RPs including CB, charnolophagy, and CS-PET biomarkers. Considerable effort is being made to develop innovative, efficient, and cost-effective, remote-controlled RPs synthesis procedures. Several carbon-carbon and carbon-heteroatom bond-forming reactions were used for the future development of novel PET-RPs. These innovative procedures can be utilized for the novel discovery of DSST charnolo-pharmacotherapeutics for the targeted, safe, and effective EBPT. Furthermore, CB based PET RPs can be utilized to evaluate the therapeutic potential of a specific microRNA as a post-transcriptional regulator in AIS and in other chronic MDR diseases. The significance of these reactions in organic chemistry as well as biomedical sciences was the basis of a Nobel Prize award (Wu et al. 2010). These unique approaches utilize Stille cross-coupling for radiofluorination with 4-fluorophenyl boronic acid for radiolabeling (Wuest et al. 2008a; Wuest et al. 2008b). A desired radiotracer could be obtained utilizing 4-[^{18}F]fluoro-1-iodobenzene. Transition metal-mediated cross-coupling reactions were also used for labeling with ^{18}F with Suzuki cross-coupling and microwave heating. Several organo-boron compounds were labeled to achieve as high as 30–90% radiochemical yield.

Click Chemistry in Basic Understanding of Spatio-Temporal Mitochondrial Bioenergetics and microRNA-Mediated ICD in Health and Disease. This procedure employs Cu(I) catalyzed 1,3 dipolar cyclo-addition between an azide and acetylene to form a triazole, which is termed as "click chemistry" and is utilized for the synthesis of ethynylbenzene-substituted glycol for radiolabeling oligonucleotides (Rostovtsev et al. 2002; Ren et al. 2014). By ^{18}F labeling, either the azide or the acetylene, peptide labeling can be achieved. Hence "click chemistry" is facilitating the synthesis of novel ^{18}F-RPs, which can be used in the investigations of DA-ergic, 5-HTergic, cholinergic, opioid, and GABA-ergic functional pathways, to assess the heterogeneity of brain regional neurotransmission in health and disease. Future development of CB, charnolophagy, and CS-specific PET imaging biomarkers and their functional association with DSST microRNA and brain regional neurotransmission and MB will provide further information regarding cognitive decline in progressive NDDs such as PD, AD, drug addiction, schizophrenia, and MDDs. Recently, we reported that accumulation of CB at the junction of the axon hillock blocks the normal axoplasmic transport of various ions, neurotransmitters, hormones, neurotrophic factors (IGF-1, BDNF), and mitochondria in the terminal end bulbs to cause initially synaptic silence followed by synaptic atrophy; whereas the accumulation of structurally and functionally-destabilized CS causes the release of toxic mitochondrial metabolites to cause synaptic degeneration, involved in early morbidity and mortality due to cognitive impairments in learning, intelligence, memory, and behavior (Sharma 2016, 2017). Hence, fusion imaging with ^{18}F or ^{11}C-labelled CB, charnolophagy, and/or CS biomarker along with a specific microRNA-labeled PET radiopharmaceutical for evaluating brain regional DAeric, cholinergic, 5-HT-ergic, GABAergic neurotransmission will provide real-time precise understanding and will establish the exact interaction between MB, charnolophagy, CPS/CS, and brain-regional neurotransmission, which is impaired in numerous NDDs and repaired during neuroregeneration. Hence, future investigations to develop labeled DSST-CB, charnolophagy, and CS biomarker will provide exact molecular dynamics of chronic diseases and their possible prevention and effective cure. Studies in this direction will provide basic molecular mechanism of CMB, ICD and their implication in regulating brain regional neurotransmission in health and disease. Hence, future development of novel PET-RPs will be exceedingly important for basic understanding of the intricate processes of NDDs, CVDs, and chronic MDR malignancies at the cellular, molecular, genetic, and epigenetic level. Indeed! This is highly promising area of research and development because currently we have very limited knowledge regarding the involvement of DSST-CMB and microRNA pharmacodynamics in CB molecular pathogenesis, ICD, and brain regional neurotransmission, which is impaired in progressive NDDs, CVDs, and MDR malignancies. Further studies in this direction are extremely important particularly for the clinical management of AIS patients because these victims lose millions of functional neurons in a matter of few seconds which could be fatal or render them crippled rest of their life due to the induction of presently uncontrolled brain regional CB molecular pathogenesis.

^{11}C-Labeled and Other PET-RPs. Routine clinical application of ^{11}C-labeled PET-RPs is currently challenging due to short half-life of this radionuclide. The synthesis time is usually between 30–40 min and the imaging time is usually 40–90 min. It is envisaged that with the improvement in computer-controlled radiosynthesis modules and image acquisition capabilities, it will be possible to utilize ^{11}C, ^{13}N, and ^{15}O-labelled PET-RPs routinely to accomplish EBPT. The radioactivity for the first patient is about five times lower than what is obtained from the cyclotron. For the second patient, it is 16–32 times less than that produced by the cyclotron, suggesting that it is presently challenging to inject ^{11}C-labeled RPs routinely for clinical applications. However, ^{11}C-labelled-RPs will be highly suitable for evaluating DSST-CMB to accomplish

EBPT. In addition, CPS/CS exocytosis/endocytosis enhancers and inhibitors will be therapeutically beneficial in MDR malignancies and other chronic diseases.

Currently, ^{11}C-PET-RPs are used primarily in clinical research and development centers. However, ^{11}C-labeled PET-RPs may play a significant role to evaluate the basic concepts and biological significance of CB, charnolophagy, and CS as compared to ^{18}F. Since the endogenous molecules do not contain ^{18}F, and it is not highly suitable to compare *in vivo* bio-distribution and confirm that the endogenous molecule retains functionally-similar properties. For example, ^{11}C-methioinine is used to study brain regional protein synthesis in tumor imaging. Other tumor imaging agents are ^{11}C-choline and ^{11}C-thymidine. These PET-RPs showed promise in detecting prostate cancer cell proliferation. Furthermore, ^{11}C-hydroephedrine was used to differentiate between heart transplant patients and myocardial hypertrophy, ^{11}C-flumazenil as a GABA/benzodiazepine receptor antagonist to assess epilepsy, and ^{11}C-raclopride to assess DA-D$_2$ receptor activity in drug addiction. However, as discussed earlier, clinical evaluation with ^{11}C-labeled RPs is possible only if the cyclotron is available adjacent to PET imaging facility. Therefore, most of the PET imaging is performed on a routine basis with ^{18}FDG. However, several studies are now going on for the future development of ^{11}C-labeled RPs for cardiology, oncology, and receptor neuroimaging because low or medium energy cyclotrons can produce at least four (^{11}C, ^{13}N, ^{15}O, ^{18}F) radionuclides in addition to ^{64}Cu.

In general, positron emitting radionuclides [(^{11}C, ^{13}N, ^{15}O, ^{18}F, ^{64}Cu, ^{68}Ga), ^{76}Br ($t_{1/2}$ = 16.2 h; Iβ+ = 54%) and ^{124}I ($t_{1/2}$ = 4.18 d; Iβ+ =22.5%)] are of considerable interest both in clinical diagnosis as well as in therapy and their production at low energy cyclotrons is now well established. Ultra-short RPs of ^{13}N ($t_{1/2}$: 10 min) and ^{15}O ($t_{1/2}$: 2 min) or less, must be synthesized concomitantly along with the cyclotron for clinical applications. However, the increasing demand for these radionuclides requires optimization of conventional methods as well as further development of radiosynthesis procedures. For instance, ^{76}Br is produced via the ^{76}Se (p,n) ^{76}Br nuclear reaction using enriched target material. Measurements of this reaction over the proton energy range of 4.6 to 20 MeV using the stacked-foil technique and enriched target material were developed and ^{76}Br production (^{78}Kr (d,α) ^{76}Br) method was established. By utilizing ^{78}Kr and the gas-cell technique, cross sections was estimated over the deuteron energy range up to 13 MeV for the formation of ^{76}Br. The target yield of ^{76}Br was 59 kBq/μA/hr, which was insufficient for clinical applications.

The radionuclide, ^{124}I is generally produced via ^{124}Te(p,n)^{124}I nuclear reaction. Although the purity is high, the yield is poor. Hence, a ^{126}Te(p,3n)^{124}I reaction was tried using enriched target material, thin source via electrolytic deposition using stacked-foil technique. The excitation function of this reaction and other competing reactions was estimated over the proton energy up to 70 MeV. However, the target impurities were very high, hence, it has limited use in routine clinical applications.

Generator-Synthesized PET-RPs for Charnoly Body and microRNA-based Personalized Theranostics

^{68}Ge-^{68}Ga Generator. Although PET-RPs are synthesized from cyclotron-generated ^{18}F and ^{11}C radionuclides because they produce minimum chemical alteration in the

biomolecule, their tedious synthesis steps and reduced half-lives limits the number of molecules that could be labeled (Prata 2012). A positron emitting radiometal, ^{68}Ga produced by a ^{68}Ge/^{68}Ga generator, can be used for PET-RPs synthesis, independent of onsite cyclotron on a routine basis if freeze-dried kit-based formulations are developed. Kit-based precursors along with the ^{68}Ge/^{68}Ga generator may be developed, like ^{99}Mo/^{99m}Tc-based RPs (Fani et al. 2008). ^{68}Ge has a $t_{1/2}$ of 271 days and ^{68}Ga has a $t_{1/2}$ of 69 min. The generator is composed of alumina (Al_2O_3)-packed glass column. ^{68}Ga is eluted using 0.005M EDTA or 1M HCl when ^{68}Ge is adsorbed in a stannous dioxide (SnO_2) column. EDTA is removed before clinical application. ^{68}Ga-EDTA was used for brain tumor imaging. Octreotide was labeled with ^{68}Ga; however, its clinical utility is still being evaluated for brain tumor imaging. Recently, basic knowledge of purification, concentration of the eluate, and ligand chemistry led to the development of ^{68}Ga-labeled RPs for EBPT. The coordination chemistry of Ga^{+3} makes it highly suitable for the synthesis of several PET-RPs. A variety of mono- and bifunctional chelators allow the formation of stable ^{68}Ga^{3+} complexes and coupling to biomolecules. Moreover, ^{68}Ga coupling to small biomolecules is an alternative to ^{18}F^{-} and ^{11}C-based RPs. Particularly, peptides targeting G-protein coupled receptors demonstrated sensitivity and specificity for tumor localization. ^{68}Ga-labeled RPs qualify all options of ^{99m}Tc, with the higher resolution of PET in comparison to SPECT. Several ^{68}Ga-based PET-RPs were synthesized for basic research, routine clinical diagnosis, novel discovery of biomarkers, specific targets and their ligands improved automation of production for EBPT (Velikyan 2013a). Particularly, identification of somatostatin receptor with ^{68}Ga labeled DOTA-derivative peptides conferred in-depth knowledge of tumor biology (Win et al. 2007). ^{68}Ga-labeled analogs of octreotide, such as ^{68}Ga-DOTATOC and ^{68}Ga-DOTANOC were used for the clinical management of neuroendocrine and neural crest tumors such as pheochromocytoma and paraganglioma with theranostic capabilities. Furthermore, it can be utilized for the meningiomas and prostate cancer theranostics (Khan et al. 2009). Similarly, ^{68}Ga can be used for radiolabeling of CB, charnolophagy, CPS/CS biomarkers, and specific microRNA agonists and antagonists to quantitatively assess *in vivo* DSST-CMB, CS exocytosis/endocytosis, ICD, and their functional association with NDDs, CVDs, and MDR malignancies to accomplish the targeted, safe, and effective EBPT.

Although pharmacopoeia of generator-produced ^{68}Ga radionuclide and ^{68}Ga-labeled somatostatin analogs are in progress, currently ^{68}Ga-RPs await FDA approval, which will further augment development of novel RPs for EBPT. ^{68}Ga can also be used for labeling small organic molecules, peptides, proteins, and oligonucleotides (including disease-specific microRNAs) as well as NPs, demonstrating its potential to become a PET analog of the generator-produced γ-emitting ^{99m}Tc but with higher sensitivity and resolution as well as quantitation and dynamic functional imaging with theranostic capabilities. Particularly, HCl-based elution provided ^{68}Ga-complexes for the synthesis of Me(III)-based RPs (Rösch 2013; Rosch and Riss 2010; Velikyan 2013b). The clinical impact of ^{68}Ga-RPs, in addition to ^{68}Ga-DOTA-octreotide derivatives for tumor localization, is due to the further development of Ga^{+3} chelating molecules. In addition, open chain complexing agents were substituted with DOTA and NOTA-derived conjugates. Recently, Rice et al. (2011) developed [^{68}Ga]DO2A-(butyl-L-tyrosine), a tumor-localizing agent for PET imaging. These investigators studied the influence of time, temperature, precursor concentrations, and pH on the radiochemical yields by comparing conventional heating method with microwave irradiation for radiolabeling. The purification of ^{68}Ga-labeled RPs via solid-phase extraction and quality control was established which may serve as a guideline for optimizing future ^{68}Ga labelling reactions. Hsiao et al. (2009) prepared the lipophilic ^{67}Ga-labeled chelates. The bio-distribution and PKs of these chelates was determined and compared with the [^{86}Rb]rubidium chloride in rats. Most of these agents, particularly [$^{67/68}$Ga] [Ga(3-MeOsal)(2)BAPDMEN](1+) are superior to bis(salicylaldimine) ligands of N,N'-bis(3-aminopropyl)ethylenediamine for PET imaging of the heart.

^{82}Rb Generator. ^{82}Rb ($t_{1/2}$ = 75 Sec) is a cationic analog of potassium which is generator-produced and does not require onsite cyclotron. ^{82}Sr ($t_{1/2}$ = 25.5 days) is decayed to ^{82}Rb, by electron capture. Generally, ^{82}Rb is produced by spallation of the target, molybednum in high-energy accelerators. The difference in the charge number between Sr and Rb and their chemical properties makes it possible to isolate ^{82}Sr from ^{82}Rb. ^{82}Sr is loaded on to SnO_2 column and can be eluted after every 15 min with saline. Due to short half-life ($t_{1/2}$ = 75 sec), it is difficult to elute ^{82}Rb from the generator, collect, and then inject to the patient by a syringe. Therefore, only direct infusion is performed by adjusting the radioactivity, flow, and pressure of the infusion system. Prior safety measures are performed to ascertain that the entire infusion system is working properly. Excessive pressure may cause vascular injury and reduced pressure may lead to poor image quality whereas too high radioactivity may lead to undesirable radiation exposure to the patient. The life span of a single generator is about one month. Hence, a regular supply will require twelve ^{82}Rb generators/year. This is practically feasible only if the generator is used in high-throughput dedicated cardiac center. ^{82}Sr-^{82}Rb Generator System (Cardiogen-82) is available from Bracco Diagnostics, NJ. ^{82}Rb-labelled CB, charnolophagy, CPS/CS biomarkers, and specific microRNAs agonists/antagonists can be utilized to image DSST-MB, CS exocytosis/endocytosis, and ICD in health and disease.

^{62}Zn-^{62}Cu Generator. ^{62}Zn ($t_{1/2}$ = 9.3 hrs) is disintegrated to ^{62}Cu ($t_{1/2}$ = 9.7 min) by electron capture. In this generator, ^{62}Zn is loaded in a Dowex 1X10X column and ^{62}Cu is eluted with 2M HCl. Due to short $t_{1/2}$ of ^{62}Cu, ^{62}Zn is shipped daily for clinical applications. Two clinically-significant PET-RPs of ^{62}Cu are ^{62}Cu-ATSM (diacetyl-bis-N4-methyesemithiocarbazone) and ^{62}Cu-PTSM (pyrualdehyde bis-N-methylthiosemicarbazone). ^{62}Cu-ATSM is used as hypoxia imaging agent whereas ^{62}Cu-PTSM, for brain and myocardial perfusion imaging (Lapi et al. 2015). ^{62}Zn-labelled CB, charnolophagy, CPS/CS, and microRNA biomarkers can be utilized to quantitatively assess DSST-MB, CS exocytosis/endocytosis, and ICD/toxification in health and disease.

^{89}Zr-Labeled RPs. There is increasing demand for PET radiotracers which allow specific accumulation in the target as well as decay characteristics based on *in vivo* PKs. To meet this criterion, the development of new targeting vectors as well as uncommon radionuclides become important (Deri et al. 2013). Certain radionuclides selectively accumulate in molecules such as peptides, antibodies, their fragments, proteins, and artificial structures for PET imaging. Among these radionuclides, ^{89}Zr is promising due to its long half-life, which enables imaging at late time-points, especially in slowly-accumulating targeting vectors. Significant developments in ^{89}Zr-labeled biomolecules, their potential application in PET imaging as well as future challenges were provided in a recent report (Fischer et al. 2013). Moreover, [89]Zr-labelled CB, charnolophagy, CPS/CS, and microRNA biomarkers can be utilized to image DSST-CMB, CS exocytosis/endocytosis, and ICD/toxification in health and disease. These PET RPs seem to have better theranostic potential compared to routinely used [18]FdG, which exhibits considerable un-specificity in the EBPT of proinflammatory diseases.

Microfluidic System. The microfluidic system has a potential for the efficient synthesis of PET-RPs for routine molecular imaging employing either cyclotron-based or generator-based radionuclides. A microfluidic system in which ^{18}F is used for fluorination of biomolecules and other agents of clinical significance was developed (Chambers and Spink 1999). The miniaturization of chemical synthesis initiated with the micro-analytical devices consisting of computer-controlled sensors, actuators, and other components is for the rapid radiochemical synthesis (Manz and Widmer 1990; Hadd et al. 1997; Kopp et al. 1998). In fact, PET-RPs industry is basically a microchemistry because the amounts used in the synthesis are in nano or microgram range. We can achieve high specific activity and explore short half-lived positron emitters to facilitate radiolabeling of a wide range of compounds. These micro-devices can be produced on a large scale, hence, could be discarded after use, thus overcoming the requirement to clean the system after every production run (Gillies et al. 2006a; Gillies et al. 2006b; Gillies et al. 2006c). Recently microfluidic system was developed to synthesize [18]FdG and [124]I-Annexin-V using ^{18}F and [124]I radionuclides, respectively. The radiochemical yields were comparable to conventional methods. Furthermore, it was used to synthesize [[124]I]-doxorubicin iodobenzoate (I-DOXIB) within 20 seconds with a labeling efficiency of 80% as accomplished with routine method. The labeling efficiency and radiochemical yield improved by further optimization to synthesize ^{11}C-doxorubicin (Elsinga et al. 1996). Microfluidic system can also be utilized to synthesize ^{18}F or ^{11}C-labelled CB, charnolophagy, CPS/CS, and specific microRNA agonists/antagonists as biomarkers for the molecular imaging of DSST-MB, CS exocytosis/endocytosis, and ICD/toxification in health and disease.

CB and microRNA-based PET-RPs in NDDs

Drug Addiction. Recently, several PET imaging RPs were developed for evaluating the brain regional physiology, biochemistry, and pharmacology in drug addiction research on nonhuman primates. A detailed report on the clinical applications of PET-RPs in nonhuman drug addiction models of cocaine, METH, and MDMA was published (Howell et al. 2011). In addition, there is an excellent report on the synthesis of PET-RPs to explore brain regional receptor activity in PD, schizophrenia, pain, epilepsy, myocardial infarction, and in cancer diagnosis (Miller et al. 2008). For instance, DAT activity can be estimated by using ^{18}F-DOPA, ^{11}C-CFT, and ^{11}C-altropane for the clinical evaluation of PD and schizophrenia. D1 receptor mapping was accomplished by ^{11}C-SCH 23390 in drug addiction, whereas D2 receptor activity was estimated by ^{11}C-raclopride and [^{18}F]-fallypride and $5HT_{1A}$ receptor activity by using ^{11}C-WAY 100635 for the clinical evaluation of schizophrenia. Furthermore, a specific benzodiazepine receptor radioligand, ^{11}C-flumazenil was synthesized to determine the epileptic focus. Three clinically important PET radioligands synthesized for pain research, were ^{11}C-flumazenil, ^{11}C-deprenorphine, and ^{11}C-carfentanil.

Alzheimer's Disease. A recent study compared brain regional glucose metabolism and amyloid-β density in patients with AD, mild cognitive impairment (MCI), and healthy elderly subjects (Bailly et al. 2015). These investigators enrolled 18 patients (including 6 AD, 5 amnestic MCI, and 7 controls) for clinical, neuropsychological, and MRI evaluations. PET images were acquired using ^{18}F-florbetapir and ^{18}F-FdG. Brain-specific SUV ratios were determined employing PMOD-3.2 software. Mean ^{18}FdG SUV ratios were significantly reduced in frontal, anterior cingulate, and temporal regions in MCI patients than in healthy controls. A global reduction in glucose metabolism was observed in AD patients, particularly in the parietal and precuneus regions as compared to healthy controls. An increased ^{18}F-florbetapir uptake was detected exclusively in the precuneus cortex of AD patients, indicating that PET imaging with ^{18}F-florbetapir provides global analysis of amyloid-β, whereas ^{18}F-FdG provides analysis of brain regional glucose metabolism and hence, CMB involving CB molecular pathogenesis, as we reported in nutritional stress and in experimental models of AD (Sharma et al. 2016).

CB and micro-RNA Based PET-RPs in CVDs

Hemodynamic and Other Studies. Usually hemodynamic function is impaired in stroke, cardiac infarct, and cancer. Estrogen receptor activity in cancer was detected by 16–α-[^{18}F]fluoro-17β-estradiol. Hemodynamic parameters including blood flow can be estimated by $C^{15}O_2$, and $H_2^{15}O$. Blood volume is estimated by $C^{15}O$ or ^{11}CO, and myocardial perfusion by $^{13}NH_3$. Body metabolism is impaired in cancer, stroke, infarct, AD, and HD and can be estimated by PET imaging with ^{18}FdG and oxygen metabolism by $^{15}O_2$ and amino acid metabolism by ^{11}C-methionine for the differential diagnosis of cancer patients. Recently, PET imaging of integrin αVβ3 expression was investigated as a biomarker in tumor angiogenesis and metastasis. For instance, [^{18}F]-glacto-RGD was developed for PET and SPECT imaging. However, it did not cross the blood brain barrier easily (Beer et al. 2011). Several other clinically-significant PET-RPs were synthesized including the ^{124}I-annexin-V to study phosphatidyl serine externalization as a biomarker of apoptosis and to quantitatively estimate CPS/CS destabilization, CS body formation, leading to the formation of apoptotic bodies and eventually neurodegenerative apoptosis (Dekker et al. 2005a; Dekker et al. 2005b; Keen et al. 2005; Sharma 2016; Sharma 2017), ^{18}FdG for metabolic studies (Fletcher et al. 2002), [^{99m}Tc]macro-aggregated albumin (MAA) for myocardial infarction studies (Kondo et al. 1998), [^{99m}Tc]HDP oxidronate and radiosynthesis of [^{99m}Tc]HDP oxidronate using the microfluidic system for bone imaging (Lary et al. 1998).

CB and micro-RNA Based PET-RPs in Cancer Theranostics

Cancer presents a significant therapeutic challenge because of its heterogeneity, uncontrolled cell proliferation, and invasive nature. Recent developments in PET-RPs facilitated novel drug discovery and multimodality imaging for *in vivo*, non-invasive diagnosis, prognosis, and personalized theranostics at the cellular, molecular, and genetic level. Cancer biomarkers including cell adhesion molecules, protein kinases, protease, growth factor receptors, hypoxia, apoptosis, and angiogenesis were evaluated employing high-resolution microPET imaging in experimental animals. A recent review discussed radio-pharmacological, radiochemical, regulatory aspects, and general guidelines for the synthesis of PET-RPs for EBPT of cancer and other diseases (Wadsak and Mitterhauser 2010). Although ^{18}FdG is currently used for the clinical evaluation of cancer owing to its sensitivity, non-traditional PET-RPs, using the transition metals such as Cu-based radionuclides were developed. For instance, ^{64}Cu has 12.7 hrs, half-life and suitable energies to accomplish successful EBPT. Its coordination chemistry permits chelation for labeling proteins, peptides, antibodies, and other biomolecules including microRNAs. Tetra-aza-macrocyclic 1,4,8,11-tetraazacyclotetradecane-1,4,8,11-tetraacetic acid (TETA) as Cu chelators are quite stable. ^{64}Cu-labeled RPs were used to study somatostatin receptors, EGF receptor, and integrin $\alpha(v)\beta$-3 as cancer biomarkers (Shokeen et al. 2009). In addition, newly-developed radiolabeled bio-mimetics are highly specific for *in vivo* molecular imaging of cancer. Although bio-mimetics are sensitive, these are less specific, involve different transporters and metabolic pathways, and are eliminated slowly from the biological system. The radiolabeled drugs and drug-like compounds confer increased specificity, limited sensitivity, and complexity. Although the translation of these PET-RPs for EBPT was attenuated owing to concerns about ionizing radiations and federal regulatory constraints; changing health care system, diagnostic accuracy, and economy, offer new hope. Hence, ^{64}Cu-labelled CB, charnolophagy, CPS/CS, and microRNA biomarkers can be developed in the future to image DSST-MB and CS exocytosis/endocytosis to evaluate ICD/toxification in health and disease.

A review published studies on the use of molecular imaging for assessing tumor proliferation, apoptosis, growth receptor expression, bone metabolism, and hypoxia (Garcia et al. 2012). The dual imaging modality provided a unique opportunity in translational research bringing molecular knowledge for patient selection, prediction of prognosis, and as a diagnostic tool for PET imaging. ^{18}FdG, which provides metabolic information, was used for the early detection and staging of breast cancer to accomplish EBPT (Bravata et al. 2011). To evaluate associations between ^{18}FdG uptake and single nucleotide polymorphisms (SNPs) in GLUT1, HIF-1a, EPAS1, APEX1, VEGFA and MTHFR genes, these investigators performed a translational imaging study with ^{18}FdG. Whole body PET/CT was performed on 26 patients with breast cancer. Human gene mutation database and dbSNP short genetic variations database were used to analyze regions with SNPs. DNA sequencing was performed by capillary electrophoresis to obtain patient genotypes. Absence of correlation between these polymorphisms and ^{18}FdG uptake, suggested further investigations. Another study evaluated 19 subjects with 25 solid malignant renal tumors who underwent ^{18}FdG-PET/CT (Nakhoda et al. 2013; Nakhoda et al. 2013). PET portion of the ^{18}FdG-PET/CT imaging had a sensitivity of 88% for the detection of solid malignant renal lesions, and differences in metabolic activity, which may be useful for EBPT. Hence, the use of PET/CT is highly significant in breast cancer staging, treatment, and follow-up because it allows detection of nano-molar quantities of radiotracer for molecules targeting of breast cancer (Bourgeois et al. 2013; Gillings 2013). Although ^{18}FdG-PET/CT imaging demonstrated significant promise not only for diagnostics but also for staging, prognosis, and relapse detection in breast cancer, novel PET-RPs demonstrating DSST-CB pathogeneis are still needed for molecular characterization of other cancers and chronic MDR diseases to accomplish the targeted, safe, and effective EBPT.

It has been reported that although [18]FdG is the most widely used radiotracer, there are certain limitations to its use (Jiang et al. 2014). These investigators described various labeling procedures, biological targets, and preclinical and clinical trial of the next generation of PET-RPs and PET radionuclides for radiolabeling: [18]F for FACBC, FDHT, choline, and Galacto-RGD; ^{11}C, for choline; ^{68}Ga, for peptides including: DOTATOC and bombesin analogs; and the long-lived radionuclides [124]I and [89]Zr, for monoclonal antibodies cG250, J591, and trastuzumab, respectively. In addition, non-[18]FdG PET-RPs that are being used in research and development were also explained in detail (Nunez et al. 2013). Many of these new PET-RPs are being investigated for the assessment of molecular functions in cancer cells, which could eventually contribute to successful EBPT.

Recently, Wu et al. (2013) reported that in addition to conventional anti-cancer therapies such as surgery, chemotherapies, and radiotherapy, neoadjuvant chemotherapies, minimally invasive treatments, and molecular-targeting may be translated into clinical practice, because a futile therapy makes a patient miss the optimum time for treatment. Conventional methods based on anatomical evidence, such as CT and MRI, have limitations in early response evaluation. Moreover, PET imaging using [18]FdG is promising especially when combined with CT or MRI. By predicting response early during radiotherapy, PET imaging confers better selection of patients who would be benefited most from treatment (Herrera and Prior 2013). These advances opened avenues to modify the way treatment is designed and the dose is delivered, based on the radiobiology of solid cancers. For example, to accomplish EBPT, DNA- or RNA-based tests of gene expression and/or immunohistochemistry are essential. Particularly, estrogen receptor (ER), progesterone receptor (PR), and human epidermal growth factor receptor 2 (HER2/neu) as breast cancer biomarkers have been evaluated. Depending on the location, invasive biopsy to detect these biomarkers could be difficult to detect. Moreover, not all tumors that express targets those are identified based on histological examination, respond to therapy. PET imaging can be used for detecting, learning molecular biology of the tumor, and predicting the prognosis of targeted therapies. How [18]FDG-PET and estrogen analogs could be used successfully in breast cancer, particularly ER-positive metastatic breast cancer, as an example to guide EBPT, was recently explained in sufficient detail (Clark et al. 2014).

Assessment of Tumor Hypoxia. Tumor hypoxia is associated with poor prognosis; therefore, patients with hypoxic tumors could benefit from intensive treatment, particularly, those with head and neck cancer. Tumor hypoxia can be evaluated by non-invasive PET imaging. Halmos et al. (2014) summarized the literature on animal and human PET imaging with ^{18}F-FAZA and future perspectives on how PET could be applied in patients with hypoxic head and neck tumors along with hypoxia sensitizers or intensity-modulated radiation therapy for better prognosis. As an alternative to the invasive polarographic needle electrode procedure, PET imaging using ^{18}F-labeled fluoromisonidazole (^{18}F-FMISO) can be performed to visualize hypoxia noninvasively. A related molecule, ^{18}F-fluoroazomycin-arabinoside (^{18}F-FAZA), has superior PKs; hence, may be a better hypoxia biomarker. A recent study performed a comparative analysis of 3 hypoxia PET radiotracers: [^{18}F]FMISO, [^{18}F]FAZA, and [^{18}F]HX4, in a tumor model of rhabdomyosarcoma R1-bearing WAG/Rij rats (Peeters et al. 2015). They evaluated the optimal time-points for imaging, tumor to blood ratios (TBR), reproducibility by voxel-to-voxel analysis, and sensitivity to oxygen modification, induced by either carbogen/nicotinamide treatment or 7% oxygen breathing. A maximum TBR was obtained at 2 hrs for [^{18}F]FAZA, at 3 hrs for [^{18}F]HX4, and at 6 hrs for [^{18}F]FMISO. Voxel-to-voxel comparisons and Dice similarity coefficients to evaluate reproducibility demonstrated 30% standard uptake volume (SUV) for [^{18}F]FMISO and [^{18}F]HX4, whereas [^{18}F]FAZA was less reproducible. Enhanced mean standardized uptake values were detected for both [^{18}F]HX4 and [^{18}F]FAZA upon modification of the hypoxia fraction (7% oxygen breathing), whereas only [^{18}F]FMISO uptakes were reversible upon exposure to nicotinamide and carbogen, suggesting that each radiotracer has its own merits and limitations. Depending on the tumor and nature of investigation, these radiotracers can be utilized for the clinical evaluation of tumor hypoxia. In addition, paraganglioma syndromes related to succinate dehydrogenase (SDH) gene mutations are rare hereditary conditions with heterogeneous symptoms difficult to classify. Recently, pathophysiological, clinical, lab, morphological, and functional imaging of SDH gene mutation PGLs, employing ^{18}F-DOPA-PET/CT and correlated clinical and genetic features of SDH-related PGLs were investigated to accomplish EBPT of paraganglioma syndromes (Marzola and Rubello 2014).

In Vivo Detection of Apoptosis in Cancer. It is known that caspases are the determinants of apoptotic signaling cascades and represent targets for molecular imaging; hence, they can be used for assessing the response to therapy. Recently, [^{18}F]FB-VAD-FMK: [^{18}F]4-fluorobenzylcarbonyl-Val-Ala-Asp(OMe)-fluoromethylketone, a peptide-probe for the quantification of apoptosis employing PET imaging was developed (Hight et al. 2014). The validity of the probe was authenticated by *in vitro* assays as well. Labeling of pan-caspase inhibitory peptide, [^{18}F]FB-VAD-FMK, using radiofluorination was confirmed in the mouse model of human colorectal cancer to predict the therapeutic response of targeted therapy employing microPET imaging. The bio-distribution of [^{18}F]FB-VAD-FMK was also performed in normal and cancer tissue. [^{18}F]FB-VAD-FMK was localized primarily in the tumor in agreement with the elevated caspase-3 activity in response to Aurora B kinase inhibition and treatment with mutant BRAF and PI3K/mTOR inhibitor. Furthermore, localization of [^{18}F]FB-VAD-FMK was enhanced in the tumors that reduced in their size in response to treatment, suggesting its potential as a novel biomarker for EBPT of cancer.

Rationale Treatment of ^{131}I. Generally, patients are followed with thyroglobulin (Tg) estimation after initial treatment of disseminated thyroid carcinoma (DTC) to detect recurrence. In case of elevated Tg and negative neck ultrasonography, patients are treated 'blindly' with ^{131}I. In up to 50% of patients, the imaging reveals no ^{131}I-targeting of tumor lesions. Such patients do not benefit from this therapy but are exposed to unnecessary ^{131}I radiotoxicity. ^{124}I-PET/CT imaging can visualize DTC lesions, whereas ^{18}FdG-PET/CT detects the recurrent DTC, which does not accumulate iodine. Hence, combined imaging with ^{124}I-PET/CT and ^{18}FdG-PET/CT can differentiate patients for successful treatment with ^{131}I. A study was performed to confirm that combined ^{124}I-PET/CT and ^{18}FdG-PET/CT imaging avoids unnecessary ^{131}I treatment planned for 'blind' therapy with ^{131}I (Kist et al. 2014). The primary objective was to reduce the number of futile ^{131}I therapies and Nation-wide introduction of ^{124}I-PET/

CT and [18]FDG-PET/CT to correlate imaging outcome with histopathological findings, compare [124]I and ^{131}I dosimetry, and [124]I-PET/CT after rhTSH treatment and after withdrawal of thyroid hormone. One hundred patients for ^{131}I treatment were subjected to both [124]I-PET/CT and [18]FdG-PET/CT imaging following rhTSH stimulation. Patients received the ^{131}I therapy after thyroid hormone withdrawal. The post ^{131}I therapeutic imaging was compared with [124]I-PET/CT and [18]FdG-PET/CT to evaluate the theranostic significance of integrated imaging. This study confirmed the significance of combination imaging to prevent futile ^{131}I therapies in patients with suspected recurrence of DTC, which is clinically significant because this treatment is costly, involves morbid toxicity; hence, it should be restricted to only those likely to benefit. Hence, [124]I and ^{131}I-labelled CB, charnolophagy, CPS/CS, and microRNA biomarkers can be utilized for molecular imaging of DSST-CMB and CS exocytosis/endocytosis to quantitatively assess ICD/toxification for the safe and effective EBPT of thyroid cancer.

Prostate Cancer. Molecular imaging is paving the way to successful accomplishment of EBPT of prostate cancer. A recent study provided information regarding the current-status and potential for future developments in the theranostic utility of PET in prostate cancer (Jadvar 2013). In view of the biologic and clinical heterogeneity of prostate cancer, molecular imaging could play a pivotal role in the evaluation of prostate cancer. The history of prostate cancer varies from a localized process to biochemical relapse after radical treatment to a lethal castrate-resistant malignancy. The complex tumor biology places molecular imaging with PET to clinically manage prostate cancer just like breast cancer to accomplish EBPT. Hence, development of PET-RPs for the evaluation of MB and ICD seems promising to accomplish the safe and effective EBPT of prostate cancer.

Neuroendocrine Tumors (NETs). It was shown that NETs are originated from neuroendocrine cells in the body (Wang et al. 2013). The detection of NETs is important for EBPT, which could be based on tumor type and clinical symptoms. Molecular imaging of NETs can be achieved by using SPECT-RPs. In addition, somatostatin receptor imaging using PET is significant for the clinical management of NETs. The somatostatin analogs labeled with β-emitters, such as ^{177}Lu or ^{90}Y, could be a therapeutic option for patients with malignant NETs. Molecular imaging can confer valuable information to improve the prognosis by achieving earlier and better EBPT for patients with NETs. Hence, ^{177}Lu or [90]Y-[177–] labelled CB, charnolophagy, and CPS/CS biomarkers can be developed for molecular imaging of DSST microRNAs, MB, and CS exocytosis/endocytosis to quantitatively assess ICD/toxification in health and disease.

CB and micro-RNA Based PET-RPs in Other Diseases

[18]FdG Dose Adjustment Based on Body Mass Index (BMI). Recently it was established that the dose of [18]FdG can be significantly reduced by measuring BMI instead of patient's weight, without compromising the image quality (Sánchez-Jurado 2014). These investigators conducted a study in > 1,800 patients undergoing PET/CT. The control group was administered based on body weight and the treatment group was administered based on BMI. A reduction of 9–20% dose was achieved in those who were injected based on BMI compared to those who were injected based on body weight with a dose reduction of 56% and 12.5% for patients and staff, respectively. The cost of study was considerably reduced while image quality was improved, suggesting that this dose reduction not only follows the ALARA principle of radiation safety but also can be performed without compromising the image quality and diagnostic accuracy.

Assessment of Implant Efficacy. It is difficult to predict cochlear implant efficacy and cortical processing of the visual component of language in deaf patients with congenital CMV infection. Early diagnosis and cochlear implantation are extremely important for speech development, and each patient needs EBPT based on etiology and brain function. The cortical activity of two children was evaluated with CMV-related hearing loss employing ^{18}FdG-PET with a visual language task before cochlear implantation (Moteki et al. 2013). Total development and auditory perception were assessed after one year. CMV-related hearing loss showed activation in the auditory association area and cortical activation as observed in patients with congenital hearing loss. Differences in verbal ability and discrimination of sentences were noticed, suggesting that the differences in cortical activities could be influenced by CMV infection that involves higher functions.

Internal Dosimetry. The main objective of internal dosimetry is to establish dose-effect correlation for EBPT. It was developed for ^{131}I-mIBG treatment for over the last 20 years. Recently, whole-body dosimetry was introduced to prevent hematological toxicity for the European multi-center trial, in which the activity of a second dose was determined based on the results obtained from the previous study (Chiesa et al. 2013). This study was conducted to assess improvement and achieve better predictive power of dosimetry by setting intrinsic radiobiological limits. The authors suggested that further development of internal dosimetry, radiobiology, and quantitative ^{124}I PET imaging may provide more precise mIBG theranostics. However, this will require multicenter trials with quality-controlled instruments and scientific approach.

Analysis of CB, Charnolophagy, CPS, CS, microRNA Biomarkers in Biological Fluids by SPR Spectroscopy

Although molecular interaction studies with ELISA and radiotracers have led to the development of many life-saving therapies, SPR spectroscopy is a further step to eliminate the need of costly markers that vary significantly between labs across the globe. Owing to its relatively high sensitivity, precision, accuracy, reproducibility, and information capability; SPR can be utilized for the development of novel charnolopharmacotherapeutics as described in this chapter and in several QC and R&D pharmaceutical labs. As a matter of fact, experimental variability in protocols generates imperfections to impede progress in biomedical research. SPR confers a more efficient and time-saving strategies to resolve important research questions, leading to the quicker development of specific charnolopharmacotherapeutics and microRNA biomarkers for EBPT and for a better quality of life.

SPR confers several benefits not achievable by conventional methods like ELISA. SPR is a label-free study of molecular binding interactions. It is cost-

Table 3: Comparison between ELISA and SPR analysis.

S.NO.	ELISA	SPR
Analysis Time:	> 5–6 hrs	1–2 hrs
Information	Yes/No Binding, Conc.	Affinity, Kinetics, Thermodyamics Concentration, Activity, Yes/No Binding
Time Information	Last Step	Real-Time On-Line Monitoring Through all steps
Number of steps	5+	2–3
Limit of Detection	ng/ml range	pg/ml
Precision (CV%) (Intra-assay)	5–10	< 1–5
Precision (Inter-assay)	7–15	~ 5
Analytes	Proteins/Peptides	Low MW compounds (< 100 DA) Peptide, Proteins, DNA, Virus, Bacteria
Type of Interaction	Only high interaction	Weak-High Interactions
Advantages		No washing, No Secondary Reagents, Real-Time data Control, Fully Automated
Disadvantages	Multiple reagents, Multiple washing steps End-point assay Difficult to optimize Plate-base denaturation	
Plate-based epitope inaccessibility	Plate-based blocking step Weak affinity antibodies are washed away	

effective and provides a detailed analysis of molecular interactions and minimizes the variables which result from fluorescent and radioactive markers. Fluorescent-labeled antibodies may cost from $50–$500 per vial and radiolabeled probes require extensive biohazard training. Moreover, fluorochrome analysis requires compensation for spectral overlap, which may provide false-positive or false-negative results, and compromise precision, accuracy, and reproducibility in data interpretation and arriving at definitive conclusions regarding CB, CPS, CS, and microRNA biomarker analysis and their exact clinical significance in EBPT. Label-free capabilities of SPR simplify experimental protocols and provide reproducible and accurate results to facilitate efficient use of financial and human resources as Zantek Biotechnologies recently introduced. The most significant advantages of SPR spectroscopy is that it enhances the integrity of data by minimizing the investigator's bias, which is introduced by fluorescent or radioactive markers, requiring post-analysis to prevent inter-assay as well as intra-assay variability between different labs. In conventional methods, lab protocols may vary and influence the reproducibility, while a consistent experimental platform can be established by SPR analysis, which confers reproducible results in different labs across the globe. Conventional methods provide only a single parameter at any given time, whereas SPR's lab-on-a-chip, label-free capabilities provide real-time manipulation of the experimental settings to save sample, labor, and time of the investigator. When radiolabeled molecules and fluorescent dyes are utilized to determine molecular binding interactions, additional parameter selection may modify the experimental data, which may compromise the accuracy and reproducibility. Moreover, fluorescent and radioactive probes require complicated data analysis and weeks or months of training to correctly interpret, whereas label-free SPR studies permit analysis of the data in real-time. Although, post-processing in SPR is necessary, it is equipped with user-friendly software, affording a reliable investigative tool, which can be adopted in the novel discovery of CB, CPS/CS, and microRNA biomarkers from various biological fluids including serum, plasma, CSF, saliva, tear, nasal fluid, urine, toe nails, and hair samples of normal and diseased subjects to accomplish EBPT (Modified from Zantek Biotechnologies).

Conclusions

This chapter proposed CB, charnolophagy, CPS/CS, and microRNA biomarkers as ligands (agonists/antagonists) to evaluate DSST-MB and ICD to accomplish the targeted, safe, and effective EBPT. Currently, the number of cyclotron-based PET-RPs centers is increasing globally. Although cyclotrons are used primarily for the bulk synthesis of ^{18}FdG and ^{18}F-DOPA, the production of other short and long-lived radionuclides will provide unique opportunities to develop novel RPs for EBPT; particularly, DSST-CB, charnolophagy, CPS/CS, and microRNA biomarkers, as described in this chapter. Although ^{11}C, ^{13}N, ^{15}O labeled RPs have shown promise in diagnosis, prognosis, and research, their routine synthesis presently poses a significant challenge due to limited availability of cyclotrons, lack of sophisticated technology, experienced PET-RPs scientists, and multi-modality imaging experts (Miller et al. 2008). Future advances in PET imaging will depend on the novel discovery of RPs which will complement ^{18}F-FdG and ^{18}F-DOPA imaging studies. Extensive efforts are being made to discover innovative procedures to develop novel PET-RPs. Future RPs development will accomplish reduced synthesis time, acceptable radionucleidic, radiochemical, and RPs purity, and increased radiochemical yield. In addition, microfluidic, multifunctional NPs, and nano-devices to radiolabel organ and DSST-CB, charnolophagy, CPS/CS, and microRNA biomarkers will revolutionize the synthesis of novel PET-RPs to accomplish EBPT of chronic MDR diseases. In summary, automated remote-controlled RPs synthesis modules, microfluidic system, innovative chemical reactions, microwave heating, solid phase extraction procedures, and advanced computer technology will facilitate novel drug discovery and superior RPs to accomplish EBPT of chronic MDR diseases. Although conventionally-used γ-emitting radionuclides such as ^{99m}Tc, ^{131}I, and ^{111m}In can be utilized for labeling CB, charnolophagy, CPS/CS, and microRNA biomarkers for molecular imaging of DSST-MB and exocytosis/endocytosis to quantitively estimate ICD, these RPs have limited spatio-temporal resolution and 3D penetration for accurate image reconstructions. However, PET radionuclides including: ^{18}F, ^{11}C, ^{13}N, ^{15}O, ^{124}I, ^{68}Ga, ^{82}Rb, ^{62}Cu, ^{64}Cu, ^{62}Zn, ^{89}Zr-labeled CB, charnolophagy, CPS/CS, and microRNA biomarkers can provide real-time functional genomics and molecular imaging of DSST-MB, CS exocytosis/endocytosis, and ICD/toxification in health and disease. Future studies in this direction along with SPR analyses promise to accomplish the targeted, safe and effective EBPT of NDDs, CVDs, MDR malignancies, and several pro-inflammatory chronic diseases beyond the scope of this chapter.

References

Adam, M.J. and S. Jivan. 1988. Synthesis and purification of L-6-[^{18}F]fluorodopa. Appl Radiat Isot 39: 1203–1210.

Antoni, G. and B. Langstrom. 2008. RPs: molecular imaging using positron emission tomography. Handb Exp Pharmacol 185: 177–201.

Bailly, M., M.J. Ribeiro, J. Vercouillie, C. Hommet, V. Gissot, V. Camus and D. Guilloteau. 2015. ^{18}F-FDG and ^{18}F-florbetapir PET in clinical practice: regional analysis in mild cognitive impairment and Alzheimer disease. Clin Nucl Med 40: e111–116.

Beer, A.J., H. Kessler, H.J. Wester and M. Schwaiger. 2011. PET imaging of integrin α-Vβ3 expression. Theranostics 1: 48–57.

Bourgeois, A.C., L.A. Warren, T.T. Chang, S. Embry, K. Hudson and Y.C. Bradley. 2013. Role of positron emission tomography/computed tomography in breast cancer. Radiol Clin North Am 51: 781–798.

Bravatà, V., A. Stefano, F.P. Cammarata, L. Minafra, G. Russo, S. Nicolosi, S. Pulizzi, C. Gelfi, M.C. Gilardi and C. Messa. 2011. Genotyping analysis and ^{18}FDG uptake in breast cancer patients: a preliminary research. J Exp Clin Cancer Res 32: 23.

Chambers, R.D. and R.C.H. Spink. 1999. Microreactors for elemental fluorine. Chem Comm 883–884.

Cherry, C., B. Thompson, N. Saptarshi, J. Wu and J. Hoh. 2016. A 'Mitochondria' odyssey. Trends in Molecular Medicine 22: 391–403.

Chiesa, C., R. Castellani, M. Mira, A. Lorenzoni and G.D. Flux. 2013. Dosimetry in ^{131}I-mIBG therapy: moving toward personalized medicine. Q J Nucl Med Mol Imaging 57: 161–170.

Clark, A.S., E. McDonald, M.C. Lynch and D. Mankoff. 2014. Using nuclear medicine imaging in clinical practice: update on PET to guide treatment of patients with metastatic breast cancer. Oncology (Williston Park) 28: 424–430.

Coenen, H.H., P.H. Elsinga, R. Iwata, M.R. Kilbourn, M.R.A. Pillai, M.G.R. Rajan, H.N. Wagner Jr and J.J. Zaknun. 2010. Fluorine-18 RPs beyond [^{18}F]FDG for use in oncology and neurosciences. Nuc Med and Biol 37: 727–740.

Cole, E.L., M.N. Stewart, R. Littich. R. Hoareau and P.J. Scott. 2014. Radiosyntheses using fluorine-18: the art and science of late stage fluorination. Curr Top Med Chem 14: 875–900.

Das, S., M. Ferlito, O.A. Kent, K.F. Talbot, R. Wang, D. Liu, N. Raghavachari, Y. Yang, S.J. Wheelan, E. Murphy and C. Steenbergen. 2012. Nuclear miRNA regulates the mitochondrial genome in the heart. Circulation Research 110: 1596–1603.

Das, S., D. Bedja, N. Campbell, B. Dunkerly, V. Chenna, A. Maitra et al. 2014. miR-181c regulates the mitochondrial genome, bioenergetics, and propensity for heart failure *in vivo*. PLoS ONE 9(5): e96820.

de Vries, E.F.J., G. Luurtsema, M. Brüssermann, P.H. Elsinga and W. Vaalburg. 1999. Fully automated synthesis module for the high yield one-pot preparation of 6-[^{18}F]Fluoro-L-DOPA. Appl Radiat Isot 51: 389–394.

Dekker, B.A., H.G. Keen, S. Lyons, L. Disley, H. Hastings, A.J. Reader, P. Ottewell, A. Watson and J. Zweit. 2005. MBP–annexin V radiolabeled directly with iodine-124 can be used to image apoptosis *in vivo* using PET. Nucl Med Biol 32: 241–252.

Dekker, B.A., H.G. Keen, D. Shaw, L. Disley, D. Hastings, J. Hadfield, A. Reader, D. Allan, P. Julyan, A. Watson and J. Zweit. 2005a. Functional comparison of annexin V analogues labeled indirectly and directly with iodine-124. Nucl Med Biol 32: 403–413.

Deri, M.A., B.M. Zeglis, L.C. Francesconi and J.S. Lewis. 2013. PET Imaging with ^{89}Zr: From radiochemistry to the clinic. Nucl Med Biol 40: 3–14.

Durate, F.V., C.M. Palmeira and A.P. Rolo. 2014. The role of microRNAs in mitochondria: Small players acting wide. Genes (Basel) 5(4): 865–886.

Ebadi, M., S. Sharma, P. Ghafourifar, H. Brown-Borg and H.E.I. Refaey. 2005. Peroxynitrite in the pathogenesis of Parkinson's disease and the neuroprotective role of metallothioneins. Methods in Enzymol 396: 276–298.

Ebadi, M. and S. Sharma. 2006. Metallothioneins 1 and 2 attenuate peroxynitrite induced oxidative stress in Parkinson's disease. J Exp Biol & Med 231: 1576–1583.

Elsinga, P.H., E.J. Franssen, N.H. Hendrikse, L. Fluks, A.M. Weemaes, W.T. Van der Graaf, E.G. De Vries, G.M. Visser and W. Vaalburg. 1996. Carbon-11-labeled daunorubicin and verapamil for probing P-glycoprotein in tumors with PET. J Nucl Med 37: 1571–1575.

Fani, M., J.P. André and H.R. Maecke. 2008. ^{68}Ga-PET: a powerful generator-based alternative to cyclotron-based PET RPs. Contrast Media Mol Imaging 3: 67–77.

Fischer, G., U. Seibold, R. Schirrmacher, B. Wängler and C. Wängler. 2013. ^{89}Zr, a radiometal nuclide with high potential for molecular imaging with PET: chemistry, applications and remaining challenges. Molecules 18: 6469–6490.

Fletcher, P.D.I., S.J. Haswell, E. Pombo-Villar, B.H. Warrington, P. Watts, S.Y.F. Wong and X. Zhang. 2002. Micro reactors: principles and applications in organic synthesis. Tetrahedron 58: 4735–4757.

Garcia, C., G. Gebhart and P. Flamen. 2012. New PET imaging agents in the management of solid cancers. Curr Opin Oncol 24: 748–755.

Gillies, J.M., C. Prenant, G.N. Chimon, G.J. Smethurst, W. Perrie, I. Hamblett, B. Dekker and J. Zweit. 2006a Microfluidic reactor for the radiosynthesis of PET radiotracers. Appl Radiat Isot 64: 325–332.

Gillies, J.M., C. Prenant, G.N. Chimon, G.J. Smethurst, B.A. Dekker and J. Zweit. 2006b. Microfluidic technology for PET radiochemistry. Appl Radiat Isot 64: 333–336.

Gillies, J.M., N. Najima and J. Zweita. 2006c. Analysis of metal radioisotope impurities generated in [^{18}O]H$_2$O during the cyclotron production of fluorine-18. Applied Radiation and Isotopes 64: 431–434.

Gillings, N. 2013. Radiotracers for positron emission tomography imaging. MAGMA 26: 149–158.

Hadd, A.G., D.E. Raymond, J.W. Halliwell, S.C. Jacobson and J.M. Ramsey. 1997. Microchip device for performing enzyme assays. Anal Chem 69: 3407–3412.

Halmos, G.B., L. Bruine de Bruin, J.A. Langendijk, B.F. van der Laan, J. Pruim and R.J. Steenbakkers. 2014. Head and neck tumor hypoxia imaging by 18F-fluoroazomycin-arabinoside (18F-FAZA)-PET: a review. Clin Nucl Med 39: 44–48.

Haug, A., C.J. Auernhammer, B. Wängler, R. Tiling, G. Schmidt, B. Göke et al. 2009. Intra-individual comparison of ^{68}Ga-DOTA-TATE and ^{18}F-DOPA PET in patients with well-differentiated metastatic neuroendocrine tumors. Eur J Nucl Med Mol Imaging 36: 765–770.

Hendrikse, N.H., G. Luurtsema, A.A. van der Veldt and M. Lubberink. 2008. Positron emission tomography for modeling pathophysiological processes *in vivo*. Curr Opin Drug Discov Devel 11: 717–725.

Herrera, F.G. and J.O. Prior. 2013. The role of PET/CT in cervical cancer. Front Oncol 3: 34.

Hight, M.R., Y.Y. Cheung, M.L. Nickels, E.S. Dawson, P. Zhao, S. Saleh, J.R. Buck, D. Tang, M.K. Washington, R.J. Coffey and H.C. Manning. 2014. A peptide-based positron emission tomography probe for *in vivo* detection of caspase activity in apoptotic cells. Clin Cancer Res 20: 2126–2135.

Howell, L.L. and K.S. Murnane. 2011. Nonhuman primate positron emission tomography neuroimaging in drug abuse research. Pharmacol Exp Ther 337: 324–334.

Hsiao, Y.M., C.J. Mathias, S.P. Wey, P.E. Fanwick and M.A. Green. 2009. Synthesis and biodistribution of lipophilic and monocationic gallium RPs derived from N,N'-bis(3-aminopropyl)-N,N'-dimethylethylenediamine: potential agents for PET myocardial imaging with ^{68}Ga. Nucl Med Biol 36: 39–45.

Hu, Y., H. Deng, S. Xu and J. Zhang. 2015. microRNAs regulate mitochondrial function in cerebral ischemia-reperfusion injury. Taguchi Y, ed. International Journal of Molecular Sciences 16: 24895–24917.

Hung, J.C. 2002. Comparison of various requirements of the quality assurance procedures for ^{18}FDG injection. J Nucl Med 43: 1495–506.

Iwata, R. 2004. Reference Book for PET RPs. Cyclotron and Radioisotope Center, Tohoku University. Japan. 4th Edition.

Jacobson, M.S., J.C. Hung, T.L. Mays and B.P. Mullan. 2002. The planning and design of a new PET radiochemistry facility. Mol Imaging Biol 4: 119–127.

Jadvar, H. 2013. Molecular imaging of prostate cancer with PET. J Nucl Med 54: 1685–1688.

Jiang, L., Y. Tu, H. Shi and Z. Cheng. 2014. PET probes beyond ^{18}F-FDG. J Biomed Res 28: 435–446.

Keen, H.G., B.A. Dekker, L. Disley, H. Hastings, S. Lyons, A.J. Reader, P. Ottewell, A. Watson and J. Zweit. 2005. Imaging apoptosis *in vivo* using ^{124}I-annexin V and PET. Nucl Med Biol 32: 395–402.

Khan, M.U., S. Khan, S. El-Refaie, Z. Win, D. Rubello and A. Al-Nahhas. 2009. Clinical indications for Gallium-68 positron emission tomography imaging. Eur J Surg Oncol 35: 561–567.

Kist, J.W., B. de Keizer, M.P. Stokkel, O.S. Hoekstra and W.V. Vogel. 2014. THYROPET study group. Recurrent differentiated thyroid cancer: towards personalized treatment based on evaluation of tumor characteristics with PET (THYROPET Study): study protocol of a multicenter observational cohort study. BMC Cancer 14: 405.

Klongpanichapak, S., P. Govitrapong, S. Sharma and M. Ebadi. 2006. Attenuation of *Cocaine* and METH neurotoxicity by coenzyme Q_{10}. Neurochem Res 31: 303–311.

Kondo, M., A. Nakano, D. Saito and Y. Shimono. 1998. Assessment of "microvascular no-reflow phenomenon" using technetium-99m macroaggregated albumin scintigraphy in patients with acute myocardial infarction. J Am Coll Card 32: 898–903.

Koopmans, K.P., A.H. Brouwers, M.N. De Hooge, A.N. Van der Horst-Schrivers, I.P. Kema and B.H. Wolffenbuttel. 2005. Carcinoid crisis after injection of 6-^{18}F-fluorodihydroxyphenylalanine in a patient with metastatic carcinoid. J Nucl Med 46: 1240–1243.

Kopp, M.U., A.J. de Mello and A. Manz. 1998. Chemical amplification: continuous flow PCR on a chip. Science 280: 1046–1047.

Långström, B., F. Karimi and Y. Watanabe. 2013. Endogenous compounds labeled with radionuclides of short half-life-some perspectives. J Labelled Comp Radiopharm 56: 251–262.

Lapi, S.E., J.S. Lewis and F. Dehdasgti. 2015. Evaluation of hypoxia with Cu-ATSM. Semin Nucl Med 45: 177–185.

Lary, A., M.D. Robinson, P.A.C. Dianne Preksto, M.C. Carlos and S.H. David. 1998. Intraoperative gamma probe-directed biopsy of asymptomatic suspected bone metastases. Ann Thoracic Surgery 65: 1426–1432.

Li, L. and C.M. Stary. 2016. Targeting glial mitochondrial function for protection from cerebral ischemia: Relevance, mechanisms, and the role of microRNAs. Oxidative Medicine and Cellular Longevity 2016: 6032306.

Li, Z. and P.S. Conti. 2010. Radiopharmaceutical chemistry for positron emission tomography. Advanced Drug Delivery Reviews 62: 1031–1051.

Loane, C. and M. Politis. 2011. Positron emission tomography neuroimaging in Parkinson's disease. Am J Transl Res 3: 323–341.

Lodi, F., A. Rizzello, A. Carpinelli, D. Di Pierro, G. Cicoria, V. Mesisca, M. Marengo and S. Boschi. 2008. Automated synthesis of [^{11}C]Meta hydroxyephedrine, a PET radiopharmaceutical for studying sympathetic innervations in the heart. Computers in Cardiology 35: 341–343.

Manz, A. and H.M. Widmer. 1990. Miniaturized total chemical analysis systems: a novel concept, for chemical sensing. Sensors Actuators B 1: 244–248.

Marzola, M.C. and D. Rubello. 2014. Molecular imaging in hereditary succinate dehydrogenase mutation-related paragangliomas. Clin Nucl Med 39: e53–58.

Miller, P.W., N.J. Long, R. Vilar and A.D. Gee. 2008. Synthesis of ^{11}C, ^{18}F, ^{15}O, and ^{13}N radiolabels for positron emission tomography. Angew Chem Int Ed Engl 47: 8998–9003.

Minn, H., S. Kauhanen, M. Seppänen and P. Nuutila. 2009. ^{18}F-FDOPA: a multiple-target molecule. J Nucl Med 50: 1915–1918.

Moteki, H., M. Suzuki, Y. Naito, K. Fujiwara, K. Oguchi, S.Y. Nishio, S. Iwasaki and S. Usami. 2013. Evaluation of cortical processing of language by use of positron emission tomography in hearing loss children with congenital cytomegalovirus infection. Int J Pediatr Otorhinolaryngol 78: 285–289.

Nakhoda, Z., D.A. Torigian, B. Saboury, F. Hofheinz and A. Alavi. 2013. Assessment of the diagnostic performance of ^{18}F-FDGPET/CT for detection and characterization of solid renal malignancies. Hell J Nucl Med 16: 19–24.

Namavari, M., A. Bishop, N. Satyamurthy, G. Bida and J.R. Barrio. 1992. Regioselective radiofluorodestannylation with [^{18}F]F2 and [^{18}F] CH3COOF: a high yield synthesis of 6-[^{18}F] fluoro-L-dopa. Appl Rad Isot 43: 989–996.

Nunez, M. and M.A. Pozo. 2011. Non-FDG PET in oncology. Clin Transl Oncol 13: 780–786.

Okarvi, S.M. 2001. Recent progress in fluorine-18 labelled peptide RPs. Eur J Nucl Med 28: 929–38.

Ouyang, Y.B., C.M. Stary, G.Y. Yang and R. Giffard. 2013. microRNAs: innovative targets for cerebral ischemia and stroke. Current Drug Targets 14(1): 90–101.

Ouyang, Y.B., M.S. Creed, R.E. White and R.G. Giffard. 2015. The use of microRNAs to modulate redox and immune response to stroke. Antioxid Redox Signal 22: 187–202.

Peeters, S.G., C.M. Zegers, N.G. Lieuwes, W. van Elmpt, J. Eriksson, G.A. van Dongen, L. Dubois and P. Lambin. 2015. A comparative study of the hypoxia PET tracers [^{18}F]HX4, [^{18}F]FAZA, and [^{18}F]FMISO in a preclinical tumor model. Int J Radiat Oncol Biol Phys 91: 351–359.

Prajapati, P., L. Sripada, K. Singh, K. Bhatelia, R. Singh and R. Singh. 2015. TNF-α regulates miRNA targeting mitochondrial complex-I and induces cell death in dopaminergic cells. Biochimica et Biophysica Acta 1852: 451–461.

Prata, M.I. 2012. Gallium-68: a new trend in PET radiopharmacy. Curr Radiopharm 5: 142–149.

Pretze, M., P. Grobe-Gehling and C. Mamat. 2011. Cross-coupling reactions as versatile tool for the preparation of PET radiotracers. Molecules 16: 1129–11263.

Ren, Q., K. Tsunaba, Y. Kitamura, R. Nakashima, A. Shibada, M. Ikeda and Y. Kitade. 2014. Synthesis of ethynylbenzene-substituted glycol as a versatile probe for labeling oligonucleotides. Bioorg Med Chem Lett 24: 1519–1522.

Rice, S.L., C.A. Roney, P. Daumar and J.S. Lewis. 2011. The next generation of positron emission tomography RPs in oncology. Semin Nucl Med 41: 265–282.

Riss, P.J., C. Burchardt and F. Roesch. 2011. A methodical ^{68}Ga-labelling study of DO2A-(butyl-L-tyrosine)2 with cation-exchanger post-processed ^{68}Ga: practical aspects of radiolabelling. Contrast Media Mol Imaging 6: 492–498.

Rosch, F. and P.J. Riss. 2010. The renaissance of the ^{68}Ge/^{68}Ga radionuclide generator initiates new developments in ^{68}Ga radiopharmaceutical chemistry. Curr Top Med Chem 10: 1633–1668.

Rösch, F. 2013. Past, present and future of ^{68}Ge/^{68}Ga generators. Appl Radiat Isot 76: 24–30.

Rostovtsev, V.V., L.G. Green, V.V. Folkin and B.K. Sharpless. 2002. A stepwise Huisgen cycloaddition process: copper(I) catalyzed regioselective "ligation" of azides and terminal alkynes. Angew Chem Int Ed 41: 2596–2599.

Sánchez-Jurado, R., M. Devis, R. Sanz, J.E. Aguilar, M. del Puig Cózar and J. Ferrer-Rebolleda. 2014. Whole-body PET/CT studies with lowered ^{18}F-FDG doses: the influence of body mass index in dose reduction. J Nucl Med Technol 42: 62–67.

Sharma, S. and M. Ebadi. 2005. Distribution kinetics of ^{18}F-DOPA in weaver mutant mice. Mol Brain Res 139: 23–30.

Sharma, S., G. Krause and M. Ebadi. 2006. Radiation safety and quality control in the cyclotron laboratory. Radiation Protection Dosimetry 118: 431–439.

Sharma, S., H.EI. Refaey and M. Ebadi. 2006. Complex-1 activity and ^{18}F-DOPA uptake in genetically engineered mouse models of Parkinson's disease and the neuroprotective role of coenzyme Q_{10}. Brain Res Bull 70: 22–30.

Sharma, S., G. Krause and M. Ebadi. 2007. Basic requirements of quality control of PET RPs. Proceedings of the International Atomic Energy Agency, Bangkok, Thailand (Extended Synopsis: IAEA-CN-157/171p, Nov 10–14).

Sharma, S. and M. Ebadi. 2008. SPECT neuroimaging in translational research of CNS disorders. Neurochemistry International 52: 352–62.

Sharma, S. and M. Ebadi. 2008. Therapeutic potential of metallothioneins in Parkinson's disease. New research in Parkinson's disease. pp. 1–41. *In*: Timothy F. Hahn and Julian Werner (eds.). New Research in Parkinson's Disease. Nova Science Publishers, Inc., USA.

Sharma, S. and M. Ebadi. 2014. *In vivo* molecular imaging in Parkinson's disease. *In*: Manuchair Ebadi and Ronald Pfiffer (eds.). Parkinson's Disease. CRC Press.

Shen, B., W. Ehrlichmann, M. Uebele, H.J. Machulla and G. Reischl. 2009. Automated synthesis of n.c.a. [^{18}F]-DOPA via nucleophilic aromatic substitution with [^{18}F]fluoride. Appl Radiat Isot 67: 51650–51653.

Shokeen, M. and C.J. Anderson. 2009. Molecular imaging of cancer with copper-64 RPs and positron emission tomography (PET). Acc Chem Res 42: 832–841.

Stary, C.M. and R.G. Giffard. 2015. Advances in Astrocyte-targeted approaches for stroke therapy: An emerging role for mitochondria and microRNAs. Neurochemical Res 40: 301–307.

Sawai, C.M., S. Babovic, S. Upadhaya, D.J.H.F. Knapp, Y. Lavin, C.M. Lau, A. Goloborodko, J. Feng, J. Fujisaki, L. Ding, L.A. Mirny, M. Merad, C.J. Eaves and B. Reizis. 2016. Hematopoietic stem cells are the major source of multilineage hematopoiesis in adult animals. Immunity 45: 597–609.

Tomasetti, M., J. Neuzil and L. Dong. 2014. microRNAs as regulators of mitochondrial function: role in cancer suppression. Biochim Biophys Acta 1840: 1441–1453.

Trivedi, M., A. Singh, M. Talekar, G. Pawar, P. Shah and M. Amiji. 2017. microRNA-34a encapsulated in hyaluronic acid nanoparticles induces epigenetic changes with altered *mitochondrial bioenergetics* and apoptosis in non-small-cell lung cancer cells. Scientific Reports 7: 3636.

Velikyan, I. 2013a. The diversity of ^{68}Ga-based imaging agents. Recent Results Cancer Res 194: 101–131.

Velikyan, I. 2013b. Prospective of ^{68}Ga-radiopharmaceutical development. Theranostics 4: 47–80.

Wadsak, W. and M. Mitterhauser. 2010. Basics and principles of RPs for PET/CT. Eur J Radiol 73: 461–469.

Wang, L., K. Tang, Q. Zhang, H. Li, Z. Wen, H. Zhang and H. Zhang. 2013. Somatostatin receptor-based molecular imaging and therapy for neuroendocrine tumors. Biomed Res Int 2013: 102819.

Win, Z., A. Al-Nahhas, D. Rubello and M.D. Gross. 2007. Somatostatin receptor PET imaging with Gallium-68 labeled peptides. Q J Nucl Med Mol Imaging 51: 244–250.

Wu, P., Y. Zhang, Y. Sun, X. Shi, F. Li and Z. Zhu. 2013. Clinical applications of ^{18}F-FDG PET/CT in monitoring anti-cancer therapies. Curr Pharm Biotechnol 14: 658–668.

Wu, X.F., P. Anbarasan, H. Neumann and M. Beller. 2010. Vom Edelmetall zum Nobelpreis: Palladiumkatalysierte Kupplungen als Schlüsselmethode in der organischen Chemie. Angew Chem 122: 9231–9234.

Wuest, F., K.E. Carlson and J.A. Katzenellenbogen. 2008a. Expeditious synthesis of steroids containing a 2-methylsulfanyl-acetyl side chain as potential glucocorticoid receptor imaging agents. Steroids 73: 69–76.

Wuest, F., T. Kniess, R. Bergmann and J. Pietzsch. 2008b. Synthesis and evaluation *in vitro* and *in vivo* of a ^{11}C-labeled cyclooxygenase-2 (COX-2) inhibitor. Bioorganic & Medicinal Chem 16: 7662–7670.

Yu, S. 2006. Review of ^{18}F-FDG synthesis and quality control. Biomed Imaging Interv J 2: e57.

CHAPTER-13

Theranostic Potential of Stem Cells from Different Biological Sources as Charnoly Body Anagonists, Charnolophagy Agonists, and Charnolosome Stabilizers

INTRODUCTION

Recently numerous types and sources of stem cells have been discovered with a potential for specific therapeutic applications depending on the natural abundance of specific biomarkers these highly specialized cells possess. Although, clinical application of iPPCs seems quite promising, risk of their tumorigenic potential is a serious concern. Hence, the theranostic potential of stem cells depends on the nature of biomarkers present in these cells.

Recently, we reported that MSCs can be derived from the bone marrow, adipose tissue, placenta, menstrual blood, cord blood, endothelial progenitor cells, peripheral blood mononuclear cells, hematopoietic stem cells, Wharton's jelly, skin cells, bursa tissue, and other sources by culturing in defined media (Sharma and Ebadi 2013). We also highlighted their therapeutic potential as CB antagonists. MSCs derived from diversified biological sources usually adhere on the surface of the culture flask within 48–72 hrs. The remaining cells can be removed and MSCs can be washed and maintained by adding fresh conditioned medium for amplification and subsequent theranostic applications. As compared to bone marrow derived MSCs, placenta-derived MSCs have several advantages of proper source, reduced immunogenicity, minimum risk of viral contamination, no ethical controversy, and thus possess a better prospect for personalized theranostic applications.

This chapter evaluates various stem cells derived from different biological sources and confers recent knowledge regarding their theranostic potential as CB antagonists, charnolophagy agonists, and CS stabilizers to accomplish DSST targeted, safe, and effective EBPT of clinical conditions where conventional treatment remains ineffective.

Theranostic Potential of Induced Pluripotent Cells. Recent developments in DNA sequencing and the advances in genome-wide association studies (GWAS) are changing the conventional concepts of our understanding of human diseases. Future studies in this direction may ultimately result in a more precise understanding of how genomic variations contribute to diseases and their effective clinical management with no or minimum adverse effects. Recently, Rossbach (2013) reported that iPSCs are now entering clinical research phases, allowing the investigation of disease pathways and the identification of new targets and potential clinical biomarkers which might have theranostic applications. The iPSCs possess all the genetic information; hence, they can be used as an experimental model of human diseases and for drug screening or discovery. The most unique feature of these highly primitive cells is that these are rich in antioxidants which scavenge free radicals to provide theranostic benefit by inhibiting CB formation, augmenting charnolophagy, and by stabilizing CS. The stem cells also facilitate CS exocytosis as a basic molecular mechanism of ICD for normal health and well-being.

By combining next generation sequencing (NGS) and GWAS, iPSCs may be used to predict adverse drug interactions and toxicity based on the induction of CB formation, charnolophagy, and CS destabilization and inhibition of its exocytosis. The emerging concepts of regenerative theranostics, iPSCs, and NGS technologies provide a powerful tool to analyze the complexity of diseases at the molecular level for better understanding of their pathophysiology. To promote the widespread use of iPSC-based approaches in drug development, it has been shown that these cells can be produced in sufficient quantity, consistency, and purity required to meet pharmaceutical standards. Particularly, combinatorial and correlative genomics, and genetic approaches have proven useful in elucidating the complexity of gene regulatory mechanisms for molecular modeling of diseases and theranostic applications. In addition, feeder-free culture of human induced pluripotent stem cells (hiPSc) is necessary to avoid adverse effects of foreign proteins. Hence, Tomizawa et al. (2013) cultured hiPS cells with combinations of activin (A), CHIR99021 (C), basic fibroblast growth factor (F), and leukemia inhibitory factor (L) under feeder-free conditions. Cultures were terminated after 12 passages or when the cell morphology changed from pluripotency (which was analyzed by estimating alkaline phosphatase (ALP) staining and immunostaining with antibodies to Oct3/4, Nanog, SSEA4, and TRA-1-60). An activin inhibitor, SB431542 (SB), was administered to observe morphology of these cells. The hiPS cells cultured with A, AC, and ACL after 12 passages were positive for ALP staining. Oct3/4 was positive in hiPS cells cultured with A, AC, and ACL. The hiPS cells were positive for Nanog when cultured with A and AC; however, Nanog signal was weaker in cells cultured with ACL, whereas, SSEA4 was positive in hiPS cells cultured with A and AC but negative in those cultured with ACL. The hiPS cells were positive for TRA-1-60 when cultured with A, AC, and ACL. At six passages, hiPS cells lost their undifferentiated morphology when cultured with A + SB, 5 passages with AC + SB, and 9 passages with ACL, suggesting that feeder-free culture of hiPS cells requires A or AC to retain pluripotency.

Theranostic Potential of Neural Progenitor Cells (NPCs). NPCs have been proposed as a therapy for CNS disorders, including NDDs and traumatic brain injuries (TBIs), however, their accessibility is a major concern. NPCs are usually derived from iPPCs. Birbrair et al. (2013) recently isolated Tuj1+ cells from skeletal muscle culture of Nestin-GFP transgenic mice; however, whether they form functional neurons in the brain remains unknown. Moreover, their isolation from non-transgenic species and identification of their ancestors remains unknown. This lacuna in the present knowledge motivated studying their role as a valuable alternative to neural progenitors. These investigators identified two pericyte subtypes, type-1 and type-2, using a double transgenic Nestin-GFP/NG2-DsRed mouse and demonstrated that Nestin-GFP+/Tuj1+ cells derived from type-2 Nestin-GFP+/NG2-DsRed+/CD146+ pericytes are localized in the skeletal muscle interstitium. These cells are bipotential as they generate either Tuj1+ cells when cultured with muscle cells or become "classical" α-SMA+ pericytes when cultured alone. In contrast, type-1 Nestin-GFP-/NG2-DsRed+/CD146+ pericytes generated α-SMA+pericytes but not Tuj1+ cells. Interestingly, type-2 pericyte derived Tuj1+ cells retained pericytic biomarkers (CD146+/PDGFRβ+/NG2+). Given the potential application of Nestin-GFP+/NG2-DsRed+/Tuj1+ cells for cell therapy, these investigators discovered NFG receptor as a surface biomarker, which is expressed specifically in these cells and can be used to identify and isolate them from mixed cell populations in non-transgenic species for theranostic applications.

Clinical Proteomic Analysis. Although there have been several technological advances in mass spectrometry in recent years, these have not resulted in similar advances in clinical proteomics. Moreover, application of proteomic biomarkers in clinical diagnosis and improvement in the disease is rare. Recently, Rodríguez-Suárez et al. (2014) discussed the issues associated with identification of specific biomarkers of clinical interest. Urine was considered as an ideal source of biomarkers, for theoretical, methodological, and practical considerations. These investigators searched for biomarkers in urine for the non-invasive assessment of diseases including urogenital tract diseases, CVDs, or appendicitis. They also discussed the importance of data validation in clinical practice and examined various examples of proteomic biomarkers discovery and their implications for the safe and effective theranostic applications.

Omic Analysis of Breast Cancer Tissue. Although significant improvements have been made in recent years in breast cancer treatment, many patients may develop metastatic complications, of which up to 70% involve bone metastasis, resulting in skeletal complications, leading to poor quality of life and early mortality. Bisphosphonates and newer bone-targeted agents have reduced the prevalence of skeletal complications, yet there is a need for the discovery of specific bio-makers for the prevention and treatment of metastatic bone disease, for the prediction of risk in individual patients, and for the evaluation of prognosis. Modern 'omic' biotechnologies have made a significant contribution in nucleic acid sequencing. In addition, mass spectrometry and metabolic profiling have made progress in genomics, transcriptomics (functional genomics), proteomics, and metabolomics of stem cell biomarkers for theranostic applications. These approaches have been applied to studies of breast cancer metastasis (particularly involving bone), with a focus on understanding how omic biotechnology may lead to therapeutic strategies and to novel biomarker discoveries with potential theranostic applications. Wood et al. (2013) recently proposed future directions of omics research, particularly micro-RNAs analyses and their role in the post-transcriptional regulation of genes, the role of cancer-stem cells, and epigenetic modifications in breast cancer metastasis involving CB molecular pathogenesis. I have proposed DSST charnolosomics along with conventional omics (genomics, proteomics, lipidomics, glycomics, matallomics) employing correlative and combinatorial bioinformatics to accomplish the targeted, safe, and effective EBPT of NDDs, CVDs, and chronic MDR malignancies with MSCs derived from different biological sources as described in this chapter.

Theranostic Potential of MSCs. Recently, MSCs generated a significant interest among researchers and clinicians due to their unique biomarkers and potential theranostic profile. MSCs are somatic cells with a dual capacity for self-renewal and differentiation, and diverse theranostic applicability, both experimentally as well as in clinical settings. These cells can be isolated from various human tissues that may differ anatomically or developmentally as described earlier. Heterogeneity due to biological origin or *in vitro* manipulation is, however, considerable and may equate to differences in qualitative and quantitative characteristics which can prove crucial for successful theranostic applications. Recently, Zhao (2013) proposed the concept of a hierarchical system which is composed of all MSCs from post-embryonic totipotent stem cells to MSC progenitors during embryonic development. MSC system is a combination of cells that are derived from different stages of embryonic development, possess differentiation potential and give rise to cells that share a similar set of biomarkers. MSCs possess following significant characteristics: (i) stem cell properties as components of tissue microenvironment and immunomodulatory functions, (ii) balancing immune responses and tissue metabolism, (iii) as a source of tissue-specific stem cells for theranostic application with high efficiency and safety, (iv) as CB antagonists and charnolophagy agonists, and (v) as CS stabilizers. By secreting growth promoting cytokines and free radical scevengers, MSCs possess great theranostic potential as intracellular detoxifiers. Moreover, MSCs improve the MB by enhancing energy (ATP)-dependent CS exocytosis.

McGuckin et al. (2013) recently reported that the increasing global birth rate, coupled with the aging population surviving into their 8th decade has increased the incidence of diseases. Particularly, brain related ischemia at birth, later in life, or during stroke, is increasing. It has been identified that reactive microglia can contribute to neuronal damage leading to compromised transplantation.

One potential treatment strategy is cellular therapy, using hMSCs, which possess immunomodulatory and cell repair properties by enhancing the MB, inhibiting CB formation, and augmenting charnolophagy during acute phase, and by stabilizing CS and its exocytosis during the chronic phase as a basic molecular mechanism of ICD for health and well-being.

Therefore, for effective therapy, basic molecular mechanisms of action of stem cells must be thoroughly understood. A multicentre international lab assessed basic molecular mechanism of action of hMSCs, their therapeutic application, and their role as reactive microglia. Modulation by hMSCs in *in vivo* and *in vitro* demonstrated that these cells decrease biomarkers of microglial activation (lower ED1 and Iba) and astrogliosis (lower GFAP) following transplantation in an Ouabain-induced brain ischemia rat model and in hippocampal cultures. The anti-inflammatory effect was CD-200 ligand-dependent with increased ligand expression by IL-4 stimulation. The hMSC transplants reduced rat microglial STAT3 gene expression and reduced activation of Y705 phosphorylated STAT3, but STAT3 in the hMSCs was increased upon grafting. The activity was dependent on heterodimerization with STAT1 activated by IL-4 and Oncostatin M, suggesting that these studies can facilitate preclinical trials with hMSC, and the involvement of non-canonical JAK-STAT signaling of un-phosphorylated STAT3 in immunomodulatory effects of hMSCs. In addition, feeder layers have been introduced to support the growth and stemness potential of cells in *in vitro* cultures. Mouse embryonic fibroblast and fibroblast cell line (SNL) was used as common feeder cells for hiPSCs cultures. Havasi et al. (2013) tested human adult bone marrow-derived MSCs as a potent feeder system. This method prevents the contamination of animal origin feeder systems. The hiPSCs transferred onto mitotically inactivated hMSCs and passaged every 5 days. The MSCs were first characterized by flow cytometry for their biomarkers and evaluation of osteogenic and adipogenic differentiation potentials. The morphology, expressions of specific pluripotency biomarkers such as SSEA-3, NANOG, and TRA-1-60, ALP activity, formation of embryoid bodies, and their differentiation potentials on SNL and MSC feeder layers were evaluated. To investigate the maintenance of pluripotency, quantitative transcriptions of some pluripotency biomarkers including OCT4, SOX2, NANOG, and REX1 were compared in the iPS clones on SNL or MSC feeders. Human iPSCs cultured on human MSCs feeder were thinner and flatter than those on the other feeder system. MSCs supported prolonged *in vitro* proliferation of hiPSCs along with maintenance of their pluripotency suggesting human iPSCs cultures for theranostic applications. Furthermore, Christodoulou et al. (2013) evaluated the proliferation kinetics and phenotypic characteristics of MSCs derived from fetal umbilical cord matrix (Wharton's jelly) and adipose tissue during prolonged *in vitro* expansion, a process necessary for obtaining cell numbers sufficient for theranostic applications. WJSC were derived with relatively high efficiency and possessed increased proliferation potential whilst sustaining the expression of specific immunophenotypic biomarkers, whereas ADSC demonstrated a reduced proliferation potential exhibiting typical signs of senescence at an early stage. By combining kinetic with phenotypic data both cell types maintained their stemness for theranostic applications.

Bone Repair by MSCs. Song et al. (2013) recently reported that rotator cuff injuries are a common clinical problem either due to overuse, or aging. Biological approaches to tendon repair that involve the use of scaffolding materials or cell-based approaches are currently being investigated. The cell-based approaches are applying multi-potent MSCs derived from bone marrow. These investigators characterized cells harvested from tissues associated with rotator cuff tendons based on an assumption that these cells would be appropriate for tendon repair. The MSCs were isolated from bursa tissue associated with rotator cuff tendons and were characterized for multilineage differentiation *in vitro* and *in vivo*. The bursa was obtained from patients undergoing rotator cuff surgery and cells were isolated using collagenase and dispase digestion and were characterized for osteoblastic, adipogenic, chondrogenic, and tenogenic differentiation. These cells exhibited MSCs characteristics as evidenced by the expression of putative cell surface biomarkers assigned to MSCs. The cells exhibited high proliferative potential and differentiated to mesenchymal lineages with high efficiency. Bursa-derived cells expressed biomarkers of tenocytes when treated with bone morphogenetic protein-12 (BMP-12) and exhibited aligned morphology in culture. Moreover, Bursa-derived cells pretreated with BMP-12 and seeded in ceramic scaffolds formed bone as well as tendon-like tissue as detected by BMP-1 immunofluorescence and collagen fibers in the tendon-like tissue. Bursa-derived cells also formed a fibro-cartilagenous tissue in the ceramic scaffolds, suggesting their theranostic potential for tendon repair.

Pancreatic Islet Transplantation. Although subcutaneous tissue has been proposed as a potential site for pancreatic islet transplantation, the microvasculature of subcutaneous tissue is poor to support transplanted islets. To overcome this limitation, Bhang et al. (2013) evaluated whether fibrin gel with human adipose-derived stem cells (hADSCs) and rat pancreatic islets could cure diabetes mellitus when transplanted into the subcutaneous space of diabetic mice. The co-transplanted islets and hADSCs exhibited normalization of the diabetic recipient's blood glucose levels. Co-treatment of fibroblast growth factor-2 (FGF2) in the fibrin gel further augmented the outcome. The hADSCs enhanced islet viability after transplantation by secreting various growth factors that could protect islets from hypoxic damage. Moreover, hADSCs maintained islet viability by recruiting new microvasculature near the transplanted islets via over-expression of VEGF. The hADSCs did not differentiate into endothelial cells but exhibited evidence of differentiation toward insulin-secreting cells. Mice receiving islet transplantation alone did not become normoglycemic suggesting that co-transplantation of fibrin gel with islets and hADSCs may enhance the islet transplant therapy in diabetes.

Theranostic Application of Placental-Derived Stem Cells. It is now known that as compared to bone marrow derived MSCs, placenta-derived MSCs have the advantages of adequate sources, low immunogenicity, minimum risk of viral contamination, no ethical controversy, and thus possess a better prospect for theranostic application. The placental tissue includes chorionic, amniotic, and decidua basalis which locate in the maternal placental surface. Recently, Han et al. (2013) investigated the biologic characteristics of placenta decidua basalis-derived MSCs. They used the short tandem repeats (STR) test to identify the cells derived from the maternal placental surface. MTT assay was performed to measure the growth rate of decidua basalis mesenchymal stem cells (DB-MSC) and flow cytometry to detect cell cycle and cell phenotype. The multipotency of DB-MSC was used to induce differentiation. For testing the immunosuppression of DB-MSC, these were co-cultured with peripheral blood mononuclear cells (PBMNC) stimulated by phytohemagglutinin (PHA) and then IFN-γ in the media was quantified by ELISA. The cells were derived from the maternal placenta by STR analysis. DB-MSC showed typical fibroblast morphology and these cells were positive for the MSC surface biomarkers including: CD90, CD73, CD105, CD44 and negative for CD45, CD11b, and CD34. DB-MSC underwent osteogenic, adipogenic and chondrogenic differentiation, and could inhibit the secretion of IFN-γ by PBMNC, suggesting that these cells possess the basic properties of MSCs, and hence could be maternal autologous MSCs for the safe and effective theranostics of immune system diseases.

Stem Cells in Corneal Tissue Engineering. Recently, Li et al. (2013) investigated the efficacy of low-temperature airlift preservation of human corneal limbal tissue for expansion and allograft kerato-limbal transplantation. Limbal tissue either was submerged or airlifted in optisol-GS medium and preserved at 4°C for 8 days. Hematoxylin and eosin, and E-cadherin staining was performed to investigate the epithelial structure and cell-cell junction. Epithelial cell differentiation and proliferation were studied using K10, K12, K14, Ki67, and p63 as biomarkers and apoptosis was detected with the TUNEL assay. The epithelial progenitor cells were evaluated by clonal culture of epithelial cells on 3T3 feeder layers. For theranostic application, kerato-limbal transplantation was performed in 3 patients with limbal stem cell deficiency, using preserved limbal tissues. Pre- and postoperative evaluations were conducted by slit-lamp microscopy and fluorescein staining. After 8 days, epithelia with structurally-intact cell-cell junctions were retained only in airlifted tissues. Airlifting maintained a normal corneal differentiation pattern, along with low proliferation and increased proliferation potential, little apoptosis, clonogenicity, and successfully reconstructed corneal and limbal surfaces in limbal stem cell-deficient patients, indicating that limbal tissues preserved under hypothermic airlift conditions maintains the intact structure, normal phenotype, and high viability. Hence, these cells may be used in eye bank tissue processing and corneal epithelial tissue engineering.

Theranostic Potential of EPCs. Bayat et al. (2013) recently described endothelial progenitor cells (EPCs) that have potential application for cell therapy; however, their biological nature is not well-understood. EPCs also possess some stemness features, such as clonogenicity and differentiation capacity. These investigators evaluated the expression of transcription factors regulating self-renewal of stem cells. The peripheral blood mononuclear cells were isolated from the fresh human blood of volunteers and were cultured in fibronectin-coated plates. EPCs were identified based on their morphology and growth characteristic. The expression of cell surface biomarkers, CD31 and CD34, and those implicated in self-renewal capacity was determined by RT-PCR and immunocytochemistry. These cells had the capability for Di-ACLDL incorporation as well as attachment to lectin-I. EPCs did not express the stem cell biomarkers, like OCT4-A, Nanog, and Sox2; however, they expressed the weaker pluripotent biomarkers, including OCT4B and OCT4-B1 spliced variants, such as Nucleostemin and ZFX. Furthermore, a decreasing pattern from days 4–11(th) was observed for Nucleostemin and ZFX genes suggesting that the main regulators of stem cell self-renewal genes, including OCT4-A, Nanog, and Sox2 are not expressed in EPCs. However, forced expression of these genes could elevate the stemness property and theranostic potential of EPCs.

Hematopoietic Stem Cell Biomarkers. The most important property of hematopoietic stem and progenitor cells (HSPCs) regarding differentiation from the self-renewing quiescent to the proliferating stage is their adhesion to the bone marrow (BM) niche. An important molecule involved in proliferation of HSPCs in the BM is the hypoxia-induced urokinase-type plasminogen activator receptor (uPAR). Nishi et al. (2013) recently reported that the soluble form (sLR11) of LR11 (also called SorLA or SORL1) modulates the uPAR-mediated attachment of HSPCs under hypoxic conditions. Immunohistochemical and mRNA expression analyses revealed that hypoxia increased LR11 expression in c-Kit(+) Lin(−) cells. In U937 cells, hypoxia induced a transient rise in LR11 transcription, production of cellular protein, and release of sLR11. Attachment to stromal cells of c-Kit(+) Lin(–) cells of lr11(–/–) mice was significantly reduced by hypoxia compared to lr11(+/+) animals. The sLR11 induced the adhesion of U937 and c-Kit(+) Lin(–) cells to stromal cells. Cell attachment was increased by sLR11 and reduced in the presence of anti-uPAR antibodies. Furthermore, the fraction of uPAR co-immunoprecipitated with LR11 in membrane extracts of U937 cells was increased by hypoxia. A chemical inducer of HIF-1α, CoCl$_2$ enhanced LR11 and sLR11 in U937 cells. The decrease in hypoxia-induced attachment of HIF-1α-knockdown cells was prevented by sLR11. Finally, hypoxia induced HIF-1α binding to a binding site in the LR11 promoter suggesting that sLR11 regulates the hypoxia-enhanced adhesion of HSPCs via an uPAR-mediated pathway that stabilizes the hematological pool size by controlling cell attachment to the BM niche. In addition, life-threatening risks associated with HLA-mismatched unrelated donor hematopoietic cell transplantation limit its application for the treatment of blood diseases. The increased risks might be explained by genetic variation within the highly polymorphic major histocompatibility complex (MHC) region. Therefore, Petersdorf et al. (2013) assessed each of the 1108 MHC region single nucleotide polymorphisms (SNPs) in 2628 patients and their HLA-mismatched donors to determine whether SNPs are associated with the risk of mortality, disease-free survival, transplant-related mortality, relapse, and acute and chronic graft-versus-host disease (GVHD). Multivariate analysis adjusted for HLA mismatching and nongenetic variables associated with each clinical endpoint. Twelve SNPs were identified as transplantation determinants. SNP-associated risks were conferred by either patient or donor SNP genotype or by patient-donor SNP mismatching.

Risks after transplantation increased with increasing numbers of unfavorable SNPs. SNPs that influenced acute GVHD were independent of those that affected risk of chronic GVHD and relapse. HLA haplotypes differed with respect to haplotype content of SNPs. Outcome after HLA-mismatched unrelated donor transplantation was influenced by MHC region variation that is undetected with conventional HLA typing. Hence, knowledge of the SNP content of HLA haplotypes can estimate risks prior to transplantation and to lower complications through proper selection of donors with favorable MHC genetics. Paroxysmal nocturnal hemoglobinuria (PNH) is a disorder caused by a PIG-A gene mutation in a stem cell clone. Its clinical picture can make challenging the distinction from other disorders, and especially from myelodysplastic syndromes (MDS), since both diseases correlate with cytopenias and morphological abnormalities of bone marrow (BM) cells. Recently, flow cytometry (FC) has been proposed to integrate the morphologic assessment of BM dysplasia to improve the theranostics of MDS. Mannelli et al. (2013) analyzed FC data of BM cells from patients with PNH and MDS. These data demonstrated abnormalities in PNH beyond the deficiency of glycosylphosphatidylinositol-linked proteins and the application of a systematic approach allowed the researchers to effectively separate MDS and PNH in a cluster analysis and to highlight disease-specific abnormalities. Indeed, the parallel evaluation of some key parameters, that is, patterns of expression of CD45 and CD10, provided information with theranostic usefulness and distinction between PNH and MDS. Moreover, the hypo-expression of CD36 that was observed on monocytes might be related to the thrombotic tendency in PNH. Thus, these investigators explored the phenotypic profile of BM cells from patients with PNH and provided useful antigenic patterns to resolve between PNH and MDS, sometimes morphologically overlapping. Furthermore, T cell precursors are an attractive target for adoptive immunotherapy. Hence, Liu et al. (2013) examined the regulation of early T lymphopoiesis by human bone marrow stromal cells to explore *in vitro* manipulation of T cell precursors in a coculture system. The generation of CD7(+)CD56(−)cy CD3(−) proT cells from hematopoietic progenitors on telomerized bone marrow stromal cells was enhanced by stem cell factor, flt3 ligand, and thrombopoietin, but these stimulatory effects were suppressed by IL-3. Expression of Notch ligands Delta-1 and -4 on stromal cells promoted T cell differentiation into the CD7(+)cyCD3(+) pre-T cell stage, while cell growth was inhibited. By combining these coculture systems, these investigators found that initial coculture with telomerized stromal cells in the presence of stem cell factor, flt3 ligand, and thrombopoietin, followed by coculture on delta-1 and -4-coexpressing stromal cells led to a higher percentage and number of pre-T cells. Adoptive immunotherapy using peripheral blood T cells transduced with a tumor antigen-specific T cell receptor (TCR) is a promising strategy but has several limitations, such as the risk of forming a chimeric TCR with the endogenous TCR. They demonstrated that incubation of TCR-transduced hematopoietic progenitors with the combination of coculture systems gave rise to CD7(+)TCR(+)CD3(+)CD1a(−) T cell precursors that proliferated and differentiated to induce mature T cells. These data demonstrated the regulatory mechanism of early T lymphopoiesis on human stromal cells and the potential utility of human stromal cells to manipulate early T cell development for theranostic application.

Bone marrow (BM) or hematopoietic stem cell (HSC) transplantation is currently used as a therapy for hematologic malignancies. Incorporation of gene therapy to drive tolerogenic expression of antigens is a promising strategy to overcome the limited long-term efficacy of autologous HSC transplantation for autoimmune diseases. HSC engraftment and tolerance induction are accomplished after myeloablative or immune-depleting conditioning regardless of the cellular compartment in which antigen is expressed. However, it remains to be resolved whether the efficiency of engraftment and tolerance induction is influenced by targeting antigen to specific cellular compartments. This is particularly important when using low-intensity conditioning aimed at preserving infectious immunity. In this situation immunologic memory exists to the autoantigen to be expressed. Coleman et al. (2013) demonstrated that under immune-preserving conditions, confining expression of a transgenically-expressed antigen to dendritic cells permits stable, long-term engraftment of genetically modified BM even when recipients are immune to the expressed antigen. In contrast, broader expression within the hematopoietic compartment leads to graft rejection and therapeutic failure because of antigen expression in HSCs. These findings are relevant to the theranostic application of genetically engineered HSCs and provide evidence that proper selection of promoters for HSC-mediated gene therapy is important, particularly where tolerance is sought under immune-preserving conditions.

Recently, Ji et al. (2013) evaluated the effect of membrane functionalization with a chemotactic factor on cell recruitment and bone formation to develop a bioactive membrane for guided bone regeneration (GBR) applications. GBR membranes were prepared by electrospinning using poly(ε-caprolactone) (PCL) blended with type B-gelatin and functionalized with stromal cell derived factor-1α (SDF-1α) via physical adsorption. These membranes were evaluated *in vitro* for SDF-1α release and chemotactic effect on BMSCs. Subsequently, *in vivo* BMSCs recruitment and bone regeneration in response to SDF-1α loaded PCL/gelatin electrospun membranes were assessed in rat cranial defects. PCL/gelatin electrospun membranes provided a diffusion-controlled SDF-1α release profile. Furthermore, the membranes loaded with different amounts of SDF-1α (50–400 ng) induced chemotactic migration of BMSCs. Eight weeks after implantation in rat cranial defects, SDF-1α-loaded membranes yielded a 6-fold increase in the amount of bone formation compared to the bare membranes. However, contribution of *in vivo* BMSCs recruitment to the bone regeneration could not be ascertained indicating the potential for using SDF-1α loaded PCL/gelatin electrospun membrane as beneficial for optimizing theranostic application of GBR strategies.

Donor T cells directed at hematopoietic system-specific minor histocompatibility antigens (mHags) are currently considered important cellular tools to induce therapeutic graft-versus-tumor (GvT) effects with low risk of graft-versus-host disease after allogeneic stem cell transplantation. Oostvogels et al. (2103) described novel mHag UTA2-1 with ideal characteristics. These investigators identified this antigen using genome-wide zygosity-genotype correlation analysis of a mHag-specific CD8(+) cytotoxic T lymphocyte (CTL) clone derived from a multiple myeloma patient who achieved a long-lasting complete remission after donor lymphocyte infusion from human leukocyte antigen (HLA)-matched sibling. UTA2-1 is a polymorphic peptide presented by the common HLA molecule HLA-A*02:01, which is encoded by the bi-allelic hematopoietic-specific gene C12orf35. Tetramer analyses demonstrated an expansion of UTA2-1-directed T cells in patient blood samples after several donor T-cell infusions that mediated clinical GvT responses. Particularly, UTA2-1-specific CTL lysed mHag (+) hematopoietic cells, including patient myeloma cells, without affecting non-hematopoietic cells. Thus, with the capacity to induce relevant immunotherapeutic CTLs, its HLA-A*02 restriction and balanced phenotype frequency, UTA2-1 is a highly valuable mHag to facilitate theranostic application of mHag-based immunotherapy.

Theranostic Potential of Adipose-Derived Stromal Cells Biomarkers. Cell-based therapies are required to meet the critical care needs of pediatrics and healthy aging in long-lived human population. The repair of compromised tissue by supporting autologous regeneration is a life changing objective uniting the fields of medical science and engineering. Human adipose-derived stromal cells (hASCs) are promising for bone tissue engineering. However, before the clinical application of hASCs for the treatment of bone defects, important questions need to be addressed, including whether pre-osteoinduction (OI) and flow cytometric purification are important steps for *in vivo* bone formation by hASCs. Liu et al. (2013) purified hASCs by flow cytometric cell sorting (FCCS). The osteogenic capabilities of hASCs and purified hASCs with or without pre-osteo-induction were examined through *in vitro* and *in vivo* experiments. Pre-OI enhanced the *in vitro* osteogenic potential of hASCs. However, there were no significant differences between hASCs and hASCs that had undergone OI (hASCs+OI) or between purified hASCs and purified hASCs+OI after 8 weeks *in vivo* implantation. Purified hASCs had an osteogenic potential as unpurified hASCs *in vitro* and *in vivo* suggesting that FCCS and *in vitro* pre-OI are not required for *in vivo* bone formation by hASCs. Furthermore, adipose tissue-derived MSCs (AT-MSCs) are an alternative for theranostic application due to their minimally invasive accessibility and availability in the body. However, the hepatic differentiation efficiency of AT-MSCs is insufficient for theranostic application and the role of extra-hepatic stem cells in liver regeneration is yet to be established. In a study, Sun et al. (2013) investigated the effects of serum from rats subjected to 70% partial hepatectomy (PH) on the differentiation ability of rat AT-MSCs *in vitro* and explored the role of AT-MSCs *in vivo* following PH injury. Cells treated with serum 24 hrs after 70% PH differentiated into hepatocyte-like cells, resembled hepatocyte-like cells with round or polygonal shape, expressed specific biomarkers including α-fetoprotein, secreted albumin, synthesized urea, and acquired CYP3A4 enzyme activity, and upregulated the expression of IL-6 and hepatocyte growth factor (HGF) *in vitro* however, the differentiation efficiency was extremely low. AT-MSC transplantation after 70% PH ameliorated liver injury and promoted liver regeneration but did not increase the serum levels of IL-6 and HGF *in vivo* suggesting that the theranostic efficacy of AT-MSCs *in vivo* after 24 hrs of 70% PH does not increase IL-6 and HGF expression.

It is being realized that adipose stem cells (adSCs) are promising candidates in cell-based therapy due to their plasticity and existence in numerous tissues. Adipose tissue contains a relatively high concentration of stem cells and is easily isolated by a minimally-invasive clinical intervention, such as liposuction. Recently, Bryan et al. (2013) utilized primary rat adipose to validate a strategy for selecting adult stem cells. They explored the use of large, very dense cell-specific antibody loaded isolation beads which overcome the problem of endocytosis and proved to be very effective in cell isolation from minimally processed primary tissue. The technique also benefited from pH mediated release, which enabled the elution of captured cells using a simple pH shift. Large beads captured and released adSCs from rat adipose, were characterized using microscopy, flow cytometry, and PCR. The purified cell population retains minimal artifact facilitating autologous reperfusion or application in *in vitro* models. This approach can be applied to isolate any cell population for which there is a characterized surface antigen. Human ASCs are currently a focus for bone tissue engineering applications. However, the *ex vivo* expansion of stem cells before theranostic application remains a challenge.

Fetal bovine serum (FBS) is generally used as a medium and exposes the recipient to infections and immunological reactions. Hence, de Paula et al. (2013) evaluated the osteogenic differentiation process of hASCs in poly-3-hydroxybutyrate-co-3-hydroxyvalerate (PHB-HV) scaffolds with the osteogenic medium supplemented with pooled allogeneic human serum (aHS). The hASCs grown in the presence of FBS or aHS did not show remarkable differences in morphology or immunophenotype. The PHB-HV scaffolds, developed by the freeze-drying technique, showed an adequate porous structure and mechanical performance as observed by micro-CT, SEM, and compression tests. The 3D structure was suitable for allowing cell colonization, which was revealed by SEM micrographs. Moreover, these scaffolds were not toxic to cells as revealed by 3-(4,5-dimethylthiazol-2-yl)-2,5-diphenyltetrazolium bromide (MTT) assay. The differentiation capacity of hASCs was confirmed by the reduction of the proliferation, the ALP activity, expression of osteogenic gene markers (ALP, collagen type I, Runx2, and osteocalcin), and the expression of bone biomarkers, such as osteopontin, osteocalcin, and collagen type I. The osteogenic capacity of hASCs on PHB-HV scaffolds indicated that this is adequate for cell growth and differentiation and that aHS is a promising supplement for the *in vitro* expansion of hASCs. This strategy seems to be useful and safe for theranostic application in bone tissue engineering.

During skin tumor progression, expression of the cutaneous cancer stem cell (CSC) biomarker CD34(+) is required for stem cell activation and tumor formation. The activation of protein kinase D1 (PKD1) is involved in epidermal tumor progression; however, the signals that regulate CSCs in skin carcinogenesis have not been characterized. Recently, Chiou et al. (2013) investigated the chemopreventive potential of peracetylated (–)-epigallocatechin-3-gallate (AcEGCG) on 7,12-dimethylbenz[a]-anthracene (DMBA)-initiated and 12-O-tetradecanoylphorbol-13-acetate (TPA)-promoted skin tumorigenesis in ICR mice and elucidated the possible mechanisms involved in the inhibitory action of PKD1 on CSCs. Topical application of AcEGCG before TPA treatment was more effective than EGCG in reducing DMBA/TPA-induced tumor incidence and multiplicity. AcEGCG not only inhibited the expression of p53, p21, c-Myc, cyclin B, p-CDK1, and Cdc25A but also restored the activation of extracellular signal-regulated kinase 1/2 (ERK1/2), which decreased DMBA/TPA-induced increases in tumor proliferation and mitotic index. To clarify the role of PKD1 in cell proliferation and tumorigenesis, these investigators studied the expression and activation of PKD1 in CD34(+) skin stem cells and skin tumors. PKD1 was expressed in CD34(+) cells and that pretreatment with AcEGCG inhibited PKD1 activation and CD34(+) expression. Pretreatment with AcEGCG suppressed NFκB, cAMP-responsive element-binding protein (CREB), and CCAAT-enhancer-binding protein (C/EBPs) activation by inhibiting the phosphorylation of c-Jun-N-terminal kinase 1/2, p38, and phosphatidylinositol 3-kinase (PI3K)/Akt and by attenuating downstream target gene expression, including inducible NOS, COX-2, ornithine decarboxylase and VEGF, demonstrating that AcEGCG is a CD34(+) and PKD1 inhibitor in the multistage mouse skin carcinogenesis mode, suggesting that AcEGCG could be developed into a novel chemo-preventive agent and that PKD1 may be a preventive and theranostic target for skin cancer.

Recent studies reported a relatively high failure rate for tendon-bone healing after rotator cuff repair. Several studies have investigated biologically-augmented rotator cuff repair; however, none has shown the theranostic application of synovial MSCs for such repair. Utsunomiya et al. (2013) demonstrated whether cells derived from shoulder tissues have MSCs properties and identified which tissue is the best source of the MSCs cells. Forty-two patients with a diagnosed rotator cuff tear preoperatively were enrolled in this study. Human mesenchymal tissues were obtained during surgery for rotator cuff tears from 19 donors who met the inclusion criteria and had investigable amounts of tissue. Colony-forming units, yield obtained, expandability, differentiation potential, epitope profile, and gene expression were compared among the cells from 4 shoulder tissues: synovium of the glenohumeral joint, subacromial bursa, margin of the ruptured supraspinatus tendon, and residual tendon stump on the greater tuberosity. The number of live cells from whole tissue was significantly higher in cells derived from the subacromial bursa as these cells retained their expandability even at passage 10. In adipogenesis experiments, the frequency of Oil Red O-positive colonies was higher for synovium- and subacromial bursa-derived cells than for tendon- and enthesis-derived cells. In studies of osteogenesis, the rate of von Kossa- and ALP-positive colonies was highest in these cells. The chondrogenic potential was highest in cells derived from the enthesis. For epitope profiling, 11 surface antigens were measured, and most had similar epitope profiles, irrespective of cell source indicating that the subacromial bursa is an excellent candidate for the MSCs in rotator cuff tears. Thus, synovial cells from the subacromial bursa in patients with rotator cuff tears are a superior cell source *in vitro*, suggesting that these cells may augment rotator cuff repair.

Theranostic Potential of Stem Cells in Chronic Lung Disease. Chronic lung diseases such as idiopathic pulmonary fibrosis and cystic fibrosis or COPD and asthma are leading causes of morbidity and mortality worldwide with considerable human, societal, and financial burden. In view of the current disappointing status of available pharmaceutical agents, there is an urgent need for alternative, more effective theranostic approaches that will not only help to relieve patient symptoms but will also affect the natural course of the disease. Regenerative medicine represents a promising option with successful theranostic potential in patients suffering from chronic lung diseases. Nevertheless, despite relative enthusiasm arising from experimental data, application of stem cell therapy in the clinical setting has been hampered by several safety concerns arising from the lack of knowledge on the fate of exogenously administered stem cells within a chronically injured lung as well as the mechanisms regulating the activation of resident progenitor cells. However, the data arising from few pilot investigations of the safety of stem cell treatment in chronic lung diseases seem promising. Tzouvelekis et al. (2013) summarized the current state of knowledge regarding the application of stem cell treatment in chronic lung diseases, addressed important safety and efficacy issues, and presented future challenges and perspectives. These investigators recommended large multicenter clinical trials as realistic goals to assess treatment efficacy and used biomarkers that reflect clinically inconspicuous alterations of the disease molecular phenotype. Tzuovelekis et al. (2013) reported that COPD is characterized by dramatic alterations in lung architecture associated to an exaggerated inflammatory process, alveolar epithelial cell apoptosis, endothelial dysfunction, and extracellular matrix destruction due to a protease and anti-protease imbalance. In addition, a significant inflammatory spillover into systemic circulation is responsible for a wide range of fatal morbidities. In view of the current disappointing status of available pharmaceutical agents, there is an urgent need for alternative more effective theranostic approaches that will fulfill the unmet need of modulating both local and systemic inflammation and accelerate alveolar epithelial and endothelial turnover intervening into disease natural course and not just relieving patient's symptoms. Regenerative medicine based on stem cells properties represents a promising option with successful theranostic applications in patients with COPD. Nevertheless, despite enthusiasm arising from experimental data, application of stem cell therapy in the clinical setting has been hampered by safety concerns arising from the lack of knowledge on the fate of exogenously administrated stem cells within the COPD lung as well as the mechanisms regulating activation of resident progenitor cells. The above evidence coupled with the disappointing results emerging from the first stem cell clinical trials in COPD patients underline the need for careful study design by setting goals to assess the efficacy of biomarkers that reflect clinically inconspicuous alterations of the disease molecular phenotype before rigid conclusions can be drawn. In this context, it will be highly prudent to discover novel DSST-CB, charnolophagy, and CS biomarkers for the targeted, safe, and effective EBPT of pulmonary diseases.

Cancer Stem Cells. Emerging knowledge about cancer stem cells (CSCs) is raising concerns about the need to provide a precise and complete diagnosis including the biomarker profile of a patient's CSCs. As opposed to simply treating the bulk of the tumor, a more complete diagnosis can lead to theranostic regimens designed to eradicate CSCs from a patient. The authors provided application of the mammosphere assay in the study of breast CSCs. Saadin and White (2013) described transition of the mammosphere assay from the research lab to the clinic by employing microsystems technology, which enables the integration of multiple functions into a single automated device. They projected that future clinical devices will be capable of isolating circulating metastatic cells from patient blood, enriching the dangerous CSCs, and providing a molecular profile of the CSCs, thus conferring physicians with the information to select a theranostic strategy that combats CSCs. *Ex vivo* expansion of CD34(+) cells has become significant to obtain sufficient hematopoietic stem cells for theranostic application. Among major regulators involved in *ex vivo* expansion, telomerase activity and apoptosis have been revealed to be linked to cell cycle progression. However, their exact role remains to be elucidated. Changes in telomerase activity and apoptosis in cord blood CD34(+) cells were evaluated together with specific cell population growth rate during *ex vivo* culture. CD34(+) cells isolated from human cord blood, were expanded over a 28-day period. Besides monitoring cell proliferation kinetics of the CD34(+) cells, changes in telomerase activity and apoptotic levels were investigated. Several relevant genes were quantified by qRT-PCR. Significant elevation of telomerase activity had close relationship to activation of cord blood CD34(+) cell expansion. Peak apoptotic level was accompanied by a decline in cell-specific growth rate, and apoptotic level of differentiated CD34(−) population was higher than that of the CD34(+) population. Although telomerase activity was activated during the culture, expansion of cord blood CD34(+) cells was more susceptible to apoptotic suppression when cultured *ex vivo*, suggesting that apoptosis may serve as a rate-limiting factor in controlling expansion efficiency (Ge et al. 2013). Furthermore, Scatena et al. (2013) reported the discovery and implementation of valid cancer biomarkers as one of the most challenging fields in oncology and particularly oncoproteomics. Moreover, it is generally accepted that an evaluation of cancer biomarkers from the blood could enable biomarker assessments by providing a relatively non-invasive source of representative tumor material. In this regard, circulating tumor cells (CTCs) isolated from the blood of metastatic cancer patients have significant promise. It has been demonstrated that localized and metastatic cancers may give rise to CTCs, which are detectable in the bloodstream. Despite technical difficulties, recent studies highlighted the prognostic significance of the presence and number of CTCs in the blood. Future studies are needed not only to detect CTCs but also to characterize them. Furthermore, another pathogenically significant type of cancer cells, known as cancer stem cells (CSCs) or more recently termed as circulating tumor stem cells (CTSCs), might have a significant role as a subpopulation of CTCs.

Recently, I proposed the involvement of cancer stem cell-specific CS (CSscs) in MDR malignancies. The CSscs is derived from the cancer stem cells and is relatively more stable as compared to a CS derived from wild type cells. The CSscs is exocytosed from the CSCs and is endocytosed in the neighboring or distant cells to induce malignant transformation in normal nonproliferating cells. Hence, therapeutic drugs should be targeted to specifically inhibit CSscs formation during the acute phase of malignant transformation, and/or inhibit CSscs exocytosis from the CSCs, or prevent their endocytosis in the neighboring or distant nonproliferating normal cells to prevent invasive maliganacy of MDR tumors during chronic phase (Sharma 2017).

Theranostic Potential of Stem Cells from Birth-Associated Tissues. Recently, Bongso and Fong (2013) reported that MSCs from bone marrow, adult organs, and fetuses have the disadvantages of invasive isolation, limited cell numbers, ethical constraints, while embryonic stem cells (ESCs) and iPSCs have the clinical hurdles of potential immunorejection and tumorigenesis, respectively. These challenges prompted interest in the evaluation of stem cells from birth-associated tissues. Hematopoietic stem cells (HSCs) harvested from cord blood have been successfully used for the treatment of hematopoietic diseases. Stem cell populations have also been reported in other compartments of the UC viz., amnion, subamnion, perivascular region, Wharton's jelly, umbilical blood vessel adventia, and endothelium. Differences in stemness between compartments have been reported and hence, protocols using whole UC pieces containing all compartments yield mixed stem cell populations with varied characteristics. Stem cells derived from the Wharton's jelly (hWJSCs) offers the best theranostic utility because of their unique beneficial properties. The use of these cells is non-controversial, can be harvested painlessly in abundance, with enhanced proliferative potential, possess stemness properties that last several passages *in vitro*, are multipotent and hypoimmunogenic, and do not induce tumorigenesis even though they have some ESC biomarkers. The hWJSCs and their extracts also possess anti-carcinogenic properties and support HSC expansion *ex vivo*. Thus, these cells are highly attractive autologous or allogeneic agents for the targeted, safe, and effective theranostics of malignant and non-malignant hematopoietic and non-hematopoietic diseases. These cells can be further evaluated by exploring their potential as CB inhibitors, MB and charnolophagy enhancers, and CS stabilizers to further establish their DSST theranostic applications in chronic MDR diseases.

Storage and Preservations of Stem Cells. Efficient transport of stem/progenitor cells without affecting their survival and function is extremely important in cell-based therapy. However, the current approach using liquid nitrogen for the transfer of stem cells requires a short delivery time window which is technically-challenging and financially-expensive. Chen et al. (2013) used semipermeable alginate hydrogels (crosslinked by strontium) to encapsulate, store, and release stem cells, to replace the conventional cryopreservation method for the transport of therapeutic cells within a global distribution time frame. Human hMSCs and mouse embryonic stem cells (mESCs) could be successfully stored inside alginate hydrogels for 5 days under ambient conditions in an air-tight sealed cryovial. The cells extracted from alginate gel, provided 74% (mESC) and 80% (hMSC) survival rates, which compared favorably to cryopreservation. The subsequent proliferation rate and detection of common stem cell biomarkers (both in mRNA and protein level) from hMSCs and mESCs retrieved from alginate hydrogels were also comparable to results gained following cryopreservation suggesting that alginate hydrogel encapsulation may offer an economical alternative to cryopreservation for the transport and storage of stem cells for both clinical and research applications.

Tumor reversion is the biological process by which highly tumorigenic cells lose their malignant phenotype. The purpose of this research was to understand the molecular program of tumor reversion and its clinical application. Amson et al. (2013) first established biological models of reversion by deriving revertant cells from different tumors. Secondly, the molecular program that could override the malignant phenotype was assessed. Differential gene-expression profiling showed that at least 300 genes are implicated in this reversion process such as SIAH-1, PS1, TSAP6, and, most importantly, translationally controlled tumor protein (TPT1/TCTP). Decreasing TPT1/TCTP is central in reprogramming malignant cells, including CSCs. Recent findings indicated that TPT1/TCTP regulates the P^{53}-MDM2-Numb axis. Notably, TPT1/TCTP and p^{53} are implicated in a reciprocal negative-feedback loop. TPT1/TCTP is a significant prognostic factor in breast cancer. Sertraline and thioridazine interfere with this repressive feedback by targeting directly TPT1/TCTP and inhibiting its binding to MDM2, restoring wildtype p^{53} function. Combining sertraline with classical drugs such as Ara-C in acute myeloid leukemia may be also beneficial.

Despite great progress in the fields of tissue engineering and stem cell therapy, the translational and preclinical studies are required to accelerate the clinical application of tissue engineered nerve grafts, as an alternative to autologous nerve grafts for peripheral nerve repair. Rhesus monkeys are clinically more relevant and suitable for scaling up to humans as compared to other mammalians. Based on this premise and considering a striking similarity in the anatomy and function between human and monkey hands, Hu et al. (2013) used chitosan/PLGA-based, autologous marrow MSCs-containing tissue engineered nerve grafts (TENGs) for bridging a 50-mm long median nerve defect in rhesus monkeys. At 12 months after grafting, locomotive activity, electrophysiological assessments, and FG retrograde tracing tests indicated that the recovery of nerve function by TENGs was more efficient than that by chitosan/PLGA scaffolds alone; histological and morphometric analyses of regenerated nerves confirmed that the morphological reconstruction by TENGs was close to that by autografts and superior to that by chitosan/PLGA scaffolds alone. In addition, blood test and histopathological examination demonstrated that TENGs featured by addition of autologous MSCs could be safely used in the primate body suggesting the efficacy of developed TENGs for peripheral nerve regeneration and their promising perspective for clinical applications. Furthermore, Uematsu et al. (2013) demonstrated that multilayered periosteal sheets prepared from the explant culture of alveolar periosteum serve as a promising osteogenic grafting material in periodontal tissue regeneration. For the preparation of more potent periosteal sheets, these investigators examined the applicability of stem-cell culture media. Compared to the control medium (Medium 199+10% FBS), periosteal sheets expanded with MesenPRO-RSTM medium exhibited these features: Cells grew three-dimensionally and deposited collagen in the extracellular spaces to form thicker multilayers of cells. Chondrocytic markers were not significantly up-regulated. Contractile force was generated in proportion with the increased thickness of the periosteal sheets and the formation of cytoplasmic α-smooth muscle actin fibers. However, myofibroblastic markers were not significantly up-regulated. The surface marker CD146 was up-regulated, while both CD73 and CD105 were down-regulated. A representative osteoblastic biomarker, ALP, was not up-regulated by osteogenic induction. However, these expanded periosteal sheets exhibited osteogenic differentiation when implanted in nude mice. Therefore, MesenPRO medium effectively expanded the cells contained in periosteal sheets to promote the formation of thicker multilayers of cells *in vitro*, and these enhanced periosteal sheets expressed osteogenic potential at implantation sites *in vivo*, indicating that CD146-positive cells are expanded and that CD146 is a biomarker for osteogenic progenitor cells in the bone marrow stroma, and that MesenPRO medium improves the quality of osteogenic periosteal sheets for theranostic application through the induction of CD146-positive cells.

Conclusion

Several biological sources of stem cells have been explored recently to establish their targeted, safe, and effective theranostic potential in chronic intractable diseases and in regenerative medicine. Stem cells from different biological sources may serve as potent CB antagonists, charnolophagy agonists, CS stabilizers, and boosters of the MB for ICD in health and disease. MSCs can be derived from various biological sources as described in this chapter. Quality of these cells can be evaluated by analyzing their theranostic potential as CB inhibitors, charnolophagy agonists, and CS stabilizers after their transplantation in the biological system as a function of time by analyzing DSST biomarkers. The MSCs derived from different biological sources have specific biomarkers, which can be used for their identification and characterization. Hence, MSCs biomarkers from different biological source determine their theranostic potential for a specific disease. Moreover, freezing, storing, and thawing may influence the biomarkers activity of stem cells. I have proposed CB, charnolophagy, and CS as DSST biomarkers of stem cells, which can be employed to clinically assess their theranostic potential in chronic diseases. In addition, CSscs can be used for the early identification, characterization, and clinical management of MDR malignancies by preventing CS exocytosis from the cancer stem cell and its endocytosis in the neighboring normal nonproliferating or distant cells to prevent MDR malignancies with minimum or no adverse effects. A further study in this direction will go a long way in the targeted, safe, and effective EBPT of MDR malignancies and other chronic diseases beyond the scope of this chapter.

References

Amson, R., J.E. Karp and A. Telerman. 2013. Lessons from tumor reversion for cancer treatment. Curr Opin Oncol 25: 59–65.

Bayat, H., F. Fathi, H. Peyrovi and S.J. Mowla. 2013. Evaluating the expression of self-renewal genes in human endothelial progenitor cells. Cell J 14: 298–305.

Bhang, S.H., M.J. Jung, J.Y. Shin, W.G. La, Y.H. Hwang, M.J. Kim, B.S. Kim and D.Y. Lee. 2013. Mutual effect of subcutaneously transplanted human adipose-derived stem cells and pancreatic islets within fibrin gel. Biomaterials 34: 7247–7256.

Birbrair, A., T. Zhang, Z.M. Wang, M.L. Messi, G.N. Enikolopov, A. Mintz and O. Delbono. 2013. Skeletal muscle pericyte subtypes differ in their differentiation potential. Stem Cell Res 10: 67–84.

Bongso, A. and C.Y. Fong. 2013. The therapeutic potential, challenges and future clinical directions of stem cells from the Wharton's jelly of the human umbilical cord. Stem Cell Rev 9: 226–240.

Bryan, N., F.C. Lewis, D. Bond, C. Stanley and J.A. Hunt. 2013. Evaluation of a novel non-destructive catch and release technology for harvesting autologous adult stem cells. PLoS ONE 8(1): e53933.

Chen, B., B. Wright, R. Sahoo and C.J. Connon. 2013. A novel alternative to cryopreservation for the short-term storage of stem cells for use in cell therapy using alginate encapsulation. Tissue Eng Part C Methods 19(7): 568–576.

Chiou, Y.S., S. Sang, K.H. Cheng, C.T. Ho, Y.J. Wang and M.H. Pan. 2013. Peracetylated (–)-epigallocatechin-3-gallate (AcEGCG) potently prevents skin carcinogenesis by suppressing the PKD1-dependent signaling pathway in CD34+ skin stem cells and skin tumors. Carcinogenesis 34: 1315–1322.

Christodoulou, I., F.N. Kolisis, D. Papaevangeliou and V. Zoumpourlis. 2013. Comparative evaluation of human mesenchymal stem cells of fetal (Wharton's Jelly) and adult (Adipose Tissue) origin during prolonged *in vitro* expansion: Considerations for cytotherapy. Stem Cells Int 2013: 246134.

Coleman, M.A., J.A. Bridge, S.W. Lane, C.M. Dixon, G.R. Hill, J.W. Wells, R. Thomas and R.J. Steptoe. 2013. Tolerance induction with gene-modified stem cells and immune-preserving conditioning in primed mice: restricting antigen to differentiated antigen-presenting cells permits efficacy. Blood 121(6): 1049–1058.

de Paula, A.C. et al. 2013. Human serum is a suitable supplement for the osteogenic differentiation of human adipose-derived stem cells seeded on poly-3-hydroxibutyrate-co-3-hydroxyvalerate scaffolds. Tissue Eng Part A.

Han, Z.B., Y.W. Wang, T. Wang, Y. Chi, Z.X. Yang, Y.R. Ji, L. Meng, P. Yang and Z.C. Han. 2013. Isolation and biological characteristics of mesenchymal stem cells derived from human placentadecidua basalis. Zhongguo Shi Yan Xue Ye Xue Za Zhi 21: 754–759.

Havasi, P., M. Nabioni, M. Soleimani, B. Bakhshandeh and K. Parivar. 2013. Mesenchymal stem cells as an appropriate feeder layer for prolonged *in vitro* culture of human induced pluripotent stem cells. Mol Biol Rep 40: 3023–3031.

Hu, N., H. Wu, C. Xue, Y. Gong, J. Wu, Z. Xiao, Y. Yang, F. Ding and X. Gu. 2013. Long-term outcome of the repair of 50 mm long median nerve defects in rhesus monkeys with marrow mesenchymal stem cells-containing, chitosan-based tissue engineered nerve grafts. Biomaterials 34: 100–111.

Katayoon, S. and M. Ian. 2013. White breast cancer stem cell enrichment and isolation by mammosphere culture and its potential diagnostic applications. Theme: Emerging Molecular Diagnostic Technologies pp. 49–60.

Li, C., N. Dong, H. Wu, F. Dong, Y. Xu, H. Du, H. He, Z. Liu and W. Li. 2013. A novel method for preservation of human corneal limbal tissue. Invest Ophthalmol Vis Sci 54: 4041–4047.

Liu, Y., Y. Zhao, X. Zhang, T. Chen, X. Zhao et al. 2013. Flow cytometric cell sorting and *in vitro* pre-osteoinduction are not requirements for *in vivo* bone formation by human adipose-derived stromal cells. PLoS ONE 8(2): e56002.

Mannelli, F., S. Bencini, B. Peruzzi, I. Cutini, A. Sanna, M. Benelli, A. Magi, G. Gianfaldoni, G. Rotunno, V. Carrai, A.M. Gelli, V. Valle, V. Santini, R. Notaro, L. Luzzatto and A. Bosi. 2013. A systematic analysis of bone marrow cells by flow cytometry defines a specific phenotypic profile beyond GPI deficiency in paroxysmal nocturnal hemoglobinuria. Cytometry B Clin Cytom 84(2): 71–81.

McGuckin, C.P., M. Jurga, A.M. Miller, A. Sarnowska, M. Wiedner, N.T. Boyle, M.A. Lynch, A. Jablonska, K. Drela, B. Lukomska, K. Domanska-Janik, L. Kenner, R. Moriggl, O. Degoul, C. Perruisseau-Carrier and N. Forraz. 2013. Ischemic brain injury: a consortium analysis of key factors involved in mesenchymal stem cell-mediated inflammatory reduction. Arch Biochem Biophys 534: 88–97.

Nishi, M., Y. Sakai, H. Akutsu, Y. Nagashima, G. Quinn, S. Masui et al. 2013. Induction of cells with cancer stem cell properties from nontumorigenic human mammary epithelial cells by defined reprogramming factors. Oncogene 10.1038/onc.2012.614.

Oostvogels, R., M.C. Minnema, M. van Elk, R.M. Spaapen, G.D. te Raa, B. Giovannone, A. Buijs, D. van Baarle, A.P. Kater, M. Griffioen, E. Spierings, H.M. Lokhorst and T. Mutis. 2013. Towards effective and safe immunotherapy after allogeneic stem cell transplantation: identification of hematopoietic-specific minor histocompatibility antigen UTA2-1. Leukemia 27(3): 642–649.

Petersdorf, E.W., M. Malkki, M.M. Horowitz, S.R. Spellman, M.D. Haagenson and T. Wang. 2013. Mapping MHC haplotype effects in unrelated donor hematopoietic cell transplantation. Blood 121(10): 1896–1905.

Rodríguez-Suárez, E., J. Siwy, P. Zürbig and H. Mischak. 2014. Urine as a source for clinical proteome analysis: from discovery to clinical application. Biochim Biophys Acta 1844: 884–898.

Rossbach, M. 2013. A comment on pluripotent stem cells in next-generation biomedical theranostics. Curr Mol Med 13: 879–883.

Saadin, K. and I.M. White. 2013. Breast cancer stem cell enrichment and isolation by mammosphere culture and its potential diagnostic applications. Expert Rev Mol Diagn Jan 13(1): 49–60.

Scatena et al. 2013. Effects of telomkerase activity and apoptosis on *ex vivo* expansion of cord blood CD34+ cells. Cell Prolif 46: 38–44.

Sharma, S. and M. Ebadi. 2013. Antioxidant Targeting in Neurodegenerative Disorders. Ed. I. Laher, Springer Verlag. Germany. Chapter 85, pp. 1–30.

Sharma, S. 2013. Fetal Alcohol Spectrum Disorders. Nova Science Publishers, New York. U.S.A.

Sharma, S. 2017. Fetal Alcohol Spectrum Disorders: Concepts, Mechanisms, and Clinical Management. Nova Science Publishers, New York, U.S.A.

Song, N., A.D. Armstrong, F. Li, H. Ouyang and C. Niyibizi. 2014. Multipotent mesenchymal stem cells from human subacromial bursa: potential for cell based tendon tissue engineering. Tissue Eng Part A 20: 239–249.

Sun, J., Y. Yufeng, Q. Haiquan, Y. Chengching, L. Weijun, Z. Jin, H. Yueming and L. Zhisu. 2013. Serum from hepatectomized rats induces the differentiation of adipose tissue mesenchymal stem cells into hepatocyte-like cells and upregulates the expression of hepatocyte growth factor and interleukin-6 *in vitro*. International Journal of Molecular Medicine 31: 667–675.

Tomizawa, M., F. Shinozaki, T. Sugiyama, S. Yamamoto, M. Sueishi and T. Yoshida. 2013. Activin A is essential for feeder-free culture of human induced pluripotent stem cells. J Cell Biochem 114: 584–588.

Tzouvelekis, A. et al. 2013. Respiration. Stem cell treatment for chronic lung diseases. Respiration 85: 179–192.

Uematsu, K., T. Kawase, M. Nagata, K. Suzuki, K. Okuda, H. Yoshie, D.M. Burns and R. Takagi. 2013. Tissue culture of human alveolar periosteal sheets using a stem-cell culture medium (MesenPRO-RS™): *In vitro* expansion of CD146-positive cells and concomitant upregulation of osteogenic potential *in vivo*. Stem Cell Res 10: 1–19.

Utsunomiya, H., U. Soshi and S. Ichiro. 2013. Isolation and characterization of human mesenchymal stem cells derived from shoulder tissues involved in rotator cuff tears. American J Sports Medicine 41.

Wood, S.L., J.A. Westbrook and J.E. Brown. 2014. Omic-profiling in breast cancer metastasis to bone: Implications for mechanisms, biomarkers and treatment. Cancer Treatment Reviews 40: 139–152.

Zhao, CH. 2013. Concept of mesenchymal stem cells: bring more insights into functional research of MSC. Zhongguo Shi Yan Xue Ye Xue Za Zhi 21: 263–267.

CHAPTER-14

Charnolopharmacotherapeutics of Chronic Multidrug Resistant Diseases by Metallothionein-induced Hypoxia Inducible Factor-1

INTRODUCTION

Recently, HIF-1α has proved beneficial for the clinical management of chronic kidney failure-induced anemia as it is involved in the induction of erythropoietin gene. HIF-1α-induced activation of erythropoietin gene at the transcriptional level is involved in the synthesis of erythropoietin, required for RBCs synthesis and alleviation of chronic kidney failure-induced anemia.

Recently, we reported that the drugs which prevent CB formation, enhance charnolophagy, and stabilize and exocytose CS; are classified as charnolopharmacotherapeutics. We also reported that MTs prevent CB formation as potent free radical scavengers. Hence, any physiological and/or pharmacological intervention to enhance MTs-induced HIF-1α will be clinically-significant MB-based CB-targeted charnolopharmacotherapeutics, as described in this chapter.

MT-1G: A Regulator of Ferroptosis in HCC Cells. Recently, Sun et al. (2016) reported that hepatocellular carcinoma (HCC) is a major cause of cancer-related death worldwide and is responsible for the increased incidence of all cancers. Sorafenib is an inhibitor of multiple oncogenic kinases and is the only approved drug for advanced HCC. However, acquired resistance to sorafenib is noticed in HCC patients, which results in poor prognosis. These investigators emphasized that MT-1G is a transcriptional regulator and promising therapeutic target of sorafenib resistance in human HCC cells. The expression of MT-1G mRNA and protein was induced by sorafenib but not by other clinically-relevant kinase inhibitors (e.g., erlotinib, gefitinib, tivantinib, vemurafenib, selumetinib, imatinib, masitinib, and ponatinib). Activation of the nuclear transcription factor (erythroid 2-related factor 2), but not p^{53} and HIF-1-α, was essential for the induction of MT-1G following sorafenib treatment. Genetic and pharmacological inhibition of MT-1G enhanced the anticancer activity of sorafenib *in vitro* and in tumor xenograft models. The molecular mechanisms underlying the action of MT-1G in sorafenib resistance involved the inhibition of ferroptosis, a form of regulated cell death. Knockdown of MT-1G by RNA interference increased glutathione depletion and lipid peroxidation, which contributed to sorafenib-induced ferroptosis. These data suggested that MT-1G is a regulator of ferroptosis in HCC cells as it inhibits CB formation and stabilizes CS to render cancer cells resistant to chemotherapy.

[Zn²⁺]ᵢ Overload and Neurological Disorders. It has been shown that $[Zn^{2+}]_i$ overload causes neuronal injury in NDDs, whereas mild levels of Zn^{2+} are beneficial to neurons. Previous reports indicated that NSAIDs, including indomethacin and aspirin, can reduce the risk of ischemic stroke. Recently, Lee et al. (2015) demonstrated that chronic pretreatment of rats with indomethacin, a non-selective Cox inhibitor, provides tolerance to ischemic injuries in an animal model of stroke by inducing moderate Zn^{2+} elevation in neurons. Consecutive injection of indomethacin (3 mg/kg/day for 28 days, i.p.) led to modest increases in intraneuronal Zn^{2+} as well as synaptic Zn^{2+} content, with no evidence of neuronal demise. Furthermore, indomethacin induced $[Zn^{2+}]_i$ homeostatic and neuroprotective proteins, rendering the brain resistant against ischemic damages and improving neurological outcomes. However, administration of a Zn^{2+}-chelator, N,N,N',N'-tetra(2-picolyl)ethylenediamine (TPEN; 15 mg/kg/day), after indomethacin administration eliminated the beneficial effects of the drug, indicating that indomethacin preconditioning can modulate intracellular Zn^{2+} availability, contributing to ischemic tolerance in the brain after stroke.

Zn²⁺ Chelating Strategies to Treat NDDs. Although, it is well-established that $[Ca^{2+}]_i$ overload is a crucial event in glutamate excitotoxicity associated neurodegeneration, the basic molecular mechanism in hypobaric hypoxia mediated neuronal damage remains enigmatic. Recently, Zn^{2+} accumulation and its neurotoxic role like Ca^{2+} was proposed. Malairaman et al. (2014) highlighted that free chelatable Zn^{2+} released during hypobaric hypoxia mediates neuronal damage and memory impairment. However, the role of free Zn^{2+} in such neuropathological condition has not been elucidated. These investigators evaluated the underlying role of free chelatable Zn^{2+} in hypobaric hypoxia-induced neuronal inflammation and apoptosis resulting in hippocampal damage. Adult male Balb/c mice were exposed to hypobaric hypoxia and treated with saline or Ca2EDTA (1.25 mM/kg i.p.) daily for 4 days. The effects of Ca2EDTA on apoptosis (caspases activity and DNA fragmentation), pro-inflammatory markers (iNOS, TNF-α and COX-2), NADPH oxidase activity, PARP activity and expressions of Bax, Bcl-2, HIF-1α, MT-3, ZnT-1 and ZIP-6 were examined in the hippocampus. Hypobaric hypoxia induced increased expression of MT-3 and Zn^{2+} transporters (ZnT-1 and ZIP-6). Hypobaric hypoxia elicited an oxidative stress and inflammatory response characterized by elevated NADPH oxidase activity and up-regulation of iNOS, COX-2, and TNF-α. Furthermore, hypobaric hypoxia induced HIF-1α protein expression, PARP activation, and apoptosis. Administration of Ca2EDTA attenuated hypobaric hypoxia induced oxidative stress, inflammation, and apoptosis. Based on these studies, these investigators proposed that hypobaric hypoxia/reperfusion instigates free chelatable Zn^{2+} imbalance in the brain associated with neuroinflammation and apoptosis. Hence, chelating strategies which inhibit Zn^{2+} mediated neuronal damage linked with cerebral hypoxia and other neurodegenerative conditions may be developed in future.

MTs in ROS Detoxification in Aquatic Animals. Aquatic animals encounter variation in O_2 tension that leads to the accumulation of ROS that can harm these organisms. Under these circumstances, some organisms have evolved to tolerate hypoxia. In mammals, MTs protect against hypoxia-generated ROS. Felix-Portillo et al. (2014) reported MT gene from the shrimp Litopenaeus vannamei (LvMT). The gene, LvMT is differentially expressed in hemocytes, intestine, gills, pleopods, heart, hepatopancreas and muscle, with the highest levels in hepatopancreas and heart. LvMT mRNA increased during hypoxia in hepatopancreas and gills after 3 hrs at 1.5 mg L(–1) dissolved oxygen. This gene structure resembled the homologs from invertebrates and vertebrates possessing 3 exons, 2 introns, and response elements for metal response transcription factor 1 (MTF-1), hypoxia-inducible factor 1 (HIF-1) and p^{53} in the promoter region. Based on this study, these investigators suggested that during hypoxia, HIF-1/MTF-1 induce MTs to develop tolerance to ROS toxicity. Hence, MTs in aquatic organisms may also include ROS-detoxifying processes.

Hypoxia, MTs, and HIF-1α Expression. To study the relationship between hypoxia and MTs expression in bladder biopsies of interstitial cystitis/painful bladder syndrome patients, Lee et al. (2014) conducted a study on 41 patients with interstitial cystitis/painful bladder syndrome, and the control group consisting of 12 volunteers without any interstitial cystitis/painful bladder syndrome symptoms. All biopsy specimens were analyzed for both proteins of HIF-1α and MTs expression by immunoblotting, immunostaining, and confocal laser scanning microscopy. An increased expression of HIF-1α and MTs was observed in the study group compared with the control group. Both proteins of HIF-1α and MTs were primarily distributed over bladder urothelium as determined by immunohistochemical staining, and their co-localization was confirmed by confocal microscopy. High expression and co-localization of MTs and HIF-1α in the bladder mucosa of patients with interstitial cystitis suggested that overexpression of MTs is associated with the bladder hypoxia related to interstitial cystitis/painful bladder syndrome.

Overexpression of HIF-1α, MTs, and SLUG in Lymph Node Metastasis. It is well established that HIF-1α is upregulated by hypoxia and is involved in tumor growth and metastasis in many malignant tumors including papillary thyroid carcinoma (PTC). MTs is a group of small molecular weight cysteine-rich proteins with diversified functions. SLUG is a member of SNAIL superfamily of Zn^{2+} finger transcriptional factors implicated in epithelial-mesenchymal transition (EMT). Therefore, Wang et al. (2013) conducted a study to examine HIF-1α, MT, and SLUG expression in PTC and assessed association of their expression with clinicopathological biomarkers. HIF-1α, MT and SLUG protein in 129 PTCs, 61 nodular hyperplasia, and 118 normal thyroid tissue specimens were analyzed using immunohistochemistry. The protein expression of these three molecules were up-regulated in PTCs. High expression of

HIF-1α, MTs, and SLUG was correlated with TNM stage and lymph node metastasis (LNM). Furthermore, HIF-1α, MTs and SLUG expressions were correlated with each other. Concomitant high expression of any two of these three molecules had stronger correlation with high TNM stage for HIF-1α/MT, MT/SLUG and HIF-1α/SLUG, respectively than did each alone, and high expression of these molecules was associated with high TNM stage and LNM, indicating that HIF-1α, MTs, and SLUG in PTC may serve as useful biomarkers in predicting the risk of LNM and high TNM stage.

Cordyceps Sinensis Increases Hypoxia Tolerance by Inducing Heme Oxygenase-1 and MTs. Cordyceps sinensis, an edible mushroom growing in Himalayan regions, was recognized in traditional system of medicine. Singh et al. (2013) reported the efficacy of Cordyceps sinensis in facilitating tolerance to hypoxia using A549 cell line as an *in vitro* experimental model. Treatment with aqueous extract of Cordyceps sinensis attenuated hypoxia induced ROS generation, oxidation of lipids and proteins, and maintained antioxidant status via induction of antioxidant genes HO1 (heme oxygenase-1), MTs, and Nrf2 (nuclear factor erythroid-derived 2-like 2). In contrast, the lower level of NFκB and TNF-α might be due to higher levels of HO1, MT, and TGF-β. Further, increase in HIF-1 and its regulated genes (crythropoietin, VEGF, and Glut-1) was observed. Interestingly, Cordyceps sinensis treatment under normoxia did not regulate the expression of HIF1 and NFκB, indicating that it does not have any effect on these transcription factors. Overall, Cordyceps sinensis treatment inhibited hypoxia induced oxidative stress by maintaining higher cellular Nrf2, HIF-1, and MTs, and lowering NFκB levels, which conferred a basis for the potential therapeutic use of Cordyceps sinensis in tolerating hypoxia.

MT-3-induced VEGF Induction. Recently, Choi et al. (2013) investigated the role of the Zn^{2+}-binding protein MT3 and cellular Zn^{2+} in a mouse model of laser-induced choroidal neovascularization (CNV) using wild-type (WT) and MT3-knockout (KO) mice. Quantitative RT-PCR was used for the detection of MT3 mRNA. CNV was induced between 8 and 12 weeks of age by disrupting the Bruch's membrane using an argon laser. Fundus photography and fluorescein angiography (FA) were performed two weeks following laser photocoagulation. The possible connection between MT3 and VEGF expression was explored by quantifying VEGF levels in WT and MT3-KO mouse retinas by ELISA. The role of Zn^{2+} in VEGF expression was tested in WT and MT3-KO cells treated with pyrithione, with or without additional Zn^{2+}, using immunoblotting and fluorescence photomicrography. Following laser-treatment, MT3-KO mice exhibited significantly reduced areas of CNV compared to WT mice. In addition, retinal angiograms revealed less severe fluorescein leakage in MT3-KO mice than in WT mice. On day 14, following the induction of CNV, VEGF expression was significantly increased in WT mice, but remained unchanged in MT3-KO mice. Consistent with the possible involvement of Zn^{2+} released from MT3, elevating intracellular Zn^{2+} increased VEGF levels and induced its receptor, Flk-1, in both WT and MT3-KO retinal cells, indicating that neural retinal cells express high levels of MT3, which might play a role in CNV development. Moreover, Zn^{2+} released from MT3 may also contribute to VEGF induction.

Cadmium-induced Lung Cancer. Cd is a well-known human lung carcinogen. Person et al. (2013) developed an *in vitro* model of Cd-induced human lung carcinogenesis by chronically exposing the peripheral lung epithelia cell line, HPL-1D, to a low level of Cd. Cells were exposed to 5-μM Cd, a noncytotoxic level, and monitored for acquired cancer characteristics. By 20 weeks of Cd exposure, lung (CCT-LC) cells showed significant increases in MMP-2 activity (3.5-fold), invasion (3.4-fold), and colony formation in soft agar (2-fold). CCT-LC cells were hyperproliferative, grew in serum-free media, and overexpressed cyclin D1. The CCT-LC cells also exhibited decreased expression of the tumor suppressor genes p16 and SLC38A3 at the protein levels. Consistent with an acquired cancer cell phenotype, CCT-LC cells showed increased expression of the oncoproteins K-RAS and N-RAS as well as the epithelial-to-mesenchymal transition marker protein Vimentin. MTs expression was increased by Cd and was overexpressed in human lung cancers. The major MT isoforms, MT-1A and MT-2A, were induced in CCT-LC cells. Oxidant adaptive response genes HO-1 and HIF-1A were also induced in CCT-LC cells. Expression of the metal transport genes ZNT-1, ZNT-5, and ZIP-8 increased in CCT-LC cells, resulting in reduced Cd accumulation, suggesting adaptation to the metal, and that exposure of human lung epithelial cells to Cd causes induction of malignant transformation, which occurs despite the cell's ability to adapt to chronic Cd exposure.

Hypoxia as a Target for Tissue-Specific Gene Therapy. Recently, Rhim et al. (2013) reported that hypoxia is a hallmark of various ischemic diseases such as ischemic heart disease, ischemic limb, ischemic stroke, and solid tumors. Gene therapies for these diseases were developed with various therapeutic genes including growth factors, anti-apoptotic genes, and toxins. However, non-specific expression of these therapeutic genes may induce serious side effects in the normal tissues. To avoid the side effects, gene expression should be strictly regulated in an O_2 concentration dependent manner. The hypoxia inducible promoters and enhancers were evaluated as transcriptional regulators for hypoxia inducible gene therapy. The hypoxia inducible UTRs were also used in gene therapy for spinal cord injury as a translational regulation strategy. In addition to transcriptional and translational regulations, post-translational regulation strategies were developed using the HIF-1α ODD domain. These studies suggested that hypoxia inducible transcriptional, translational, and post-translational regulations are useful for tissue specific gene therapy of ischemic diseases.

Effect of Hypobaric Hypoxia on Oxidative Stress in Rat Heart. Recently, Singh et al. (2013) examined the effect of subchronic hypobaric hypoxia on rat hearts. These investigators exposed adult male Sprague-Dawley rats at 25,000 ft for different time periods (2 and 5 days) and evaluated the susceptibility of their hearts to mitochondrial oxidative stress as well as modulation in gene expression. Their results demonstrated a crosstalk between ROS and NO. The initial response was accompanied by increase in ROS generation and development of oxidative stress as confirmed by increased lipid peroxidation, protein oxidation, and accumulation of 2, 4-dinitrophenyl hydrazine and 4-hydroxy-2-nonenal adducts. Simultaneously, glutathione decreased; however, antioxidant enzymatic activities of SOD, glutathione-S-transferase, and glutathione peroxidase increased in response to 5-days hypoxia. Although, NO level increased till 5 days, ROS decreased after 5 days, suggesting that ROS/NO balance plays an important role in cardio-protection. This was further supported by upregulation of antioxidant genes MTs and heme-oxygenase (HO-1). In addition, hypoxia also induced upregulation of HIF-1α, which induced the expression of adaptive genes erythropoetin, VEGF, Glut-1, and NOS, suggesting a reciprocal regulation of ROS and NO and that this effect is mediated by the increase in antioxidant proteins MTs and HO-1. In addition, HIF-1-mediated induction of various cardioprotective genes plays a crucial role in acclimatization during hyperbaric hypoxia-induced oxidative stress in the rat heart.

Anti-Apoptotic Effect of Fucoxanthin on CCl$_4$-induced Hepatoxicity. In a recent study, Kaneko et al. (2013) evaluated the anti-apoptotic activity of fucoxanthin in CCl$_4$-induced hepatotoxicity. An *in vitro* study using the MTT assay demonstrated an attenuation of CCl$_4$-induced hepatotoxicity with fucoxanthin. This effect was dose-dependent; 25 μM of fucoxanthine was more effective than 10 μM in attenuating the hepatotoxicity induced by 5 mM of CCl$_4$. Acute CCl$_4$-hepatotoxicity in rats, with cells positive for the terminal deoxynucleotidyl-transferase (TdT)-mediated deoxyuridine triphosphate-digoxigenin (dUTP) nick-end labeling (TUNEL) assay were detected in the pericentral area of the hepatic lobule. Oral pretreatment of CCl$_4$-injected rats with fucoxanthin reduced hepatocyte apoptosis. Fucoxanthin increased HO-1 expression in the cultured liver cells of Hc cells and TRL1215 cells. By oral pretreatment of CCl$_4$-injected rats with fucoxanthin, the hepatic HO-1 protein levels were significantly increased compared to those not pretreated with fucoxanthin. HO-1 mRNA expression after CCl$_4$ injection was higher in the CCl$_4$+ fucoxanthin group than in the CCl$_4$ group, suggesting that fucoxanthin attenuates hepatocyte apoptosis through HO-1 induction in CCl$_4$-induced acute liver injury.

MTs-induced HIF-1 Provides Cardioprotection for the Diabetic Heart. It is well-established that MTs protect against heavy metal-induced cellular damage and may participate in other basic physiological and pathological processes, such as antioxidation, proliferation, and cell survival. Xue et al. (2012) showed that elevation of MTs by transgene or by induction with Zn^{2+} protects the heart against diabetic cardiomyopathy by mechanisms such as anti-diabetes-induced oxidative stress and inactivation of glycogen synthase kinase-3, which mediates glucose metabolism. These investigators also highlighted that MT overexpression rescues the diabetes-induced reduction of HIF-1α, which plays an important role in glucose utilization and angiogenesis and showed that overexpression of MT increased hexokinase (HK)-II expression and attenuated diabetes-induced decrease in HK-II expression. Glycolytic flux assay demonstrated that MT increased glycolysis output in high glucose-containing media-cultured H9c2 cells. The diabetes-induced reduction in cardiac capillaries was also attenuated by MT overexpression. Furthermore, MTs induction increased HIF-1 expression under both control and diabetic conditions. Moreover, MTs-enhanced HIF-1α activity occurred through a mechanism of protein nuclear translocation, suggesting that MTs induce HIF-1α expression, leading to increased HK-II in the diabetic heart. We reported that MTs, as potent free radical scavengers, provide protection as potent CB antagonists, charnolophagy agonists, and as CS stabilizers.

Increased Expression of HIF-1 and MTs in Varicocele and Vericose Vein. The increased blood stasis and venous volume pressure causing tissue hypoxia are observed in both varicocele and varicose veins. MT, a metal-binding protein, protects against apoptosis under hypoxic stress. MTs also plays an important role in collateral flow recovery and angiogenesis. Lee et al. (2012) studied the distribution of HIF-1α and MT in varicocele and varicose veins. Study specimens consisted of 1 cm venous segments and were obtained from 12 male patients during vascular stripping surgery for varicose veins and 1 cm of internal spermatic vein (ISV) obtained from 12 patients during left varicocele repair. The control samples of 1 cm ISV were obtained from 10 male patients who underwent left inguinal herniorrhaphy. In both venous diseases, the increased expression of HIF-1α and MT compared with the control group and most of the proteins distributed over smooth muscle layers were detected by IHC staining: HIF-1α and MTs in the muscle layer with co-localization, and MTs overexpression in the endothelium of venous diseases under confocal microscopy. These studies revealed the higher expression of HIF-1α and MT in varicocele and varicose veins than in the control group; MT overexpression in the muscle layer of both diseased vessels and especially located in the endothelium under confocal microscopy. As MT protects vascular cells from apoptosis under hypoxia as CB antagonists, charnolophagy agonists, and CS stabilizers, it may decrease vascular cell apoptosis and contribute to the dilated and thickened walls of varicocele and varicose veins.

Correlation of HIF-1 and MTs in Inflammatory Bowel Disease. A positive-feedback mechanism between HIF-1α and MTs was identified in different diseases. Both proteins were proposed in the pathogenesis of inflammatory bowel disease (IBD); however, their relation has not been studied in the gut. Devisscher et al. (2012) investigated the interaction between HIF-1α and MTs in colonic epithelial cells and in experimental colitis. Dimethyloxalylglycine (DMOG) was used to subject colonocytes to hydroxylase inhibition and HIF-1α stabilization in 3 experimental models (*in vitro*, *in vivo*, and *ex vivo*). Small interfering RNA targeting HIF-1α (siRNA-HIF) and MT (siRNA-MT) together with Zn^{2+}-mediated MT induction were used to study the interaction between HIF-1α and MT in HT29 cells. Acute colitis was induced in C57BL/6 mice using dextran sulphate sodium. MT expression and HIF-1α protein levels were measured by qRT-PCR and ELISA, respectively. VEGF expression was quantified as an indirect measure of HIF-1 transcriptional activity. DMOG down-regulated MT expression in HT29 cells, in freshly isolated human colonocytes, and in colonocytes isolated from mice treated with DMOG. siRNA-HIF-treated cells displayed higher MT levels and an attenuated MT down-regulation after DMOG treatment. The HIF-1α stabilization was lower in Zn^{2+}-treated control cells, displaying high MT levels, compared to siRNA-MT cells treated with DMOG. In experimental colitis, MT and VEGF mRNA expression were inversely related. MTs expression was induced in the acute phase and down-regulated during recovery. Opposing results were observed for VEGF expression. This study highlighted the inverse relation between HIF-1α and MT expression in colonocytes and during experimental colitis and suggested that the manipulation of MTs may represent a novel therapeutic strategy for patients suffering from IBD.

Hypoxia-induced Metal-Responsive Transcription Factor-1 (MTF-1). MTF-1 is essential for the induction of genes encoding MTs by metals and hypoxia. Dubé et al. (2011) studied the mechanism controlling the activation of MTF-1 by hypoxia. Hypoxia activation of MT gene transcription was dependent on the presence of metal regulatory elements (MREs) in the promoter regions of MTs genes. These investigators showed that MREa and MREd are the main elements controlling mouse MT-1 gene induction by hypoxia. Transfection experiments in MTF-1-null cells showed that MTF-1 is essential for induction by hypoxia. Chromatin immunoprecipitation showed that MTF-1 DNA-binding activity is enhanced in the presence of Zn^{2+} but not by hypoxia. HIF-1α was recruited to the MT-1 promoter in response to hypoxia but not to Zn^{2+}. MTF-1 activation was inhibited by PKC, JNK, and PI3K inhibitors and by the electron transport chain inhibitors rotenone and myxothiazol, but not by the antioxidant N-acetylcysteine. These investigators also demonstrated that prolyl-hydroxylase inhibitors can activate MTF-1, but this activation required the presence of HIF-1α. HIF-dependent transcription was enhanced in the presence of MTF-1 and the induction of the MRE promoter was stimulated by HIF-1α, indicating cooperation between these two factors. However, coimmunoprecipitation experiments did not support direct interaction between MTF-1 and HIF-1α.

Toxicological Applications of Primary Hepatocyte Cultures. Fish primary hepatocyte cultures are frequently used for toxicological assessment of contaminants. Søfteland et al. (2010) described an experiment in which they isolated intact hepatocytes from mature individuals. Hepatic CYP1A expression was evaluated by *in situ* hybridization after an i.p. injection of the potent CYP1A inducer ss-naphthoflavone (BNF). Cod hepatocytes were exposed to 1,2,3,7,8-polychlorinated dibenzo-p-dioxin (PCDD) and Cd. Transcriptional responses of 11 genes were quantified (CYP1A, MT, aryl hydrocarbon receptor 2 (AhR2), UDP-glucuronosyltransferase (UGT), glutathione S-transferase (GST), vitellogenin B (VTGB), HIF1, HO-1, transferrin, glutathione peroxidase (GPx), and HSP70). The immunohistochemisty evaluation showed elevated CYP1A mRNA expression in primary hepatocytes isolated from BNF-exposed fish. The transcriptional results showed that PCDD exposure causes a 311-fold up-regulation of CYP1A and Cd a 1.82-fold increase in MT. AhR2 and UGT mRNA levels were not significantly up-regulated in PCDD-exposed cod hepatocytes. HO-1 and transferrin demonstrated a dose-dependent transcriptional response to Cd exposure. Cd served as an endocrine-disrupting metal in primary Atlantic cod hepatocytes. This study authenticated the use of Atlantic cod primary hepatocyte cultures in toxicological research.

HIF-1 and MTs in Aggressive Colorectal Carcinoma. It is well-established that HIF-1α is a hypoxia-induced transcription factor that regulates gene expression in critical pathways involved in tumor growth and metastasis. MTs is a group of small molecular weight cysteine-rich proteins with diversified functions. Schmitz et al. (2009) analyzed the prognostic impact of HIF-1α and MT expression in colorectal cancer to evaluate a possible link of combined HIF-1α and MT expression with colorectal cancer progression. They examined the relationship of HIF-1α and MT with each other and clinicopathological parameters including proliferative activity (Ki67) and apoptosis (TUNEL). HIF-1α expression was identified as a prognostic parameter in multivariate survival analysis and characterized an aggressive cancer phenotype. In addition, HIF-1α was linked to an increased expression of MTs, suggesting that these are involved in the biological pathways induced by hypoxia in human cancer tissue.

Ischemia-induced Angiogenesis by Benzo[a]pyrene. Ichihara et al. (2009) investigated the effect of benzo[a]pyrene (B[a]P), a carcinogen of tobacco smoke and an agonist for the aryl hydrocarbon receptor (AHR), on hypoxia-induced angiogenesis. Ischemia was induced by femoral artery ligation in wild-type and AHR-null mice, and the animals were subjected to oral administration of B[a]P (125 mg/kg) once a week. Exposure to B[a]P up-regulated MTs expression in the ischemic hind limb and inhibited ischemia-induced angiogenesis in wild-type mice. The amounts of IL-6 and of VEGF mRNA in the ischemic hind limb of wild-type mice were reduced by exposure to B[a]P. These effects of B[a]P were attenuated in AHR-null mice, suggesting that the loss of the inhibitory effect of B[a]P on ischemia-induced angiogenesis in AHR-null mice may be attributable to maintenance of IL-6 expression and induction of angiogenesis through up-regulation of VEGF expression.

Hypoxic Preconditioning Facilitates Acclimatization to Hypobaric Hypoxia in Rat Heart. It is known that acute systemic hypoxia induces delayed cardioprotection against ischemia-reperfusion injury in the heart. As $CoCl_2$ is known to elicit hypoxia-like responses, it was used to mimic the preconditioning effect and facilitate acclimatization to hypobaric hypoxia in the rat heart. In this study, Singh et al. (2010) treated male Sprague-Dawley rats with distilled water or $CoCl_2$ (12.5 mg Co/kg for 7 days). The animals were exposed to simulated altitude at 7622 m for different time periods (1, 2, 3 and 5 days). Hypoxic preconditioning with Co attenuated hypobaric hypoxia-induced oxidative damage as observed by a reduction in free radical (ROS) generation, oxidation of lipids and proteins. The protective effect was due to increased expression of the antioxidant proteins HO-1 and MTs, as no significant change was observed in antioxidant enzyme activity. Hypoxic preconditioning with Co increased HIF-1α expression as well as HIF-1 DNA binding activity, which further increased expression of HIF-1-regulated genes (*Erythropoietin, VEGF, and Glut-1*). A significant decrease was observed in LDH activity and lactate levels in the heart of preconditioned animals compared with non-preconditioned animals exposed to hypoxia, suggesting that hypoxic preconditioning with Co induces acclimatization by up-regulation of *HO-1 and MT-1 via HIF-1* stabilization.

Hypoxic Preconditioning with Cobalt (Co) Attenuates Hypobaric Hypoxia-induced Oxidative Damage in Rat Lungs. It is known that hypoxic preconditioning (HPC) provides protection against injury from subsequent prolonged hypobaric hypoxia, which is a characteristic of high altitude and induces oxidative injury to the lung by increasing the generation of ROS and decreasing the effectiveness of the antioxidant defense system. Shukla et al. (2009) hypothesized that HPC with Co might protect the lung from subsequent hypobaric hypoxia-induced lung injury. HPC with Co can be achieved by oral feeding of $CoCl_2$ (12.5 mg kg(−1)) in rats for 7 days. Nonpreconditioned rats responded to hypobaric hypoxia (7619 m) by increased ROS generation and a decreased GSH/GSSG ratio. They also showed increase in lipid peroxidation, heat-shock proteins (HSP32, HSP70), MTs, levels of inflammatory cytokines (TNF-α, IFN-γ, MPC-1), and SOD, GPx, and GST enzyme activity. In contrast, rats preconditioned with Co were far less impaired by severe hypobaric hypoxia, as observed by decreased ROS generation, lipid peroxidation, and inflammatory cytokine release and an increased GSH/GSSG ratio. Increased expression of antioxidative proteins Nrf-1, HSP-32, and MT was also observed in Co-preconditioned animals. A significant increase in the protein expression and DNA binding of HIF-1α and its regulated genes, such as erythropoietin (EPO) and glut-1, was observed after HPC with Co, suggesting that it enhances antioxidant status in the lung and protects from subsequent hypobaric hypoxia-induced oxidative stress.

Cobalt Chloride-mediated Neuroprotection in Hypobaric Hypoxia-induced Oxidative Stress. Hypobaric hypoxia, characteristic of high altitude increases the formation of reactive oxygen and nitrogen species (RONS), and decrease effectiveness of antioxidant enzymes. RONS play a causative role in high altitude related ailments (i.e., pulmonary edema, chronic kidney failure). The brain is highly susceptible to hypoxic stress and is involved in physiological responses that follow. Shrivastava et al. (2008) discovered that exposure of rats to hypobaric hypoxia (7619 m) resulted in increased oxidation of lipids and proteins due to increased RONS and decreased reduced to oxidized glutathione (GSH/GSSG) ratio. A significant increase in SOD, glutathione peroxidase (GPx), and glutathione-S-transferase (GST) levels was observed. Increase in HO-1 and HSP70 was also noticed along with MT-2 and MT-3. Administration of Co attenuated the RONS generation, oxidation of lipids and proteins, and maintained GSH/GSSH ratio like that of control cells via induction of HO-1 and MT providing efficient neuroprotection. These studies indicated that Co reduces hypoxia oxidative stress by maintaining higher cellular HO-1 and MT levels via induction of HIF-1α signaling mechanisms. These findings provided a basis for the potential use of Co for the prevention of hypoxia-induced oxidative stress involving CB molecular pathogenesis.

MTs are Upregulated by Hypoxia and Stabilize the HIF in the Kidney. Earlier studies highlighted that chronic hypoxia in the tubule-interstitium is a final common pathway to progression to end-stage renal failure regardless of etiology. Kojima et al. (2009) conducted a microarray analysis of rat kidneys made hypoxic by unilateral renal artery stenosis to measure transcriptomic events and clarify pathophysiological mechanisms of renal injury induced by chronic hypoxia. Many genes were upregulated in the kidney by chronic hypoxia, but these investigators focused on MTs due to their antioxidative properties. Using tubular epithelial cells transfected with a reporter construct of luciferase, driven by the hypoxia-responsive elements (HRE), they found that the addition of MTs to the culture media increased luciferase activity. This was associated with upregulation of the target genes of HIF, such as VEGF, and Glut-1. Stimulation of the HIF-HRE pathway by MTs was confirmed by MTs-overexpression. Hypoxia and exogenous MTs increased HIF-1α protein without changes in its mRNA levels, suggesting protein stabilization. Upregulation of the HIF-HRE system by MTs was associated with phosphorylation of ERK but not Akt. In addition, MEK inhibition and rapamycin decreased MTs-induced HIF activity, suggesting that induction of MTs expression by hypoxia activates the HIF-HRE system through the ERK/mTOR pathway and may be a novel defense against hypoxia.

Cooperative Interactions Between Metal-Responsive Transcription Factor-1 and HIF-1α. Mammalian MTs genes are transcriptionally activated by the essential metal Zn^{2+} as well as by environmental stresses, including toxic metal overload and redox fluctuations. In addition to playing a key role in Zn^{2+} homeostasis, MTs can protect against metal- and oxidant-induced cellular damage and may participate in other fundamental physiologic and pathologic processes such as cell survival, proliferation, and neoplasia. In their earlier studies, Murphy et al. (2008) reported the requirement for MTF-1 in hypoxia-induced transcription of mouse MT-I and human MT-IIA genes. They provided evidence that the pro-tumorigenic HIF-1α is essential for induction of MT-1 by hypoxia, but not zinc. Chromatin immunoprecipitation assays revealed that MTF-1 and HIF-1α are both recruited to the mouse MT-I promoter in response to hypoxia, but not Zn^{2+}. In the absence of HIF-1α, MTF-1 was recruited to the MT-I promoter but failed to activate MT-1 gene expression in response to hypoxia. Thus, HIF-1α seemed to function as a coactivator of MT-1 gene transcription by interacting with MTF-1 during hypoxia. Co-immunoprecipitation studies suggested the interaction between MTF-1 and HIF-1α, either directly or as mediated by other factors. It was proposed that association of these transcription factors in a multiprotein complex represents a common strategy to control hypoxia-inducible genes in both normal and diseased tissue.

MT-3-induced HIF-1α Enhances VEGF Expression in Brain Endothelial Cells. It is well established that MT-3, a metal-binding protein, is associated with resistance to neuronal injury. However, the underlying mechanism for its effects remains unclear. Therefore, Kim et al. (2008) examined whether MT-3 can induce VEGF expression and promote neuroprotective effects in brain endothelial bEND.3 cells. MT-3 induced VEGF mRNA and protein expression in bEND.3 cells in a dose- and time-dependent manner. Furthermore, MT-3 treatment augmented the stability of HIF-1α and stimulated transcription of a reporter gene under the control of the VEGF promoter. MT-3 also increased the accumulation of HIF-1α in nuclei and increased HIF-1α-binding to the VEGF promoter. MT-3 increased PI3K/Akt and ERK1/2 phosphorylation. However, pretreatment with PD98059 and LY294002 (ERK1/2 and Akt inhibitors) inhibited MT-3-induced stimulation of HIF-1α protein expression and VEGF production, suggesting that MT-3 enhances VEGF production in brain endothelial cells by HIF-1α-dependent mechanism.

Hypoxia Pre-conditioning Genes Involved in Neuroprotection. Retinal degeneration is a main cause of blindness in humans. Neuroprotective therapies may be used to rescue retinal cells and preserve vision. Hypoxic preconditioning stabilizes the transcription factor HIF-1α in the retina and protects photoreceptors in an animal model of light-induced retinal degeneration. To address the molecular mechanisms of the protection, Thiersch et al. (2008) analyzed the transcriptome of the hypoxic retina using microarrays and real-time PCR. Hypoxic exposure induced a marked alteration in the retinal transcriptome with significantly different expression levels of 431 genes immediately after hypoxic exposure. The normal expression profile was restored within 16 hrs of reoxygenation. Among the differentially regulated genes, several candidates for neuroprotection were identified like MT-1 and -2, the HIF-1 target gene adrenomedullin, and the gene encoding the antioxidative and cytoprotective enzyme paraoxonase-1. The upregulated cyclin dependent kinase inhibitor p^{21} was excluded from being essential for neuroprotection, suggesting that neuroprotection after hypoxic preconditioning occurs due to the differential expression of several genes which may act in concert to protect visual cells against a toxic insult.

MT-3 as a Highly Hypoxia-Inducible Gene in Human Adipocytes. In a study, Wang et al. (2008) used hypoxia-signaling pathway PCR arrays to examine the response of human adipocytes to low O_2 tension. Incubation of adipocytes in 1% O_2 for 24 hrs resulted in no change in the expression of 63 of the 84 genes on the arrays, a reduction in expression of 9 genes (including uncoupling protein 2), and increased expression of 12 genes. Significant induction (> 10-fold) in leptin, angiopoietin-like protein-4, VEGF, and GLUT-1 mRNA were observed. Particularly, the expression of MT-3, was dramatically (> 600-fold) and rapidly (within 60 min) induced by hypoxia. MT-3 gene expression was also induced by hypoxia mimetics ($CoCl_2$, desferrioxamine, dimethyloxalylglycine), indicating transcriptional regulation through HIF-1 involved in CB inhibition, charnolophagy induction, and CS stabilization to augment MB and ICD for normal cellular function and homeostasis to remain healthy. Hypoxia induced MT-3 expression in preadipocytes, and MT-3 mRNA were detected in obese human subcutaneous and omental adipose tissue, suggesting that MT-3 is a hypoxia-inducible gene which may protect adipocytes from hypoxic damage.

MTs Rescue HIF-1α Transcriptional Activity in Cardiomyocytes in Diabetes. MTs are effective in the prevention of diabetic cardiomyopathy, and HIF-1 controls VEGF gene expression and regulates angiogenesis in diabetic hearts. Therefore, Feng et al. (2007) examined whether MT affects HIF-1 activity in the heart of diabetic mice and in the cardiac cells cultured in high glucose (HG) media. Diabetes was induced by streptozotocin in a cardiac-specific MT_{trans} mouse model. The primary cultures of neonatal cardiomyocytes and the embryonic rat cardiac H9c2 cell line were cultured in HG media. HIF-1 and VEGF were determined by immunofluorescent staining and ELISA, respectively. The H9c2 cells were transfected with HRE-dependent reporter plasmid and the HIF-1 transcriptional activity was measured by the luciferase reporter assay. MT overexpression increased HIF-1α in diabetic hearts. HG suppressed $CoCl_2$-induced VEGF expression in primary cultures of neonatal cardiomyocytes and MT overexpression suppressed the inhibition. The addition of MT into the cultures of H9c2 cells relieved the HG suppression of hypoxia-induced luciferase activity, indicating that MTs can rescue HIF-1 transcriptional activity in cardiomyocytes in diabetes.

A Chimeric Promoter that is Highly Responsive to Hypoxia and Metals. To develop a potent hypoxia-inducible promoter, Lee et al. (2006) evaluated the usefulness of chimeric combinations of the (Egr-1)-binding site (EBS) from the Egr-1 gene, the metal-response element (MRE) from the MTs gene, and the HRE from the phosphoglycerate kinase 1 gene. In transient transfection assays, combining 3 copies of HRE (3 × HRE) with either EBS or MRE increased hypoxia responsiveness. When a 3-enhancer combination was tested, the EBS-MRE-3 × HRE (E-M-H) gave a hypoxia induction ratio of 69. The expression induced from E-M-H-pGL3 was 2.4-fold higher than that induced from H-pGL3 and surpassed the expression from a human cytomegalovirus (CMV) promoter-driven vector. The high inducibility of E-M-H was confirmed in different cells and by expressing other cDNAs. Gel shift assays together with functional overexpression studies suggested that increased levels of HF\IF-1α, MTF-1, and Egr-1 may be associated with the high inducibility of the E-M-H chimeric promoter. E-M-H was also induced by hypoxia mimetics such as Co^{2+}, DFX, and by H_2O_2. Gene expression from the E-M-H was reversible as shown by the reduced expression of the transgene upon removal of inducers such as hypoxia and DFX. *In vivo* evaluation of the E-M-H in ischemic muscle revealed that erythropoietin secretion and luciferase and LacZ expression were higher in the E-M-H group than in a control or H group, indicating that with its high induction capacity and versatile means of modulation, this novel chimeric promoter should find wide application in the treatment of ischemic diseases and cancer.

Effect of Metal Ions on IRP-1 HIF-α Genes. Several carcinogenic metal ions affect cellular iron homeostasis by competing with iron transporters or iron-regulated enzymes. Some metal ions can mimic a hypoxia response in cells under normal oxygen tension and induce expression of HIF-1α-regulated genes. Hence, Li et al. (2006) investigated whether 12 metal ions altered iron homeostasis in human lung carcinoma A549 cells as measured by an activation of IRP-1 and ferritin level. They also studied hypoxia signaling by measuring HIF-1α protein levels, hypoxia response element (HRE)-driven luciferase reporter activity, and Cap43 protein level (an HIF-1α responsive gene). These results showed the following: (i) Ni(II), Co(II), V(V), Mn(II), and to a lesser extent As(III) and Cu(II) activated the binding of IRP-1 to IRE after 24 hrs, while the other metal ions had no effect; (ii) 10 of 12 metal ions induced HIF-1α protein but to different degrees. Two of these metal ions, Al(III) and Cd(II), did not induce HIF-1α protein; however, only Ni(II), Co(II), and to lesser extent, Mn(II) and V(V), activated HIF-1α-dependent transcription. The combined effects of both [Ni(II) + As(III)] and [Ni(II) + Cr(VI)] on HIF-1α protein were synergistic; (iii) Addition of Fe(II) with Ni(II), Co(II), and Cr(VI) attenuated the induction of HIF-1α after 4 hrs of treatment; (iv) Ni(II), Co(II), and Mn(II) decreased ferritin level after 24 hrs exposure; (v) Ni(II), Co(II), V(V), and Mn(II) activated the HRE reporter gene after 20 hrs treatment; (vi) Ni(II), Co(II), V(V), and Mn(II) increased the HIF-1-dependent Cap43 protein level after 24 hrs of treatment. Only Ni(II), Co(II), and to a lesser extent Mn(II) and V(V) stabilized HIF-1α protein, activated IRP, decreased the levels of ferritin, induced the transcription of the HIF-dependent reporter, and increased the expression of Cap43 protein levels (HIF-dependent gene). The mechanism for the stabilization and elevation of HIF-1α protein which drives these other parameters involve a loss of cellular Fe as well as inhibition of HIF-1α-dependent prolyl hydroxylases which target the binding of VHL ubiquitin ligase and degrade HIF-1α. Even though there were small effects of some of the other metals on IRP and HIF-1α, downstream effects of HIF-1α activation and hence, robust hypoxia signaling were only observed with Ni(II), Co(II), and to much lesser extents, with Mn(II) and V(V) in human A549 lung cells. The metal ions that were most effective in activating hypoxia signaling were the ones that were poor inducers of MTs and decreased ferritin levels, since both these proteins can bind metal ions and protect the cell against toxicity in human lung cells. Hence, it is highly prudent to study effects of these metals on human lung cells since this represents a major route of human environmental and occupational exposure to these metal ions.

Effects of Short-Term Cu Exposure on Gill Structure, MTs, and HIF-1α in Rainbow Trout. van Heerden et al. (2004) exposed rainbow trout (Oncorhynchus mykiss) to 1.65 μM of waterborne Cu for 24 hrs. Fish were then transferred to metal-free water. The induction of MTs mRNA in liver and gill tissue, HIF-1α accumulation in the gill tissue, and thickness of gill epithelium (Har) were determined at 4 and 24 hrs as well as 48 hrs after transfer to metal-free water. The arithmetic mean distance from water to blood was significantly elevated after both 4 and 24 hrs of exposure (Har was 4.67 and 4.66 μm, respectively in exposed fish, compared to 3.81 and 3.62 μm for the corresponding control fish). During the 48 hrs recovery, Har returned towards the control values; the recovery value of 4.21 μm was lower than values during exposures. There was also increase in gill MT mRNA after the 4 hrs exposure with MT/GAPDH ratio of 1.288 versus the control value of 0.988. In the liver, MTs induction was not observed. HIF-1α protein showed an increased accumulation in gills after 4 hrs, with the HIF-1α/α-tubulin ratio of 0.562 being higher than the 24 hrs. Exposure value of

0.232, suggested that exposure to Cu for 4 hrs causes hypoxia in the gill epithelium for the activation of HIF-1α.

Inhibition of the Transcription of CYP1A1 Gene by the Upstream Stimulatory Factor-1 in Rabbits. Takahashi et al. (1997) demonstrated that a xenobiotic-responsive element (XRE)-binding factor(s) other than the AhR. Arnt complex inhibited the transcription of CYP1A1 gene in the liver from adult rabbits, known to be nonresponsive to CYP1A1 inducers. The constitutive factor(s) in liver nuclear extracts were bound to the core sequence of XRE. The binding was eliminated by the presence of an excess amount of the AhR. Arnt complex synthesized *in vitro*. To identify the constitutive factor(s), a sequence like rabbit XRE was sought. The sequence of rabbit XRE overlapped with that of the upstream stimulatory factor 1 (USF1)-binding site in the mouse MT-I promoter. A super shift assay using a specific antibody against human USF1 indicated that it was capable of binding to rabbit XRE. In addition, the AhR.Arnt-mediated activation of XRE-TK/Luc reporter gene in RK13 cells was blocked by the transfection with a USF1 expression vector with the amounts of the expression vector transfected, indicating that the XRE of the rabbit CYP1A1 gene is recognized by the basic helix-loop-helix proteins to regulate the expression of CYP1A1 in both an agonistic (AhR.Arnt) and an antagonistic (USF1) manner.

Conclusion

In this chapter, a brief description of an important gene transcription factor, HIF1α and its clinical significance, in various chronic diseases including high altitude pulmonary edema, chronic kidney failure and in anemia is highlighted. HIF1α induces two important antioxidant genes, MTs and HO-1, to provide genetic resistance in various MDR malignancies as CB inhibitor and CS stabilizer. MTs also provide protection by serving as free radical scavengers and by inhibiting CB formation, by enhancing charnolophagy, and by stabilizing labile CPS/CS membranes. In addition, MTs promote CPS/CS exocytosis as a basic molecular mechanism of ICD to maintain normal cellular function to remain healthy even during aging. Hence, DSST charnolopharmacotherapeutics to promote HIF-1α-induced HO-1 and MTs will be therapeutically beneficial for NDDs and CVDs and vice versa for the personalized theranostics of MDR malignancies.

References

Choi, J.A., J.U. Hwang, Y.H. Yoon and J.Y. Koh. 2013. Methallothionein-3 contributes to vascular endothelial growth factor induction in a mouse model of choroidal neovascularization. Metallomics 5: 1387–1396.

Devisscher, L., P. Hindryckx, K. Olievier, H. Peeters, M. De Vos and D. Laukens. 2011. Inverse correlation between metallothioneins and hypoxia-inducible factor 1 alpha in colonocytes and experimental colitis. Biochem Biophys Res Commun 416: 307–312.

Dubé, A., J.F. Harrisson, G. Saint-Gelais and C. Séguin. 2011. Hypoxia acts through multiple signaling pathways to induce metallothionein transactivation by the metal-responsive transcription factor-1 (MTF-1). Biochem Cell Biol 89: 562–577.

Felix-Portillo, M., J.A. Martinez-Quintana, A.B. Peregrino-Uriarte and G. Yepiz-Plascencia. 2014. The metallothionein gene from the white shrimp Litopenaeus vannamei: characterization and expression in response to hypoxia. Mar Environ Res 101: 91–100.

Feng, W., Y. Wang, L. Cai and Y.J. Kang. 2007. Metallothionein rescues hypoxia-inducible factor-1 transcriptional activity in cardiomyocytes under diabetic conditions. Biochem Biophys Res Commun 360: 286–289.

Ichihara, S., Y. Yamada, F.J. Gonzalez, T. Nakajima, T. Murohara and G. Ichihara. 2009. Inhibition of ischemia-induced angiogenesis by benzo[a]pyrene in a manner dependent on the aryl hydrocarbon receptor. Biochem Biophys Res Commun 381: 44.

Kaneko, M., T. Nagamine, K. Nakazato and M. Mori. 2013. The anti-apoptotic effect of fucoxanthin on carbon tetrachloride-induced hepatotoxicity. J Toxicol Sci 38: 115–126.

Kim, H.G., Y.P. Hwang and H.G. Jeong. 2008. Metallothionein-III induces HIF-1alpha-mediated VEGF expression in brain endothelial cells. Biochem Biophys Res Commun 369: 666–671.

Kojima, I., T. Tanaka, R. Inagi, H. Nishi, H. Aburatani, H. Kato, T. Miyata, T. Fujita and M. Nangaku. 2009. Metallothionein is upregulated by hypoxia and stabilizes hypoxia-inducible factor in the kidney. Kidney Int 75: 268–277.

Lee, J.D., C.H. Lai, W.K. Yang and T.H. Lee. 2012. Increased expression of hypoxia-inducible factor-1α and metallothionein in varicocele and varicose veins. Phlebology 27: 409–415.

Lee, J.D. and M.H. Lee. 2014. Metallothionein overexpression of bladder biopsies associated with tissue hypoxia in patients with interstitial cystitis/painful bladder syndrome. Int J Urol 21: 719–723.

Lee, J.Y., Y.S. Lee, J.M. Kim, K.L. Kim, J.S. Lee, H.S. Jang, I.S. Shin, W. Suh, E.S. Jeon, J. Byun and D.K. Kim. 2006. A novel chimeric promoter that is highly responsive to hypoxia and metals. Gene Ther 13: 857–868.

Lee, J.Y., S.B. Oh, J.J. Hwang, N. Suh, D.G. Jo, J.S. Kim and J.Y. Koh. 2015. Indomethacin preconditioning induces ischemic tolerance by modifying zinc availability in the brain. Neurobiol Dis 81: 186–195.

Li, Q., H. Chen, X. Huang and M. Costa. 2006. Effects of 12 metal ions on iron regulatory protein 1 (IRP-1) and hypoxia-inducible factor-1 alpha (HIF-1alpha) and HIF-regulated genes. Toxicol Appl Pharmacol 213: 245–255.

Malairaman, U., K. Dandapani and A. Katyal. 2014. Effect of Ca2EDTA on zinc mediated inflammation and neuronal apoptosis in hippocampus of an *in vivo* mouse model of hypobaric hypoxia. PLoS One 9: e110253.

Murphy, B.J., T. Kimura, B.G. Sato, Y. Shi and G.K. Andrews. 2008. Metallothionein induction by hypoxia involves cooperative interactions between metal-responsive transcription factor-1 and hypoxia-inducible transcription factor-1alpha. Mol Cancer Res 6: 483–490.

Person, R.J., E.J. Tokar, Y. Xu, R. Orihuela, N.N. Ngalame and M.P. Waalkes. 2013. Chronic cadmium exposure *in vitro* induces cancer cell characteristics in human lung cells. Toxicol Appl Pharmacol 273: 281–288.

Rhim, T., D.Y. Lee and M. Lee. 2013. Hypoxia as a target for tissue specific gene therapy. J Control Release 172: 484–494.

Schmitz, K.J., C.I. Müller, H. Reis, H. Alakus, G. Winde, H.A. Baba, J. Wohlschlaeger, B. Jasani, J. Fandrey and K.W. Schmid. 2009. Combined analysis of hypoxia-inducible factor 1 alpha and metallothionein indicates an aggressive subtype of colorectal carcinoma. Int J Colorectal Dis 24: 1287–1296.

Shrivastava, K., D. Shukla, A. Bansal, M. Sairam, P.K. Banerjee and G. Ilavazhagan. 2008. Neuroprotective effect of cobalt chloride on hypobaric hypoxia-induced oxidative stress. Neurochem Int 52: 368–375.

Shukla, D., S. Saxena, P. Jayamurthy, M. Sairam, M. Singh, S.K. Jain, A. Bansal and G. Ilavazaghan. 2009. Hypoxic preconditioning with cobalt attenuates hypobaric hypoxia-induced oxidative damage in rat lungs. High Alt Med Biol 10: 57–69.

Singh, M., D. Shukla, P. Thomas, S. Saxena and A. Bansal. 2010. Hypoxic preconditioning facilitates acclimatization to hypobaric hypoxia in rat heart. J Pharm Pharmacol 62: 1729–1739.

Singh, M., P. Thomas, D. Shukla, R. Tulsawani, S. Saxena and A. Bansal. 2013. Effect of subchronic hypobaric hypoxia on oxidative stress in rat heart. Appl Biochem Biotechnol 169: 2405–2419.

Singh, M., R. Tulsawani, P. Koganti, A. Chauhan, M. Manickam and K. Misra. 2013. Cordyceps sinensis increases hypoxia tolerance by inducing heme oxygenase-1 and metallothionein via Nrf2 activation in human lung epithelial cells. Biomed Res Int 2013: 569206.

Søfteland, L., E. Holen and P.A. Olsvik. 2010. Toxicological application of primary hepatocyte cell cultures of Atlantic cod (Gadus morhua)-effects of BNF, PCDD and Cd. Comp Biochem Physiol C Toxicol Pharmacol 151: 401–411.

Sun, X., X. Niu, R. Chen, W. He, D. Chen, R. Kang and D. Tang. 2016. Metallothionein-1G facilitates sorafenib resistance through inhibition of ferroptosis. Hepatology 64: 488–500.

Takahashi, Y., K. Nakayama, S. Itoh, Y. Fujii-Kuriyama and T. Kamataki. 1997. Inhibition of the transcription of CYP1A1 gene by the upstream stimulatory factor 1 in rabbits. Competitive binding of USF1 with AhR.Arnt complex. J Biol Chem 272: 30025–30031.

Thiersch, M., W. Raffelsberger, R. Frigg, M. Samardzija, A. Wenzel, O. Poch and C. Grimm. 2008. Analysis of the retinal gene expression profile after hypoxic preconditioning identifies candidate genes for neuroprotection. BMC Genomics 9: 73.

van Heerden, D., A. Vosloo and M. Nikinmaa. 2004. Effects of short-term copper exposure on gill structure, metallothionein and hypoxia-inducible factor-1alpha (HIF-1alpha) levels in rainbow trout (Oncorhynchus mykiss). Aquat Toxicol 69: 271–280.

Wang, B., I.S. Wood and P. Trayhurn. 2008. PCR arrays identify metallothionein-3 as a highly hypoxia-inducible gene in human adipocytes. Biochem Biophys Res Commun 368: 88–93.

Wang, N., C.R. Dong, R. Jiang, C. Tang, L. Yang, Q.F. Jiang, G.G. Chen and Z.M. Liu. 2013. Overexpression of HIF-1α, metallothionein and SLUG is associated with high TNM stage and lymph node metastasis in papillary thyroid carcinoma. Int J Clin Exp Pathol 7: 322–330.

Xue, W., Y. Liu, J. Zhao, L. Cai, X. Li and W. Feng. 2012. Activation of HIF-1 by metallothionein contributes to cardiac protection in the diabetic heart. Am J Physiol Heart Circ Physiol 302: H2528–2535.

Part-III

Charnoly Body Molecular Pathogenesis

Clinical Significance of Disease-Specific Charnoly Body Formation and other Biomarkers in Chronic Diseases

(Recent Update on Evidence-based Personalized Theranostics)

CHAPTER-15

Disease-Specific Charnoly Body Formation

INTRODUCTION

It is now well-established that CB appears as a pleomorphic, multi-lamellar, quasi-crystalline, electron-dense stacks of degenerated mitochondrial membranes in the most vulnerable cell in response to nutritional and environmental stress due to free radical overproduction. Free radicals are generated in the mitochondria as a byproduct of oxidative phosphorylation during ATP synthesis in the electron transport chain. CB is the pre-apoptotic biomarker of CMB and is formed due to free radical over-production in response to malnutrition, environmental toxins, drugs, and/or infection. Free radicals are highly reactive oxygen species ($\cdot$OH, $\cdot$ON, CO$\cdot$) with a half-life of 10^{-13} to 10^{-14} seconds and induce lipid peroxidation by causing structural and functional breakdown of polyunsaturated fatty acids in the plasma membranes, particularly in the brain, heart, liver, muscle, and adipose tissue.

Mitochondria are highly essential for intracellular drug detoxification, sperm motility, and fertilization. Recently, we reported that inefficient charnolophagy following conception in the oocytes may induce zygotic death and/or craniofacial abnormalities in the intrauterine alcohol-nicotine, or ZIKV-exposed developing embryo (Sharma et al. 2015). A cell may possess between 120–1000 mitochondria depending on the metabolic and physiological demand of an organ. For example, skeletal muscles of birds used for the flight are highly rich in mitochondria. The genetic susceptibility of the mitochondrial genome in response to DPCI induces CB formation as a universal biomarker of cell injury (Sharma 2017; Sharma et al. 2016; Sharma 2014; Sharma and Ebadi 2014; Sharma et al. 2013a; Sharma et al. 2013b). Moreover, there are several genetic diseases derived from the maternal mitochondrial DNA.

Experimental Models of CB Formation

There are primarily two experimental approaches to study CB formation: (*a*) *In vivo*, and (b) *In vitro*.

In Vivo Model of CB Formation. CB formation can be studied *in vivo* in experimental animals like mice and rats, particularly during the prenatal or immediate postnatal period in the developing brain or in aging animals. We discovered CB formation in the Purkinje neurons of developing 15 days postnatal rats those were exposed to nutritional stress during the gestational and postnatal period. We also discovered selective CB formation in the hippocampal CA-3 and dentate gyrus regions in the intrauterine DOM-exposed mice. CB formation in these highly vulnerable regions was associated with loss of memory and cognitive impairment as noticed in AD patients.

In Vitro Cellular Model of CB Formation

(i) Mitochondrial genome knockout (RhO_{mgko}) cultured human dopaminergic (SK-N-SH) neurons.

(ii) Monoamine oxidase and Parkinsonian neurotoxin, MPP^+-exposed cultured SK-N-SH neurons.

(iii) We also examined the therapeutic benefit of a selective MAO-B inhibitor, selegiline, via MTs induction and inhibition of MPP^+-induced CB formation.

RhO_{mgko} Cells as an In Vitro Model of Aging. The mitochondrial genome is relatively more vulnerable compared to nuclear genome to DPCI because it is intron-less, nonhelical, and devoid of histones and protamines, whereas nuclear DNA is double-stranded super-helical coil with introns, histones, and protamines, which provide structural and functional stability to the nuclear genome, whereas, the mitochondrial genome remains in a hostile microenvironment of free radicals (such as OH, CO, NO), generated as a byproduct of oxidative phosphorylation during ATP synthesis. The rate limiting enzyme (ubiquinone-NADH) oxidoreductase (complex-1) in the oxidative phosphorylation is specifically down-regulated in PD patients. To develop RhO_{mgko} cells as cellular model of aging and AD, we used 5 ng/l ethidium bromide in Dulbecco's modified Eagle's Medium (DMEM), with high glucose, glutamine, and sodium bicarbonate for 6–8 weeks. The medium was changed after 72 hrs. The RhO_{mgko} neurons were authenticated by digital fluorescence microscopic analyses, using JC-1 as a fluorochrome to assess $\Delta\Psi$. Inhibition or down-regulation of complex-1 occurs in the RhO_{mgko} neurons, which was authenticated by RT-PCR analysis of gene encoding complex-1 and by immunoblotting of complex-1 protein using a specific antibody. Down-regulation of complex-1 confirmed that these cells can be used as cellular model of aging and AD to further explore the effects of various toxins and/or drugs involving CB molecular pathogenesis. Usually, CB formation in response to DPCI in the vulnerable cells occurs as an initial attempt of ICD and as a defensive mechanism in the perinuclear region to protect nuclear DNA from the further deleterious attack of free radicals.

The mitochondria remain structurally and functionally viable during fission and fusion; however, during CB formation these are destroyed and require eradication for ICD. Charnolophagy is an energy-consuming process and requires ATP from neighboring mitochondria during ICD. RhO_{mgko} cells exhibit elliptical appearance and stunted growth. Neuritogenesis, tubulinogenesis, myelinogenesis, axonogenesis, and synaptogenesis are significantly compromised. Although RhO_{mgko} neurons reduce their potential to differentiate due to CMB, their potential to divide remains intact, suggesting the structural and functional integrity of nuclear DNA as confirmed by the multiple fluorochrome comet assay which serves as a bridge between cell biology and molecular biology. We can differentiate structurally-intact, condensed, partially condensed, partially fragmented, and fully fragmented DNA quantitatively by performing this sensitive method. Transfection of RhO_{mgko} neurons with mitochondrial complex-1 gene transformed these cells to appear like neurons as determined by multiple fluorochrome confocal microscopic analysis (Sharma et al. 2004).

Multiple Fluorochrome Comet Assay. A multiple fluorochrome comet assay was developed to evaluate the neurotoxic action of the Parkinsonian neurotoxin, MPP$^+$, on the control wild type and RhO_{mgko} neurons. By performing this assay, we established that MPP$^+$ (1-μM, overnight) selectively causes oxidation of highly sensitive and vulnerable mtDNA, without inducing any damage to the nuclear DNA.

Primary Events in CB Formation. As described above, normal healthy mitochondria remain actively engaged in oxidative phosphorylation and in TCA cycle for ATP synthesis. Usually, we obtain 34 ATP molecules from one glucose molecule. Physiologically-active mitochondria maintain proper $\Delta\Psi$. Certain fluorescent dyes such as JC-1 dihydro-fluorescein, or rhodamine can be used to determine $\Delta\Psi$. Under the confocal or epifluorescence microscope, mitochondria appear as crimson-red colored tiny entities (like *Christmas lights*) at 1000X magnification. On repeated exposure to UV light, the crimson-red fluorescence is changed green due to $\Delta\Psi$ collapse. When the $\Delta\Psi$ is reduced to zero, even the green fluorescence is quenched. At this stage, the mega-pores open and Ca^{2+} ions enter inside the mitochondria. Increased intra-mitochondrial Ca^{2+} and Na^+ causes entry of water to induce hypotonicity and electrolyte imbalance. The swollen mitochondria are also named as mega-mitochondria with significantly reduced and blunt cristae. The swollen mitochondria lose their potential to divide and proliferate as their Cyt-C is completely delocalized. At this stage lot of free radicals are generated which cause oxidation of the mtDNA to synthesize 8-OH, 2dG, which is significantly increased in the plasma and urine samples of patients suffering from progressive NDDs such as PD, AD, drug addiction, MDD, CVDs, and many others. Free radicals enhance lipases, proteases, and nucleases to cause lipolysis, proteolysis, and nuclear DNA damage, respectively. The mitochondrial membranes are subsequently fragmented and degenerated to form electron-dense multi-lamellar structures, named as CBs.

It is important to emphasize that mitochondrial fission as well as fusion are normal physiological events and should not be misinterpreted as CBs. CB formation is a pathological event and becomes intracellular inclusion, if not eradicated immediately by energy (ATP)-driven charnolophagy. It remains unknown whether these degenerated pleomorphic mitochondrial membrane stacks (CBs) can be recycled in the biological system. However, E.M. analyses provided evidence that CBs are phagocytosed by lysosomes as a basic molecular mechanism of ICD during the acute phase. The number of lysosomes was also significantly increased during nutritional stress as an attempt to eradicate CBs from the physico-chemically-injured susceptible cells. Usually, we detected 8–12 mature CBs in the developing UN Purkinje neurons. There are primarily 4 major stages of CB life cycle: (i) origin, (ii) development, (iii) maturation, and (iv) degradation which we explained in detail in our publications (Sharma and Ebadi 2014; Sharma et al. 2013a; Sharma et al. 2013b).

Table 4: Comparative analysis of lysosome and charnolosome.

S. No.	Lysosome	Charnolosome
1.	Intracellular organelle	Intracellular organelle
2.	Structurally and functionally stable	Structurally and functionally labile
3.	Independent organelle	Lysosome-derived organelle
4.	Energy (ATP) dependent	Energy (ATP) dependent
5.	**Biomarker**	**Biomarkers**
	Enzymes	Metabolites of mitochondrial metabolism
	Lipases	Cytochrome-C, Acetaldehyde
	Proteases	Ammonia, H_2O_2, Lactate
	Nucleases	8-OH, 2dG, 2,3 Dihydroxy Nonenal
		TSPO (18 kDa), MAOs, GAPDH, TRPCs, Caspase-3, AIF-1, MTs, HSPs, HIF-1α, Cholesterol, Ca^{2+}
6.	Does not form lysosome bodies	Forms CS bodies
7.	Is not exocytosed	CS is exocytosed to maintain ICD
8.	The lysosomal enzymes can be detected in circulation	CS biomarkers can be detected in circulation
9.	Does not follow typical PKs	Follows typical PKs and detoxification in the liver and elimination by kidneys
10.	Is involved in autophagy as a basic molecular mechanism of ICD	A byproduct of charnolophagy exocytosed efficiently, maintains ICD involved in chronic degenerative diseases
11.	Involved in lysosomal storage diseases	Involved in charnolosomal storage, and can be destabilized by free radicals.
12.	It can be destabilized by free radicals	
13.	Relatively less cytotoxic	Extremely cytotoxic and involved in chronic MDR NDDs, CVDs, and cancer
14.	Rich in acid phosphatase	Rich in many toxins such as Cyt-C, iron, $ONOO^-$, lactate, acetate, ammonia, H_2O_2, Ca^{2+}

Disease-Specific CB Formation. Disease-specific CB formation is also cell-specific and occurs in specific cells in response to disease, toxin/drug exposure, and/or infection. For instance, CB formation in the hippocampal CA-3 and dentate gyrus region due to intrauterine KA and DOM exposure causes memory loss in AD and MDDs in schizophrenia; in the striatal region, it causes PD; in the hypothalamic medio-basal nuclei, it causes eating disorders (anorexia nervosa and bulimia); in the cerebellar Purkinje neurons, it causes delayed motor learning and loss of co-ordination; in the cardiomyocytes, it causes myocardial infarction (MI) and atherosclerosis; in the oligodendrocytes, it causes MS; in the pancreatic β-cells, it causes insulin-resistant Type-2 diabetes, in the adipocytes, it causes obesity; and in the hyper-proliferating cancer stem cells, it causes MDR malignancies.

Charnolophagy. In general, CB is phagocytosed efficiently by lysosomes as a basic molecular mechanism of ICD for normal cellular function. The number of lysosomes is significantly increased during malnutrition, infection, and toxic and/or drug exposure in a vulnerable cell. This forms the basis of selective and targeted toxicity of certain anti-infective (anti-bacterial, anti-viral, antifungal, anti-malarial, and anti-amoebic) drugs. Charnolophagy is highly efficient in MDR cancers due to MTs induction. Hence, these cells are difficult to eradicate even with aggressive multi-drug combination protocols.

CB Sequestration. In general, MDR cancers and infections are difficult to eradicate because CB sequestration occurs in these cells when they become highly resistant to lysosomal phagocytosis. When the lysosomes phagocytose a considerable number of CBs, they appear swollen and electron dense and are named as phagolysosomes as we observed in nutritionally stressed Purkinje neurons, in serum-deprived cultured SK-N-SH neurons and NFG-1015 cell lines, and in O_2 and glucose-deprived cortical neurons. Hence, the lysosomal-resistant CBs are an integral part of the degenerating cells. Upon sequestration, CBs release highly cytotoxic substances including Cyt-C, caspase-3, AIF, Bax, and Bak, to trigger an apoptotic cascade to cause further degeneration, which usually occurs during atherosclerotic plaque rupture. We demonstrated zone of growth inhibition due to Cyt-C release from cultured vascular smooth muscle cells derived from de-endothelialized pig coronary arteries. Persistent myocardial infarction can cause dilated cardiomyopathy ventricular thinning, and eventually ventricular rupture due to volume overload, if remained uncontrolled and untreated. CB sequestration can also be demonstrated in hyper-proliferating cancer cells, which lack contact inhibition and induce angiogenesis. The hyper-proliferating tumor cells may be subjected to hypoxia, ischemia, and nutritional stress. A further study is needed to elucidate the precise role of DSST-CB formation and CS destabilization and its targeting for novel drug development of various NDDs, CVDs, and cancer.

References

Sharma, S., M. Kheradpezhou, S. Shavali, H.El. Refaey, J. Eken, C. Hagen and M. Ebadi. 2004. Neuroprotective actions of coenzyme Q_{10} in Parkinson's disease. Methods in Enzymology 382: 488–509.

Sharma, S., A. Rais, R. Sandhu, W. Nel and M. Ebadi. 2013. Clinical significance of metallothioneins in cell therapy and nanomedicine. International Journal of Nanomedicine 8: 1477–1488.

Sharma, S., C.S. Moon, A. Khogali, A. Haidous, A. Chabenne, C. Ojo, M. Jelebinkov, Y. Kurdi and M. Ebadi. 2013. Biomarkers of Parkinson's disease (Recent Update). Neurochemistry International 63: 201–229.

Sharma, S. 2014. Nanotheranostics in evidence based personalized medicine. Current Drug Targets 15: 915–930.

Sharma, S. and M. Ebadi. 2014. Charnoly body as a universal biomarker of cell injury. Biomarkers and Genomic Medicine 6: 89–98.

Sharma, S. and M. Ebadi. 2014. Significance of metallothioneins in aging brain. Neurochemistry International 65: 40–48.

Sharma, S., J. Choga, V. Gupta et al. 2016. Charnoly body as novel biomarker of nutritional stress in Alzheimer's disease. Functional Foods in Health and Disease 6: 344–377.

Sharma, S. and W. Lippincott. 2017. Emerging biomarkers in Alzheimer's disease (Recent Update). Current Alzheimer Research 14 (in press).

CHAPTER-16

Charnoly Body in Fetal Alcohol Syndrome

INTRODUCTION

The adverse effects of prenatal alcohol consumption have long been known; however, a formal description and clinical diagnosis of these effects was not introduced until 1973. Since then, the distinction of the wide range of effects that can be induced by prenatal alcohol exposure (PAE), and, consequently, the terminology to describe these effects has continued to evolve. Although much progress has been made in understanding the consequences of PAE, challenges remain in properly identifying all affected individuals as well as their individual patterns of alcohol-induced deficits. Also, as the large numbers of women who continue to drink during pregnancy indicate, prevention efforts still require further refinement to enhance their effectiveness. In addition, the mechanisms underlying alcohol-induced damage have not yet been fully elucidated; as knowledge of the mechanisms underlying alcohol-induced deficits continues to grow, the possibility of minimizing potential harm by intervening during PAE is enhanced. Finally, researchers are exploring additional ways to improve or fully restore behavioral and cognitive functions disrupted by PAE by treating the individuals with fetal alcohol spectrum disorder (FASD), thereby reducing the heavy burden for affected individuals and their families.

Exposure to alcohol *in utero* is considered a leading cause of developmental disabilities. The most severe consequence of such exposure, fetal alcohol syndrome (FAS), is characterized by distinct facial anomalies, growth retardation, and CNS dysfunction. Both animal and human studies, however, suggest that there may be considerable variability in the manifestations of *in utero* alcohol exposure across individuals, and, consequently, the term FASD has come into usage to reflect the entire continuum of effects associated with such exposure. In addition to FAS, this term encompasses the conditions of partial FAS, alcohol-related neurodevelopmental disorders (ARND), and alcohol-related birth defects (ARBD). Despite extensive evidence of cognitive, behavioral, and social deficits in people with FASD, research on behavioral interventions for FASD has lagged-behind. However, in recent years there has been a phenomenal increase in efforts to design and test interventions for this population. Neurotrophic factors influence cell metabolism and growth, proliferation, differentiation, migration and maturation of cells, and apoptotic cell death. Alcohol exposure during development may impair neurotrophic factor production, leading to CMB and CB molecular pathogenesis.

In 2005, the Surgeon General's office updated the advisory on alcohol use and pregnancy. The new advisory reads: "We do not know what, if any, amount of alcohol is safe. However, we do know that the risk of a baby being born with any of the FASD increases with the amount of alcohol a pregnant woman drinks, as does the likely severity of the condition. And when a pregnant woman drinks alcohol, so does her baby. Therefore, it is in the child's best interest for a pregnant woman to simply not drink alcohol" Considerable efforts to educate women not to abuse alcohol during pregnancy have failed to reduce the incidence of FAS. Therefore, other approaches to limit the effects of PAE are under consideration, including the development of prevention programs and interventions. It is important to improve methods for identifying affected children. The use of animal models in PAE research is critical because of the practical and ethical limitations of using human subjects for such studies. The use of animal models in 3 areas of research: addressing basic questions about alcohol exposure during development; improving the identification of affected individuals; and developing approaches to reduce the impact of PAE. The various animal-model systems that have been used to study FASD have provided new findings that have been extrapolated to human subjects, resulting in advancement in our understanding of FASD. It is important to continue to investigate the effects of developmental ethanol exposure on modulators of neurotransmission including CB formation, charnolophagy, and CS destabilization, as these clinically-significant biomarkers of CMB may be key targets for the development of effective theranostic interventions against FASD as described in this chapter.

Clinical Biomarkers of FAS. Chronic intake of ethanol during pregnancy can cause primarily 4 major clinical conditions, including FAS, autism, trout syndrome, and sudden infant death syndrome (SIDS), in addition to still birth, abortion, or pre-eclampsia. Clinical biomarkers can be sub-divided into (i) anatomical biomarkers, (ii) developmental biomarkers, (iii) neurological biomarkers, (iv) impaired handwriting, and (v) delayed motor learning. Anatomical biomarkers include (i) facial abnormalities, (ii) micrognathia, (iii) small size lips, (iv) reduced frontal lobe development, and (v) reduced eye blinking. Neurological biomarkers of FAS include primarily: (i) mental retardation, (ii) slow learning, (iii) reduced intelligence, (iv) reduced memory retention, (v) abnormal behavior, and (vi) aggressive behavior. All these biomarkers become evident due to ethanol-induced CMB in the NPCs involved in the normal growth and development of the brain as described in detail in my recently published books "Fetal Alcohol Spectrum Disorders: Concepts, Mechanisms, and Cure, and Zika Virus Disease: Prevention and Cure" Nova Science Publishers, New York.

Molecular Biomarkers of FAS. Although several molecular and genetic biomarkers have been discovered, none of them is selective. Omics biomarkers of the FAS can be divided into (a) proteomic biomarkers, (b) metabolomic biomarkers, (c) lipidomic biomarkers, (d) glycomic biomarkers, and (e) genomic biomarkers. In addition, urinary ethyl sulfate can be estimated to determine the severity of FAS. Although knowledge of the dangers of alcohol consumption during pregnancy isn't a new issue, the recent evidence of ethyl-glucuronide and ethyl-sulfate in meconium as novel biomarkers of prenatal ethanol exposure opens new perspectives for the early diagnosis of ARBD. This is crucial for a better developmental outcome of the affected pediatric population and for preventing additional cases in at risk families. Coca-ethylene is an active metabolite of changes in how drugs are absorbed, distributed, metabolized, and eliminated (i.e., pharmacokinetics: PKs) may help explain why multiple drug use is dangerous to fetal development. PKs interaction is the process that occurs when two or more drugs interact in the system simultaneously. Although the PKs of individual drugs may be well-characterized, when the drugs are combined, one drug can unpredictably alter the concentration, bioavailability (the rate of a drug entering the bloodstream), and net effect of the other drug. I have now proposed a combinatorial bioinformatic approach to precisely determine the CMB of NPCs involving charnolosomics in response to FAE.

Temporal Assessment of FAS Biomarkers. The concentrations of the FAS biomarkers depends on the severity and duration of maternal ethanol abuse. Usually < 1 drink/day is considered low, 2 drinks/day moderate, and > 14 drinks/week or binge-drinking episodes are considered severe. There exists a temporal relationship for the detection of FAS biomarkers. For example, within hrs of birth, breath alcohol, blood alcohol, and urine alcohol can be estimated to assess the severity of maternal ethanol abuse. Urinary ethyl glucuronide can be detected within the first five days of delivery, whereas %CDT, phosphatidyle-ethanolamine can be detected within < 3 weeks. MCV, γ-glutamyl transferase (GGT) can be detected within < 3 weeks. Hair analysis of FAEE, EtG, and PEth can be done within < 3 months. Generally, weeks and months arc the target areas for the development of better biomarkers of FAS. In this respect, biomarkers of CMB involving CB molecular pathogenesis seem promising.

Terminology used to Describe Alcohol's Effects. The evolution in the understanding of alcohol's effects on the fetus has resulted in a variety of (sometimes overlapping) terms that have been used to characterize the range of alcohol's potential effects. These include FAS, partial FAS (pFAS), fetal alcohol effects (FAE), alcohol-related birth defects (ARBD), alcohol-related neurodevelopmental disorder (ARND), and fetal alcohol spectrum disorders (FASD). A diagnosis of full FAS is made if the following 3 primary defining features are present: (i) documentation of characteristic facial abnormalities (smooth philtrum, thin vermillion border, and short palpebral fissures); (ii) documentation of prenatal and postnatal growth deficits; and (iii) documentation of CNS abnormalities (i.e., structural, neurological, or behavioral, or a combination thereof).

Facial Characteristics Associated with FAS. Typical Symptoms of FAS: low nasal bridge, minor ear abnormalities, indistinct philtrum, micrognathia, epicanthal folds, short palpabral fissures, flat midface and short nose, and thin upper lip.

Binge Drinking and Severity of FASD Quantity and Frequency

Table 5: Cases of FAS and partial FAS (pFAS) in various population studies by frequency, percent, and ratio.

Community Studies Organized from Top to Bottom by Proportion of Binge Drinking	FAS n (%)	pFAS n (%)	Ratio of FAS
South Africa I	40 (91)	4 (9)	10 to 1
South Africa II	37 (56)	29 (44)	1.3 to 1
South Africa III	55 (75)	18 (25)	3.1 to 1
Total South Africa*	132 (72)	51 (28)	2.6 to 1
Plains USA**	56 (45)	69 (55)	0.81 to 1
Western City, USA (1 & 2)*	6 (33)	12 (67)	0.5 to 1
Italy (1 & 2)*	8 (18)	36 (82)	0.22 to 1

Notes: All of these were school-based studies in which all consenting first-grade children were screened if their growth in height, weight, and head circumference was below the 10th percentile or they were picked randomly from the entire first-grade population as control subjects. *All of these studies were school-based studies in which all consenting first-grade children were screened if their growth in height, weight, and head circumference was found to be below the 10th centile or they were picked randomly from the entire first-grade population as control subjects. **Plains USA was an active-case ascertainment study in which children (birth to age 18 years) were recruited from seven communities to referral clinics for FASD and related developmental disabilities if they had physical features, behavior, or learning problems similar to those characteristics of FASD.

For example, the key facial features that are commonly used to diagnose FAS and pFAS include short eye openings, thin border between the upper lip and facial skin, flat middle groove in the upper lip (i.e., philtrum), underdeveloped midface, wide distance between the right and left inner corners of the eyes (i.e., inner canthal distance), and droopy eyelid (i.e., ptosis). Each of these conditions develops during the 6th through the 9th week of gestation. If a woman's drinking produces high BACs during this window of fetal gestation, then one or more of these features may be negatively affected and abnormal.

Molecular Imaging in FAS. The imaging techniques including MRI, diffusion tensor imaging (DTI), and MRS provide valuable tools for studying brain structure and neurochemistry in FASD. Although the application of MR-based methodologies in the study of FASD in animal models is in its infancy, it has provided clinically-relevant insights and holds significant promise to further extend our understanding of alcohol's effects on the developing fetus. Animal studies using MR-based imaging technologies, including MRI, DTI, and MRS provide important insight into alcohol's early effects on the fetal brain. This chapter presents how these valuable tools have been applied to the study of FASD in animal models. Compared with clinical studies of the effects of alcohol on development, using animal models allows greater control over dose, duration, and pattern of alcohol exposure. For example, research examining the effects of alcohol at different developmental stages and at various doses has helped highlight the vulnerability of the prenatal brain to very early alcohol-mediated damage. This research has important implications for clinical practice and ongoing research. The application of MR-based technologies to the study of FASD in animal models promises to facilitate the definition of the full spectrum of alcohol-induced birth defects along with their developmental stage and dosage dependency. Recognition of the entire range of consequences is essential for accurate diagnosis and prevention. With respect to the latter, MRI-based rodent studies have highlighted the vulnerability of the brain to alcohol-mediated damage resulting from alcohol exposure at developmental stages that occur in humans prior to the time that pregnancy is recognized, emphasizing the importance of pre-pregnancy counseling. In addition to the *ex vivo* analyses, evolving MRI technologies are expected to allow longitudinal studies of both the brain and behavior. These MR-based animal studies are expected to provide data that will inform clinical practice and ongoing research. It has been proposed that FASD victims should be evaluated for at least 6 years after their birth.

Because changes in the pattern of DNA methylation in many cases might be related to changes in gene expression, such alcohol-induced hypomethylation might alter gene expression that could contribute to the developmental abnormalities seen in FASD. Future studies focused on both genetic and epigenetic mechanisms on potential links between the two will help to illuminate central mechanisms through which alcohol interacts with critical target pathways to reprogram genes. Studies focused on genetic variation in the gene encoding an enzyme called methylenetetrahydrofolate reductase (MTHFR), which is a key enzyme in the methionine–homocysteine cycle, are a good example of this type of research.

FAS and FASD are underdiagnosed in general treatment settings. Among the factors involved in identifying the effects of PAE are (1) the evidence for PAE; (2) the effects of the postnatal, caregiving environment; (3) comorbidities; and (4) differential diagnosis, which includes identifying the neurodevelopmental effects of alcohol and discriminating these effects from those characterizing other conditions. This chapter illustrates findings on the neurodevelopmental effects of PAE, including learning and memory, motor and sensory/motor effects, visual/spatial skills, and executive functioning and effortful control. Encouraging clinicians to discriminate the effects of PAE from other conditions may require more education and training but ultimately will improve outcomes for affected children.

Functional Measures of Brain Dysfunction. Children prenatally exposed to alcohol with and without the physical features of FAS demonstrate similar deficits in neurobehavior, including impairments in memory, attention, reaction time, visuospatial abilities, fine and gross motor skills, social and adaptive functioning, abnormal activity, reactivity, hyperactivity, attention deficits, lack of inhibition, impaired learning, reduced habituation, feeding difficulties, gait abnormalities, developmental delays, impaired motor skills, hearing abnormalities, and poor state regulation (sleep, jitteriness, and arousal abnormalities). For detailed information of CB molecular pathogenesis in FAS and FASD, readers are requested to refer to my recently published manuscripts and book "Fetal Alcohol Spectrum Disorders: Concepts, Mechanisms, and Cure", Nova Science Publishers, New York, U.S.A.

Novel Therapeutic Strategies in FAS. Novel therapeutic strategies in FAS can be developed by employing CB as biomarker of theranostic significance. Nutritional rehabilitation, Zn^{2+}, and MTs provide neuroprotection in drug addiction, malnutrition, and in response to general anesthetics, toxins, and anti-epileptic drugs. Hence, carcinotherapeutic drugs may be developed as CB agonists and charnolophagy antagonists, whereas neuro and cardioprotective drugs may be developed as CB inhibitors and charnolophagy agonists as illustrated in Fig. 38.

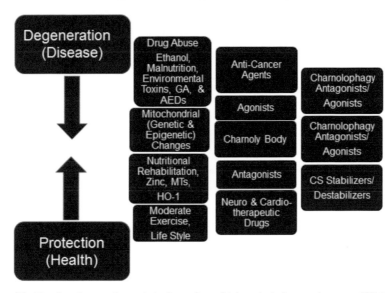

Fig. 38: Novel therapeutic strategies in fetal alcohol syndrome (CB-targeted charnolopharmacotherapeutics).

References

Sharma, S., S. Gawande, A. Jagtap, R. Abeulela and Z. Salman. 2014. Fetal alcohol syndrome, prevention, diagnosis, & treatment. In Alcohol Abuse: Prevalence, Risk Factors. Nova Science Publishers, New York, pp. 1–45.

Sharma, S. 2017. Fetal Alcohol Spectrum Disorder: Concepts, Mechanism, and Cure. Nova Science Publishers, New York, U.S.A.

Sharma, S. 2017. Zika Virus Disease: Prevention and Cure. Nova Science Publishers, New York, U.S.A.

CHAPTER-17

Charnoly Body in Nicotinism

INTRODUCTION

Recently, I described the novel concept of DSST-charnolopharmacotherapeutics for the safe and effective EBPT of progressive NDDs, CVDs, and MDR malignancies in multiple drug addiction, and in microbial infections including ZIKV disease in my books entitled "Personalized Medicine, Beyond PET Biomarkers; "Zika Virus Disease, Prevention and Cure," and "Fetal Alcohol Disorders: Concepts, Mechanism, and Clinical Management" released by the Nova Science Publishers, New York, U.S.A. These novel charnolopharmacotherapeutics of CMB can also have EBPT significance in the clinical management of nicotinism.

There are primarily two major types of acute vs chronic addiction and their deleterious consequences on the developing new born infant during intrauterine life. I have emphasized that inhibition of AgNOR (involved in ribosomal synthesis) by nicotine-induced CS body formation prevents protein synthesis to cause apoptosis due to CB formation and CS destabilization, which is represented by its enhanced permeabilization, sequestration, and/or fragmentation to increase intracellular toxicity and hence, MDR diseases. This chapter describes, basic molecular mechanism of nicotine-induced MDR malignancies. In addition, the deleterious effect of environmental pollutants on metal ion speciation of MTs is presented to further elucidate their influence on Zn^{2+}-induced transcriptional regulation of genes involved in DNA cell cycle, cell growth, proliferation, migration, differentiation, and invasion during malignant transformation through AgNOR activation. That MTs inhibit CB formation and augment charnolophagy during the acute phase, and stabilize CS and augment CS exocytosis, during the chronic phase to prevent apoptosis render immortalization to cancer stem cells in MDR malignancies, are novel and presented for the first time. The uncontrolled release of toxic metabolites from nicotine-induced CSscs body and concomitant induction of antioxidant proteins (MTs, HSPs, P[53], BCL[2], glutathione, SOD, catalase) in MDR malignancies are described to highlight the therapeutic potential of MTs in nicotine-induced NDDs, CVDs, and their undesirable role in MDR malignancies, particularly when their metal ion speciation is impaired due to malnutrition, environmental pollution, heavy metal ions (Hg, Pd, Cd, As, Cr, Co, Ni) exposure, and/or microbial (bacteria, viral, fungal) infection.

The chapter also highlights the detailed pharmacology of nicotinism in relation to specific neurotransmitters and their receptors, psychiatric comorbidity in nicotinism, and the detection of DSST biomarkers from biological fluids for early theranostic interventions of chronic MDR malignancies and other illnesses.

Three Major Types of Addiction. Three are primarily three major types of addiction: These include (a) food addiction, (b) sex addiction, and (c) drug addiction. Out of these 3 types of addictions, drug addiction has devastating consequences involving poor quality of life, socio-economic stigma, early morbidity, and mortality. Drug addiction has significantly deleterious consequences on the health and wellbeing of a person. In fact, a chronic drug addict suffers from early morbidity and mortality due to CMB of NPCs derived from iPPCs particularly during intrauterine life and adolescence. Drugs of abuse, including nicotine induce CB formation in these highly vulnerable cells to induce charnolopathies implicated in diversified embryopathies. Simultaneously, charnolophagy is induced as a cytoprotective mechanism. Charnolophagy is highly orchestrated energy (ATP)-driven process involved in ICD. A lysosome containing phagocytosed CB is named as charnolophagosome (CPS). The CPS is transformed to CS, when CB is hydrolyzed by the lysosomal enzymes. The CS is a single layered, highly labile intracellular organelle. It is efficiently eliminated from the cell by energy (ATP)-driven exocytosis as a basic molecular mechanism of ICD. Although, charnolophagy occurs during the acute phase of drug addiction as an efficient molecular mechanism of ICD, chronic drug addiction destabilizes CS and it buds off to synthesize CS bodies. CS bodies subsequently coalesce with the plasma membrane to form apoptotic bodies, which enhance membrane permeabilization. Thus, chronic drug addiction (nicotine) induces CS destabilization, represented by permeabilization, sequestration, and fragmentation which ultimately releases toxic mitochondrial metabolites to cause non-nuclear DNA-dependent neurodegenerative apoptosis.

Acute vs Chronic Nicotine in Intrauterine Life. Intrauterine exposure to nicotine can have acute as well as chronic effects. Acute exposure of nicotine to the developing fetus can induce mitochondrial oxidative stress to cause free radical overproduction. The energy (ATP) requirements are significantly increased in the NPCs during nicotine exposure. Free radicals-induced lipid peroxidation causes degeneration of mitochondrial membranes. The degenerated mitochondrial membranes condense to form electron-dense penta or hepta-lamellar structures. These quasi-crystalline intra-cellular inclusions are named as CB, which is efficiently phagocytosed by energy (ATP)-driven lysosome-dependent charnolophagy. The lysosome containing phagocytosed CB is named as CPS. CPS is transformed to CS when CB is hydrolyzed by the lysosomal enzymes. During the acute phase, the CS is subjected to energy (ATP)-dependent exocytosis as an efficient basic molecular mechanism of ICD. The CS is structurally and functionally labile intracellular organelle and can be easily destabilized by a subsequent free radical attack, which causes lipid peroxidation of CS membranes to trigger structural and functional breakdown of PUFA. At certain weak points, CS membrane exhibits protubrances in the form of CS bodies, which coalesce with the plasma membranes to cause apoptotic bodies to induce membrane perforations. Thus, free radicals-induced permeabilization, sequestration, and degradation of CS bodies releases highly toxic substances, such as Cyt-C, 8-OH-2dG,

2,3 dihydroxy nonenal, iron, acetaldehyde, H_2O_2, and ammonia to cause degenerative apoptosis.

Inhibition of AgNOR by Nicotine-induced CS Body Prevents Protein Synthesis to Cause Apoptosis. Inhibition of AgNOR by nicotine-induced CS body formation prevents protein synthesis to cause degenerative apoptosis. Ribosomes are involved in protein synthesis for cell growth and proliferation in MDR malignancies even in the presence of anticancer drugs. In addition to BCl_2, HSP, SOD, and catalase, CSscs releases MTs in the nucleus. MTs release Zn^{2+} to induce transcriptional activation of genes involved in DNA cell cycle, growth, proliferation, migration, and development in MDR malignancies. MTs are induced in severe malnutrition, in response to environmental toxins (nicotine, ethanol, Cd, Pb, Hg, As, Cr), microbial infections, and in numerous physico-chemical injuries as a defensive mechanism. Nuclear translocation of MTs through CS bodies renders MDR malignancies refractory to conventional therapeutic interventions, because MTs-induced release of Zn^{2+} is involved in the transcriptional regulation of genes involved in cell growth, proliferation, migration, and development of malignant tumors even in the presence of anticancer drugs. MTs also serve as potent free radical scavengers to prevent AgNOR down-regulation in MDR malignancies. Hence, conventional protein synthesis inhibitors are unable to inhibit protein synthesis due to MTs-mediated attenuation of AgNOR down-regulation and CS stabilization in the malignant cells.

Nicotine and Ethanol-induced CS Destabilization. Nicotine and ethanol-induced CS destabilization induce inhibition of Purkinje cell AgNOR to cause SIDS. CS are highly labile single layered organelles and can be easily destabilized to form CS bodies. The endonucleosis of CS bodies causes the release of toxic substances including Cyt-C, iron, and acetaldehyde, ammonia, and H_2O_2 to inhibit AgNOR, which synthesizes ribosomes depending on the transcriptional regulation of Zn^{2+}-induced microRNA-mediated activation of nuclear genes involved in DNA cell cycle, growth, proliferation, migration, and development. Blockade of AgNOR-induced ribosomal production, inhibits protein synthesis (involved in the cell survival) to cause apoptotic degeneration.

Molecular Mechanism of Nicotine-induced MDR Malignancies. The nicotine-induced CSscs body is highly rich in antioxidant proteins such as BCl_2, MTs, HSPs, SOD, and catalase, which protect AgNOR from free radical attack and from protein synthesis inhibitors used for cancer chemotherapy, in addition to antibacterial, antifungal, and antiviral therapy. The therapeutic efficacy of various protein synthesis inhibitors is nullified by nicotine abuse because nicotine inhibits AgNOR to prevent ribosomes required for the protein synthesis. The cancer stem cell-specific CSscs are rich in MTs, which store, donate, and buffer Zn^{2+} ions for the transcriptional activation of genes involved in the induction of AgNOR to synthesize ribosomes involved in proteins synthesis for growth, proliferation, and development of MDR malignancies.

Environmental Pollution and Metal Ion Speciation of MTs. MTs are primarily Zn^{2+}-binding proteins and under normal physiological conditions store, buffer, donate, and release Zn^{2+}. Zn^{2+} is translocated from the mitochondria to the nucleus, where it is involved in the transcriptional regulation of genes to enhance DNA cell cycle, cell growth, proliferation, migration, differentiation, and development particularly in highly proliferating and metabolically-active cells. Environmental pollution of heavy metals such as Cd, Hg, Lead, Cr, As, Fe can also bind with MTs which render them either non-functional in several NDDs and CVDs, where cellular differentiation is very crucial, or these proteins may induce malignant transformation in MDR malignancies. Hence, metal ion speciation of these anti-apoptotic, anti-inflammatory, and free radical scavenging antioxidant proteins is extremely important to determine their exact pathophysiological significance in health and disease. Impaired metal ion speciation of MTs is unable to prevent CB formation, CPS induction, and CS destabilization or disintegration. Metal ion speciation of MTs can be determined precisely by metallomic analyses utilizing ICP-MS as described earlier.

MTs Stabilize CS to Prevent Apoptosis and Render Immortalization to Cancer Stem Cells in MDR Malignancies. There are primarily 4 major types of CSs depending on the level of MTs these structurally and functionally labile intracellular organelles possess. These include (a) MTs-deficient CS; (b) MTs-inadequate CS; (c) MTs-normal CS; and (d) MTs-over-expressing CS. MTs are low molecular weight (6–7 kDa), cysteine-rich, metal (Zn^{2+})-binding proteins, which serve as antioxidant, antiapoptotic, and anti-inflammatory proteins. MTs inhibit CB formation, and stabilize CS by serving as potent free radical scavengers. The translocation of MTs in the nucleus triggers genes involved in cell proliferation, cell migration, and cell differentiation by donating Zn^{2+} ions resulting in hyperproliferation of cells. The structural and functional integrity of CS depends on the levels of MTs in these intracellular organelles. MTs-deficient CS are highly unstable and vulnerable to free radicals-induced permeabilization, sequestration, and disintegration. Free radical-induced lipid peroxidation causes structural and functional breakdown of PUFA in the CS membranes, resulting in the formation and rupture of CS bodies to enhance CS membrane permeabilization and release highly toxic substances such as Cyt-C, acetate, ammonia, H_2O_2, acetone, iron, Bax, and Bak. These molecular events induce further apoptotic neurodegeneration.

Free radicals are partially scavenged around the *CS* having inadequate MTs. MTs over-expressing *CS* remain structurally and functionally stable because these can readily scavenge free radicals. CS-MTs interaction renders the cancer cells either susceptible or resistant to anticancer therapy. Hence:

(a) MTs-deficient CS can be readily disintegrated by free radical overload due to MTs deficiency.

(b) MTs-inadequate CS are susceptible to free radicals.

(c) MTs-normal CS are relatively stable because these organelles can scavenge free radicals to a certain extent.

(d) CS possessing high levels of MTs are resistant to free radical attack and confer MDR malignancies and adverse effects.

(e) MTs-over-expressing CS render structural and functional stability to CS to trigger MDR malignancies in a nonproliferating cell.

Nicotine-induced CSscs Body Antioxidant Proteins Augment MDR Malignancies. Nicotine-induced CSscs body antioxidant proteins trigger MDR malignancies in nonproliferating cells. AgNOR in the nucleolus maintains and sustains protein synthesis by producing ribosomes, required for the cell growth, development, proliferation and development in MDR malignancies even in the presence of protein synthesis inhibitors prescribed as anticancer agents. CSscs release antioxidant proteins such as MTs, HSPs, BCl_2, SOD, and catalase to protect AgNOR. Therefore, it goes on synthesizing ribosomes for protein synthesis during MDR malignancy. Translocation and/or release of MTs from CSscs in the nucleus donates Zn^{2+} to induce transcriptional activation of genes involved in the induction of DNA cell cycle, cell proliferation, migration, development, and invasion in MDR malignancies. MTs are induced in DPCI to the most vulnerable cell as a basic molecular mechanism of cell repair and growth. Uncontrolled induction of MTs in response to nicotine or ethanol-induced cell injury is involved in malignant transformation due to CS_{scs} destabilization. MDR malignancies develop because of uncontrolled induction of AgNOR in the nucleolus goes on synthesizing ribosomes for the growth and proliferation of MDR tumors even in the presence of protein synthesis inhibitors used conventionally for the chemotherapy of MDR malignancies. Hence, anticancer drugs should be developed to inhibit specifically CSscs for the safe and effective eradication of nicotine and/or ethanol-induced MDR malignancies.

Detailed Pharmacology of Nicotine Addiction

The 1988 Surgeon General's Report, The Health Consequences of Nicotine Addiction, concluded that "Nicotine is the drug in tobacco that causes addiction" (USDHHS 1988, p. 9). Studies show that animals self-administer or prefer nicotine over saline and that many people smoke to regulate blood concentrations of nicotine. For example, if smokers are given cigarettes with lower nicotine yields than their usual brands, they tend to smoke more intensely or to cover the filter ventilation holes to increase their nicotine intake. VTA and the meso-cortico-limbic DA-ergic neurons are primarily responsible for the positive reinforcing aspects of nicotine. An increase in the levels of DA is mediated by nicotine directly stimulating nAChRs, primarily α7 homomeric and α4β2-containing nAChRs within the ventral tegmental area (VTA), thus increasing activity of VTA neurons projecting to the nucleus accumbens and the frontal cortex. Nicotine stimulates α7 nAChRs on glutamatergic terminals that release glutamate, an excitatory neurotransmitter, which results in increased release of DA in the nucleus accumbens, amygdala, and frontal cortex. Nicotine also excites nAChRs on GABA-releasing terminals. Thus, levels of GABA, an inhibitory neurotransmitter, are also increased by nicotine. However, the interaction between quick desensitization of nAChRs on the GABA neuron and higher doses of nicotine required to desensitize nAChRs on the glutamatergic neuron result in a greater increase in DA levels. The neurophysiology associated with withdrawal symptoms may be based on the type of symptoms experienced (e.g., somatic versus affective). It appears that nAChRs differ in their involvement in both the somatic and affective components of nicotine withdrawal and dependence. As seen in animal studies, β4 nAChRs play an important role in the somatic signs of withdrawal, whereas β2 nAChRs play an important role in the affective aspects of withdrawal. The role of α4 nAChRs is unclear, but these receptors may play a role in both the affective and somatic withdrawal effects of nicotine addiction. The α7 nAChRs is involved only in some of the somatic signs of nicotine withdrawal.

The amount and speed of nicotine delivery also plays a critical role in the potential for abuse of tobacco products. The speed and amount of nicotine delivered to the brain depend on the amount of nicotine in the product, the alkalinity of the product, and the route of administration. Nicotine, 3-(1-methyl-2-pyrrolidinyl) pyridine, is a volatile alkaloid in the tobacco plant, and its absorption and renal secretion is dependent on pH. Products with higher alkalinity are associated with greater amounts of nicotine in the non-ionized or free base state, which can vaporize more easily into the gas phase, can be deposited directly on the lung tissues, and crosses cell membranes more rapidly than ionized nicotine. Tobacco products may contain ammonia to increase the conversion of nicotine to the nonionized or free base state. Physical design features such as filter-tip ventilation also increase the free base fraction of nicotine. The fastest rate of nicotine delivery is through smoking cigarettes. Nicotine, when inhaled, enters the lungs, which present a large surface area of small airways and alveoli, undergoes dissolution in pulmonary fluid at a high pH, is transported to the heart, and then immediately enter in the brain. This rapid and bolus delivery of nicotine through cigarettes leads to greater control over the amount of nicotine delivered to the brain and in higher abuse potential than do other tobacco- or nicotine-containing products.

Nicotine in the tobacco product and its kinetic profile are not the only factors that might contribute to a tobacco product's potential for addiction. Other constituents may also serve as re-inforcers or may enhance blood levels of nicotine or its effects. For example, animal studies have shown that nor-nicotine, a secondary tobacco alkaloid, functions as a reinforcer at less potency than nicotine. The effect of nor-nicotine in humans, remains uncertain. Acetaldehyde in tobacco smoke from burning sugars and in the tobacco leaf, may play an important role in increasing the reinforcing effects of nicotine. In animal studies, acetaldehyde enhanced the acquisition of nicotine self-administration among adolescent rats but not in adult rats. Extracts from flue-cured tobacco that appear to inhibit MAO activity in the brain may be another contributory factor to the reinforcing effects of cigarettes. Increased MAO inhibition results in increased levels of catecholamines. Current smokers have lower levels of MAO than do nonsmokers or former smokers.

Tobacco product design and ingredients contribute to the risk of addiction by reducing noxious effects such as the unpleasant taste of nicotine and unpleasant sensory effects. Such designs include ventilation to cool the smoke and ingredients such as menthol and chocolate that make nicotine inhalation more pleasant. Other non-nicotine factors can also contribute to addiction potential. These factors include the associative learning processes (internal and environmental cues linked with nicotine administration) that develop with repeated tobacco use. This associative learning can be as powerful as the direct effects of nicotine. For example, presenting smokers with sensory aspects of smoking without nicotine results in a decrease in craving for cigarettes, a decreased subset of withdrawal symptoms, and short-term reinforcing efficacy like that of cigarettes containing nicotine.

Typically, smoking initiation occurs during adolescence. Research shows that adolescent smokers report symptoms of dependence even at low levels of cigarette consumption, and animal studies show that sensitivity to nicotine in adolescents differs from that in adults. For example, from the paradigms of self-administration and conditioned place preference in rats, demonstrate that adolescence may be at a stage of development with higher sensitivity to nicotine exposure than that in adults. Using mixture modeling, longitudinal studies have identified multiple age-related trajectories of smoking behavior. These trajectories include smokers with early initiation of smoking and steep acceleration of smoking, persons who engage in experimental or light smoking, smokers with late initiation and accelerated progression of smoking, persons who stopped smoking, and those who never smoked. The group with early initiation and steeply escalating and persistent smoking has been associated with familial smoking, which reflects genetic and/or environmental risk factors, less parental support, and a risk for chronic heavy smoking in adulthood. Ethnic differences have also been observed for the age at initiation of smoking and the speed of progression in smoking. These studies showed that African Americans were more likely to have slower progression of smoking and a lower number of cigarettes smoked than do Whites. Studies that have looked at predictors for developing nicotine addiction or heavy smoking suggest the importance of both genes and environmental influences. Parental smoking and substance abuse disorders, and externalizing disorders (attention-deficit/hyperactivity, disruptive behavior, and alcohol and drug abuse) have been found to be predictive of nicotine dependence and/or daily smoking.

It has been hypothesized that the sensitization to the locomotor-activating effects of drugs, including effects observed after repeated nicotine administrations, reflect a progressive augmentation in the motivation to self-administer the drug (Robinson and Berridge 1993). (The locomotor-activating effects consist of progressively increased locomotor responses to repeated drug-challenge injections). However, no direct evidence suggests that sensitization to the locomotor-activating effects of nicotine reflects any aspect of dependence on nicotine. If sensitization to the reinforcing effects of nicotine develops, it will most likely be relevant to early phases of tobacco use involving the acquisition of tobacco smoking as a continuing behavior. The focus has been on the comorbidity of nicotine dependence and psychiatric disorders in the context of shared substrates that mediate nicotine dependence and depression-like aspects of psychiatric disorders (Markou et al. 1998; Markou and Kenny 2002; Paterson and Markou 2007). The predominant role of nAChRs in the brain is the modulation of neurotransmitter release, because nAChRs are situated primarily on presynaptic terminals (Wonnacott 1997). Nevertheless, nAChRs are also found at somato-dendritic, axonal, and postsynaptic sites (Sargent 1993). As a result of actions at the nAChR sites, nicotine stimulates the release of most neurotransmitters throughout the brain (Kenny et al. 2000; Grady et al. 2001). Therefore, various transmitter systems are involved in the rewarding effects of nicotine and in the adaptations that occur in response to chronic exposure to nicotine, which give rise to dependence and withdrawal symptoms.

Neuro-substrates of Nicotine Reinforcement. The meso-cortico-limbic brain system in the midbrain of mammals is composed of brain structures involved in the effects of drugs of abuse (Koob 2008). Among the main components of this system are the DAergic neurons originating in the ventral tegmental area (VTA) and projecting to the nucleus accumbens and the frontal cortex. The activity of these VTA-DA neurons is regulated by the release of the excitatory neurotransmitter glutamate from neuronal projections originating from several sites, including the nucleus accumbens and the frontal cortex. Other inputs that also regulate activity of the mesolimbic system are (1) γ-aminobutyric acid (GABA) inhibitory interneurons located within the VTA and the nucleus accumbens and (2) cholinergic projections from brainstem nuclei to the VTA. These cholinergic projections release ACh, which acts on excitatory nAChRs located on glutamate and GABA neuronal terminals in the VTA. Extensive studies have demonstrated a critical role of the meso-cortico-limbic system and its connections in several behavioral and affective responses to drugs of abuse, including nicotine.

DA and Nicotinic Acetylcholine Receptors. As with other drugs of abuse, it has been demonstrated that the mesolimbic DAergic system and nAChRs within that system are involved in the reinforcing properties of nicotine (Watkins et al. 2000; Picciotto and Corrigall 2002; Balfour 2004). Acute administration of nicotine increased the firing rate of DAergic neurons in the VTA (Pidoplichko et al. 1997) and elevated dialysate levels of DA in the shell of the nucleus accumbens (Nisell et al. 1997; Carboni et al. 2000). These effects of nicotine may occur through excitatory actions at nAChRs on the mesolimbic DAergic neurons in both the VTA and the nucleus accumbens and at nAChRs located on local neuronal circuitry within these brain regions (Teng et al. 1997). The nAChRs in the VTA plays more important role in the nucleus accumbens than the effect of nicotine on the release of DA from the nucleus accumbens (Nisell et al. 1997).

Several findings support that nAChRs located within the VTA are involved in nicotine reinforcement. I.V. nicotine self-administration is a procedure that allows assessment of the reinforcing effects of nicotine by measuring the number of infusions a rat chooses to receive i.v. through an indwelling permanent catheter by pressing a lever during 1 hr daily sessions in a testing chamber. Each of the 4 factors decreased i.v. nicotine self-administration in rats (Picciotto and Corrigall 2002). The factors were (1) injections of the competitive nAChR antagonist DHβE into the VTA (Williams and Robinson 1984) but not the nucleus accumbens (Corrigall et al. 1994), (2) development of lesions of the mesolimbic DA-ergic projections from the VTA to the nucleus accumbens (Corrigall et al. 1992), (3) development of cholinergic lesions of the brainstem pedunculo-pontine tegmental nucleus that project to the VTA (Lança et al. 2000), and (4) systemic administration of DA receptor antagonists (Corrigall and Coen 1991b). Studies suggest an involvement of the nAChR subtypes containing α4β2 in both the nicotine-induced release of DA and nicotine reinforcement (Grillner and Svensson 2000; Sharples et al. 2000). In addition, mutant mice with hypersensitive α4 nAChRs demonstrated a 50-fold increase in sensitivity to the reinforcing effects of nicotine measured by a place-preference procedure (Tapper et al. 2004). A place-preference procedure assesses the rewarding effects of a drug by measuring the preference for a compartment previously associated with the effects of a drug instead of a compartment associated with an injection of saline. The place-preference finding further indicated a critical role of α4 nAChRs in nicotine reinforcement. The α7 homomeric receptors may be involved in the reinforcing effects of nicotine. Methyllycaconitine, an antagonist with limited selectivity for the α7 nAChR, decreased the i.v. nicotine self-administration procedure in rats (Markou and Paterson 2001), although another study with rats showed no effects of this antagonist on nicotine-induced hyperactivity or nicotine self-administration (Grottick et al. 2000). Finally, both the α4β2 and α7 subtypes have been implicated in the effects of nicotine on memory (Bancroft and Levin 2000) and the anxiolytic effects of nicotine which also contribute to persistent tobacco use (Cheeta et al. 2001).

Glutamate. Other mechanisms by which nicotine may elevate striatal DA levels include increases in excitatory glutamatergic inputs from the frontal cortex to the nucleus accumbens and/or excitatory glutamatergic inputs to VTA DAergic neurons projecting to the striatum. Nicotine increases the release of glutamate by agonist actions at excitatory presynaptic nAChRs on glutamatergic terminals in various brain sites, including the VTA (Mansvelder and McGehee 2000), nucleus accumbens (Reid et al. 2000), prefrontal cortex (Gioanni et al. 1999), and hippocampus (Gray et al. 1996). In the VTA, nicotine acts at presynaptic $\alpha7$ nAChRs located on glutamate neurons (neurons that release glutamate as the primary neurotransmitter). Activation of these $\alpha7$ nAChRs on glutamate neurons (Mansvelder and McGehee 2000) increases the release of glutamate in the VTA. This activity, in turn, stimulates the release of DA in the nucleus accumbens (Fu et al. 2000). This increased release of glutamate acts on metabotropic and ionotropic glutamate receptors located on postsynaptic DA-ergic neurons (neurons that have DA as the primary neurotransmitter). Activation of these glutamate receptors leads to the excitation of the DAergic neurons that results in increased release of DA in terminal brain sites where these neurons project, as the nucleus accumbens, the amygdala and the frontal cortex.

Ionotropic antagonists of N-methyl-D-aspartate (NMDA) receptors blocked (prevented) tolerance to the locomotor depressant effects of acute nicotine administration (Shoaib et al. 1994) and blocked sensitization to the locomotor stimulant effects of chronic nicotine administration (Shoaib and Stolerman 1992). Blockade of the postsynaptic metabotropic glutamate receptor subtype 5 (mGluR5) with 2-methyl-6-(phenyl-ethynyl)pyridine (MPEP) decreased i.v. nicotine self-administration in rats and mice (Paterson et al. 2003) and decreased the motivation to self-administer nicotine (Paterson and Markou 2005). These effects were mediated by decreasing the Nicotine-stimulated release of DA in the mesolimbic system. In doses that blocked nicotine self-administration, MPEP had no effect on response for food. The progressive-ratio schedule of reinforcement, which gradually increases the response requirements after each earned reward, allows the assessment of the motivation for reinforcers, such as nicotine or food, by evaluating the maximal number of responses emitted by the rat (i.e., breaking point) to receive a single i.v. infusion of nicotine or a single food reward. In this schedule, MPEP had a greater effect on motivation for nicotine than on motivation for food, even when the magnitudes of reinforcer value were equated to support equal breaking points for nicotine and food under baseline conditions. This selectivity of the MPEP effects for nicotine reinforcement versus food reinforcement suggested that MPEP selectively blocks the reinforcing effects of nicotine without affecting motor performance or food reinforcement. Furthermore, evidence suggested a potential role of ionotropic glutamate receptors in the effects of nicotine. Animals that self-administered nicotine chronically exhibited an increase in ionotropic glutamate receptor subunits in brain regions, such as the VTA and the frontal cortex, that are implicated in the reinforcing effects of nicotine (Wang et al. 2007).

Molecular Mechanisms of Nicotinism. Activated nAChRs are permeable to both Na^+ ions and Ca^{2+}, which lead to activation of the neurons and thus the release of many neurotransmitters (Wonnacott et al. 2005). The widespread brain activation induced by acute or long-term administration of nicotine is shown by the expression of C-FOS in areas such as the amygdala, bed nucleus of the stria terminalis, lateral septum, hypothalamic nuclei, striatum, parts of the cortex, superior colliculus, optic tract, interpeduncular nucleus, supra-mammillary nucleus, periaqueductal gray matter, nucleus of the solitary tract, and locus coeruleus (Merlo Pich et al. 1999). C-FOS-related antigens are C-FOS proteins that heterodimerize with C-JUN proteins to produce complexes of activator protein-1 (AP-1) and transcriptionally regulate large numbers of genes related to plasticity (Merlo Pich et al. 1997). Another protein that researchers have studied extensively is the cyclic adenosine monophosphate–response element binding protein (CREB), because it is part of the signaling cascade for several receptors, including nAChRs (Nestler 2001). Acute treatment with nicotine had no effect on levels of total CREB or phosphorylated CREB (p-CREB). However, 18 hrs after the withdrawal from long-term administration of nicotine, the total concentrations of CREB and p-CREB decreased in the shell but not in the core of the nucleus accumbens (Pluzarev and Pandey 2004) and in the medial and basolateral amygdala but not in the central amygdala (Pandey et al. 2001; Pandey et al. 2007). The high Ca^{2+} permeability of nAChRs also stimulates additional intracellular messenger systems such as calmodulin-dependent protein kinases, including Ca^{2+} calmodulin-dependent protein kinase II (CaMKII), which is the most abundant kinase in the brain (Schulman and Hanson 1993). Acute administration of nicotine in mice induced increases in CaMKII expression in the spinal cord that was involved in the antinociceptive effects of nicotine (Damaj 2000). These are a few examples of the molecular changes observed after acute or long-term administration of nicotine and on withdrawal from long-term administration, suggesting that nicotine induces changes in molecular mechanisms involved in long-term plasticity. Such molecular effects are likely to mediate several aspects of nicotinism.

Psychiatric Comorbidity in Nicotinism

Antidepressant and Antipsychotic Drugs and Nicotine Withdrawal. Another experimental approach used to identify systems that mediate nicotine withdrawal and dependence is a study of pharmacologic manipulations that reverse spontaneous nicotine withdrawal. Inferences can be made regarding the underlying abnormality associated with withdrawal through the mechanisms associated with the pharmacotherapy. Based on the phenomenological similarities among depression, the depression-like aspects of nicotine withdrawal, and the negative symptoms of schizophrenia, researchers hypothesize that overlapping neurobiological substrates may mediate these depressive symptoms and that antidepressant and atypical antipsychotic treatments would alleviate the depression-like symptoms of nicotine withdrawal (Markou and Kenny 2002). Such common substrates mediating nicotine dependence and psychiatric disorders may explain the high prevalence of tobacco smoking among psychiatric populations. Compared with the percentage of smokers in the general population (20–30%), a higher percentage of mentally ill patients were smokers (26–88%, depending on the mental illness) (Lasser et al. 2000), particularly those with schizophrenia, depression, or addiction to alcohol or other drugs (Hughes et al. 1986; Glassman et al. 1990; Breslau 1995).

DSST-CS Biomarkers from Biological Fluids for Early Theranostics of Chronic MDR Malignancies and other Disease. DSST biomarkers for an early EBPT of chronic MDR diseases can be determined by performing simple lab procedures such as microtiter protein determination, colorimetric ELISA, immunoblotting, and RT-PCR. For example, DSST-CSF biomarkers will facilitate in the early detection of compromised brain regional MB and early detection and clinical management of PD, AD, HD, dementia, multidrug addiction, schizophrenia, epilepsy, MDDs, MS, and stroke. The most significant CS biomarkers are Cyt-C, iron, acetaldehyde, H_2O_2, ammonia, 2, 3 dihydroxy nonenal, 8-OH, 2dG, GAPDH, Bax, lactate, caspase-3, cholesterol regulator TSPO (18 KDa), MAOs, and Ca^{2+} channel regulators (TRPCs), which can be estimated by multiplex fluorescence ELISA, antibody microarray, and by pathways specific cDNA microarrays. In a cell free system, DSST-CS biomarkers can be analyzed from the peripheral blood and hematopoietic tissue by multiple fluorochrome flow cytometric analysis equipped with a sorting facility. The quantitative analysis of DSST-CS biomarkers from tears can be utilized for the early theranostics of various ocular diseases such as cataracts, glaucoma, and macular degeneration associated with diabetic neuropathies. DSST-CS biomarkers from saliva can help in the early theranostics of oral diseases, cancer, gastrointestinal and hepatic diseases accompanied with nicotinism and other drugs of abuse. DSST-CS biomarkers analysis from nasal discharge can be helpful in the early theranostics of various pulmonary diseases including lung cancer, COPDs (asthma, emphysema, and bronchitis) linked to nicotine abuse by employing combinatorial and correlative charnosomic analysis. Similarly, blood serum and plasma samples can be utilized to determine DSST-CS biomarkers for the early theranostics of NDDs, CVDs, and MDR malignancies associated with nicotinism and other diseases. DSST-CS biomarker analysis of urine samples can help in the early theransotics of renal diseases linked to chronic tobacco abuse. The analysis of DSST-CS biomarkers from semen samples can help in detecting prostate cancer and the basic molecular mechanism of infertility associated with nicotinism in males and from the vaginal and menstrual fluids of females to early detect fibroids, and endometrial and uterine/ovarian carcinoma. The analysis of DSST-CS biomarkers from hair samples can help in determining dermatological diseases and steroid hormone related abnormalities associated with alopecia and hypertrichosis. DSST-CS biomarkers from the ear wax can help in the early theranostics of hearing impairments. DSST-CS biomarker analysis of stool samples can help in determining liver and GIT diseases linked to nicotinism.

The major hypothesis is that all diseases initiate because of free radical-induced intracellular toxicity which is the primary cause of CMB, mitochondrial degeneration, and CB formation. Charnolophagy is an immediate and early attempt of ICD followed by CS formation, CS stabilization, and CS exocytosis/endocytosis. However, CS is a structurally and functionally highly labile intracellular organelle. A subsequent free radical attack due to chronic nicotinism can induce CS destabilization, characterized by permeabilization, sequestration, and fragmentation as described and explained with simple pictorial diagrams in this book. Hence, DSST-CS biomarkers-targeted charnolopharmacotherapeutics employing novel combinatorial and correlative charnolosomics developed to prevent or inhibit CB formation and augmentation of charnolophagy will be therapeutically-beneficial during acute phases, whereas CS stabilizers and CS exocytosis enhancers will be helpful during the chronic phase of disease progression. Thus, DSST biomarkers can be analyzed employing conventional omics and newly-introduced combinatorial and correlative charnolosomics to precisely evaluate the extent of CMB of human body in health and disease to accomplish the targeted, safe, and effective EBPT of nicotinism and associated illnesses.

Charnolosomics in Personalized Theranostics of MDR Diseases. Charnolosomics (CB-omics) can be utilized to precisely determine DSST mitochondrial bioenergetics (MB) and ICD utilizing modern biotechnologies (such as cDNA microarrays, antibody microarrays, microRNA microarrays, LC-MS, capillary electrophoresis, DNA sequencing, multiple fluorochrome flow cytometry, multiplex ELISA, SPR spectroscopy, and molecular imaging) along with combinatorial and correlative bioinformatics to accomplish the targeted, safe, and effective EBPT of NDDs, CVDs, MDR malignancies, and several other chronic diseases for human health, happiness, and better quality of life (BQL). CS is a byproduct of CB and charnolosomics refers to detailed molecular genetic and epigenetic analysis of CB biomarkers as highlighted in Fig. 39.

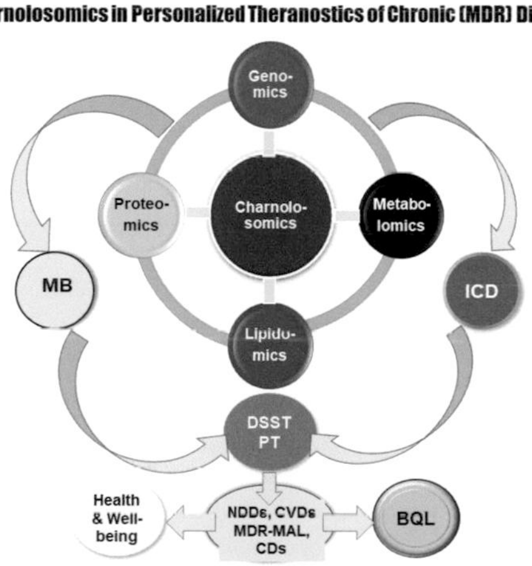

Charnolosomics in Personalized Theranostics of Chronic (MDR) Diseases

Fig. 39: Charnolosomics in personalized theranostics of chronic (MDR) diseases.

References

Balfour, D.J.K. 2004. The neurobiology of tobacco dependence: a preclinical perspective on the role of the DA projections to the nucleus accumbens. *Nicotine* & Tobacco Research 6: 899–912.

Bancroft, A. and E.D. Levin. 2000. Ventral hippocampal α4β2 nicotinic receptors and chronic *Nicotine* effects on memory. Neuropharmacology 39: 2770–2778.

Breslau, N., M.M. Kilbey and P. Andreski. 1994. DSM-III-R *Nicotine* dependence in young adults: prevalence, correlates and associated psychiatric disorders. Addiction 89: 743–754.

Carboni, E., L. Bortone, C. Giua and G. Di Chiara. 2000. Dissociation of physical abstinence signs from changes in extracellular DA in the nucleus accumbens and in the prefrontal cortex of *Nicotine* dependent rats. Drug and Alcohol Dependence 58: 93–102.

Cheeta, S., S. Tucci and S.E. File. 2001. Antagonism of the anxio-lytic effect of *Nicotine* in the dorsal raphé nucleus by dihydro-β-erythroidine. Pharmacology, Biochemistry, and Behavior 70: 491–496.

Corrigall, W.A. and K.M. Coen. 1991a. Opiate antagonists reduce *Cocaine* but not *Nicotine* self-administration. Psychopharmacology 104: 167–170.

Corrigall, W.A. and K.M. Coen. 1991b. Selective DA antagonists reduce *Nicotine* self-administration. Psychopharmacology 104: 171–176.

Corrigall, W.A., K.B.L. Franklin, K.M. Coen and P.B.S. Clarke. 1992. The mesolimbic DAergic system is implicated in the reinforcing effects of *Nicotine*. Psychopharmacology 107: 285–289.

Corrigall, W.A., K.M. Coen and K.L. Adamson. 1994. Self-administered *Nicotine* activates the mesolimbic DA system through the ventral tegmental area. Brain Research 653: 278–284.

Damaj, M.I. 2000. The involvement of spinal Ca^{2+}/calmodulin-protein kinase II in *Nicotine*-induced antinociception in mice. European Journal of Pharmacology 404: 103–110.

Fu, Y., S.G. Matta, W. Gao, V.G. Brower and B.M. Sharp. 2000. Systemic *Nicotine* stimulates DA release in nucleus accumbens: re-evaluation of the role of *N*-methyl-d-aspartate receptors in the ventral tegmental area. Journal of Pharmacology and Experimental Therapeutics 294: 458–465.

Glassman, A.H., J.E. Helzer, L.S. Covey, L.B. Cottler, F. Stetner, J.E. Tipp and J. Johnson. 1990. Smoking, smoking cessation, and major depression. JAMA: The Journal of the American Medical Association 264: 1546–1549.

Gioanni, Y., C. Rougeot, P.B. Clarke, C. Lepousé, A.M. Thierry and C. Vidal. 1999. Nicotinic receptors in the rat prefrontal cortex: increase in glutamate release and facilitation of mediodorsal thalamo-cortical transmission. Eur J Neurosci Jan 11(1): 18–30.

Grady, S.R., N.M. Meinerz, J. Cao, A.M. Reynolds, M.R. Picciotto, J.P. Changeux, J.M. McIntosh, M.J. Marks and A.C. Collins. 2001. Nicotinic agonists stimulate acetylcholine release from mouse interpeduncular nucleus: a function mediated by a different nAChR than DA release from striatum. Journal of Neurochemistry 76: 258–268.

Gray, R., A.S. Rajan, K.A. Radcliffe, M. Yakehiro and J.A. Dani. 1996. Hippocampal synaptic transmission enhanced by low concentrations of nicotine. Nature 383(6602): 713–736.

Grillner, P. and T.H. Svensson. 2000. *Nicotine*-induced excitation of midbrain DA neurons *in vitro* involves ionotropic glutamate receptor activation. Synapse 38: 1–9.

Grottick, A.J., G. Trube, W.A. Corrigall, J. Huwyler, P. Malherbe, R. Wyler and G.A. Higgins. 2000. Evidence that nicotinic α7 receptors are not involved in the hyperlocomotor and rewarding effects of *Nicotine*. Journal of Pharmacology and Experimental Therapeutics 294: 1112–1119.

Hughes, J.R., D.K. Hatsukami, J.E. Mitchell and L.A. Dahlgren. 1986. Prevalence of smoking among psychiatric outpatients. American Journal of Psychiatry 143: 993–997.

Kenny, P.J., S.E. File and M.J. Neal. 2000. Evidence for a complex influence of nicotinic acetylcholine receptors on hippo-campal serotonin release. Journal of Neurochemistry 75: 2409–2414.

Koob, G.F. 2008. Neurobiology of addiction. pp. 3–16. *In*: Galanter, M. and H.D. Kleber (eds.). The American Psychiatric Publishing. Textbook of Substance Abuse Treatment. 4th Edition. Arlington (VA): American Psychiatric Publishing.

Lança, A.J., K.L. Adamson, K.M. Coen, B.L.C. Chow and W.A. Corrigall. 2000. The pedunculopontine tegmental nucleus and the role of cholinergic neurons in *Nicotine* self-administration in the rat: a correlative neuroanatomical and behavioral study. Neuroscience 96: 735–742.

Lasser, K., J.W. Boyd, S. Woolhandler, D.U. Himmelstein, D. McCormick and D.H. Bor. 2000. Smoking and mental illness: a population-based prevalence study. JAMA: The Journal of the American Medical Association 284: 2606–2610.

Mansvelder, H.D. and D.S. McGehee. 2000. Long-term potentiation of excitatory inputs to brain reward areas by *Nicotine*. Neuron 27: 349–357.

Markou, A., T.R. Kosten and G.F. Koob. 1998. Neurobiological similarities in depression and drug dependence: a self-medication hypothesis. Neuropsychopharmacology 18: 135–174.

Markou, A. and N.E. Paterson. 2001. The nicotinic antagonist methyl-lycaconitine has differential effects on *Nicotine* self-administration and *Nicotine* withdrawal in the rat. *Nicotine* and Tobacco Research 3: 361–373.

Markou, A. and P.J. Kenny. 2002. Neuroadaptations to chronic exposure to drugs of abuse: relevance to depressive symptomatology seen across psychiatric diagnostic categories. Neurotoxicity Research 4: 297–313.

Markou, A. 2006. Neural pathways for γ-aminobutyric acid, glutamate, DA, and excitatory neurotransmitters (Wiley-Blackwell).

Merlo Pich, E., C. Chiamulera and L. Carboni. 1999. Molecular mechanisms of the positive reinforcing effect of *Nicotine*. Behavioral Pharmacology 10: 587–596.

Merlo Pich, E., S.R. Pagliusi, M. Tessari, D. Talabot-Ayer, R. Hooft van Huijsduijnen and C. Chiamulera. 1997. Common neural substrates for the addictive properties of *Nicotine* and *Cocaine*. Science 275(5296): 83–86.

Nestler, E.J. 2000. Genes and addiction. Nature Genetics 26: 277–281.

Nisell, M., M. Marcus, G.G. Nomikos and T.H. Svensson. 1997. Differential effects of acute and chronic *Nicotine* on DA output in the core and shell of the rat nucleus accumbens. Journal of Neural Transmission 104: 1–10.

Pandey, S.C., A. Roy, T. Xu and N. Mittal. 2001. Effects of protracted nicotine exposure and withdrawal on the expression and phosphorylation of the creb gene transcription factor in rat brain. J Neurochem 77(3): 943–952.

Panday, S., S.P. Reddy, R.A.C. Ruiter, E. Bergstrom and H. DeVries. 2007. *Nicotine* dependence and withdrawal symptoms among occasional smokers. Journal of Adolescent Health 40: 144–150.

Paterson, N.E., S. Semenova, F. Gasparini and A. Markou. 2003. The mGluR5 antagonist MPEP decreased *Nicotine* self-administration in rats and mice. Psychopharmacology 167: 257–264.

Paterson, N.E., A.W. Bruijnzeel, P.J. Kenny, C.D. Wright, W. Froestl and A. Markou. 2005a. Prolonged *Nicotine* exposure does not alter GABA$_B$ receptor-mediated regulation of brain reward function. Neuropharmacology 49: 953–962.

Paterson, N.E., W. Froestl and A. Markou. 2005b. Repeated administration of the GABA$_B$ receptor agonist CGP44532 decreased *Nicotine* self-administration, and acute administration decreased cue-induced reinstatement of *Nicotine*-seeking in rats. Neuropsychopharmacology 30: 119–128.

Paterson, N.E. and A. Markou. 2007. Animal models and treatments for addiction and depression co-morbidity. Neurotox Res 11: 1–32.

Picciotto, M.R. and W.A. Corrigall. 2002. Neuronal systems underlying behaviors related to *Nicotine* addiction: neural circuits and molecular genetics. Journal of Neuroscience 22: 3338–3341.

Pidoplichko, V.I., M. DeBiasi, J.T. Williams and J.A. Dani. 1997. *Nicotine* activates and desensitizes midbrain DA neurons [letter]. Nature 390: 401–404.

Pluzarev, O. and S.C. Pandey. 2004. Modulation of CREB expression and phosphorylation in the rat nucleus accumbens during *Nicotine* exposure and withdrawal. Journal of Neuroscience Research 77: 884–891.

Reid, M.S., L. Fox, L.B. Ho and S.P. Berger. 2000. Nicotine stimulation of extracellular glutamate levels in the nucleus accumbens: neuropharmacological characterization. Synapse 35(2): 129–136.

Robinson, T.E. and K.C. Berridge. 1993. The neural basis of drug craving: an incentive-sensitization theory of addiction. Brain Res Brain Res Rev 18: 247–291.

Sargent, P.B. 1993. The diversity of neuronal nicotinic acetylcholine receptors. Annu Rev Neurosci 16: 403–443.

Schulman, H. and P.I. Hanson. 1993. Multifunctional Ca^{2+}/calmodulin-dependent protein kinase. Neurochemistry Research 18: 65–77.

Sharma, S. 2017. Zika Virus Disease: Prevention and Cure. Nova Science Publishers, New York, U.S.A.

Sharma, S. 2017. Fetal Alcohol Spectrum Disorders: Concepts, Mechanisms, and Clinical Management. Nova Science Publishers, New York, U.S.A.

Sharma, S. 2017. Personalized Medicine: Beyond PET Biomarkers. Nova Science Publishers, New York, U.S.A.

Sharples, C.G.V., S. Kaiser, L. Soliakov, M.J. Marks, A.C. Collins, M. Washburn, E. Wright, J.A. Spencer, T. Gallagher, P. Whiteaker et al. 2000. UB-165: a novel nicotinic agonist with subtype selectivity implicates the α4β2 subtype in the modulation of DA release from rat striatal synaptosomes. Journal of Neuroscience 20: 2783–2791.

Shoaib, M. and I.P. Stolerman. 1992. MK801 attenuates behavioral adaptation to chronic *Nicotine* administration in rats. British Journal of Pharmacology 105: 514–515.

Shoaib, M., M.E.M. Benwell, M.T. Akbar, I.P. Stolerman and D.J.K. Balfour. 1994. Behavioural and neurochemical adaptations to *Nicotine* in rats: influence of NMDA antagonists. British Journal of Pharmacology 111: 1073–1080.

Tapper, A.R., S.L. McKinney, R. Nashmi, J. Schwarz, P. Deshpande, C. Labarca, P. Whiteaker, M.J. Marks, A.C. Collins and H.A. Lester. 2004. *Nicotine* activation of α4* receptors: sufficient for reward, tolerance, and sensitization. Science 306: 1029–1032.

Teng, L., P.A. Crooks, S.T. Buxton and L.P. Dwoskin. 1997. Nicotinic-receptor mediation of S(-)nor *Nicotine*-evoked [³H] overflow from rat striatal slices preloaded with [³H]dopamine. Journal of Pharmacology and Experimental Therapeutics 283: 778–787.

Wang, F., H. Chen, J.D. Steketee and B.M. Sharp. 2007. Upregulation of ionotropic glutamate receptor subunits within specific mesocorticolimbic regions during chronic *Nicotine* self-administration. Psychopharmacology 32: 103–109.

Watkins, S.S., L. Stinus, G.F. Koob and A. Markou. 2000. Reward and somatic changes during precipitated *Nicotine* withdrawal in rats: centrally and peripherally mediated effects. Journal of Pharmacology and Experimental Therapeutics 292: 1053–1064.

Williams, M. and J.L. Robinson. 1984. Binding of the nicotinic cholinergic antagonist, dihydro-β-erythroidine, to rat brain tissue. Journal of Neuroscience 4: 2906–2911.

Wonnacott, S. 1997. Presynaptic nicotinic ACh receptors. Trends in Neurosciences 20: 92–98.

Wonnacott, S., N. Sidhpura and D.J.K. Balfour. 2005. *Nicotine*: from molecular mechanisms to behavior. Current Opinion in Pharmacology 5: 53–59.

CHAPTER-18

Charnoly Body in ZIKA Virus Disease

INTRODUCTION

Usually a neuron may have anywhere between 200–1000 mitochondria, depending on its function and metabolic activity. Therefore, we should expect anywhere between 200–250 CBs in a physico-chemically-injured neuron such as Pukinje neuron. However, at any given time, we identified 10–12 mature CBs. The rest remained in different stages of origin, development, maturation, degradation, and elimination by charnolophagy depending on the nutritional status of the animal.

Brain is highly rich in mitochondria and is constantly dependent on TCA cycle-dependent energy (ATP) supply for its normal function. Two physiologically-significant events, "mitochondrial fusion & fission", occur during normal brain development in well-fed intrauterine microenvironment. The mtDNA and its redox balance remains structurally and functionally intact to sustain normal brain development in the well-nourished embryo. ZIKV infection during intrauterine life can cause progressive neurodegeneration due to free radical-induced CB formation which triggers apoptosis to cause microcephaly in the developing brain. This occurs due to the incorporation of viral genome with the host cell nuclear genome. Brain regional CB formation in response to ZIKV infection in highly vulnerable NPCs triggers apoptosis to cause microcephaly in the developing embryonic brain *in utero*. In developing embryonic brain particularly during first trimester (gastrulation) ZIKV infection can enhance lipid peroxidation, anti-inflammatory cytokine, IL-10 down-regulation, and pro-inflammatory cytokine IL-6 upregulation to cause further neurodegeneration due to CB formation leading to the inhibition of energy-driven charnolophagy and induction of lysosomal-resistant CB sequestration, which enhance intracellular toxicity to induce microcephaly. In adults, ZIKV infection remains localized and restricted to only mitochondrial degeneration. The incorporation of viral genome with the mitochondrial genome can only compromise MB and/or induce CB formation to cause milder symptoms such as (i) fatigue, (ii) fever, (iii) pain, rashes, and in rare cases, Guillian Barre' Syndrome as I have described in detail in my book: "Zika Virus Disease: Prevention and Cure".

In this chapter, I have described ZIKV-induced microcephaly by mitochondrial degeneration in the most vulnerable NPCs, derived from iPPCs through CB formation, charnolophagy induction, and CS destabilization.

ZIKV belongs to the Flaviviridae family of positive-strand RNA viruses that includes human pathogens, such as the mosquito-transmitted (i) Dengue virus (DENV), (ii) West Nile virus (WNV), (iii) Japanese encephalitis virus (JEV), (iv) Yellow fever virus (YFV), and (v) Tick-borne encephalitic virus. Due to the cutting of 50% Amazon trees, climate change, and global warming, the outbreak of Aedes mosquito in Brazil increased tremendously in the recent past. The center for disease control (CDC) issued a warning to the Central and South American countries regarding the deleterious consequences of ZIKV infection in developing embryo to cause microcephaly in the neonates. There are primarily two types of mosquitos: (i) Aedes aegypti and (ii) Aedes elbopictus. The estimated range of Aedes aegypti is less as compared to Aedes elbopictus. However, Aedes aegypti has been reported to cause maximum incidences of microcephaly. Some sporadic cases of ZIKV infection have also been reported in the US in 2015–2016. It is now realized that ZIKV disease and ZIKV congenital infection are nationally notifiable conditions. This update from the CDC Arboviral Disease Branch includes provisional data reported to ArboNET for January 01, 2015–June 08, 2016. In the US, travel-associated cases reported: 691; locally acquired vector-borne cases reported: 0 (Total: 691); sexually transmitted: 11; Guillain-Barré Syndrome: 2. In US Territories, travel-associated cases reported: 4; locally acquired cases reported: 1,301 (Total: 1,305); Guillain-Barré Syndrome: 7. The ZIKV infection cases have been reported in 62 countries. The ZIKV is now distributed not only in Americas, but has a global distribution, which has raised a serious concern among WHO authorities. In fact, WHO declared a ZIKV infection as a global emergency. Laboratory-confirmed ZIKV disease cases have been reported to ArboNET by state or territory-United States, 2015–2016.

In this chapter, I have highlighted the clinical significance of CB formation in the pathogenesis of ZIKV-induced microcephaly and is prevention and/or treatment with diet rich in proteins, vitamins, and antioxidants to prevent microcephaly because the development of vaccine will take at least couple of years according to WHO and CDC report.

Transmission of ZIKV Infection. It is now realized that transmission of ZIKV in developing brain occurs readily due to the absence of mature biological barriers including immunological, biochemical, and physiological barriers. The brain development occurs ~ 200 times faster in the utero particularly during gastrulation period of first trimester, which is the highly vulnerable to nicotine, alcohol and/or other drugs such as anesthetics, antidepressants, antipsychotic, and aminoglycoside in addition to microbial (bacteria, viral, and fungal) infection, including ZIKV.

Early and Delayed Consequences of CB Formation and Microcephaly. We reported that CB formation in highly-susceptible cells is associated with MAOs down-regulation/delocalization (depletion of 5-HT, NE, and DA) due to MAO-A-CB and MAO-B-CB formation [GIT and adrenal gland]; TSPO down-regulation/delocalization (depletion of mitochondrial steroidogenesis) [membrane destabilization & pro-inflammation]. CB formation in pediatric and geriatric population can induce acute diarrhea/acute constipation. Hippocampal CB formation is associated with loss of social, physical, mental, economical, sexual, and psychological drive, leading to early morbidity and mortality.

Structural Details of ZIKV. Recently Sirohi et al. (2016) determined the structural details of ZIKV by cryo-EM analyses. Its 3.8Å resolution Cryo-EM structure was elucidated. ZIKV possesses a single glycosylation site in the E protein (Asn154), whereas DENV is glycosylated at two sites within the E protein (Asn67 and Asn153). The structure is like other known flaviviruses, except ~ 10 amino acids that surround the Asn154 glycosylation site in each of the 180 envelope glycoproteins that make up the icosahedral shell. The carbohydrate moiety associated with this residue acts as an attachment site of the virus to host cells. This region also varies in other flaviviruses suggesting that differences in this region may influence virus transmission and disease. These structural details can help in developing a vaccine against ZIKV.

Clinical Symptoms of ZIKV Infection. ZIKV infection in adults is usually associated with very mild symptoms such as high fever, arthralgia, fatigue, red hot eyes, rhinorrhea; whereas in developing embryos, it can cause microcephaly. In adults, it is represented by febrile flu-like symptoms and neurological abnormalities (Gullan Barre' Syndrome). In addition to transmission by mosquitoes, ZIKV may be sexually and vertically transmitted. The structure, tropism, and pathogenesis of ZIKV remain unknown. However, there is a dire need for rapid development of vaccines and therapy for ZIKV infection. Microcephaly can be estimated by measuring the head circumference. The peripheral symptoms of ZIKV infection are very rare with certain evidence of folded skin in the foot pads. The mother's reaction is associated with anger, fear, worry, sorrow, and guilt.

Mechanism of Zika Viral Microcephaly. The exact peripheral symptoms are not yet fully established. Moreover, the exact cellular and molecular mechanism of microcephaly remains unknown. I have proposed that ZIKV compromises MB by down-regulating highly-vulnerable mitochondrial genome, which augments CB formation to cause apoptosis and eventually, microcephaly. Furthermore, ZIKV impairs normal function of endothelial progenitor cells involved in angiogenesis to cause severe damage to NPCs involved in early neurogenesis, that is, development of brain regional neurocircuitry in the developing brain. Although the delayed consequences of ZIKV microcephaly remain unknown, it will have significant impact on learning, intelligence, memory, behavior, and early morbidity associated with cognitive impairments and mortality. These children will suffer from severe cognitive impairments and/or delayed sensory-motor learning. Basic cellular and molecular events such as: tubulinogenesis, axonogenesis, neuritogenesis, myelinogenesis, synaptogenesis, and neurogenesis, gliogenesis, angiogenesis, and BBB formation are all compromised due to ZIKV infection *in utero*, which ultimately induce microcephaly. ZIKV infection through mosquito bite can even infect sperms to cause CMB and enhance oxidative stress and free radical overproduction to enhance CB formation, apoptosis, and eventually infertility. In addition, ZIKV compromises the MB, which augments CB formation to cause neuroapoptosis and eventually, microcephaly, with deleterious consequences.

CMB in ZIKV Microcephaly. Based on the electrophysiological and PET neuroimaging studies, we developed a kinetic equation to describe the CMB in the developing undernourished, MTs gene-manipulated, and wv/wv mice. ΔE was determined quantitatively by estimating the differences in the brain regional ^{18}FDG uptake in N and UN rats. ΔT was determined by estimating the differences in the duration of intracellular electrical activity of N and UN rat Purkinje neurons. Based on these electrophysiological and PET neuroimaging findings, a kinetic equation was developed as follows: $\Delta E = K\Delta T$, where K is a constant and depends on the nature of the neuron or any vulnerable cell during gastrulation phase.

Genetic Susceptibility of mtDNA. We proposed mitochondrial hypothesis of ZIKV microcephaly because the mtDNA is highly vulnerable to environmental and ZIKV-induced toxins. The mtDNA is uncoiled ring, GC-rich, intron less (that means it is devoid of any non-coding (introns), which renders it highly susceptible to almost any environmental and/or toxic insult). It has only coding regions (exons) and always remains unprotected in a hostile microenvironment of free radicals, generated as a byproduct of oxidative phosphorylation during ATP synthesis in the electron transport chain. The energy requirement for the intramitochondrial and intracellular compartment are significantly elevated during oxidative and nitrative stress and following toxic exposure. The mtDNA is devoid of histones and protamines which provide structural and functional stability to the nDNA during transcriptional activation of genes involved in growth, proliferation, differentiation, and development. The mtDNA is highly susceptible to methylation as it remains naked and exposed to methyl residues available from S-adenosyl methionine (SAM) involved in DNA methylation. On the other hand, nDNA is double helical elongated coil with coding (exons) and non-coding (introns) regions and a protected free radical-independent micro-environment. Gene transcription is regulated by adequate microenvironment and inducers. In the mitochondria, the microenvironment remains hostile and the inducers constantly influence the sensitive mtDNA. The nDNA remains protected by the double nuclear wall, nucleoplasm, and further strength is provided by histones and protamines which are acetylated during epigenetic changes due to neurotoxic insult such as ZIKV infection. Epigenetic changes with miRNA can also influence nDNA to cause changes in gene expression. This was confirmed by preparing RhO_{mgko} neurons, which demonstrate stunted neuritogenesis, elliptical appearance, reduced metabolic activity, and de-differentiation. However, their proliferative potential remains structurally and functionally intact while their complex-1 gene is significantly down-regulated, indicating that the down-regulation of the complex-1 gene can significantly compromise the MB and these cells cannot synthesize sufficient ATP to perform normal physiological activity.

Main Hypothesis. (i) The mtDNA remains structurally and functionally-intact during mitochondrial fission as well as fusion, while it is destroyed during free-radical-induced CB formation involved in neurodegenerative apoptosis and microcephaly, as we confirmed in RhO_{mgko} cells. (ii) The Zika viral genome can destroy mtDNA but cannot replicate when its genome gets incorporated with the mitochondrial genome.

Various Other Causes of Microcephaly. In addition to ZIKV, cytomegalovirus, rubella virus, toxoplasma, undernutrition, Zn^{2+} deficiency, folate deficiency, drug (nicotine, alcohol) addiction, neurotoxic drugs, anesthetics, anti-epileptics, antipsychotics, antidepressants, can also cause microcephaly involving CB molecular pathogenesis during intrauterine life.

Therapeutic Potential of Nutrition. We have reported that the brain to body weight ratio is significantly increased in severe malnutrition, whereas nutritional rehabilitation reduces brain/body weight ratio as well as eliminates CB formation in the highly vulnerable developing neurons to prevent microcephaly.

Correlation of ZIKV Microcephaly with Drug Abuse. It has been noticed that there is high prevalence of drug abuse and ZIKV infection in Central and South America, where the maximum number of children have been born with microcephaly. Hence, there were potential risk factors even in Olympic Games in Rio de Janeiro, Brazil. These included but were not limited to stress (which can increase circulating cortisol levels to induce microglial activation and cytokine TNFα and NFκβ-mediated neurodegeneration), infection, inadequate nutritional status, susceptible reproductive age (18–35 years), susceptibility to drug abuse, insanitation, indulgence in unprotected sex, excessive intake of coffee, nicotine, alcohol, and fat. We proposed that ZIKV infection + alcohol abuse during pregnancy may induce synergistic microcephaly by triggering CB molecular pathogenesis. Thus, synergistic consequences of ZIKV infection and fetal alcohol will cause not only craniofacial abnormalities but also microcephaly. Hence, ZIKV+alcohol-induced CMB augments lysosome-resistant CB formation to induce deleterious consequences on the developing embryo. Hence, microcephaly can be assessed by evaluating the following equation: $\Delta E = K\Delta T$

Development of CB-Targeted Drugs to Prevent/Treat Microcephaly. As we proposed the mitochondrial hypothesis of ZIKV-induced microcephaly, various antioxidants as free radical scavengers will find their pivotal role in EBPT of these victims. As potent free radical scavengers, MTs prevent and/or inhibit different phases of CB formation. Hence, charnolo-pharmaco-therapeutic agents inhibiting CB formation and/or inducing charnolophagy during the acute phase of ZIKV infection can prevent apoptosis and hence, microcephaly. Charnolophagy is an efficient basic molecular mechanism of ICD, which is an energy driven process and requires ATP and structurally and functionally intact mitochondria. Hence, ICD escapes microcephaly.

ZIKV-induced Neurodegeneration Causes Microcephaly. The ZIKV-induced neurodegeneration can be systematically described in following systematic steps: A: Random Distribution of Mitochondria, B: Virus Attachment and Endocytosis, C: Perinuclear Mitochondrial Aggregation, D: Viral Attachment with Mitochondria, E: CB formation due to Incorporation of Viral Genome with Nuclear Genome and Apoptosis, F: Microcephaly and/or Morbidity, Impaired Neuro-Cybernetics, and Cognition. Normal Developing Vulnerable Neuron-ZIKV-Infected Neuron-Viral Endocytosis-Viral-Induced Mitochondrial Degeneration-CB formation Nuclear DNA Damage and Apoptosis (Neurodegeneration)-Microcephaly, Malnutrition, Zinc Deficiency, Folate Deficiency, Environmental Toxins, Toxoplasma, Rubella, Alcohol, Anesthetics and Anti-epileptics (ZIKV Infection).

Prevention of Intrauterine Neurotoxic Insult (Microcephaly)

Therapeutic Interventions in Microcephaly. Several antioxidants can provide therapeutic benefit by preventing and/or treating ZIKV-induced microcephaly. These antioxidants include: MTs, CoQ_{10}, melatonin, resveratrol, quercetin, surtuins, rutins, polyphenol, lycopene, catechin, LSDs, and many more. The antioxidants inhibit CB formation as free radical scavengers and may enhance neuro-regeneration. In addition, refraining from drugs of abuse can also prevent the deleterious consequences of ZIKV microcephaly. The most significant drugs of abuse are alcohol, nicotine, and coffee. Moderate exercise by ZIKV-infected pregnant mother can also help in maintaining the normal physiological status of the developing fetal brain. Although antioxidants available from natural sources are efficacious, their reduced potency remains a significant challenge. It is now realized that cortisol, BDNF, IGF-1, and NGF can also influence normal brain development. In addition, specific CB antagonists, charnolophagy agonists, inhibitors of microglial activation, apoptosis, and neurodegeneration can prevent or attenuate deleterious consequences of ZIKV-induced microcephaly. Particularly, resveratrol available from grapes will be more beneficial rather than from wine as its levels in a 120-ml volume of wine is hardly 120 µg, whereas we need 250–450 mg resveratrol every day.

CB as a Universal Biomarker for Personalized Theranostics in Microcephaly. We need to have preventive as well as therapeutic interventions during acute and chronic phase of ZIKV-induced microcephaly. These interventions can prevent the progression of devastating deleterious consequences of ZIKV microcephaly. We need to establish preventive and therapeutic interventions to tackle acute vs chronic ZIKV toxicity to prevent craniofacial abnormalities. CB can be used as a novel biomarker for theranostic interventions in microcephaly. During the acute phase, drugs inhibiting CB formation and enhancing charnolophagy will be highly beneficial for an early escape from ZIKV-induced microcephaly. During the chronic phase, lysosome-resistant CB sequestration can cause apoptosis via CB formation to induce further microcephaly during this phase. Hence, it will be highly prudent to develop novel DSST charnolopharmacotherapeutic agents which could inhibit CB sequestration, and induce CS stabilization and its exocytosis to prevent further progressive neurodegeneration in severe microcephaly.

Clinical Management of Microcephaly. We established that MTs provide neuroprotection as free radical scavengers and CB inhibitors. Hence, physiological and/or pharmacological interventions augmenting brain regional MTs or other antioxidants may provide neuroprotection to prevent ZIKV microcephaly.

Experimental Model of Microcephaly and Progressive Neurodegeneration. We raised wv/wv mice as an experimental model of progressive neurodegeneration and microcephaly. These experimental genotypes exhibit point mutation in the inward rectifying K^+ channel, and, as a result, increased $[Ca^{2+}]_i$ occurs which causes apoptosis through CB formation. About 40% of these genotypes exhibit early mortality and the rest exhibit signs of morbidity and mortality. These genotypes exhibit neurodegeneration in the hippocampal CA-3 and dentate gyrus region which is a seat of memory, in the striatum, which is a seat of motor activity, and in the cerebellar Purkinje neurons which is involved in co-ordination of muscular activity and motor learning. All these sensory modalities are impaired in microcephaly and chronic drug addiction. MTs are down-regulated in wv/wv mice and they exhibit progressive DA-ergic neurodegeneration. Since these genotypes exhibit typical symptoms of Parkinsonims due to loss of striatal neurons, we proposed to microinject mesencephalic stem cells derived from MT_{trans} embryos and evaluate the structural and functional integrity of these cells with the host cells by performing microPET neuroimaging with ^{18}F-DOPA. Although this procedure has theranostic significance; due to ethical issues regarding stem cell applications, we adopted a unique and novel approach. To confirm that indeed MTs provide neuroprotection as free radical scavengers and hence, CB antagonists, we developed a colony of wv/wv-MTs mice by crossbreeding MT_{trans} male mice with female wv/wv mice, because wv/wv male mice are infertile. The progeny was screened by tail DNA PCR analysis. The wv/wv-MTs mice exhibited prevention of microcephaly and the MB was regained. We confirmed these findings by microPET neuroimaging with ^{18}F-DOPA and ^{18}FDG as sensitive molecular biomarkers of brain regional DA-ergic neurotransmission and MB respectively.

Prevention of Microcephaly. We determined ΔE by calculating the difference in the brain regional radioactivity from C57Bl/6J, $control_{wt}$, and wv/wv and wv/wv-MTs mice, and simultaneously recording the difference in the duration of intracellular electrical discharge activity to determine ΔT to generate the following kinetic equation: $\Delta E = K\Delta T$. Both ΔE and ΔT approached almost zero in wv/wv/MT mice when compared with normal wild type controls. Similar results were obtained in the nutritionally-rehabilitated developing UN and vitamin B_6-deficient rats. In nutritionally-rehabilitated rats, ΔE and ΔT approached zero suggesting that nutritional stress, antioxidant imbalance, and vitamin-deficiency can induce progressive neurodegeneration in the developing brain; hence, well-nourished protein-rich diet, antioxidants, and vitamins are highly essential to prevent and/or treat microcephaly. CB formation compromises mitochondrial bioenergetics to induce apoptosis and eventually microcephaly, whereas MTs avert microcephaly by preventing CB formation. MTs-mediated neuroprotection is routed through its action as potent free radical scavengers to inhibit CB formation and prevent microcephaly. MTs also provide protection from microcephaly by regulating the transcriptional activity of genes involved in growth, proliferation, differentiation, and development by donating Zn^{2+} ions in the nucleus (Sharma and Ebadi 2013). We also discovered that MTs provide ubiquinone (CoQ_{10})-mediated neuroprotection in PD and chronic drug addiction.

MTs-mediated Neuroprotection. MTs-mediated neuroprotection was confirmed by estimating the striatal CoQ_{10}, ATP, TH, dopamine, and neuromelanin which were significantly increased and MAOs and Fe^{3+} levels were reduced by MTs over-expression in wv/wv-MTs mice, indicating that MTs prevent microcephaly by inhibiting CB formation.

Different Stages of ZIKV Infection. ZIKV infection can be divided in different phases. Phase-1 is associated with induction which triggers microcephaly. The release of proinflammatory cytokines such as IL-6 and downregulation of anti-inflammatory cytokine IL-10 in the cortical neurons causes microcephaly. We discovered for the first time IL-10 receptors on the cortical neurons. Most probably, ZIKV infection inhibits IL-10 receptors on the cortical neurons to prevent their growth, proliferation, and differentiation. We reported that IL-10 receptors mediate IP3/AKT signaling involved in anti-inflammatory and anti-apoptotic activity.

Prevention/Therapeutics of ZIKV-induced Microcephaly. ZIKV-mediated free radical overproduction enhances, whereas antioxidants inhibit CB formation. Hence, free radical scavengers, CB inhibitors, and antioxidants can be used for the prevention/ therapeutics of ZIKV-induced microcephaly. Furthermore, vaccine and/or drugs may be developed to prevent and/or inhibit CB formation involved in microcephaly and progressive neurodegeneration in the developing brain.

Personalized Theranostics of ZIKV-Microcephaly. Although there is no specific guideline to treat ZIKV-induced microcephaly, based on experimental studies on developing UN mice, and MTs gene-manipulated mice, we provided the following recommendations: (i) prevention (drug-free: coffee, nicotine, ethanol), (ii) mosquito eradication, (iii) symptomatic treatment, and (iv) environmental control, proper nutrition, antioxidants, sanitation, personal hygiene, protected sex and vaccination can help in the effective EBPT of ZIKV microcephaly. In addition, avoiding tobacco, alcohol, cannabis, METH, cocaine, and opioids (morphine, heroin) could also help maintain normal brain during embryonic development.

MTs Inhibit CB Formation. MTs inhibit CB formation by serving as potent free radical scavengers. Free radicals are generated as a byproduct of mitochondrial oxidative phosphorylation and provide ubiquinone (CoQ_{10})-mediated mitochondrial neuroprotection by inhibiting CB formation involved in apoptosis, neurodegeneration, and early morbidity and mortality. Glutathione and MAO inhibitors also provide neuroprotection in AD as illustrated in Fig. 40.

ZIKV-induced Microcephaly. ZIKV infected pregnancy can induce microcephaly in the developing brain *in utero* by causing severe oxidative and nitrative stress to cause free radical overproduction which cause lipid peroxidation to induce structural and functional breakdown of PUFA in the plasma membranes and mtDNA downregulation by oxidation of guanosine to synthesize 8-OH, 2DG as a mtDNA oxidative product. 8-OH, 2dG can be determined in the serum, plasma, saliva, CSF, and urine samples of

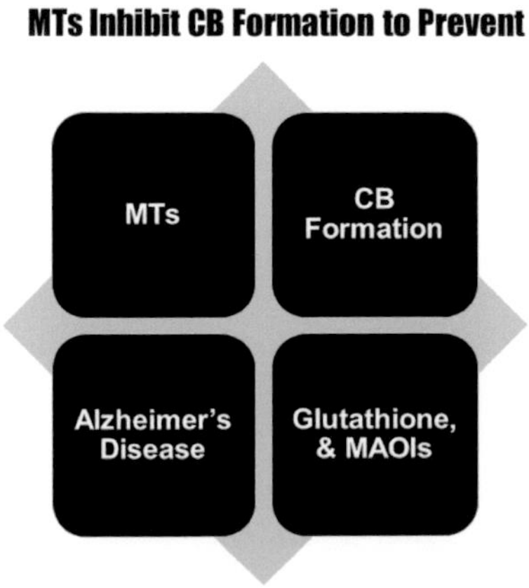

MTs Inhibit CB Formation to Prevent AD

Fig. 40: MTs inhibit CB formation to prevent AD.

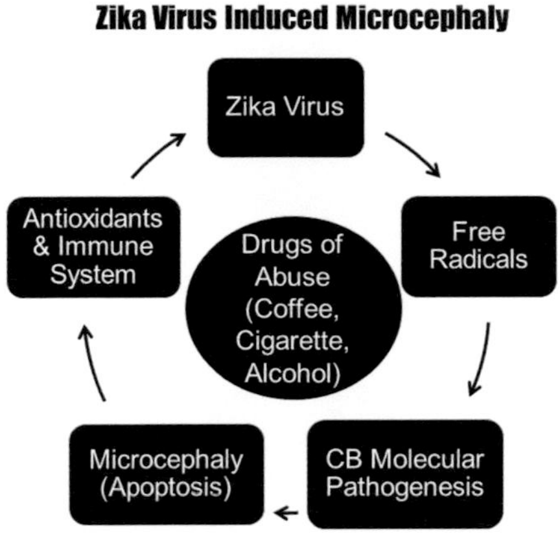

Zika Virus Induced Microcephaly

Fig. 41: Zika virus-induced microcephaly.

victims suffering from progressive neurodegeneration due to ZIKV-induced or other types of microcephaly due to CB formation and CMB. The CMB can be estimated quantitatively by estimating electrophysiological and microPET imaging parameters to derive the kinetic equation which determines the precise threshold of CB formation in a susceptible cell. It is now well established that CB formation triggers apoptosis/necrosis to cause microcephaly. The extent of microcephaly will depend on the nutritional and antioxidants and redox status of a cell under investigation. Hence, antioxidants and robust immune system will prevent and/or inhibit CB formation, whereas drugs of abuse including coffee, cigarette, and alcohol will augment ZIKV and/or other forms of microcephaly as illustrated in Fig. 41.

Mosquito Eradication. (Mosquito-borne ZIKV infection) ZIKV eradication in Brazil workers disinfected the Sambadrome in Rio de Janeiro, Brazil, ahead of the beginning of Rio's Carnival parade. Brazilian officials mobilized 220,000 troops to help eradicate the Aedes mosquito (Marcelo Sayao/EPA).

Prevention and Treatment of ZIKV Microcephaly. ZIKV microcephaly can be prevented by (i) augmenting MB and (ii) preventing/inhibiting/eradicating CB formation. Clinical management of microcephaly can be made by novel drug discovery which could prevent ZIKV entry in the developing brain. It can be prevented by developing novel CB antagonists, and vaccine. Treatment of ZIKV microcephaly is possible by developing novel charnolophagy agonists, CS stabilizers, and CB sequestration inhibitors.

Synergistic and Antagonistic Microcephaly. Based on our recent and previous findings, we proposed two types of microcephaly: (a) synergistic microcephaly and (b) antagonistic microcephaly. Drug of abuse (alcohol, coffee, cigarettes, and others) enhance mitochondrial oxidative and nitrative stress to generate excessive free radicals which can induced lipid peroxidation to cause structural and functional breakdown of PUFA to cause degeneration of plasma membranes. These deleterious intracellular events induce mtDNA and membrane degeneration to cause CB formation, involved in apoptosis, and progressive neurodegeneration to induce synergistic microcephaly, whereas antioxidants, well-nourished diet, and robust immune system prevents inflammatory apoptosis to prevent CB formation in the developing brain, which can be evaluated by performing *in vivo* molecular imaging to quantitatively assess antagonistic microcephaly.

ZIKV-induced Microcephaly. ZIKV infected pregnancy can induce microcephaly in the developing brain *in utero* by free radical-induced lipid peroxidation involved in structural and functional breakdown of PUFA in the plasma membranes and mtDNA oxidation. The oxidation of mtDNA occurs at the guanosine residues to synthesize 8-OH, 2DG which can be estimated in the serum, plasma, saliva, CSF, and urine samples of victims suffering from neurodegeneration due to ZIKV-induced or other types of microcephaly due to CB formation due to CMB. The MB can be estimated by electrophysiological and microPET imaging parameters to derive the kinetic equation and determine the precise threshold of CB formation in a susceptible cell. It is now well established that CB formation triggers apoptosis/necrosis to cause microcephaly. The extent of microcephaly will depend on the nutritional, antioxidants, and redox status of a cell under investigation. Hence, antioxidants and robust immune system can prevent and/or inhibit CB formation, whereas drugs of abuse including coffee, cigarette, alcohol, and improper dietary and physical habits will augment ZIKV and/or other forms of microcephaly.

ZIKV Surveillance and Preparedness. ZIKV rapidly spread through the WHO's Region of the Americas since being identified in Brazil in early 2015. Transmitted primarily through the bite of infected Aedes species mosquitoes, ZIKV infection during pregnancy can cause spontaneous abortion and birth defects, including microcephaly. Lee et al. (2016) recently reported that New York City (NYC) is the home of large number of persons who travel frequently to areas with active ZIKV transmission, including immigrants from these areas. In Nov 2015, the NYC Department of Health and Mental Hygiene (DOHMH) began developing and implementing plans for managing ZIKV and on Feb 1, 2016, activated its incident command system. During Jan 1–June 17, 2016, DOHMH coordinated diagnostic lab testing for 3,605 persons with travel-associated exposure, 182 (5.0%) of whom had confirmed ZIKV infection. Twenty (11.0%) confirmed patients were pregnant at the time of diagnosis. In addition, two cases of ZIKV-associated Guillain-Barré syndrome were diagnosed. DOHMH's response focused on (1) identifying and diagnosing suspected cases; (2) educating the public and medical providers about ZIKV risks, transmission, and prevention strategies, particularly in areas with large populations of immigrants from areas with ongoing ZIKV transmission; (3) monitoring pregnant women with ZIKV infection and their fetuses and infants; (4) detecting local mosquito-borne transmission through both human and mosquito surveillance; and (5) modifying existing Culex mosquito control measures by targeting Aedes species of mosquitoes through the use of larvicides and adulticides.

ZIKV Infection Symptoms and Prevention. Abbasi (2016) recently reported that ZIKV infection presents as a mild illness with symptoms lasting for several days to a week after the bite of an infected mosquito. Majority of the patients have low grade fever, rash, headaches, joints pain, myalgia, and flu like symptoms. Pregnant women are more vulnerable to ZIKV infection and serious congenital anomalies can occur in fetus through trans-placental transmission. ZIKV infection acquired in early pregnancy poses greater risk. There is no evidence so far about transmission through breast milk. Fetal microcephaly, Guillian Barre' Syndrome, and other neurological and autoimmune syndromes have been reported in areas where ZIKV outbreaks have occurred. As infection is usually mild so no specific treatment is required. Pregnant women may be advised to take rest and get plenty of fluids. For fever and pain, they can take antipyretics like paracetamol. So far, no specific drugs or vaccines are available against ZIKV infection; so prevention is the mainstay against this disease. As ZIKV infection is a vector borne disease, prevention can be a multi-pronged strategy: These entail vector control interventions, personal protection, environmental sanitation, and health education among others.

Prenatal Brain MRI of Fetuses with ZIKV Infection. An outbreak of ZIKV was observed in French Polynesia in 2013–2014. Maternal ZIKV infection is associated with fetal microcephaly and severe cerebral damage. To analyze the MRI cerebral findings in fetuses with intrauterine ZIKV infection, Guillemette-Artur et al. (2016) retrospectively analyzed prospectively collected data. Inclusion criteria comprised cases with (1) estimated conception date between June 2013 and May 2014, (2) available US and MRI scans revealing severe fetal brain lesions, and (3) positive PCR for ZIKV in the amniotic fluid. These investigators recorded the pregnancy history of ZIKV infection and analyzed US and MRI scans. Three out of 12 cases of severe cerebral lesions fulfilled all inclusion criteria. The history of maternal ZIKV infection had been documented in two cases. Calcifications and ventriculomegaly were present at US in all cases. MRI revealed microcephaly (n = 3), low cerebellar biometry (n = 2), occipital subependymal pseudocysts (n = 2), polymicrogyria with laminar necrosis and opercular dysplasia (n = 3), absent (n = 1) or hypoplastic (n = 1) corpus callosum, and hypoplastic brainstem (n = 1). Severe cerebral damage was observed, with indirect findings suggesting that the germinal matrix is the principal target for ZIKV. The lesions are like severe forms of congenital cytomegalovirus and lymphocytic choriomeningitis virus infections.

Screening of Blood Donations for ZIKV Infection. Recently, Kuehnert et al. (2016) reported transfusion-transmitted infections for several arboviruses, including West Nile and Dengue viruses. ZIKV, a flavivirus transmitted primarily by Aedes aegypti mosquitoes that has been identified as a cause of congenital microcephaly and other serious brain defects, became recognized as a potential threat to blood safety after reports from a 2013–2014 outbreak in French Polynesia. Blood safety concerns were based on very high infection incidence in the population during epidemics, the high percentage of persons with asymptomatic infection, the high proportion of blood donations with evidence of ZIKV nucleic acid upon retrospective testing, and an estimated 7–10-day period of viremia. At least one instance of transfusion transmission of ZIKV was documented in Brazil after the virus emerged there, likely in 2014. A rapid epidemic spread has followed to other areas of the Americas, including Puerto Rico.

Initial Detection and Management for ZIKV Patients. ZIKV is a vector-borne disease transmitted primarily by the Aedes aegypti mosquito. Male to female sexual transmission has been reported and there is potential for transmission via blood transfusions. After an incubation period of 2–7 days, symptomatic patients develop rapid onset fever, maculopapular rash, arthralgia, and conjunctivitis, often associated with headache and myalgias. Emergency department (ED) personnel must be prepared to address concerns from patients presenting with symptoms consistent with acute ZIKV infection, especially those who are pregnant or planning travel to ZIKV-endemic regions, as well as those women planning to become pregnant and their partners. The identify-isolate-inform (3I) tool, originally conceived for initial detection and management of Ebola virus disease patients in the ED, and later adjusted for measles and Middle East Respiratory Syndrome, can be adapted for real-time use for any emerging infectious disease. Koenig et al. (2016) reported a modification of the 3I tool for initial detection and management of patients under investigation for ZIKV. Following an assessment of epidemiologic risk, including travel to countries with mosquitoes that transmit ZIKV, patients are further investigated if clinically indicated. If after a rapid evaluation, ZIKV or other arthropod-borne diseases are the only concern, isolation (contact, droplet, airborne) is unnecessary. Zika is a reportable disease and thus, the appropriate health authorities must be notified. These investigators emphasized that the modified 3I tool will facilitate rapid analysis and appropriate actions for patients presenting to the ED at risk for ZIKV disease.

Polyphenol, EGCG in Green Tea Inhibits ZIKV Entry in the Cultured Cells. During ZIKV, the outbreak in Brazil, observed an increase of ~ 20 times the number of reported cases of microcephaly in newborn babies was obsorbed. There is no vaccine or approved drug available for the treatment and prevention of infections by this virus. EGCG, a polyphenol present in green tea has been shown to have an antiviral activity for many viruses. In view of the need for the development of a drug against a Brazilian strain of ZIKV, Carneiro et al. (2016) assessed the effect of EGCG on ZIKV entry in Vero E6 cells. The drug inhibited the virus entry by at least 1-log (> 90%) at higher concentrations (> 100 μM). The pre-treatment of cells with EGCG did not show any effect on virus attachment. This was the first study to demonstrate the effect of EGCG on ZIKV indicating that this drug might be used for the prevention of ZIKV infection.

Request for Abortion. Recently, Aiken et al. (2016) highlighted that on Nov 17, 2015, the Pan American Health Organization (PAHO) issued an epidemiologic alert regarding ZIKV in Latin America. Several countries subsequently issued health advisories, including cautions about microcephaly, declarations of national emergency, and unprecedented warnings urging women to avoid pregnancy. Yet in most Latin American countries, abortion is illegal or highly restricted, leaving pregnant women with few options. For several years, one such option for women in Latin America has been Women on Web (WoW), a nonprofit organization that provides access to abortion medications (mifepristone and misoprostol) outside the formal health care setting, through online means.

Vector-Borne Challenge to Cambat ZIKV Outbreak. Recently, Shoaib et al. (2016) reported that ZIKV is a single-stranded RNA virus of the Flaviviridae family. It is known to transmit to humans primarily through the bite of an infected Aedes species mosquito which is also known to carry dengue, chikungunya, and yellow fever virus. Transmission is anthroponotic (human-to-vector-to-human) during outbreaks, perinatally *in utero*, sexually, and via infected blood transfusion. It is a mild and self-limiting infection lasting for several days to a week. However, it is suspected as a cause of Guillain Barre' Syndrome. There is a teratogenic association of ZIKV causing congenital birth defects like microcephaly and neurologic abnormalities. Treatment is generally supportive and for symptomatic relief. No specific antiviral treatment or vaccine is yet available for ZIKV disease. It highlights importance of preventive public health measures at the community level and avoids travelling to the endemic areas.

Development of Vaccine. Three months after the WHO declared the epidemic of ZIKV infections to be a Public Health Emergency of International Concern, we can look back at what we have learned and the prospects of controlling the disease. Martinez-Palomo (2016) emphasized that although ZIKV infections may explain many cases of brain damage in newborns, it may not be the only cause. These investigators suggested that we need a clear association between confirmed cases of ZIKV infections in pregnant women and microcephaly in newborns. Until we reach a firm conclusion, past-experience with another virus that causes damage to newborns offers some hope. The development and universal use of rubella vaccine has all but eliminated the congenital rubella syndrome in the world. Rapid development of ZIKV vaccine might well do the same for this epidemic.

ZIKV Structural Biology for Intervention. There are currently no treatment options available for ZIKV infection. This virus is a part of the flavivirus genus and closely related to Dengue Fever Virus, West Nile Virus, and Japanese Encephalitis Virus. Like other flaviviruses, the ZIKV genome encodes 3 structural proteins (capsid, precursor membrane, and envelope) and 7 nonstructural proteins (NS1, NS2A, NS2B, NS3, NS4A, NS4B, and NS5). Currently, no structural information exists on these viral proteins to facilitate vaccine design and rational drug discovery. Recently, Cox et al. (2016) predicted structures for all ZIKV viral proteins using templates available from closely related viruses using the online Swiss Model server. These homology models were compared to drug targets from other viruses using Visual Molecular Dynamics Multiseq software. Sequential alignment of all ZIKV polyproteins was performed using Clustal Omega to identify mutations in specific viral proteins implicated in pathogenesis. The precursor membrane, envelope, and NS1 proteins are unique to ZIKV highlighting possible challenges in vaccine design. Sequential differences between ZIKV strains occur at critical positions on precursor membrane, envelope, NS2A, NS3, NS4B, and NS5 as potential loci for differential pathogenesis. Druggable pockets in Dengue Fever Virus and West Nile Virus NS3 and NS5 are retained in predicted ZIKV structures. Lead candidates for ZIKV can be established using NS3 and NS5 inhibitors from other flaviviruses, and the structures presented can provide opportunities for ZIKV intervention strategies.

Viral Polymerase Inhibitor 7-Deaza-2'-C-Methyladenosine as a Potent Inhibitor of ZIKV Replication. ZIKV is an emerging flavivirus typically causing a dengue-like febrile illness, but neurological complications, such as microcephaly in newborns, have been linked to this viral infection. Zmurko et al. (2016) established a panel of *in vitro* assays to allow the identification of ZIKV inhibitors and demonstrate that the viral polymerase inhibitor 7-deaza-2'-C-methyladenosine (7DMA) inhibits replication. Infection of AG129 (IFN-α/β and IFN-γ receptor knock-out) mice with ZIKV resulted in acute neutrophilic encephalitis with viral antigens accumulating in neurons of the brain and spinal cord. Additionally, high levels of viral RNA were detected in the spleen, liver, and kidney, and levels of IFN-γ and IL-18 were increased in serum of ZIKV-infected mice. Interestingly, the virus was also detected in testicles of infected mice. In line with its *in vitro* anti-ZIKV activity, 7DMA reduced viremia and delayed virus-induced morbidity and mortality in infected mice, which also validated this animal model to assess the *in vivo* efficacy of novel ZIKV inhibitors. Since AG-129 mice can generate an antibody response, and have been used in dengue vaccine studies, this model can also be used to assess the efficacy of ZIKV vaccines.

Conclusions

ZIKV compromises MB of early NPCs by triggering CB formation to cause neurodegenerative apoptosis implicated in microcephaly. Hence, there is a dire need for rapid development of a vaccines and therapy for ZIKV infection. The incorporation of viral genome with host cell nuclear genome in developing NPCs induces progressive neurodegeneration to cause microcephaly. ZIKV-induced brain regional CB formation in highly vulnerable cells triggers neuronal apoptosis to cause microcephaly in the developing brain *in utero*. Although, incorporation of viral genome with mitochondrial genome occurs in adults, it cannot replicate; hence, the ZIKV genome can induce down-regulation of only mitochondrial genome in adults. Hence, it is represented by only mild symptoms such as (i) fatigue, (ii) fever, (iii) pain, and lipid peroxidation by down regulating IL-10 and upregulating IL-6. Moreover, efficient charnolophagy does not let ZIKV cause more harm in adults. Hence, its effect remains very mild and restricted in adults. The mtDNA remains structurally and functionally-intact during fission as well as fusion, while it is destroyed during free-radical-induced CB formation involved in apoptosis and microcephaly as we confirmed in RhO_{mgko} cells and in fetal alcohol induced craniofacial abnormalities. Thus, ZIKV genome can destroy mtDNA but cannot replicate when it gets incorporated with the mitochondrial genome in adults. Nutritional rehabilitation eliminates CB formation and reduces brain/body weight ratio to prevent microcephaly, whereas CMB augments CB formation. CB formation triggers neural apoptosis, and neuronal apoptosis triggers microcephaly. Thus, charnolophagy during the acute phase of ZIKV infection prevents apoptosis and hence, microcephaly. Charnolophagy is an efficient basic molecular mechanism of ICD, which is an energy driven process and requires ATP synthesis and structurally and functionally intact mitochondria, Golgi body, E.R., and lysosomes. ZIKV triggers CB pathogenesis to cause microcephaly in developing infants. CB formation compromises MB to induce microcephaly, whereas MTs avert microcephaly by preventing CB formation, augmenting charnolophagy, and stabilizing CS. In adult males, ZIKV infection can induce infertility by enhancing CB formation in the spermatocytes. In rare situations, mengoencephalitis was noticed with ZIKV infection in an old person due to impaired blood brain barrier and immune-compromised situation. In general, ZIKV-mediated free radical overproduction enhances, whereas antioxidants inhibit CB formation. Hence, vaccine and/or drugs may be developed to prevent and/or inhibit CB formation involved in neurodegeneration and microcephaly in the developing brain. CB is a pleomorphic, multi-lamellar, electron-dense, quasi-crystalline structure that is generated in the most vulnerable degenerating cell (NPCs) due to ZIKV-induced CMB. Intrauterine nutritional stress, environmental, toxins, and ZIKV infection alone or in combination enhances free radical overproduction leading to lipid peroxidation and apoptosis by CB formation. Hence, ZIKV-induced CB formation in the developing neurons and osteoblasts is involved in microcephaly. Protein and vitamin-rich diet with antioxidants such as glutathione and MTs prevent/inhibit CB formation as free radical scavengers and by activating Zn^{2+}-mediated transcriptional regulation of genes involved in growth, proliferation, differentiation, and development. Neuron replacement therapy and/or neurosurgical ablation has limited neurotherapeutic potential. Hence, drugs and/or antioxidants may be developed to inhibit CB formation to prevent and/or inhibit ZIKV-induced or other forms of microcephaly. A detailed description of the pathophysiological role of CB formation in various progressive NDDs and ZIKV-induced microcephaly is provided in my recently published books "(i) Monoamine Oxidase Inhibitors (Clinical Applications), (ii) Progress in PET RPs, and (iii) Personalized Medicine (Beyond PET Biomarkers), (iv) Zika Virus Disease: prevention and Cure, and (v) Fetal Alcohol Spectrum Disorders: Concepts, Mechanisms, and Cure" by Nova Science Publishers, New York, U.S.A.

References

Abbasi, A.U. 2016. *ZIKV* infection: Vertical transmission and foetal congenital anomalies. J Ayub Med Coll Abbottabad 28: 1–2.

Adibi, J.J., Y. Zhao, A.R. Cartus, P. Gupta and L.A. Davidson. 2016. Placental mechanics in the Zika-*microcephaly* relationship. Cell Host Microbe 20: 9–11.

Aiken, A.R., J.G. Scott, R. Gomperts, J. Trussell, M. Worrell and C.E. Aiken. 2016. Requests for abortion in Latin America related to concern about *ZIKV* exposure. N Engl J Med 375: 396–398.

Alfaro-Murillo, J.A., A.S. Parpia, M.C. Fitzpatrick, J.A. Tamagnan, J. Medlock, M.L. Ndeffo-Mbah, D. Fish, M.L. Ávila-Agüero, R. Marín, A.I. Ko and A.P. Galvani. 2016. A cost-effectiveness tool for informing policies on *ZIKV* control. PLoS Negl Trop Dis 10: e0004743.

Aliota, M.T., E.A. Caine, E.C. Walker, K.E. Larkin, E. Camacho and J.E. Osorio. 2016. Characterization of lethal *ZIKV* infection in AG129 mice. PLoS Negl Trop Dis 10(4): e0004682.

Anderson, K.B., S.J. Thomas and T.P. Endy. 2016. The emergence of *ZIKV*: A narrative review. Ann Intern Med 165: 175–183.

Annomous. 2016. Public health authorities race to contain fast-moving Zika outbreak. ED Manag 28: 37–41.

Annonmous. 2016. Clinical features and neuroimaging (CT and MRI) findings in presumed *ZIKV* related congenital infection and *microcephaly*: retrospective case series study. BMJ 353: i3182.

Annonmous. 2016. Zika must remain a high priority. Nature 533: 291.

Araujo, A.Q., M.T. Silva and A.P. Araujo. 2016. *ZIKV*-associated neurological disorders: a review. Brain 139: 2122–2130.

Barba-Spaeth, G., W. Dejnirattisai, A. Rouvinski, M.C. Vaney, I. Medits, A. Sharma, E. Simon-Lorière, A. Sakuntabhai, V.M. Cao-Lormeau, A. Haouz, P. England, K. Stiasny, J. Mongkolsapaya, F.X. Heinz, G.R. Screaton and F.A. Rey. 2016. Structural basis of potent Zika-dengue virus antibody cross-neutralization. Nature 536: 48–53.

Beckham, J.D., D.M. Pastula, A. Massey and K.L. Tyler. 2016. *ZIKV* as an emerging global pathogen: Neurological complications of *ZIKV*. JAMA Neurol 73: 875–879.

Belfort, R. Jr, B. de Paula Freitas and J.R. de Oliveira Dias. 2016. *ZIKV*, *microcephaly*, and ocular findings-reply. MMWR Morb Mortal Wkly Rep 65: 514–519.

Bonaldo, M.C., I.P. Ribeiro, N.S. Lima, A.A. Dos Santos, L.S. Menezes, S.O. da Cruz, I.S. de Mello, N.D. Furtado, E.E. de Moura, L. Damasceno, K.A. da Silva, M.G. de Castro, A.L. Gerber, L.G. de Almeida, R. Lourenço-de-Oliveira, A.T. Vasconcelos and P. Brasil. 2016. Isolation of infective *ZIKV* from urine and saliva of patients in Brazil. PLoS Negl Trop Dis 10(6): e0004816.

Brett-Major, D.M. and C.E. Roth. 2016. *ZIKV*, emergencies, uncertainty and vulnerable populations. J R Coll Physicians Edinb 46: 3–6.

Buekens, P., J. Alger, F. Althabe, A. Bergel, A.M. Berrueta, C. Bustillo, M.L. Cafferata, E. Harville, K. Rosales, D.M. Wesson and C. Zuniga. 2016. ZIPH Working Group. *ZIKV* infection in pregnant women in Honduras: study protocol. Reprod Health 13: 82.

Bullerdiek, J., A. Dotzauer and I. Bauer. 2016. The mitotic spindle: linking teratogenic effects of *ZIKV* with human genetics? Mol Cytogenet 9: 32.

Burke, R.M., S. Candfield and P. Gothard. 2016. *ZIKV* and *microcephaly*—more questions than answers? BJOG 123: 1265–1269.

Carneiro, B.M., M.N. Batista, A.C. Braga, M.L. Nogueira and P. Rahal. 2016. The green tea molecule EGCG inhibits *ZIKV* entry. Virology 496: 215–218.

Chowell, G., D. Hincapie-Palacio, J. Ospina, B. Pell, A. Tariq, S. Dahal, S. Moghadas, A. Smirnova, L. Simonsen and C. Viboud. 2016. Using phenomenological models to characterize transmissibility and forecast patterns and final burden of Zika epidemics. May 31: 8.

Cordeiro, M.T., L.J. C.A. Brito, L.H. Gil and E.T. Marques. 2016. Positive IgM for *ZIKV* in the cerebrospinal fluid of 30 neonates with *microcephaly* in Brazil. Lancet 387: 1811–1812.

Cox, B.D., R.A. Stanton and R.F. Schinazi. 2015. Predicting *ZIKV* structural biology: Challenges and opportunities for intervention. Antivir Chem Chemother 24: 118–126.

Cugola, F.R., I.R. Fernandes, F.B. Russo, B.C. Freitas, J.L. Dias, K. Guimarães, C. Benazzato, N. Almeida, G.C. Pignatari, S. Romero, C.M. Polonio, I. Cunha, C.L. Freitas, W.N. Brandão, C. Rossato, D.G. Andrade, D.P. Faria, A.T. Garcez, C.A. Buchpigel, C.T. Braconi, E. Mendes, A.A. Sall, P.M. Zanotto, J.P. Peron, A.R. Muotri and P.C. Beltrão-Braga. 2016. The Brazilian *ZIKV* strain causes birth defects in experimental models. Nature 534: 267–271.

Culjat, M., S.E. Darling, V.R. Nerurkar, N. Ching, M. Kumar, S.K. Min, R. Wong, L. Grant and M.E. Melish. 2016. Clinical and imaging findings in an infant with Zika embryopathy. Clin Infect Dis May 18. pii: ciw324.

D'Alò, G.L., M. Ciabattini, L. Zaratti and E. Franco. 2016. *ZIKV*: a public health overview on epidemiology, clinical practice and prevention. Ig Sanita Pubbl 72: 161–180.

Dang, J., S.K. Tiwari, G. Lichinchi, Y. Qin, V.S. Patil, A.M. Eroshkin and T.M. Rana. 2016. *ZIKV* depletes neural progenitors in human cerebral organoids through activation of the innate immune receptor TLR3. Cell Stem Cell 9: 258–265.

Dasti, J.I. 2016. *ZIKV* infections: An overview of current scenario. Asian Pac J Trop Med 9: 621–625.

De Carvalho, N.S., B.F. De Carvalho, C.A. Fugaça, B. Dóris and E.S. Biscaia. 2016. *ZIKV* infection during pregnancy and *microcephaly* occurrence: a review of literature and Brazilian data. Braz J Infect Dis 20: 282–289.

De Góes Cavalcanti, L.P., P.L. Tauil, C.H. Alencar, W. Oliveira, M.M. Teixeira and J. Heukelbach. 2016. *ZIKV* infection, associated *microcephaly*, and low yellow fever vaccination coverage in Brazil: is there any causal link? J Infect Dev Ctries 10: 563–566.

de Laval, F., I. Leparc-Goffart, J.B. Meynard, H. Daubigny, F. Simon and S. Briolant. 2016. *ZIKV* infections. Med Sante Trop 26: 145–150.

Dejnirattisai, W., P. Supasa, W. Wongwiwat, A. Rouvinski, G. Barba-Spaeth, T. Duangchinda, A. Sakuntabhai, V.M. Cao-Lormeau, P. Malasit, F.A. Rey, J. Mongkolsapaya and G.R. Screaton. 2016. Dengue virus sero-cross-reactivity drives antibody-dependent enhancement of infection with *ZIKV*. Nat Immunol 17: 1102–1108.

Del Carpio-Orantes, L. 2016. Zika, a neurotropic virus? Rev Med Inst Mex Seguro Soc 54: 540–543.

Dirlikov, E., K.R. Ryff, J. Torres-Aponte, D.L. Thomas, J. Perez-Padilla, J. Munoz-Jordan, E.V. Caraballo, M. Garcia, M.O. Segarra, G. Malave, R.M. Simeone, C.K. Shapiro-Mendoza, L.R. Reyes, F. Alvarado-Ramy, A.F. Harris, A. Rivera, C.G. Major, C.G. Mayshack, L.I. Alvarado, A. Lenhart, M. Valencia-Prado, S. Waterman, T.M. Sharp and B. Rivera-Garcia. 2016. Update: Ongoing *ZIKV* transmission—Puerto Rico, November 1, 2015–April 14, 2016. MMWR Morb Mortal Wkly Rep 65: 451–455.

Dowall, S.D., V.A. Graham, E. Rayner, B. Atkinson, G. Hall, R.J. Watson, A. Bosworth, L.C. Bonney, S. Kitchen and R. Hewson. 2016. A susceptible mouse model for *ZIKV* infection. PLoS Negl Trop Dis 10: e0004658.

Duarte Dos Santos, C.N. and S. Goldenberg. 2016. *ZIKV* and *microcephaly*: Challenges for a long-term agenda. Trends Parasitol 32: 508–511.

Ekins, S., D. Mietchen, M. Coffee, T.P. Stratton, J.S. Freundlich, L. Freitas-Junior, E. Muratov, J. Siqueira-Neto, A.J. Williams and C. Andrade. 2016. Open drug discovery for the *ZIKV*. F1000Res. 5: 150.

Epelboin, L., M. Douine, G. Carles, N. Villemant, M. Nacher, D. Rousset, F. Djossou and E. Mosnier. 2016. *ZIKV* outbreak in Latin America: what are the challenges for French Guiana in April 2016? Bull Soc Pathol Exot 109: 114–125.

Fact sheet on *ZIKV* disease. 2016. Wkly Epidemiol Rec 91: 314–316.

Fajardo, A., M. Soñora, P. Moreno, G. Moratorio and J. Cristina. 2016. Bayesian coalescent inference reveals high evolutionary rates and diversification of *ZIKV* populations. J Med Virol 88: 1672–1676.

França, G.V., L. Schuler-Faccini, W.K. Oliveira, C.M. Henriques, E.H. Carmo, V.D. Pedi, M.L. Nunes, M.C. Castro, S. Serruya, M.F. Silveira, F.C. Barros and C.G. Victora. 2016. Congenital *ZIKV* syndrome in Brazil: a case series of the first 1501 livebirths with complete investigation. Lancet 388: 891–897.

Gong, Z., Y. Gao and G.Z. Han. 2016. *ZIKV*: two or three lineages? Trends Microbiol 24: 521–522.

Grills, A., S. Morrison, B. Nelson, J. Miniota, A. Watts and M.S. Cetron. 2016. Projected *ZIKV* importation and subsequent ongoing transmission after travel to the 2016 olympic and paralympic games—country-specific assessment. MMWR Morb Mortal Wkly Rep 65: 711–715.

Grischott, F., M. Puhan, C. Hatz and P. Schlagenhauf. 2016. Non-vector-borne transmission of *ZIKV*: A systematic review. Travel Med Infect Dis 14: 313–302016.

Guerbois, M., I. Fernandez-Salas, S.R. Azar, R. Danis-Lozano, C.M. Alpuche-Aranda, G. Leal, I.R. Garcia-Malo, E.E. Diaz-Gonzalez, M. Casas-Martinez, S.L. Rossi, S.L. Del Río-Galván, R.M. Sanchez-Casas, C.M. Roundy, T.G. Wood, S.G. Widen, N. Vasilakis and S.C. Weaver. 2016. Outbreak of *ZIKV* infection, Chiapas State, Mexico, 2015, and first confirmed transmission by Aedes aegypti mosquitoes in the Americas. J Infect Dis 214: 1349–1356.

Guideline: Infant Feeding in Areas of *ZIKV* Transmission. Geneva: World Health Organization; 2016. WHO Guidelines Approved by the Guidelines Review Committee.

Guillemette-Artur, P., M. Besnard, D. Eyrolle-Guignot, J.M. Jouannic and C. Garel. 2016. Prenatal brain MRI of fetuses with *ZIKV* infection. Pediatr Radiol 46: 1032–1039.

Guo, J. 2016. Studies using IPS cells support a possible link between ZIKA and *microcephaly*. Cell Biosci 6: 28.

Gyawali, N., R.S. Bradbury and A.W. Taylor-Robinson. 2016. The global spread of *ZIKV*: is public and media concern justified in regions currently unaffected? Infect Dis Poverty 5: 37.

Hajra, A., D. Bandyopadhyay and S.K. Hajra. 2016. *ZIKV*: A global threat to humanity: A comprehensive review and current developments. N Am J Med Sci 8: 123–128.

Hanners, N.W., J.L. Eitson, N. Usui, R.B. Richardson, E.M. Wexler, G. Konopka and J.W. Schoggins. 2016. Western *ZIKV* in human fetal neural progenitors persists long term with partial cytopathic and limited immunogenic effects. Cell Rep 15: 2315–2322.

Harrison, T. 2016. Effects of *ZIKV*. Emerg Nurse 24: 17.

Heukelbach, J. and G.L. Werneck. 2016. Surveillance of *ZIKV* infection and *microcephaly* in Brazil. Lancet 388: 846–847.

Hughes, B.W., K.C. Addanki, A.N. Sriskanda, E. McLean and O. Bagasra. 2016. Infectivity of immature neurons to *ZIKV*: A link to congenital zika syndrome. EBio Medicine 10: 65–70.

Jamil, Z., Y. Waheed and T.Z. Durrani. 2016. *ZIKV*, a pathway to new challenges. Asian Pac J Trop Med 9: 626–629.

Jampol, L.M. and D.A. Goldstein. 2016. *ZIKV*, *microcephaly*, and ocular findings-reply. JAMA Ophthalmol 134: 946.

Jang, H.C., W.B. Park, U.J. Kim, J.Y. Chun, S.J. Choi, P.G. Choe, S.I. Jung, Y. Jee, N.J. Kim, E.H. Choi and M.D. Oh. 2016. First imported case of *ZIKV* infection into Korea. J Korean Med Sci 31: 1173–1177.

Kass, D.E. and M. Merlino. 2016. *ZIKV*. N Engl J Med 375: 294.

Kekulé, A. 2016. How dangerous is the *ZIKV*? Dtsch Med Wochenschr 141: 969–972.

Kim, K. and S. Shresta. 2016. Neuroteratogenic viruses and lessons for *ZIKV* models. Trends Microbiol 24: 622–636.

Koenig, K.L., A. Almadhyan and M.J. Burns. 2016. Identify-isolate-inform: A tool for initial detection and management of *ZIKV* patients in the emergency department. West J Emerg Med 17: 238–244.

Kostyuchenko, V.A., E.X. Lim, S. Zhang, G. Fibriansah, T.S. Ng, J.S. Ooi, J. Shi and S.M. Lok. 2016. Structure of the thermally stable *ZIKV*. Nature 533: 425–428.

Kucharski, A.J., S. Funk, R.M. Eggo, H. Mallet, W.J. Edmunds and E.J. Nilles. 2016. Transmission dynamics of *ZIKV* in island populations: A modelling analysis of the 2013–14 French polynesia outbreak. PLoS Negl Trop Dis 10: e0004726.

Kuehnert, M.J., S.V. Basavaraju, R.R. Moseley, L.L. Pate, S.A. Galel, P.C. Williamson, M.P. Busch, J.O. Alsina, C. Climent-Peris, P.W. Marks, J.S. Epstein, H.L. Nakhasi, J.P. Hobson, D.A. Leiby, P.N. Akolkar, L.R. Petersen and B. Rivera-Garcia. 2016. Screening of blood donations for *ZIKV* infection-Puerto Rico, April 3–June 11, 2016. MMWR Morb Mortal Wkly Rep 65: 627–628.

Ladner, J.T., M.R. Wiley, K. Prieto, C.Y. Yasud, E. Nagle, M.R. Kasper, D. Reyes, N. Vasilakis, V. Heang, S.C. Weaver, A. Haddow, R.B. Tesh, L. Sovann and G. Palacios. 2016. Complete genome sequences of five *ZIKV* isolates. Genome Announc Lancet 387: 1993.

Larocca, R.A., P. Abbink, J.P. Peron, P.M. Zanotto, M.J. Iampietro, A. Badamchi-Zadeh, M. Boyd, D. Ng'ang'a, M. Kirilova, R. Nityanandam, N.B. Mercado, Z. Li, E.T. Moseley, C.A. Bricault, E.N. Borducchi, P.B. Giglio, D. Jetton, G. Neubauer, J.P. Nkolola, L.F. Maxfield, R.A. Barrera, R.G. Jarman, K.H. Eckels, N.L. Michael, S.J. Thomas and D.H. Barouch. 2016. Vaccine protection against *ZIKV* from Brazil. Nature 536: 474–478.

Lazić, S. 2016. Another emerging pathogen—*ZIKV*. Vojnosanit Pregl 73: 225–227.

Leão, J.C., L.A. Gueiros, G. Lodi, N.A. Robinson and C. Scully. 2016. *ZIKV*: oral healthcare implications. Oral Dis 23: 12–17.

Lednicky, J., V.M. Beau De Rochars, M. El Badry, J. Loeb, T. Telisma, S. Chavannes, G. Anilis, E. Cella, M. Ciccozzi, M. Rashid, B. Okech, M. Salemi and J.G. Morris Jr. 2016. *ZIKV* outbreak in Haiti in 2014: Molecular and clinical data. PLoS Negl Trop Dis 10: e0004687.

Lee, C.T., N.M. Vora, W. Bajwa, L. Boyd, S. Harper, D. Kass, A. Langston, E. McGibbon, M. Merlino, J.L. Rakeman, M. Raphael, S. Slavinski, A. Tran, R. Wong and J.K. Varm. 2016. NYC Zika Response Team; Division of Disease Control; New York City Department of Health and Mental Hygiene; New York City Department of and Mental Hygiene; Epidemic Intelligence Service; CDC; Division of Epidemiology; Office of Public Health Preparedness and Response, CDC; Office of Emergency Public Health Preparedness and Response; Division of Environmental Health; New York City Department of Health; Mental Hygiene; Office of Emergency Preparedness and Response; Division of Informatics and Information Technology; Division of Prevention and Primary Care; Division of Disease Control, New York City Department of Health and Mental Hygiene. *ZIKV* Surveillance and Preparedness—New York City, 2015–2016. MMWR Morb Mortal Wkly Rep 65: 629–635.

Lessler, J., L.H. Chaisson, L.M. Kucirka, Q. Bi, K. Grantz, H. Salje, A.C. Carcelen, C.T. Ott, J.S. Sheffield, N.M. Ferguson, D.A. Cummings, C.J. Metcalf and I. Rodriguez-Barraquer. 2016. Assessing the global threat from *ZIKV*. Science 353: aaf8160.

Li, C., D. Xu, Q. Ye, S. Hong, Y. Jiang, X. Liu, N. Zhang, L. Shi, C.F. Qin and Z. Xu. 2016. *ZIKV* disrupts neural progenitor development and leads to *microcephaly* in mice. Cell Stem Cell 19: 120–126.

Liuzzi, G., V. Puro, S. Lanini, F. Vairo, E. Nicastri, M.R. Capobianchi, A. Di Caro, M. Piacentini, A. Zumla and G. Ippolito. 2016. *ZIKV* and *microcephaly*: is the correlation causal or coincidental? New Microbiol 39: 83–85.

Lu, G.Y., Y.Y. Su and N. Wang. 2016. Several issues on the epidemiology of *ZIKV* disease. Zhonghua Liu Xing Bing Xue Za Zhi 37: 450–454.

Machado-Alba, J.E., M.E. Machado-Duque, A. Gaviria-Mendoza and V.A. Orozco-Giraldo. 2016. Hormonal contraceptive prescriptions in Colombia and *ZIKV*. Lancet 387: 1993.

Maharajan, M.K., A. Ranjan, J.F. Chu, W.L. Foo, Z.X. Chai, E.Y. Lau, H.M. Ye, X.J. Theam and Y.L. Lok. 2016. *ZIKV* infection: Current concerns and perspectives. Clin Rev Allergy Immunol 2016 May 28.

Malkki, H. 2016. CNS infections: Mouse studies confirm the link between *ZIKV* infection and *microcephaly*. Nat Rev Neurol 12: 369.

Martines, R.B., J. Bhatnagar, A.M. de Oliveira Ramos, H.P. Davi, S.D. Iglezias, C.T. Kanamura, M.K. Keating, G. Hale, L. Silva-Flannery, A. Muehlenbachs, J. Ritter, J. Gary, D. Rollin, C.S. Goldsmith, S. Reagan-Steiner, Y. Ermias, T. Suzuki, K.G. Luz, W.K. de Oliveira, R. Lanciotti, A. Lambert, W.J. Shieh and S.R. Zaki. 2016. Pathology of congenital Zika syndrome in Brazil: a case series. Lancet 388: 898–904.

Martinez-Palomo, A. 2016. Revisiting Zika (and Rubella). J Public Health Policy 2016 Jun 15.

Mawson, A.R. 2016. Pathogenesis of *ZIKV*-associated embryopathy. Biores Open Access 5: 171–176.

Messina, J.P., M.U. Kraemer, O.J. Brady, D.M. Pigott, F.M. Shearer, D.J. Weis, N. Golding, C.W. Ruktanonchai, P.W. Gething, E. Cohn, J.S. Brownstein, K. Khan, A.J. Tatem, T. Jaenisch, C.J.

Murray, F. Marinho, T.W. Scott and S.I. Hay. 2016. Mapping global environmental suitability for *ZIKV*. Elife 5: pii: e15272.

Mikrobiyol Bul. 2016 Apr; 50(2): 333–351.

Miner, J.J. and M.S. Diamond. 2016. Understanding How *ZIKV* enters and infects neural target cells. Cell Stem Cell 18: 559–560.

Miner, J.J., B. Cao, J. Govero, A.M. Smith, E. Fernandez, O.H. Cabrera, C. Garber, M. Noll, R.S. Klein, K.K. Noguchi, I.U. Mysorekar and M.S. Diamond. 2016. *ZIKV* infection during pregnancy in mice causes placental damage and fetal demise. Cell 165: 1081–1091.

Miranda, H.A. 2nd, M.C. Costa, MA. Frazão, N. Simão, S. Franchischini and D.M. Moshfeghi. 2016. Expanded spectrum of congenital ocular findings in *microcephaly* with presumed Zika infection. Ophthalmology 123: 1788–1794.

Miscellanées récréatives et virologiques, pharmaceutiques et catholiques. 2016. Rev Med Suisse 12: 622–623.

Mo, Y., B.M. Alferez Salada and P.A. Tambyah. 2016. *ZIKV*—a review for clinicians. Br Med Bull 119: 25–36.

Moron, A.F., S. Cavalheiro, H. Milani, S. Sarmento, C. Tanuri, F.F. de Souza, R. Richtmann and S.S. Witkin. 2016. *Microcephaly* associated with maternal *ZIKV* infection. BJOG 123: 1265–1269.

Moshfeghi, D.M. H.A. de Miranda 2nd and M.C. Costa. 2016. *ZIKV*, *microcephaly*, and ocular findings. JAMA Ophthalmol Jun 2.

Mysorekar, I.U. and M.S. Diamond. 2016. Modeling *ZIKV* infection in pregnancy. N Engl J Med Jul 13.

Nau, J.Y. 2016. Miscellanées Spermatiques Et Virologiques, Cutanées Et Éthiques. Rev Med Suisse 12: 862–863.

Nishiura, H., K. Mizumoto, K.S. Rock, Y. Yasuda, R. Kinoshita and Y. Miyamatsu. 2016. A theoretical estimate of the risk of *microcephaly* during pregnancy with *ZIKV* infection. Epidemics 15: 66–70.

Noronha, L.D., C. Zanluca, M.L. Azevedo, K.G. Luz and C.N. Santos. 2016. *ZIKV* damages the human placental barrier and presents marked fetal neurotropism. Mem Inst Oswaldo Cruz 111: 287–293.

Olagnier, D., M. Muscolini, C.B. Coyne, M.S. Diamond and J. Hiscott. 2016. Mechanisms of *ZIKV* infection and neuropathogenesis. DNA Cell Biol Jun 27.

Pacheco, O., M. Beltrán, C.A. Nelson, D. Valencia, N. Tolosa, S.L. Farr, A.V. Padilla, V.T. Tong, E.L. Cuevas, A. Espinosa-Bode, L. Pardo, A. Rico, J. Reefhuis, M. González, M. Mercado, P. Chaparro, M. Martínez Duran, C.Y. Rao, M.M. Muñoz, A.M. Powers, C. Cuéllar, R. Helfand, C. Huguett, D.J. Jamieson, M.A. Honein and M.L. Ospina Martínez. 2016. *ZIKV* disease in colombia—preliminary report. N Engl J Med Jun 15.

Panchaud, A., M. Stojanov, A. Ammerdorffer, M. Vouga and D. Baud. 2016. Emerging role of *ZIKV* in adverse fetal and neonatal outcomes. Clin Microbiol Rev 29(3): 659–694.

Paploski, I.A., A.P. Prates, C.W. Cardoso, M. Kikuti, M.M. Silva, L.A. Waller, M.G. Reis, U. Kitron and G.S. Ribeiro. 2016. Time lags between exanthematous illness attributed to *ZIKV*, guillain-barré syndrome, and *microcephaly*, salvador, Brazil. Emerg Infect Dis 22: 1438–1444.

Piorkowski, G., P. Richard, P. Baronti, P. Gallian, R. Charrel, I. Leparc-Goffart and X. de Lamballerie. 2016. Complete coding sequence of *ZIKV* from Martinique outbreak in 2015. New Microbes New Infect 11: 52–53.

Płusa, T. 2016. [*ZIKV* as a new threat to the health and life]. Pol Merkur Lekarski 40: 149–152.

Porrino, P. 2016. *ZIKV* infection and once again the risk from other neglected diseases. Trop Doct 46: 159–165.

Possas, C. 2016. Zika: what we do and do not know based on the experiences of Brazil. Epidemiol Health 38: e2016023.

Pylro, V.S., F.S. Oliveira, D.K. Morais, S. Cuadros-Orellana, F.S. Pais, J.D. Medeiros, J.A. Geraldo, J. Gilbert, A.C. Volpini and G.R. Fernandes. 2016. *ZIKV*-CDB: A collaborative database to guide research linking SncRNAs and *ZIKV* disease symptoms. PLoS Negl Trop Dis 10: e0004817.

Qian, X., H.N. Nguyen, M.M. Song, C. Hadiono, S.C. Ogden, C. Hammack, B. Yao, G.R. Hamersky, F. Jacob, C. Zhong, K.J. Yoon, W. Jeang, L. Lin, Y. Li, J. Thakor, D.A. Berg, C. Zhang, E. Kang, M. Chickering, D. Nauen, C.Y. Ho, Z. Wen, K.M. Christian, P.Y. Shi, B.J. Maher, H. Wu, P. Jin, H.

Tang, H. Song and G.L. Ming. 2016. Brain-region-specific organoids using mini-bioreactors for modeling *ZIKV* exposure. Cell 165: 1238–1254.

Quicke, K.M., J.R. Bowen, E.L. Johnson, C.E. McDonald, H. Ma, J.T. O'Neal, A. Rajakumar, J. Wrammert, B.H. Rimawi, B. Pulendran, R.F. Schinazi, R. Chakraborty and M.S. Suthar. 2016. *ZIKV* infects human placental macrophages. Cell Host Microbe 20: 83–90.

Rabaan, A.A., A.M. Bazzi, S.H. Al-Ahmed, M.H. Al-Ghaith and J.A. Al-Tawfiq. 2017. Overview of Zika infection, epidemiology, transmission and control measures. J Infect Public Health 10: 141–149.

Ramos da Silva, S. and S.J. Gao. 2016. *ZIKV*: An update on epidemiology, pathology, molecular biology, and animal model. J Med Virol 88: 1291–1296.

Reefhuis, J., S.M. Gilboa, M.A. Johansson, D. Valencia, R.M. Simeone, S.L. Hills, K. Polen, D.J. Jamieson, L.R. Petersen and M.A. Honein. 2016. Projecting month of birth for at-risk infants after *ZIKV* disease outbreaks. Emerg Infect Dis 22: 828–832.

Ribeiro, L.S., R.E. Marques, A.M. Jesus, R.P. Almeida and M.M. Teixeira. 2016. Zika crisis in Brazil: challenges in research and development. Curr Opin Virol 18: 76–81.

Rolfe, A.J., D.B. Bosco, J. Wang, R.S. Nowakowski, J. Fan and Y. Ren. 2016. Bioinformatic analysis reveals the expression of unique transcriptomic signatures in *ZIKV* infected human neural stem cells. Cell Biosci 6: 42.

Rossi, S.L. and N. Vasilakis. 2016. Modeling *ZIKV* infection in mice. Cell Stem Cell 19: 4–6.

Şahiner, F. 2016. [Global spread of *ZIKV* epidemic: current knowledges and uncertainties].

Saiz, J.C., A. Vázquez-Calvo, A.B. Blázquez, T. Merino-Ramos, E. Escribano-Romero and M.A. Martín-Acebes. 2016. *ZIKV*: the latest newcomer. Front Microbiol 7: 496.

Salinas, S., V. Foulongne, F. Loustalot, C. Fournier-Wirth, J.P. Molès, L. Briant, N. Nagot, P. Van de Perre and Y. Simonin. 2016. *ZIKV*, an emerging threat. Med Sci (Paris) 32: 378–386.

Sam, J.I., Y.F. Chan, I. Vythilingam and W.Y. Wan Sulaiman. 2016. *ZIKV* and its potential re-emergence in Malaysia. Med J Malaysia 71: 66–68.

Saxena, S.K., A. Elahi, S. Gadugu and A.K. Prasad. 2016. *ZIKV* outbreak: an overview of the experimental therapeutics and treatment. Virus disease 27: 111–115.

Schuler-Faccini, L., M. Sanseverino, F. Vianna, A.A. da Silva, M. Larrandaburu, C. Marcolongo-Pereira and A.M. Abeche. 2016. *ZIKV*: A new human teratogen? Implications for women of reproductive age. Clin Pharmacol Ther 100: 28–30.

Scudellari, M. 2016. How iPS cells changed the world. Nature 534: 310–312.

Shah, A. and A. Kumar. 2016. *ZIKV* infection and development of a murine model. Neurotox Res 30: 131–134.

Sharma, S. and M. Ebadi. 2013. Antioxidant-Targeting in Neurodegenerative Disorders. Ed. I. Laher, Springer Verlag. Germany. Chapter 85, pp. 1–30.

Sharma, S., C.S. Moon, A. Khogali, A. Haidous, A. Chabenne, C. Ojo, M. Jelebinkov, Y. Kurdi and M. Ebadi. 2013. Biomarkers in Parkinson's disease (Recent Update). Neurochem Int 63: 201–29.

Sharma, S., A. Rais, R. Sandhu, W. Nel and M. Ebadi. 2013. Clinical significance of metallothioneins in cell therapy and nanomedicine. Int J Nanomedicine 8: 1477–1488.

Sharma, S. and M. Ebadi. 2014. The charnoly body as a universal biomarker of cell injury. Biomarkers & Genomic Medicine 6: 89–98.

Sharma, S. 2014. Nanotheranostics in evidence based personalized medicine. Curr Drug Targets 15: 915–930.

Sharma, S. and M. Ebadi. 2014. Significance of metallothioneins in aging brain. Neurochem Int 65: 40–48.

Sharma, S. 2015. Charnoly body as a novel biomarker in drug addiction. 4th International & Exhibition on Addiction Research and Therapy Aug 3–5.

Sharma, S. 2015. Charnoly body as a novel biomarker of drug discovery in nanomedicine. BIT's 12th International Drug Discovery Conference, At Suzhou, China, Nov 20–25.

Sharma, S. 2015. Charnoly body as a universal biomarker in nanomedicine. 2nd International Conference on Translational Nanomedicine, Boston, MASS, U.S.A. July 25–27.

Sharma, S., J. Choga, V. Gupta, P. Doghor, A. Chauhan, F. Kalala, A. Foor, C. Wright, J. Renteria, K. Elliott-Theberge and S. Mathur. 2016. Charnoly body as a novel biomarker of nutritional stress in Alzheimer's disease. 20th International Conference on Functional Foods. Boston, Mass, USA Sep 22–23.

Shoaib, M., A. Faraz and S.A. Ahmed. 2016. Another vector borne challenge to combat *Zikv* outbreaks. J Ayub Med Coll Abbottabad 28: 210–211.

Silveira, F.P. and S.V. Campos. 2016. The Zika epidemics and transplantation. J Heart Lung Transplant 35: 560–563.

Simeone, R.M., C.K. Shapiro-Mendoza, D. Meaney-Delman, E.E. Petersen et al. 2016. Possible ZIKV infection among pregnant women—United States and Territories, May. MMWR Early Release. May.

Sirohi, D., Z. Chen, L. Sun, T. Klose, T.C. Pierson, M.G. Rossmann and R.J. Kuhn. 2016. The 3.8 Å resolution cryo-EM structure of *ZIKV*. Science 352: 467–470.

Slenczka, W. 2016. *ZIKV* disease. Microbiol Spectr Jun; 4(3).

Song, H., J. Qi, J. Haywood, Y. Shi and G.F. Gao. 2016. *ZIKV* NS1 structure reveals diversity of electrostatic surfaces among flaviviruses. Nat Struct Mol Biol 23: 456–458.

Spong, C.Y. 2016. Understanding *ZIKV* pathogenesis: an interview with catherine spong. BMC Med 14: 84.

Stagg, D. and H.M. Hurst. 2016. *ZIKV* and pregnancy. Nurs Womens Health 20: 299–304.

Swanstrom, J.A., J.A. Plante, K.S. Plante, E.F. Young, E. McGowan, E.N. Gallichotte, D.G. Widman, M.T. Heise, A.M. de Silva and R.S. Baric. 2016. Dengue virus envelope dimer epitope monoclonal antibodies isolated from dengue patients are protective against *ZIKV*. MBio 7(4). pii: e01123-16.

Tang, B.L. 2016. *ZIKV* as a causative agent for primary microencephaly: the evidence so far. Arch Microbiol Jul 13.

Tian, H., X. Ji, X. Yang, Z. Zhang, Z. Lu, K. Yang, C. Chen, Q. Zhao, H. Chi, Z. Mu, W. Xie, Z. Wang, H. Lou, H. Yang and Z. Rao. 2016. Structural basis of *ZIKV* helicase in recognizing its substrates. Protein Cell Jul 18.

Valentine, G., L. Marquez and M. Pammi. 2016. *ZIKV*-associated *microcephaly* and eye lesions in the newborn. J Pediatric Infect Dis Soc Jul 11.

Valerio Sallent, L., S. Roure Díez and G. Fernández Rivas. 2016. [*ZIKV* infection or the future of infectious diseases]. Med Clin (Barc).

van Hemert, F. and B. Berkhout. 2016. Nucleotide composition of the *ZIKV* RNA genome and its codon usage. Virol J 13: 95.

Ventura, C.V., M. Maia, S.B. Travassos, T.T. Martins, F. Patriota, M.E. Nunes, C. Agra, V.L. Torres, V. van der Linden, R.C. Ramos, M.A. Rocha, P.S. Silva, L.O. Ventura and R. Jr Belfort. 2016. Risk factors associated with the ophthalmoscopic findings identified in infants with presumed *ZIKV* congenital infection. JAMA Ophthalmol May 26.

Visovsky, C., S. McGhee, J.M. Clochesy and C. Zambroski. 2016. *ZIKV*: emergency and aftercare of patients. Emerg Nurse 24: 20–23.

Voelker, R. 2016. Miami obstetrician uses evidence to quell Zika fears. JAMA 315: 2051–2052.

Vogel, G. 2016. Infectious disease. Experts fear Zika's effects may be even worse than thought. Science 352: 1375–1376.

Vorou, R. 2016. *ZIKV*, vectors, reservoirs, amplifying hosts, and their potential to spread worldwide: what we know and what we should investigate urgently. Int J Infect Dis 48: 85–90.

Walsh, B. and A. Sifferlin. 2016. Zika's toll. Time 187: 42–47.

Wang, Z. and P. Wang. 2016. An J *ZIKV* and Zika fever. Virol Sin 31: 103–109.

Wikan, N. and D.R. Smith. 2016. *ZIKV*: history of a newly emerging arbovirus. Lancet Infect Dis 16: e119–126.

Wu, K.Y., G.L. Zuo, X.F. Li, Q. Ye, Y.Q. Deng, X.Y. Huang, W.C. Cao, C.F. Qin and Z.G. Luo. 2016. Vertical transmission of *ZIKV* targeting the radial glial cells affects cortex development of offspring mice. Cell Res 26: 645–654.

Zé-Zé, L., M.B. Prata, T. Teixeira, N. Marques, A. Mondragão, R. Fernandes, J. Saraiva da Cunha and M.J. Alves. 2016. *ZIKV* infections imported from Brazil to Portugal, 2015. Ann Intern Med. 2016 May 3. ID Cases 4: 46–49.

Zhang, S. and D. Li. 2016. *ZIKV* and Zika viral disease. Bing Du Xue Bao 32: 121–127.

Zmurko, J., R.E. Marques, D. Schols, E. Verbeken, S.J. Kaptein and J. Neyts. 2016. The viral polymerase inhibitor 7-Deaza-2'-C-Methyladenosine is a potent inhibitor of *in vitro* ZIKV replication and delays disease progression in a robust mouse infection model. PLoS Negl Trop Dis 10: e0004695.

CHAPTER-19

Charnoly Body in Malnutrition
(Mitochondrial Bioenergetics in Health and Disease)

INTRODUCTION

In earlier studies, we investigated the influence of undernutrition on the electrophysiological and neuromorphological parameters of the developing rat cerebellar Purkinje neurons. Undernutrition was induced by increasing the liter size to 16 pups and simultaneously restricting the mother's dietary intake of protein, casein to 50% of her daily requirement; while normal animals were reared in the litters of 8 and their mothers were fed an *ad libitum* diet as described by Widdowson and McCance (1957). Lactating mothers in both experimental groups received a high protein diet containing 25% casein. This experimental model was utilized because the rat cerebellar Purkinje neurons develop postnatally and are highly vulnerable to the deleterious effects of undernutrition. The cerebellar tissue was processed for light and E.M. study as described in our earlier publications (Sharma et al. 1986; Sharma et al. 1987).

This chapter highlights malnutrition-induced CB formation in the most vulnerable developing rat cerebellar Purkinje neurons and the clinical significance of MB in ICD for normal cellular function. The chapter also briefly describes CB molecular pathogenesis in chronic NDDs, CVDs, and MDR malignancies.

Body Weight vs Brain Weight

The brain to body weight ratio of 5–30 days developing N and UN rats was determined. At any given postnatal period, this ratio was significantly high in the UN rats as compared to N rats, indicating that the ratio of brain weight vs body weight may be used as an index of severity of nutritional stress. The brain to body weight ratio reduced as a function of nutritional rehabilitation. Severely UN rats exhibited significantly high brain to body weight ratio which was directly proportional to CB formation. Hence, we reported that CB formation and brain/body weight ratio may be clinically used as theranostic biomarkers of nutritional stress and rehabilitation or neurodegeneration/neuro-regeneration (Sharma and Ebadi 2014).

The CB formation was detected in the Purkinje neurons of 15–30 days old postnatal rats which is the most critical period of rat cerebellar development. Any nutritional and/or toxic insult during this critical period of cerebellar development induces CB formation in these highly vulnerable mitochondrial-rich neurons. Since brain weight in experimental animals was not significantly affected during postnatal undernutrition, some investigators proposed brain sparing hypothesis, which was subsequently challenged when brain region-specific neurochemistry, electrophysiology, and the ultra-structural studies were conducted by several other investigators. The novel discovery of CB formation in the developing UN Purkinje neurons further challenged the brain sparing hypothesis. Subsequently, hippocampal and hypothalamic CB formation was reported in MDDs and eating disorders (Anorexia and Bulimia) respectively (Sharma 2015). CB formation in the developing cerebellar Purkinje neurons was also associated with a significant electrophysiological deficit in the UN rat brain (Sharma et al. 1987).

Experimental Studies on Developing Rat Brain

Electrophysiological studies were conducted in developing N and UN rats as follows: (i) Spontaneous unit activity of Purkinje neurons in the cerebellum including extracellular, intracellular, and evoked unit activity, (ii) mossy fiber evoked responses (MFR), and (iii) morphological studies at the light and EM level.

Electrophysiological Studies. Electrophysiological studies were carried out in the N and UN rats during 5th to 30 days of postnatal life. UN animals were studied at five different age groups namely 5th, 10th, 15th, 20th, and 30th days. In N animals, the postnatal development of the spontaneous unit activity of Purkinje neurons was first established from 5th to 21st day of postnatal life. The mean firing frequency of simple spikes increased as a function of aging reaching a value of 37 spikes/sec in adult animals, whereas intracellular unit activity increased from 12 spikes/sec to 25 spikes/sec in N and from 11 spikes per/sec to 19 spikes/sec in UN animals. As the age advanced, not only the firing frequency of simple and complex spikes of Purkinje neurons increased, the pattern of firing and the duration of spikes also decreased from 5 mSec to 1 mSec by 20th postnatal day. In the UN animals, the mean firing frequency of the Purkinje neurons was reduced, and the spike duration was prolonged as compared to their normal age-matched controls.

The postnatal development of MFR was first established in young developing N rats during first 20 days of postnatal life, by stimulating the sciatic nerve ipsilaterally, and picking up MFR from the anterior vermis region. MFR activity could be recorded on the 10th postnatal day and thereafter. During maturation, MFR showed a gradual reduction in the latency and the duration of response, while the number of functional components increased with advancing age. The stimulus threshold to elicit MFR also reduced as a function of aging. In the UN animals, MFR exhibited prolonged latency, reduction in the number of functional components, and increased duration of MF response with typical immature developmental characteristics compared to their age-matched controls, in all the age groups studied. Even the stimulus threshold required to elicit MF response was elevated in the UN animals as compared to N controls. A typical phenomenon of MFR fatigue was observed in the Purkinje cell evoked unit activity and in the MFR at relatively higher stimulus intensities and at higher stimulus frequencies, confirming CMB in the developing UN rats (Sharma et al. 1987; Sharma et al. 1993).

Usually, major depressive patients are subjected to ECT when the pharmacotherapy becomes ineffective. ECT is required to activate the neurons to increase their responsiveness to external stimuli. Lower stimulus intensities, increased MFR linearly, the medium stimulus intensity did not alter the response, whereas higher stimulus intensities reduced MFR in UN animals, indicating CMB at higher stimulus intensities. The MFR was inhibited at higher stimulus intensities and at higher stimulus frequencies in UN animals, suggesting that these electrophysiological deficits occur due to CB formation in the developing Purkinje neurons, which is involved in the delayed or impaired synaptic neurotransmission and sensory motor development due to CMB in UN children.

Neuromorphological Studies. At the light microscopic level, persistence in the external granular layer, reduced molecular layer thickness, accumulation of the cytoplasm in the Purkinje neurons, and increased cell packing density in the internal granular layer were the most significant findings in the UN rat cerebelli. At the E.M. level, Purkinje neuron cytoplasm exhibited a free ribosomal pool, immature developmental characteristics of ER, increased incidence of lysosomes, and typical electron-dense membrane stacks (Charnoly body: CBs) were observed at 15–30 days of postnatal life. The CBs were phagocytosed by energy (ATP)-driven lysosomal phagocytosis to form a CPS. The CPS was transformed to CS, when the CB was phagocytosed by the lysosomal enzymes (hydrolases, lipases, proteases, and nucleases). The protein synthesis was inhibited due down-regulation of AgNOR involved in ribosomal synthesis and due to increased release of toxic substances from the CS due to free radicals-induced destabilization of their membranes to cause the formation of CS bodies. This was followed by CS permeabilization, sequestration, and disintegration during tertiary free radical attack as a function of severity of malnutrition. Thus, CB was frequently subjected to charnolophagy to form CPS and CS in severe undernutrition. The CS was exocytosed as a basic molecular mechanism of ICD for normal growth and development of the brain. However, secondary and tertiary free radical attack to CS membranes rendered them highly susceptible to destabilization and eventual degradation to release highly toxic mitochondrial metabolites to induce neurodegenerative apoptosis involved in progressive NDDs. These morphological deficits reduced the Purkinje neurons electrical activity (required for motor learning) in under-nutrition and suggested that undernutrition severely affects the structural and functional maturation of the developing neurons. Thus, immature developmental characteristics of the brain regional neurocircuitry due to CMB in undernutrition was primarily responsible for the prolongation of electrical conduction times, increased latent periods, and abnormalities in the response pattern in term of reduced frequency, amplitude, and waveforms. These delayed developmental characteristics of the cerebellar cortex may induce deleterious effects on the motor learning of the developing UN child.

Electrophysiological Correlates of CB Formation. Mean total duration of Purkinje neuron evoked unit activity recorded from 20 day N and UN rats was subtracted to determine ΔT and was plotted as a function of difference in the rate of ^{14}C-glucose uptake in the cerebellar cortex between N and UN rats to determine ΔE. ΔE was calculated to determine the difference in the MB between N and UN rats. Regression analysis revealed a positive linear correlation in the duration of Purkinje neuron evoked unit activity (Δ-T) and ^{14}C-glucose uptake (Δ-E). The electrophysiological impairments correlated with the neuro-morphological deficits at the light and EM levels. The amplitude, duration, and frequency of Purkinje neuron electrical activities of N and UN animals were compared to determine ΔT (difference in the duration of electrical activity between age-matched N and UN animals) and ΔE was determined by estimating the cerebellar ^{14}C-glucose utilization in the vermis region from where the Purkinje neuron intracellular unit activity was recorded. To determine difference in the MB between N and UN brain, the following kinetic equation was derived:

$$\Delta T \; \alpha \; \Delta E \text{ or } \Delta T = k\Delta E$$

where k is a constant and depends on the nature of the cell (neuron) under investigation. The frequency of CB formation was proportional to the severity of nutritional stress, whereas nutritional rehabilitation of 80 days eliminated (via charnolophagy; as a basic molecular mechanism of intraneuronal detoxification) almost all CBs from the developing 30 days UN rats and ΔT and ΔE approached to zero during nutritional rehabilitation (Sharma et al. 1986; Sharma et al. 1987; Sharma et al. 1993a; Sharma et al. 1993b; Sharma and Ebadi 2014a).

Several terms have been used to describe autophagy such as endophagy, cytophagy, and endo-parasitism as a basic molecular mechanism of ICD in DPCI due to free radical overproduction. The number of lysosomes is significantly increased in the developing UN Purkinje neurons. Lysosomes are involved in the phagocytosis of degenerated mitochondria. However, Mother Nature has provided more number of mitochondria to sustain MB as compared to lysosomes. During oxidative and nitrative stress of malnutrition, lysosomes are increased to phagocytose CBs to a certain extent. However, charnolophagy occurs less frequently as compared to transformation of CB to functional mitochondria during nutritional rehabilitation. Hence, charnolophagy seems appropriate to describe CB autophagy in any metabolically-active mitochondria-rich living cell.

In our earlier studies we discussed how to prevent CB formation for maintaining healthy nervous system and cardiovascular system and induce it in cancer stem cells to eradicate MDR malignancies, with minimum or no side effects. Hence, CB formation, charnolophagy, and CS have direct clinical significance in health and disease. Moreover, natural abundance and increased sensitivity and susceptibility of the mitochondrial genome qualifies CB as a universal pre-apoptotic biomarker of DPCI. These original discoveries have tremendous theranostic applications in biomedical field to develop novel antioxidant-loaded NPs for mitochondrial protection and hence, MB for disease control and health promotion. Any physiological and/or pharmacological intervention augmenting MTs can inhibit CB formation to prevent progressive NDDs and CVDs. For example, balanced diet and moderate exercise can augment MTs to inhibit CB formation in the most vulnerable cells of our body. We emphasized primarily the therapeutic potential of nutritional rehabilitation, physiological Zn^{2+}, and MTs regulation in preventing and/or inhibiting CB molecular pathogenesis in a patient suffering from chronic malnutrition, NDDs, CVDs, and MDR malignancies (Sharma and Ebadi 2014).

Neurotoxins in Developing N and UN Brain

An environmental neurotoxin "domoic acid" (amnesic shellfish poison, DOM) is a rigid structural analog of excitatory amino acids, kainic acid (KA) and glutamic acid. Accidental ingestion of DA in some blue mussels caused DOM toxicity and fatalities in Montreal, Canada. Quantitative estimation of DOM and its isomers from sea food and body fluids was made by Zhao et al. (1997) using capillary electrophoresis, while microtiter glutamate receptor assay was developed by Van Dolah et al. (1997). By employing competitive ELISA, Osada et al. (1997) estimated DA levels in the sea food (Osada et al. 1995). A competitive ELISA was also developed from human body fluids by Smith and Kitt (1995). These methods for quantitative estimation of DOM from different biological sources could assess the safety and toxicity of DOM and provided evidence of its natural abundance. DOM has been used extensively to discover the basic molecular mechanism of disease-specific apoptosis and its possible prevention by pharmacological or dietary interventions. We reported DOM-induced CB formation and apoptosis in vascular smooth muscle cells and its association with cardiac arrhythmia, atherosclerotic plaque rupture, stroke, epilepsy, AD, and depression (Sharma and Dhalla 2001). Since both KA as well as DOM induce hippocampal CB formation and selective apoptosis in the CA3 and dentate gyrus neurons as observed in AD and depression; these environmental neurotoxins and sea food contaminants could be used to study the basic cellular, molecular, and genetic basis of CMB in sensory-motor impairments and depression in future.

Recently, we reported molecular pharmacology of KA and DOM to elucidate the basic molecular mechanism of neurodegeneration in AD, PD, and depression (Sharma et al. 2014). The KA and domoate models were used to examine the therapeutic benefits of various anti-epileptic drugs in developing N and UN rats. Experimental epilepsy was induced in developing N, UN, and nutritionally-rehabilitated rats by locally injecting graded doses of KA (an environmental neurotoxin from algae, Digenia simplex) in the right frontal cortex. The frequency and power spectral analysis of EEG was recorded to assess progressive changes in the computerized EEG during KA or DOM-epileptogenesis. The UN animals were highly susceptible to seizure discharge. They exhibited generalized tonic-clonic seizure discharge activity of prolonged duration and frequent episodes of clinical seizures even after temporary neuronal recovery. The generalization of seizure discharge activity occurred at lower doses of KA in UN rats and they exhibited considerable background electrical inhibition in their basal EEG records. Increase in δ and θ and decrease in α and β spectral frequencies was observed in the compressed spectral array (CSA) of UN animals. Delayed neuronal recovery with reduced background EEG and marked electro-silence in response to intra-rectal sodium valproate was observed in the UN animals due to significant CMB, implicated in CB molecular pathogenesis. Nutritionally-rehabilitated animals exhibited partial neuronal recovery as was evident by their body weight gain. Spike frequency, spike amplitude, and neuronal recovery times were not significantly different between N and UN animals at lower doses of KA (7.5–60 ng), whereas at higher doses

(120–500 ng), marked differences were observed in these parameters. The relative dominance of low frequency δ rhythm, particularly in response to either local KA or DA in the hippocampal CA-3 and dentate gyrus regions of UN rats, further confirmed CMB in undernutrition. ^{3}H-Glycine uptake was significantly higher than N rats in the hippocampus and spinal cord and lower in the cerebellum indicating that undernutrition significantly influences the therapeutic response to various antiepileptic drugs due to CB-induced CMB (Sharma et al. 1990).

Further studies were conducted to examine the neurotoxic effects of KA as well as DOM in developing rat cerebral cortex and mice hippocampus employing computerized EEG and NMR analyses to confirm CMB in undernutrition. KA as well as DOM produced reductions in α and β and increases in δ and θ EEG frequencies. A reverse trend was noticed while following antiepileptic treatment. DOM enhanced KCl-induced glutamate release from the rat hippocampal slices and increased Ca^{2+} influx in the neuroblastoma/glioma (NG108/15) cells. HPLC and NMR analyses revealed a typical reduction in GABA and increase in glutamate levels in DOM-treated mice hippocampus. DOM-induced dose and time-dependent induction of proto-oncogenes (c-fos and c-jun) was inhibited following prophylactic or therapeutic antiepileptic treatment with sodium valproate, pyridoxine, 5-α-pragnan-3 α-ol-20-one, nimodipine, or 8-(OH)-DPAT. High energy phosphorylated metabolites were not significantly affected with the sub-convulsive doses of DOM. However, reductions in N-acetyl aspartate (NAA), phosphocreatine (PCr), and ATP were observed with direct exposure of DOM to NG-108/15 cells in culture. CB formation in the developing UN hippocampus and Purkinje neurons was enhanced in intrauterine KA or DOM-exposed mice. MR imaging revealed a progressive increase in the T_2 intensities following sub-convulsive doses of DOM at the level of hippocampus, which was confirmed histologically as CA3 and dentate gyrus regions; however, the CA1 layer remained relatively preserved. CA-1 layer is particularly degenerated in hypoxia or in ischemic brain injury, which was noticed at significantly higher doses of either KA or DOM. Based on these findings, we confirmed that environmental neurotoxins (such as KA and DOM) enhance glutamate release, Ca^{2+} influx, and proto-oncogenes expression to accelerate neuro-apoptosis via CB formation which increases the after-hyperpolarization (AHP) duration of developing neurons during severe nutritional stress due to increased $[Ca^{2+}]_i$ overloading, CMB, and eventually mitochondrial degeneration triggering CB formation to cause progressive NDDs, such as AD, PD, MDDs, and drug addiction involving impaired cognitive performance (Sharma et al. 1986; Sharma et al. 1987; Dakshinamurti et al. 1993; Sharma and Dakshinamurti 1993; Sharma et al. 1993; Sharma and Ebadi 2014).

Brain to Body Weight Ratio during Nutritional Rehabilitation. We determined a ratio of brain weight vs body weight between developing 5–30 days postnatal N and UN rats. At any given age, this ratio was significantly ($p < 0.01$) high in the UN rats as compared to N rats. The brain to body weight ratio reduced as a function of nutritional rehabilitation. The data were analyzed by multiple measures two-way analysis of variance. The ratio of the squares of standard deviations (SDs) were calculated to obtain the F values which were used to determine the p values to evaluate the level of significance between N and UN brain weights and body weights. These data were derived from 12 animals in each experimental group. One-way ANOVA was performed on 30 days UN rats to quantitatively determine the incidence of

CBs formation as a function of nutritional rehabilitation of 80 days at different time intervals. CB formation was practically eliminated from 30 days UN rats which were subsequently rehabilitated for 80 days, suggesting CB recycling. Since brain weight in experimental animals was not significantly affected during postnatal undernutrition, some investigators proposed brain sparing hypothesis, which was challenged when brain regional neurochemistry, electrophysiology, and ultra-structural details were explored (The discovery of CB formation in the developing UN Purkinje neurons further challenges the brain sparing hypothesis).

CB Molecular Pathogenesis in UN Rat Purkinje Neurons. The degenerated mitochondrial membranes condense to form quasi-crystalline, pleomorphic, multi-lamellar, electron-dense intracellular inclusions. Initially, these multi-lamellar stacks are loosely arranged and subsequently, are condensed to form a mature CB. A mature CB is phagocytosed by lysosomes. The phagocytosis of CB by lysosomes is named as charnolophagy. The cell initially attempts to eliminate CB by ATP-driven lysosomal-dependent charnolophagy. The process of elimination of CB by charnolophagy depends on the size of the CB. If the size of CB is abnormally enlarged, the lysosomes phagocytose only a portion of CB to prevent the dissemination of toxic substances in a cell. A lysosome containing phagocytosed CB (partially or complete) is called charnolophagosome (CPS). The CPS is transformed to CS when the phagocytosed CB is hydrolyzed by the lysosomal enzymes. A portion of the CB becomes resistant to the hydrolysis of the lysosomal enzymes, which is aggregated near the CS. These aggregates are nonfunctional inclusions and can impair the normal metabolism and ICD. Thus, CS is involved in apoptotic degeneration due to the release of highly toxic mitochondrial metabolites as highlighted in this book.

Light Microscopic Analysis of N and UN Rat Cerebellar Cortex. A light microscopic picture of 10 days (left panel) and 20 days (right panel) normal and UN rat cerebellar cortex illustrates abnormal development of Purkinje neurons in the undernourished conditions. The Apical dendrite exhibited stunted growth in the UN rat cerebellar Purkinje neurons. The size of the Purkinje neurons was also significantly reduced due to CMB in undernutrition. The external granular layer remained persistent even after 20 days in the UN rat cerebellar cortex, indicating CMB. A light microscopic analysis of N and UN rat cerebellar cortex is presented in Fig. 42.

Light Microscopic Analysis of 30 Days N and UN Rat Cerebellar Cortex. Purkinje neurons exhibited normal appearance in N rat cerebellar cortex as compared to dehydrated appearance in the UN rat cerebellar cortex Purkinje neurons. A light microscopic analysis of 30 day N and UN rat cerebellar cortex is presented in Fig. 43.

TEM Analysis of Rat Purkinje Neuron Cytomorphology. The cytomorphology of the 10 days old N Purkinje cells was characterized by an increased number of mitochondria and well-developed RER representing normal protein synthesis as compared to UN rat cerebellar Purkinje neurons exhibiting a significantly reduced number of mitochondria as well as RER (a site of intracellular protein synthesis). These differences in the number of mitochondria as well as RER were more pronounced in the 30 days UN developing rat cerebellar Purkinje neurons. The RER membranes were sparse and disorganized in the UN rat cerebellar cortex. The Purkinje

Rat Cerebellar Cortex
Light Microscopic Analysis

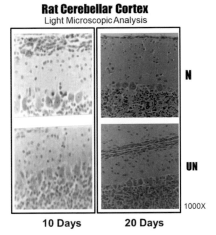

10 Days   20 Days

Fig. 42: Rat cerebellar cortex (Light microscopic analysis) (10 and 20 days).

Rat Cerebellar Cortex
Light Microscopic Analysis

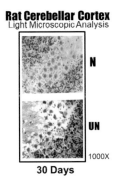

30 Days

Fig. 43: Rat cerebellar cortex (Light microscopic analysis) 30 days.

neurons were characterized by CS formation and destabilization. The RER synthesis was significantly down-regulated particularly near the *CS*, indicating that the release of toxic mitochondrial metabolites is involved in the inhibition of intracellular protein synthesis in UN conditions due to the down-regulation of AgNOR and RER synthesis. Purkinje neuron cytomorphology of 10 and 30 days N and UN rat cerebellar cortex is presented in Fig. 44.

Intracellular Morphology of 30 Days UN Rat Purkinje Neuron. In the 30-day severely UN rat cerebellar Purkinje neuron, the incidence of CB formation was significantly increased. Several pleomorphic CBs were identified. The incidence of lysosomes was also simultaneously increased as a function of nutritional stress. Consequently, charnolophagy became highly predominant during this period. This EM picture illustrates a significantly enlarged pleomorphic CB, a CPS (arrow), and a CS (square). A CS is formed when the phagocytosed CB is hydrolyzed by the lysosome as noticed in this EM picture. The ultrastructural morphology of the developing 30 days UN rat Purkinje neuron is presented in Fig. 45.

Rat Purkinje Neuron Cytomorphology
TEM Analysis

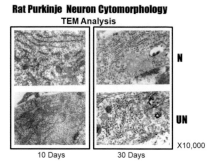

10 Days   30 Days

Fig. 44: Rat Purkinje neuron cytomorphology (TEM analysis) 10 days and 30 days.

Intracellular Morphology of Rat Purkinje Neuron
TEM Analysis

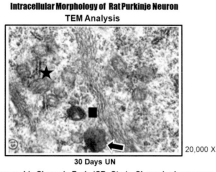

30 Days UN
Pleomorphic Charnoly Body (CB: Star); Charnolophagosome
(CPS: Arrow), and Charnolosome (CS: Square)

Fig. 45: Intracellular morphology of Purkinje neuron (30 days UN).

Rat Cerebellar Neuropil in N and UN Rats. A TEM analysis of the developing rat cerebellar neuropil revealed swollen mitochondria in the UN rat cerebellar cortex as compared to a normal rat (Fig. 46). Some degenerated mitochondrial membranes were condensed to form dense inclusions in the developing UN rat cerebellar cortex neuropil, as observed in this picture.

Cerebellar Myelination in N and UN Rat. The myelin exhibited immature developmental characteristics and was loosely wound around the axons in the UN rat cerebellum as compared to myelinated axons in the normal brain. Myelin was thin and displayed immature developmental characteristics due to CMB. The myelinated axons exhibited a significantly reduced number of microtubules in the UN rat cerebellum as compared to normal rat myelinated axons. A significant reduction in the number of microtubules in the UN rat cerebellum suggested impaired protein synthesis due to CMB and AgNOR down-regulation. Microtubules are involved in maintaining the structural and functional integrity of the developing axons for a normal axoplasmic flow. Significantly-reduced microtubules in the UN rats rendered the axons highly susceptible to deformation and further free radical attack. Myelinogenesis requires mitochondrial energy (ATP), which was significantly reduced in UN rat cerebellum. Myelinogenesis in the UN cerebellum was reduced due to CMB. E.M. pictures of 20 days N and UN rat cerebellum are presented in Fig. 47.

Rat Cerebellar Neuropil

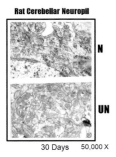

N

UN

30 Days   50,000 X

Fig. 46: Rat cerebellar neuropil (30 days N and UN).

Cerebellar Myelination
20 Days

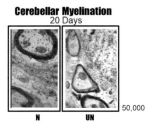

50,000

N   UN

Fig. 47: Cerebellar myelination (20 days) N and UN.

Synaptogenesis in UN Rat Cerebellar Cortex. In order to confirm the hypothesis that accumulation of CB at the junction of axon hillock can impair normal axoplasmic transport of various ions, neurotransmitters, hormones, neurotrophic factors (BDNF, and NGF-1, IGF-1), and mitochondria at the synaptic terminals to cause synaptic atrophy as noticed in AD patients, we examined the ultrastructural morphology of N and UN rat Purkinje neuron synaptic terminals. The accumulation of destabilized CS at the junction of the axon hillock releases numerous toxic substances to cause synaptic degeneration as seen in the synaptic terminal of UN rat cerebellar Purkinje neurons. This type of synaptic atrophy and degeneration occurs due to the toxic mitochondrial metabolites released from the destabilized and permeabilized CS as seen in the degenerating UN synaptic terminals and in patients suffering from severe malnutrition, chronic drug addiction, and AD. These findings confirmed our original hypothesis that: "synaptic terminal atrophy occurs due to accumulation of CB at the junction of axon hillock, whereas accumulation of destabilized CS at the junction of axon hillock releases toxic substances of mitochondrial metabolism to cause synaptic degeneration involved in reduced eye blinking, impaired motor learning, and other sensorimotor deficits of cognitive performance in UN children, chronic *drug* addiction, aging, and in AD". A TEM picture to demonstrate synaptic atrophy and synaptic degeneration in UN rat cerebellar Purkinje neurons is presented in Fig. 48.

Rat Purkinje Neuron Axonal Neurotubules in N and UN Rat Cerebellar Cortex.
The E.M. analysis of the rat Purkinje neuron axonal neurotubules in N rat cerebellar cortex demonstrated a roughly parallel arrangement of neurotubules. The neurotubules exhibited a twisted appearance in the UN rat Purkinje neuronal axons, confirming impaired axoplasmic transport of enzymes, hormones, proteins, growth factors,

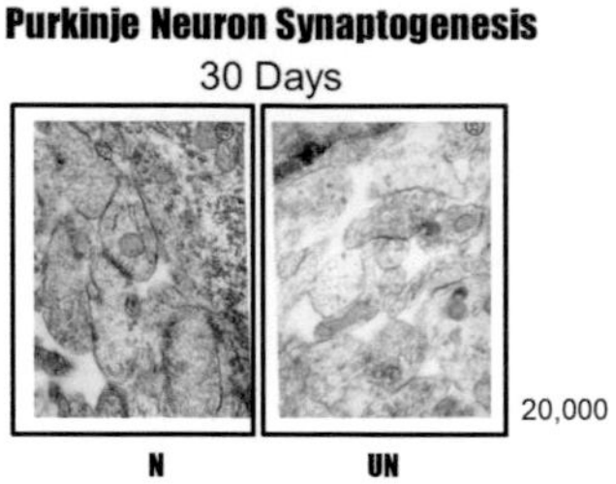

Purkinje Neuron Synaptogenesis
30 Days

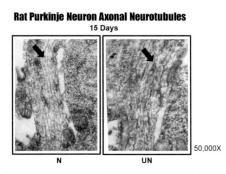

20,000

N   UN

Fig. 48: Purkinje neuron synaptogenesis (30 days N, UN).

Rat Purkinje Neuron Axonal Neurotubules
15 Days

50,000X

N   UN

Neurotubules appeared parallel in the normal and twisted
in the axons of undernourished rat Purkinje neurons

Fig. 49: Rat Purkinje neuron axonal neurotubules (15 days N and UN).

trophic factors, and mitochondria, needed for the normal brain regional synaptic neurotransmission and cybernetics involved in learning, intelligence, memory, and behavior. The E.M. analysis of the rat Purkinje neuron axonal neurotubules in N and UN rat cerebellar cortex is presented in Fig. 49.

Purkinje Neuron Synaptogensis in UN Rat Cerebellar Cortex. The E.M. analysis demonstrated synaptic atrophy and synaptic degeneration in UN rat cerebellar Purkinje neurons. This observation authenticated the hypothesis that accumulation of CB at the junction of the axon hillock impairs normal axoplasmic transport of various ions, neurotransmitters, hormones, neurotrophic factors (BDNF, and NGF-1, IGF-1), and mitochondria at the synaptic terminals to cause synaptic atrophy (as noticed in this picture and in the autopsy brain samples of AD patients). The accumulation of destabilized CS at the junction of the axon hillock releases toxic substances to cause synaptic degeneration as seen in UN rat cerebellar Purkinje neurons. This type of synaptic atrophy and synaptic degeneration occurs due to the release of toxic mitochondrial metabolites from the destabilized and permeabilized CS as seen in the synaptic terminal of degenerating UN Purkinje neurons. Thus, synaptic terminal atrophy occurs due to the accumulation of CB at the axon hillock, whereas accumulation of destabilized CS at this site releases toxic substances to cause synaptic degeneration involved in reduced eye blinking, impaired motor learning, and other cognitive and sensorimotor deficits in UN children, aging, and AD. Thus, CB molecular pathogenesis at the synaptic terminals induces early morbidity and mortality due to synaptic degeneration, as noticed in severe malnutrition, binge drinking, or morphine overdose.

References

Dakshinamurti, K., S.K. Sharma and M. Sundaram. 1991. Domoic acid induced seizure activity in normal rat. Neurosci Lett 127: 193–197.

Dakshinamurti, K., S.K. Sharma, M. Sundaram and T. Watanabe. 1993. Hippocampal changes in developing postnatal mice following intra-uterine exposure to domoic acid. J Neurosci 13: 4486–4495.

Dakshinamurti, K., S.K. Sharma, M. Sundaram and T. Watanabe. 1993. Hippocampal changes in developing postnatal mice following intra-uterine exposure to domoic acid. J Neurosci 13: 4486–4495.

Ebadi, M., H. Brown-Borg, S. Garrett, B. Singh, S. Shavali and S. Sharma. 2005. Metallothionein-mediated neuroprotection in genetically-engineered mice models of Parkinson's disease and aging. Molecular Brain Research 134: 67–75.

Jagtap, A., S. Gawande and S.K. Sharma. 2015. Biomarkers in vascular dementia 6 (A Recent Update). Bomarkers in Genomic Medicine 7: 43–56.

Osada, M. and J.E. Stewart. 1995. Determination of domoic acid by two different versions of a competitive enzyme-linked immunosorbent assay (ELISA). Bulletin of Environmental Contamination and Toxicology 54: 797–804.

Sharma, S., M. Kheradpezhou, S. Shavali, H.EI. Refaey, J. Eken, C. Hagen and M. Ebadi. 2004. Neuroprotective actions of coenzyme Q_{10} in Parkinson's disease. Methods in Enzymology 382: 488–509.

Sharma, S., C.S. Moon, A. Khogali, A. Haidous, A. Chabenne, C. Ojo, M. Jelebinkov, Y. Kurdi and M. Ebadi. 2013. Biomarkers of Parkinson's disease (Recent Update). Neurochemistry International 63: 201–229.

Sharma, S., A. Rais, R. Sandhu, W. Nel and M. Ebadi. 2013. Clinical significance of metallothioneins in cell therapy and nanomedicine. International Journal of Nanomedicine 8: 1477–1488.

Sharma, S. 2014. Molecular pharmacology of environmental neurotoxins. *In*: Kainic Acid: Neurotoxic Properties, Biological Sources, and Clinical Applications. Nova Science Publishers, New York. pp. 1–47.

Sharma, S. 2014. Nanotheranostics in evidence based personalized medicine. Current Drug Targets 15: 915–930.

Sharma, S., B. Nepal, C.S. Moon, A. Chabenne, A. Khogali, C. Ojo, E. Hong, R. Goudet, A. Sayed-Ahmad, A. Jacob, A. Murtaba and M. Firlit. 2014. Psychology of craving. Open Jr of Medical Psychology 3: 120–125.

Sharma, S. 2014. Beyond Diet and Depression (*Volume-1*). Nova Science Publishers, New York, U.S.A.

Sharma, S. 2014. Beyond Diet and Depression (*Volume-1*). Book Nova Sciences Publishers, New York, U.S.A.

Sharma, S. 2014. Beyond Diet and Depression (*Volume-2*). Nova Science Publishers, New York, U.S.A.

Sharma, S. and M. Ebadi. 2014a. Charnoly body as a universal biomarker of cell injury. Biomarkers and Genomic Medicine 6: 89–98.

Sharma, S. and M. Ebadi. 2014b. Significance of metallothioneins in aging brain. Neurochemistry International 65: 40–48.

Sharma, S. 2015. Alleviating Stress of the Soldier & Civilian. Nova Science Publishers, New York, U.S.A.

Sharma, S. 2015. Monoamine Oxidase Inhibitors: Clinical Pharmacology, Benefits, & Adverse Effects. Nova Science Publishers, New York, U.S.A.

Sharma, S., J. Choga, V. Gupta et al. 2016. Charnoly body as novel biomarker of nutritional stress in Alzheimer's disease. Functional Foods in Health and Disease 6: 344–377.

Sharma, S. 2017. Translational multimodality neuroimaging. Current Drug Targets 18: 1039–1050.

Sharma, S. and W. Lippincott. 2017. Emerging biomarkers in Alzheimer's disease (Recent Update). Current Alzheimer Research 14 (in press).

Sharma, S. 2017. *ZIKV* Disease (Prevention and Cure). Nova Science Publishers, New York, U.S.A.

Sharma, S.K., U. Nayar, M.C. Maheshwari and G. Gopinath. 1986. Ultrastructural studies of P-cell morphology in developing normal and undernourished rat cerebellar cortex. Electrophysiological Correlates Neurology India 34: 323–327.

Sharma, S.K., U. Nayar, M.C. Maheshwari and B. Singh. 1987. Effect of undernutrition on developing rat cerebellum: Some electrophysiological and neuromorphological correlates. J Neurol Sciences 78: 261–272.

Sharma, S.K., W. Selvamurthy, M.C. Maheshwari and T.P. Singh. 1990. Kainic acid induced epileptogenesis in developing normal and undernourished rats—A computerized EEG analysis. Ind Jr Med Res 92: 456–466.

Sharma, S.K., M. Behari, M.C. Maheshwari and W. Selvamurthy. 1990. Seizure susceptibility and intra-rectal sodium valproate induced recovery in developing undernourished rats. Ind J Med Res 92: 120–127.

Sharma, S.K. and K. Dakshinamurti. 1993. Suppression of domoic acid-induced seizures by 8-(OH)-DPAT. J Neural Transmission 93: 87–89.

Sharma, S.K., W. Selvamurthy and K. Dakshinamurti. 1993. Effect of environmental neurotoxins in the developing brain. Biometeorology 2: 447–455.

Sharma, S.K. and N.S. Dhalla. 2001. Domoic acid as a tool in molecular pharmacology. pp. 130–137. *In*: Gupta, S.K. (ed.). Pharmacology and Therapeutics in New Millinium. Narosa Publishing House, New Delhi (India). Chapter 12.

Smith, D.S. and D.D. Kitts. 1995. Enzyme immunoassay for the determination of domoic acid in mussel extracts. J Agric Food Chem 43(2): 367–371.

Van Dolah, F.M., T.A. Leighfield, L.H. Bennie, D.R. Hampson and J. Ramsdell. 1997. A microplate receptor assay for the amnesic shellfish poisoning toxin, domoic acid, utilizing a cloned glutamate receptor. Analytical Biochemistry 245: 102–105.

Widdowson, E.M. and R.A. McCance. 1957. Effect of a low-protein diet on the chemical composition of the bodies and tissues of young rats. Br J Nutr 11(2): 198–206.

Zhao, J.Y., P. Thibault and M.A. Quilliam. 1997. Analysis of domoic acid isomers in seafood by capillary electrophoresis. Electrophoresis 18: 268–276.

Chapter-20

Charnoly Body Formation in Drug Addiction and Other Chronic Multi-Drug-Resistant Diseases
(Therapeutic Potential of MTs)

INTRODUCTION

In general, craving may be divided into two categories: (i) craving for survival and (ii) craving to seek pleasure irrespective of deleterious life-threatening consequences. Typical examples of the pediatric population, kwashiorkor and/or marasmus, are associated with a craving for survival, whereas the adolescent population suffers from anorexia nervosa and bulimia due to psycho-neuroendocrinological disturbances and malnutrition during puberty. The Obese and adolescent population can be easily trapped in a vicious circle of craving for carbohydrates and a fat-rich diet to accomplish adequate amounts of the brain's region-specific serotonergic, DArgic, glutamatergic, and GABA-ergic neurotransmission to seek pleasure and combat mood swings (depression/anxiety). Moreover, diet has significant impact on immunocompromised chronic drug addicts, psychotic patients, HIV/AIDs patients, cancer patients, astronauts, war-wounded soldiers with post-traumatic stress disorder (PTSD), post-operative patients, premenstrual and post-partum women, and several clinical conditions where craving to eat a proper meal is significantly diminished due to CMB and the induction of brain regional neurodegenerative processes involving CB formation, charnolophagy induction, and CS destabilization involving uncontrolled release of highly toxic degenerated mitochondrial metabolites such as Cyt-C, iron, 8-OH, 2dG, dihydroxy nonenal, acetaldehyde, H_2O_2, and ammonia to impair ICD required for normal cellular function to remain healthy. To prevent and/or combat CMB involved in CB formation, charnolophagy induction, and CS destabilization, we need to provide hygienic and specialized well-nourished meals to this vulnerable group of patients not only to sustain their health and well-being but also for their ultimate survival.

We discovered that chronic abuse of cocaine and METH causes progressive reduction in the striatal DArgic neurotransmission, which is further abrogated by ethanol consumption. Thus, in addition to nicotine, ethanol abuse is the gateway to multiple drug abuse which may cause improper and unhealthy dietary craving resulting in impaired learning, intelligence, memory, behavior, early morbidity and mortality due to brain regional CB formation, charnolophagy induction, and CS destabilization. In addition, improper dietary, sex, drug craving, needle exchange, and HIV/AIDs may also impair physical, cognitive, and mental performance with a devastating impact on the overall personality of an individual. The accumulation of CB at the junction of the axon hillock causes a blockade in the axoplasmic transport of various enzymes, neurotransmitters, hormones, neurotrophic factors (i.e., IGF-1, BDNF, NGF) and mitochondria to cause synaptic atrophy, whereas CS destabilization and its sequestration can release afore-mentioned toxic substances to cause synaptic degeneration involved in impaired brain regional neurocybernetics and hence, abnormal cognitive performance as a function of time. Hence, basic knowledge of craving involving brain region-specific CB formation, charnolophagy induction, and CS destabilization, and nutritional rehabilitation involved in boosting the MB, will go a long way in the theranostic management of complicated cases of food, sex, and drug addiction as discussed in this chapter. Although sex and sleep, like eating, are essential components of life, these may become obsessions.

The term craving refers to strong desire or intense longing, is a hallmark of addiction, and characterized by obsessive thoughts and compulsive urges to use a substance whereas addiction is a compulsion to repeat a behavior regardless of its deleterious life-threatening consequences. Craving is often recognized as a feature of addiction, but the role of craving in the addictive process remains uncertain. Recently, the meaning of the craving has been extended to include all aspects of dependent individuals to use the addictive substance. Craving may be defined as an urge or desire to abuse substances, is a significant predictor of substance abuse, substance abuse disorder, and relapse following treatment. Typical examples are craving for a specific habit such as biblioholics, chocoholics, workaholics, medicine addiction, akrasia, alcoholism, alcohol-related traffic crashes, alcohol tolerance, alcoholics anonymous, cold turkey, computer addiction, craving for drug addiction, drug usage, ibogaine, internet addiction, chronic gambling, food addiction, pornography, and sex addiction. Various experimental models of craving have been proposed from biological, cognitive, and/or affective perspectives, which have improved treatment of addictive behaviors. In general, craving happens due to substance abuse during abstinence. Bowen et al. (2009) discussed how mindfulness-based relapse prevention (MBRP) may be effective in reducing substance craving by analyzing data from a randomized controlled trial that examined MBRP as an aftercare treatment for substance abuse disorders. Individuals who received MBRP reported lower levels of craving following treatment, in comparison to a treatment-as-usual control group, which mediated subsequent substance use outcomes. Thus, the mediation is consistent with the goals of MBRP and emphasizes the importance of interventions that increase acceptance and awareness and help foster a nonjudgmental attitude toward their experience.

Hence, understanding these processes may target both the experience of and response to craving (Kang et al. 2012; Kang et al. 2013).

It has been shown that the psychostimulant METH and MDMA can damage brain DAergic neurons by causing oxidative stress; however, its relevance to human METH users remains uncertain. METH is a drug of abuse and neurotoxin that may cause temporary or permanent impairments in the DA-ergic system, predisposing individuals to Parkinsonism. In earlier studies, Ajjimaporn et al. (2007) showed that METH causes DAergic cell death by increasing ROS synthesis and by depleting ATP levels by compromising brain regional MB. These effects were attenuated by pretreatment with $ZnCl_2$, which enhanced the expression of the zinc binding, antioxidant, anti-inflammatory, and anti-apoptotic protein, MT. Subsequently, these investigators studied the effects of $ZnCl_2$ on α-synuclein expression in METH-treated SK-N-SH cells in culture. METH increased α-synuclein expression and induced oxidative stress, whereas pretreatment with $ZnCl_2$ (50 μM) reversed this stimulatory effect, suggesting that Zn^{2+} provides neuroprotection through MTs induction. Furthermore, Ajjimaporn et al. (2005) examined the role of ROS in METH-induced SK-N-SH cell apoptosis and evaluated the therapeutic potential of Zn^{2+} and MT in METH-induced neurotoxicity. METH increased ROS synthesis, decreased ATP, and reduced the cell viability. Pre-treatment with Zn^{2+} attenuated METH-induced loss of cell viability. Zn^{2+} pre-treatment increased the expression of MTs and prevented METH-induced ROS generation and ATP depletion. Chelation of Zn^{2+} by CaEDTA induced a significant decrease in MT expression and depletion of protective effects of MTs against METH toxicity, suggesting that Zn^{2+}-induced MT induction protects DAergic neurons by preventing ROS synthesis and by inhibiting ATP depletion. It was also proposed that MTs may prevent METH-induced mitochondrial dysfunction, and, as a potent free radical scavenger, may provide neuroprotection in METH addiction and PD. By performing microPET neuroimaging with ^{18}F-DOPA, we established that CoQ_{10}, as an antioxidant and mitochondrial Complex-1 rejuvenator, provides neuroprotection against cocaine-induced neurotoxicity in C57BL/6J mice (Klongpanichapak et al. 2006). Alcohol augmented cocaine and METH-induced neurotoxicity, as determined by microPET neuroimaging in C57BL/6J mice (Sharma and Ebadi 2007). These observations provided evidence that alcohol may serve as a gateway to multiple drug abuse. Furthermore, MTs and Zn^{2+} as CB inhibitors, charnolophagy enhancers, and CS stabilizers, confer neuroprotection not only in METH neurotoxicity, but also in other neurotoxicities associated with alcohol, nicotine, and cocaine (Sharma 2017).

It has been demonstrated that in mice, the recreational drug MDMA ("ecstasy") causes degeneration of the mouse DA-ergic neurons. Xie et al. (2004) conducted cDNA microarray analysis to identify genes involved in MDMA-induced toxicity in DAergic neurons. Of the 15,000 mouse cDNA fragments studied, MT-1 and MT-2 emerged as candidate genes involved in MDMA-induced toxicity. Northern blot analysis confirmed the microarray findings and revealed upregulation of MT-1 and MT-2 mRNA in the ventral midbrain within 4–12 hrs following MDMA treatment. Immunoblotting also confirmed a similar increase in MT protein levels, with peak times occurring following increases in mRNA levels. MT-1-2 double knock-out mice were more vulnerable to MDMA-induced toxicity to DAergic neurons than wild-type mice. Endogenous induction of MTs with Zinc acetate conferred full protection against MDMA-induced toxicity, and exogenous MTs afforded partial protection, indicating that MDMA-induced toxicity to DAergic neurons is associated with increased MTs gene expression to provide neuroprotection at the transcriptional and translational level, confirming the therapeutic potential of MTs as CB antagonists, charnolophagy agonists, and CS stabilizers in MDMA-induced DA-ergic neurotoxicity. We reported that MTs provide mitochondrial protection by preventing CB formation and by augmenting charnolophagy during acute phase and by stabilizing CS and enhancing its exocytosis as a basic molecular mechanism of ICD to sustain normal cellular function. MTs serve as CB inhibitors, CPS/CS stabilizers, and charnolophagy and CS exocytosis enhancers in nicotine addiction during chronic phase (Sharma et al. 2013a; Sharma et al. 2013b; Sharma and Ebadi 2014; Sharma 2015; Sharma 2016; Sharma 2017a; Sharma 2017b).

Studies in mice proposed MT-2 as a potential candidate gene for ethanol (EtOH) preference (EP). Loney et al. (2006) performed RT-PCR to determine brain regional mRNA levels of MT-1 and MT-3 in 4 inbred mouse strains with variable EP and co-segregation of MT-2 brain expression with EP in F2 mice from 2 intercrosses (C57BL/6J × BALB/cJ and C57BL/6J × DBA/2J). Studies on MT_{dko} mice suggested that MT-1 is responsive to EtOH, with no evidence of differences between strains. MT-3 did not exhibit EtOH response yet indicated a strain-specific feature with C57BL/6J having the lowest levels of brain MT-3. MT-2 expression co-segregated with EP in F2 mice from a C57BL/6J (preferring) and DBA/2J (avoiding) intercross. Although, F2 mice from a cross with C57BL/6J and BALB/cJ (avoiding) strains followed a similar pattern, the results were insignificant. MT_{dko} mice had smaller litter sizes as well as increased weight compared to controls (129S1/SvImJ) and exhibited a slight increase in EP indicating that MT-2 is the candidate of the mouse MT gene family for EP; however, its effect on EP was dependent on the genetic background. Evidence also pointed to shared neural pathways involved in weight gain and obesity. However, the complex interaction between MT-2, EP, and weight gain/obesity is yet to be established.

This chapter describes MTs as CB inhibitors, charnolophagy enhancers, and CPS/CS stabilizers in multiple drug addiction, the role of NAC-1 gene in cocaine addiction, and the recent development of a monoclonal antibody 15A10 for the treatment of cocaine addiction. The chapter also describes the protective role of MTs and HSP-70 as CB inhibitor, charnolophagy enhancer, and CS stabilizer in alcohol liver disease (ALD) as confirmed by cDNA microArray analyses. That Maotai-induced MTs prevents hepatic fibrosis in the Chinese population and the role of MTs in cardiovascular protection are described briefly. The manner through which MTs induce cellular, molecular, and genetic resistance to anti-cancer therapy by inhibiting CB formation, augmenting charnolophagy, and by CPS/CS stabilization through the induction of tobacco-smoking-induced MDR proteins involved in MDR malignancies are also described.

MTs as CB Inhibitors, CPS/CS Stabilizers, and Charnolophagy and CS Exocytosis Enhancers in Nicotine Addiction

Post et al. (1984) autopsied male heavy smokers within 3 days of their postmortem. Samples from kidney, liver, and lung were taken for the analysis of Cd and protein binding within the cytosolic fraction. The levels in lung, liver, and kidney were 0.50 +/– 0.35, 2.21 +/– 0.63, and 17.4 +/– 8.8 µg Cd/g wet weight tissue, respectively. In the liver and kidney, ~ 75% was bound to a low-molecular-weight protein whereas the corresponding figure for the lung cytosolic fraction was 56%. After concentration of the low-molecular-weight Cd-binding protein(s) (CdBP) by ultrafiltration and preparative isoelectric focusing in a granulated gel, the Cd appeared in one single band with pI 5.8 (lung and liver) and 6.0 (kidney), respectively, suggesting that human lung exposed to Cd, via cigarette smoke, contains a CdBP, which binds Cd. The binding was less in the lungs than in liver or kidney, suggesting that Cd could be more toxic to the lung than to liver or kidney, as the protein serves a role in its detoxification. Of 1361 liver biopsy specimens, 24% contained orcein-positive granules. The highest positivity was found in biliary disease (90.9%), long before cirrhosis, whereas in chronic non-primarily biliary disease, positive results were noticed in patients with well-established cirrhosis. Orcein-positive granules were not found in acute liver disease. These granules were also demonstrated in tumor cells of primary hepatocellular carcinoma, while all the secondary tumor deposits were negative (Guarscio et al. 1983).

A study was designed to determine the placental Zn and Cd levels in mothers who were smokers, mothers who were exposed to air pollution, and those who were non-smokers, to establish a relationship between the expression of placental MT binding these metals and blood progesterone level. Placental Zn and Cd levels were measured by atomic absorption spectrometry. MT was determined immunohistochemically. Among 92 mothers, 33 were smokers (Group I), 29 had been exposed to air pollution (Group II), and 30 were non-smoker rural residents who had never been exposed to air pollution (Group III). Mean off-spring birth weight of 3198.62 +/– 380.01 g and mean placenta weight of 561.38 +/– 111.55 g of Group II was lower when compared with those of other two groups. In Group I, mean placental Cd and Zn were 0.063 +/– 0.022 µg/g and 39.84 +/– 15.5 µg/g, respectively. In Group II, mean placental Cd and Zn levels were higher than those of Group III. Blood progesterone levels of subjects in Group I (121 ng/ml) were the lowest of all groups. While the mean count of villi was the highest in Group III, the highest mean count of syncytial knots was in Group II. Thickening of vasculo-syncytial membrane was most prominent in Group I. Similarly, MT staining was positive and very dense in 72.7% (24/33) of cases in Group I. MT staining was positive in 69.0% (29/20) and denser in Group II cases compared to 36% (11/30) in Group III. This study showed that smoking increased Cd levels in placenta. The effects of exposure to air pollution were equally harmful as smoking related effects (Sorkun et al. 2007).

It has been reported that diabetes may increase the risk of Cd-induced kidney damage. The presence of MT antibody (MT-Ab) increased the susceptibility for tubular damage among Cd workers. This study focused on the relationships between levels of MT-Ab, urinary Cd, and kidney function in a Chinese type 2 diabetic population. Chen et al. (2006) performed a cross-sectional study on 229 type 2 diabetic patients (92 men and 137 women) who were recruited from two community centers in one district of Shanghai in China. Information was obtained from interviews, health records, and blood and urine analysis. The tubular biomarker β-2-microglobulin increased when MT-Ab and urinary Cd were elevated in male and female subjects; in contrast, urinary albumin, a glomerular biomarker, did not display such a pattern. This study proved that

MT-Ab can potentiate tubular dysfunction among diabetic subjects and that patients with high MT-Ab levels are more prone to develop tubular damage.

It has been recognized that esophageal squamous cell carcinoma (ESCC) in the Indian population is associated with poor nutritional status, low socioeconomic conditions, bidi smoking, and consumption of smokeless tobacco, besides alcohol drinking, and cigarette smoking. To determine the impact of these risk factors on molecular pathogenesis of ESCC, Kumar et al. (2007) determined the global gene expression profiles of 7 paired samples of ESCC and confirmed nonmalignant esophageal tissues using 19.1K cDNA microarrays. The most salient finding was 19 differentially-expressed genes encoding Zn^{2+} binding or modulating proteins associated with transcriptional regulation, ubiquitin-protein degradation, and the maintenance of Zn^{2+} homeostasis. The validation of differential expression of specific genes by real-time QRT-PCR in specimens of ESCC, esophageal dysplasia, and histologically nonmalignant esophageal tissues and tissue microarrays confirmed the data and demonstrated upregulation of Zn^{2+} finger proteins, cellular modulator of immune recognition (c-MIR), snail homolog 2 (SLUG), Zn^{2+} transporter (ZnT7), and downregulation of the Zn^{2+} metabolizing protein, MT1G. These investigators also observed the upregulation of mitogen activated protein kinase kinase-3 (MAP3K3/ MEKK3), a kinase anchor protein 13 (AKAP13), and transglutaminase2 (TG2). Interestingly, upregulation of ZnT7 transcripts in ESCC cells (TE13) grown in a Zn^{2+} deficient condition, indicated the deregulation of genes associated with Zn^{2+} homeostasis in ESCC.

A study estimated the concentration of MT, β-2-microglobuline (BMG), and II-6 in the amniotic fluid of smoking women during their pregnancy complicated by idiopathic oligohydramnios or premature rupture of the membranes (PROM). The amniotic fluid of 30 patients, complicated by oligohydramnios, during 20–42 weeks of their pregnancy was obtained. PROM was diagnosed in 15 patients. The degree of exposure to tobacco smoke was estimated based on cotinine levels in the serum of patients by ELISA (Serex). In the amniotic fluid MT, BMG and II-6 were measured by the "Cd/Heme assay" method using ^{109}Cd, immunoenzyme assay IMx, and ELISA (R&D), respectively. The results were divided into two groups according to gestational age: group A (20–30 weeks of gestation) and group B (31–42 weeks of gestation). A higher concentration of MT, BMG, and II-6 was determined in the earlier stage of pregnancy (group A), however, the highest concentration was noticed in women with idiopathic oligohydramnios. A positive correlation between concentrations of proteins MT/BMG was found in both groups of women. Based on this study, it was recommended that the determination of MT, β-2 microglobulin, and II-6 concentrations in the amniotic fluid could be useful in the assessment of the placental functions and fetal growth in the conditions of exposure to tobacco smoke. The correlation of MTs with Cu and Zn confirmed a lower access of these metals to fetal ovum in the conditions of exposure to tobacco smoke xenobiotics, which were different in PROM and idiopathic oligohydramnios cases (Milnerowicz and Darul 2005).

It has been shown that metal constituents of tobacco contribute to CVDs. In a study, Bernhard et al. (2006) determined serum concentrations of Al, Cd, Co, Cu, Fe, Mn, Ni, PB, Sr, and Zn of young nonsmokers, passive smokers, and smokers. Cd and Sr were increased in smokers compared with nonsmokers. The effects of these metals on primary arterial endothelial cells were assessed using microarray and RT-PCR. Sr did not interfere with endothelial cell transcription. In contrast, the effects of Cd in amounts delivered to the human body by smoking were dramatic. Arterial endothelial cells responded to Cd by upregulating MTs and by downregulating transcription factors. In addition, the mRNA of the intermediate filament protein Vimentin for the maintenance of cellular shape, was reduced. Surprisingly, pro-inflammatory genes were down-regulated in response to Cd, suggesting that by delivering Cd to the human body, smoking down-regulates transcription, exerts stress, and damages vascular endothelium. In contrast to the effects of cigarette smoke as a whole Cd seems to possess anti-inflammatory properties.

Effect of Smoking on Placental MTs. To assess the influence of smoking on the level of total protein, MT, albumin and lactoferrin in human breast milk, Milnerowicz and Schmarek (2005) analyzed samples of whole milk and supernatants of milk after centrifugation at 10000 x g and 105000 x g. Cd was determined by graphite furnace atomic absorption spectrometry. The concentrations were measured by the following methods: total protein by Lowry, albumin by colorimetry, cotinine and lactoferrin by ELISA, and MTs by ^{109}Cd/hemoglobin assay. The assessment of tobacco smoke exposure was based on concentrations of cotinine in breast milk (197 +/– 98 ng/ml in smokers and 23 +/– 11 ng/ml in non-smokers) and serum (179 +/– 87 ng/ml and 32 +/– 19 ng/ml, respectively). The level of Cd was 4X higher in the milk of smoking women than in non-smokers. The total protein was lower in smoking (37.3 +/– 10.6 mg/ml) than in non-smoking mothers (51.8 +/– 13.8 mg/ml). No significant differences between albumin and lactoferrin were observed. The MT was over twice as low in smokers (5.1 +/– 1.9 μg/ml) than in non-smokers (13.4 +/– 3.0 μg/ml), and an inverse correlation between MT and Cd was noticed. It was suggested that the breast milk of smoking mothers might be of lower nutritive value. As the amount of MT transported by milk to the mammary gland was smaller in smokers than in non-smokers, it may be advantageous to an infant because of the higher toxicity of the Cd-MT complex than that of inorganic Cd salts. In a similar study, Ronco et al. (2005) compared MT, Zn^{2+}, and Cd levels in human placentas of smoking and non-smoking women. Smoking was assessed by self-reported cigarette consumption and urine cotinine levels before delivery. Smoking pregnant women with urine cotinine levels > 130 ng/ml were included in the smoking group. Placental MT was determined by immunoblotting after tissue homogenization and saturation with $CdCl_2$ (1000 ppm). MT was analyzed with a monoclonal antibody raised against MT-1 and MT-2 and with a second anti mouse antibody conjugated to the alkaline phosphatase. Zn^{2+} and Cd were determined by neutron activation analysis and atomic absorption spectrometry, respectively. Smokers showed higher placental MT and Cd levels, together with decreased newborn birth weights, as compared to non-smokers, confirming that cigarette smoking increases Cd in placenta and suggested that this element has a stimulatory effect on placental MT production. Ronco et al. (2006) reported higher levels of MTs in placentas of smokers compared to non-smokers. They designed experiments to separate and evaluate MT-1 and MT-2 in placentas of smokers and non-smokers. MTs were extracted and separated by ion-exchange HPLC, previously saturated with $CdCl_2$. Two peaks eluting at 6 and 12.5 min, corresponding to MT-1 and MT-2, respectively, were obtained. MTs in both peaks was identified by immunoblotting using a monoclonal antibody against MT-1 and MT-2. Each isoform was calculated after measuring its Cd content by atomic absorption spectrometry (AAS) and with the ICP-MS. In placentas of smokers, MT-2 levels increased by 7X compared to non-smokers, whereas MT-1, remained unchanged. Total placental Cd and Zn concentrations, determined by AAS and neutron activation analysis, respectively, were higher in smokers. MTs were in excess to bind all Cd ions present in placentas. However, most of the placental Zn remained unbound to MTs, although a twice as many Zn ions could be bound to MT in smokers. Thus, MT-2 was the main isoform induced by smoking, suggesting that this isoform could be involved in placental Cd and Zn retention, which could contribute to reduce the transfer of Zn to the fetus, and may be associated to detrimental effects on fetal growth and development.

Smoking and the Influence MTs on Fetal Development. Normal trophoblast function, including implantation, hormone production, and formation of the selectively permeable maternofetal barrier, is essential for the establishment and maintenance of the fetoplacental unit and proper fetal development. Maternal cytotoxicant exposure causes the destruction of these cells, especially the terminally-differentiated syncytiotrophoblasts, and results in poor pregnancy outcomes. These outcomes range from intrauterine growth retardation and malformation to spontaneous abortion or stillbirth. There is evidence that the metal-binding protein, MT, is involved in the protection of human trophoblastic cells from heavy metal-induced apoptosis and severe oxidative stress-induced apoptosis. MT, with its unique biochemical structure, can both bind essential metal ions, such as the transcription modulator Zn, and yet allow their ready displacement by toxic nonessential metal ions or damaging free radicals, suggesting that MTs may be responsible not only for sequestering the cytotoxic agents, but also for altering signal transduction in the affected cells. McAleer and Tuan (2004) reviewed several causes of adverse pregnancy outcomes (specifically, prenatal exposure to cigarette smoke and alcohol, gestational infection, and exposure to environmental contaminants), and discussed the role of Zn in modulating the cellular response to these toxic insults, and proposed how MTs may function to mediate this protective response. We reported that MTs provide mitochondrial protection by preventing CB formation and augmenting charnolophagy during the acute phase and by stabilizing CS and by enhancing its exocytosis as a basic molecular mechanism of ICD to sustain normal cellular function during chronic phase (Sharma et al. 2013a; Sharma et al. 2013b; Sharma and Ebadi 2014; Sharma 2015; Sharma 2016; Sharma 2017a; Sharma 2017b).

MTs and Zinc as CB Inhibitors, Charnolophagy Enhancers, and CPS/CS Stabilizers in METH Addiction

Free Radical-induced METH Neurotoxicity. In an earlier study, samples from illicit preparations of amphetamine and METH were investigated by combined gas chromatography-mass spectrometry (GC/MS) to detect and identify contaminants, excipients, and by-products from manufacture. These samples were also subjected to energy-dispersive X-ray (EDX), and it was determined that the preparations of these compounds were made in the presence of Zn^{2+}, probably as a reductant. In addition to identifying polycondensation products, the illicit origin of amphetamine-type drugs can be determined by the detection of contaminants and by-products. Thus, a multidisciplinary analytical approach yielded data for comparative examinations and legal purposes (Lomonte et al. 1976).

Simonick and Watts (1992) applied the Abbott TDx Urine Amphetamine/ METH-II fluorescence polarization immunoassay technique to determine D-METH in hemolyzed whole blood. The assay had 100% cross-reactivity with D-METH and only 8% cross-reactivity with L-METH. Whole blood was fortified with D-METH at concentrations ranging from 25 to 1000 ng/mL. The whole blood calibrators were used to evaluate the following sample preparation techniques: direct, diluted, and buffer, and precipitated using methanol, acetone, sulfosalicylic acid, trichloroacetic acid, and zinc sulfate. Calibrators and samples were prepared by mixing 200 μL of whole blood and 200 μL precipitation reagent and centrifuging at 10,000 rpm for 5 min (9600 × g). A 50-μL aliquot of the supernatant was used for the assay. Using the zinc sulfate precipitation, blood calibration curves showed a linear range of 25–1000 ng/mL. The within-run precision for the 25-, 60-, and 200-ng/mL D-METH blood controls showed percent coefficients of variation of 17.8, 17.0, and 5.4, respectively. The TDx results were compared to RIA and GC/MS assays for the METH controls and for 8 positive case specimens and found reliable for screening of hemolyzed whole blood.

Evidence has accumulated to suggest that METH neurotoxicity is mediated via the overproduction of the superoxide radicals. Hirata et al. (1995) showed that METH-induced DA depletion is attenuated in CuZnSOD transgenic (Tg) mice. They used autoradiographic studies of $[^{125}I]$-RTI-55 labeled serotonin (5-HT) uptake sites to evaluate the effect of a two-dosing schedule (5 mg/kg or 10 mg/kg × 4) of METH on striatal 5-HT uptake sites in nontransgenic (Non-Tg), heterozygous (Hetero), and homozygous (Homo) SOD-Tg mice. The low dose of METH caused no significant changes in striatal 5-HT uptake sites in any of the groups, whereas a high dose caused marked decreases (–74%) in striatal 5-HT uptake sites in Non-Tg mice. In contrast, 5-HT uptake sites showed only a 31% decrease in homozygous SOD-Tg mice whereas heterozygous SOD-Tg mice showed 63% depletion, suggesting that increased SOD activity can protect against METH-induced neurotoxicity in the striatal 5-HTergic terminals, which provide further evidence for a role of oxidative stress in the neurotoxic effects of METH.

It is now well established that administration of METH to animals causes loss of DAergic terminals in the brain. Cadet et al. (1995) tested the effects of METH in CuZn-SOD transgenic (SOD Tg) mice, which express the human CuZnSOD gene. In nontransgenic (non-Tg) mice, acute METH administration caused significant decreases in DA and DOPAC in the striata of non-Tg mice. METH caused decreases in striatal DA and DOPAC in the non-Tg mice, but not in the SOD-Tg mice. Similar studies were carried out with MPTP, which also induced striatal DA and DOPAC depletion. As noticed in METH neurotoxicity, MPTP induced significant depletion of DA and DOPAC in the non-Tg mice, but not in the SOD Tg mice, suggesting that the mechanisms of toxicity of both METH and MPTP involved superoxide radical formation. To evaluate the role of oxyradicals in METH-induced neurotoxicity, Cadet et al. (1994) tested its effects in CuZn-SOD transgenic (Tg) mice, which express the human CuZnSOD gene. In non-Tg mice, acute METH administration induced decreases in levels of DA and DOPAC in the striatal and cortical regions of non-Tg mice. In contrast, there were no significant decreases in cortical or striatal DA in the SOD-Tg mice. The effects of METH on DOPAC were also attenuated in both structures of these SOD-Tg mice. Chronic METH administration caused reduction in the striatal DA and DOPAC in the non-Tg mice, whereas the SOD-Tg mice were not affected, suggesting that, METH-induced DAergic toxicity may be secondary to increased production of ROS such as the superoxide radical.

Wang et al. (1995) studied the effects of a single dose of the indirect DA agonists amphetamine and METH on the behavior and mRNA expression of c-fos, a member of the leucine zipper family, zif/268 (NGFI-A, egr1, and Krox-24), a member of the Zn^{2+} finger family, and the opioid peptide, preprodynorphin, in various regions of rat forebrain with quantitative *in situ* hybridization histochemistry 1, 2, 3, 6, or 30 hrs after injection. A qualitatively different behavioral syndrome was induced following METH (15 mg/kg, i.p.) as compared with that observed after amphetamine (5 mg/kg, i.p.). Similarly, METH induced a different pattern of c-fos and zif/268 m RNA in sensory/motor cortex, dorsal striatum (caudate-putamen), and ventral striatum (nucleus accumbens) than did amphetamine. The increase in c-fos mRNA expression peaked at 1 hr and returned to basal levels in all regions within 3 hrs. In contrast, the increase in zif/268 mRNA expression in the cortical regions was also significantly high at 1 and 2 hrs, gradually returning to basal levels by 6 hrs after either drug. However, in the striatum, zif/268 mRNA levels peaked at 1 hr and declined gradually to basal levels by 6 hrs. Interestingly, METH caused suppression of zif/268 gene expression (> 50%) in both caudate-putamen and nucleus accumbens within 3 hrs. Preprodynorphin mRNA expression was increased in a patchy motif in the caudate-putamen and nucleus accumbens beginning at 2 hrs and returning to basal levels by 30 hrs after injection of either drug. The induction of preprodynorphin mRNA in the caudate 3, 6, and 18 hrs after amphetamine or METH injection, provided a detailed dynamic description of the differential modulation of c-fos, zif/268, and preprodynorphin in the cerebral cortex and striatum by amphetamines as a function of time. These data implicate immediate early gene and preprodynorphin gene expression in the differential response of medium spiny striatal neurons to METH and amphetamine. Jayanthi et al. (1998) investigated the effects of METH-induced toxicity on brain cortical and striatal antioxidant defense systems. As METH-induced toxicity is attenuated in Cu/Zn-SOD-Tg mice, these investigators determined if METH had a differential effect on antioxidant enzymes on these mice. METH (4×1) mg/kg induced decrease in Cu/Zn-SOD activity in the cortical region without altering striatal enzymatic activity in non-Tg mice; whereas homozygous SOD-Tg mice showed a significant increase in the striatum. In addition, METH induced a decrease in catalase (CAT) activity in the striatum of non-Tg mice and increase in the cortex of homozygous SOD-Tg mice. METH also decreased glutathione peroxidase (GSH-Px) in both cortical and striatal regions of non-Tg mice and in the striatum of heterozygous SOD-Tg mice. Lipid peroxidation was increased in both cortices and striata of non-Tg and heterozygous SOD-Tg, mice, whereas the homozygous SOD-Tg mice were not affected, suggesting the predominant role for oxygen-based radicals in METH-induced toxicity.

It has been demonstrated that the administration of METH to mammals causes deleterious effects in their brain monoaminergic systems due to oxidative stress. Acute administration of METH causes the activation of immediate-early genes (IEGs) such as c-fos and Zif268 mRNA in rodent brains. However, the exact mechanisms involved in these changes have not been completely explored. As a first step towards assessing a possible role for free radicals in METH-induced changes in IEGs, Hirato et al. (1998) used CuZn SOD transgenic (Tg) mice and evaluated the effects of METH on c-fos and Zif268 mRNAs by *in situ* hybridization. Mice were injected with 25 mg/kg of METH and sacrificed at various time points afterwards. There were significant increases in both c-fos and Zif268 mRNAs in the frontal cortex and striatum of both strains of animals. The increases in Zif268 were attenuated in the CuZn SOD-Tg mice; the increases in *c-fos* were also attenuated, indicating that superoxide radicals might play an important role in the activation of Zif268 following METH administration. This is because IEGs are modulators of gene expression, suggesting that oxidative mechanisms might be important in neuroadaptive changes triggered by stimulant drug.

It is known that the use of METH leads to neurotoxic effects in mammals. These neurotoxic effects are related to the production of free radicals. Oxidative stress, ROS, and nitrogen (RNS) species are involved in various *NDDs* such as PD, AD, and ALS. Both ROS and RNS have very short half-lives, thereby making their identification difficult as a cause of neurodegeneration. To assess the role of ONOO$^-$ in METH-induced DAergic neurons, Imam et al. (2001) investigated the production of 3-nitrotyrosine (3-NT) in the mouse striatum. 3-NT increased in the striatum of wild-type mice treated with multiple doses of METH (4×10 mg/kg, 2 hrs interval) as compared with the controls. However, no significant production of 3-NT was observed either in the striata of nNOS $-/-$ or SOD-Tg mice treated with similar doses of METH. The DAergic degeneration induced by METH was also attenuated in nNOS $-/-$ or SOD-Tg mice, confirming that METH triggers its neurotoxic effects via the production of ONOO$^-$. Administration of METH induced significant increases in TUNEL-positive cells, in PARP cleavage, and in caspase-3 activity in the striata of C57BL/6J mice. These deleterious effects were attenuated in the Cu /Zn-SOD transgenic mice, indicating that superoxide radicals are involved in METH-induced cell death (Deng and Cadet 2000).

Mirecki et al. (2004) measured levels of key antioxidant defenses [reduced (GSH) and oxidized (GSSG) glutathione, six major GSH system enzymes, Cu/Zn superoxide dismutase (CuZnSOD), (and uric acid)] that are altered following exposure to oxidative stress, in autopsied brain of human METH abusers. Changes in the total (n = 20) METH group were limited to the DA-rich caudate (the striatal subdivision with the most severe DA loss) in which only activity of CuZnSOD and GSSG levels were altered. In the six METH abusers with severe caudate DA loss, caudate CuZnSOD activity and uric acid levels were increased with a trend for decreased GSH, suggesting that the brain levels of many antioxidant systems are preserved in METH abusers, and that GSH depletion, during severe oxidative stress, might occur only with severe DA loss. Increased CuZnSOD and uric acid might reflect compensatory responses to oxidative stress. Imam et al. (2001) developed an HPLC/EC method to identify 3-nitrotyrosine (3-NT), an *in vitro* and *in vivo* biomarker of ONOO$^-$ in cell cultures and the brain to evaluate if agent-driven neurotoxicity is produced by the generation of ONOO$^-$. A single, or multiple injections of METH produced increase in 3-NT in the striatum, which correlated with the striatal DA depletion. PC12 cells treated with METH had significantly increased 3-NT and DA depletion. Pretreatment with antioxidants such as Se and Melatonin protected against 3-NT and depletion of striatal DA. Pretreatment with ONOO$^-$ decomposition catalysts such as 5, 10, 15, 20-tetrakis(N-methyl-4'-pyridyl)porphyrinato iron III (FeTMPyP) and 5, 10, 15, 20-tetrakis (2,4,6-trimethyl-

3,5-sulfonatophenyl) porphinato iron III (FETPPS) protected against METH-induced 3-NT and striatal DA depletion. These investigators used pharmacological manipulation and transgenic animal models to further investigate the role of ONOO⁻. A selective neuronal nNOS inhibitor, 7-nitroindazole (7-NI), protected against 3-NT formation as well as striatal DA depletion. Similar results were observed with nNOS knockout and Cu/Zn superoxide dismutase (CuZnSOD)-overexpressed transgenic mice models. By using the protein data bank crystal structure of tyrosine hydroxylase, these investigators postulated the nitration of specific tyrosine moiety in the enzyme that is responsible for DAergic neurotoxicity, supporting the hypothesis that the ROS, RNS, and ONOO⁻, play a major role in METH-induced DA-ergic neurotoxicity and that antioxidants and ONOO⁻ decomposition catalysts can protect against METH-induced neurotoxicity. These antioxidants and decomposition catalysts may have therapeutic potential in the treatment of psychostimulant addictions because they prevent METH-induced CB formation and augment charnolophagy to provide neuroprotection (Sharma 2017). In addition, Imam et al. (2001) studied METH-induced alterations in the expression of p^{53} and Bcl-2 protein in the striatum of wild type, neuronal NOS knockout (nNOS –/–) and Cu/Zn-SOD-Tg mice. METH treatment up-regulated p^{53} and down-regulated BCl_2 expression in the striatum of wild type mice. No significant alterations were observed in the expression of these proteins in the nNOS –/– or SOD-Tg mice, suggesting that METH induces neurotoxic effects via the production of free radicals and secondary disruptions in the expression of genes involved in apoptosis and cell death machinery through CB formation and CS destabilization.

Genetic Correlates of Addiction. It is known that Cu and Zn are trace nutrients essential for normal brain function, yet an excess of these elements can be toxic. It is important therefore that these metals be closely regulated. Jones et al. (2006) conducted a quantitative trait loci (QTL) analysis to identify chromosomal regions in the mouse containing possible regulatory genes. The animals came from 15 strains of the BXD/Ty recombinant inbred (RI) strain panel and the brain regions analyzed were the frontal cortex, caudate-putamen, nucleus accumbens, and ventral midbrain. Several QTL were identified for Cu and/or Zn, most notably on chromosomes 1, 8, 16, and 17. Genetic correlational analysis also revealed associations between these metals and DA, Cocaine responses, saccharine preference, immune response, and seizure susceptibility. Particularly, the QTL on chromosome 17 was also associated with seizure susceptibility and contained the histocompatibility H2 complex, indicating that regulation of Zn and Cu is under polygenic influence and is related to CNS function. Based on these findings, these investigators recommended that future work will reveal genes underlying the QTL and how they interact with other genes and the environment. More importantly, the genetic underpinnings of Cu and Zn brain homeostasis will aid the understanding of neurological diseases that are related to Cu and Zn dyshomeostasis.

The Role of NAC-1 Gene in Cocaine and METH Addiction. NAC1 cDNA was identified as a novel transcript induced in the nucleus accumbens from rats chronically treated with cocaine. NAC1 is a member of the Bric-a-brac Tramtrac Broad complex/ Pox virus and Zn^{2+} finger family of transcription factors and has been shown by overexpression studies to prevent the development of behavioral sensitization resulting from repeated cocaine treatment. NAC1 is a cocaine-regulated POZ/BTB

(Pox virus and Zn^{2+} finger/Bric-a-brac Tramtrack Broad complex) protein and is increased by cocaine selectively in the nucleus accumbens, a CNS region important for drug addiction. Each of the two NAC1 isoforms, sNAC1 (short NAC1) and lNAC1 (long NAC1), may serve as corepressors for other POZ/BTB proteins. Levels of the mRNA NAC-1 are increased in the rat forebrain weeks after cocaine exposure. This long-term neuroadaptation occurs during the expression of behavioral sensitization, a model of psychostimulant-induced paranoia. NAC-1, the protein encoded by this cocaine-regulated mRNA, contains a Pox virus and Zn^{2+}-finger/bric-a-brac tramtrack broad complex (POZ/BTB) motif, which mediates interactions among several transcriptional regulators. Mackler et al. (2000) demonstrated that NAC-1 acts as a transcription factor. NAC-1 was localized to the nucleus of neurons in the brain. Transfection of NAC-1 in cell culture repressed transcription of a reporter gene. NAC-1 was also influenced by the actions of other POZ/BTB proteins in mammalian two-hybrid studies; these interactions required the presence of the POZ/BTB domain. However, NAC-1 appeared to be a unique POZ/BTB transcriptional regulator because it does not contain any Zn^{2+} finger regions found in these other DNA-binding proteins. Adenoviral-mediated overexpression of NAC-1 protein in the rat nucleus accumbens prevented the development but not the expression of behavioral sensitization induced by repeated administration of cocaine, indicating that NAC-1 may modify the long-term behaviors of psychostimulant abuse by regulating gene transcription in the mammalian brain.

NAC1 is a novel member of the POZ/BTB (Pox virus and Zn^{2+} finger/Bric-a-bracTramtrack Broad complex) but varies from other proteins of this class in that it lacks the characteristic DNA-binding motif, suggesting a novel role. In a study, Mackler et al. (2003) reported the cloning and characterization of the corresponding gene. The mouse Nac1 gene consist of 6 exons, with exon 2 containing an alternative splice donor, providing a molecular explanation of the splice variants observed in a mouse and a rat. Transcripts of Nac1 were detected in different mouse tissues with prominent expression in the brain. The mouse Nac1 gene was localized to chromosome 8, suggesting a highly plausible candidate gene to explain differences in cocaine-induced behaviors between C57BL6/J and DBA/2J mice that had previously been mapped to the area. In addition, a functional AP1 binding site was identified in an intron 1 enhancer of the Nac1 gene that plays an essential role in the activation of the gene in differentiation of neuroblastoma cells. Co-transfection with immediate early genes c-jun and c-fos expression plasmids, which encode the two subunits of AP1, activated the wild type Nac1 intron 1 enhancer two-fold over basal, nearly at the level of the NAC1 enhancer activity seen in differentiated N2A cells. Mutation of the AP1 completely abrogated all activation of the NAC1 enhancer in differentiated N2A cells. Activation of c-fos and c-jun following chronic drug treatments has been well characterized. These data described one potential regulatory cascade involving these transcription factors and activation of NAC1. Hence, the identification of drug-induced alterations in gene expression is key to understanding the types of molecular adaptations underlying addiction. In a similar study, Korutla et al. (2005) investigated whether sNAC1 and NAC1 demonstrated protein-protein interactions with other corepressors. Histone deacetylase (HDAC) inhibition reversed sNAC1 and lNAC1 repression of Gal4 luciferase, but only in neuronal-like cultures. As these inhibitors do not distinguish among histone deacetylases, two histone deacetylases were selected for further study. HDAC 3 and 4 both demonstrated protein-protein interactions with sNAC1 and lNAC1. This was demonstrated using coimmunoprecipitations, glutathione-S-transferase (GST) pulldowns, and mammalian two-hybrids. Importantly, either the POZ domain or NAC1 without the POZ domain can bind these two HDACs. Other corepressors, particularly, NCoR (nuclear receptor corepressor), SMRT (silencing mediator for retinoid and thyroid hormone receptor), and mSin3a, did not exhibit protein-protein interactions with sNAC1 and lNAC1. None showed protein-protein interactions in GST pulldowns or mammalian two-hybrids. The results of these experiments indicated sNAC1 and lNAC1 recruit histone deacetylases for transcriptional repression, further enhancing POZ/BTB protein mediated repression in cocaine and METH addiction. Mackler et al. (2007) employed constitutive gene deletion to elucidate the role of NAC1 *in vivo*. Nac1 mutant mice remain viable with no obvious developmental or physiological impairments. Earlier studies suggested a role for NAC1 in cocaine-mediated behaviors. Therefore, these investigators evaluated behaviors associated with psychomotor stimulant effects in Nac1 mutant mice. Acute locomotor activating effects of cocaine or amphetamine were absent in Nac1 mutant mice; however, longer exposure to these stimulants resulted in the development of behavioral sensitization. Acute rewarding properties of cocaine and amphetamine were also blunted in mutant mice, yet repeated exposure resulted in conditioned place preference, as observed in wild-type mice. Increases in extracellular DA in the nucleus accumbens, which accompany acute cocaine administration, were blunted in mutant mice, but following chronic cocaine extracellular DA levels, were increased to the same extent as in wild-type mice, suggesting the involvement of NAC1 in the acute behavioral and neurochemical responses to psychomotor stimulants.

In a report, Korutla et al. (2007) identified CoREST as a protein that interacts with NAC1. NAC1 is a cocaine-regulated Pox virus and Zn^{2+} finger/Bric-a-brac Tramtrack Broad complex (POZ/BTB) repressor protein, which mediates interactions among several other transcriptional regulators. These investigators detected an interaction between NAC1 and CoREST in neuro-2A cells and HEK293T cells and found that the POZ/BTB domain was necessary for interaction with CoREST. Only one of five mutations in the POZ/BTB domain that disrupts the homodimer assembly interfered with NAC1 and CoREST interactions, indicating that POZ/BTB homodimer formation is not required for NAC1-CoREST interaction. CoREST demonstrated protein-protein interactions with both isoforms of NAC1, sNAC1, and lNAC1. Coimmunoprecipitation studies revealed that NAC1 and CoREST are physically bound together. To further support the results, a direct interaction was demonstrated in glutathione-S-transferase pull down assays. siRNA directed against NAC1 mRNA reduced NAC1 protein expression and resulted in the reversal of CoREST-mediated repression in cells. This interaction between NAC1 and CoREST was not found for other POZ/BTB proteins. Endogenous interaction was demonstrated in lysates from rat brain samples. This was the first report to demonstrate that a POZ/BTB protein interacts with CoREST, suggesting that CoREST may be part of the NAC1 repressor mechanism. However, the exact role of NAC1 in CB molecular pathogenesis of drug addiction is yet to be established.

HSP-70 as CB Inhibitor, Charnolophagy Enhancer, and CS Stabilizer in Drug Addiction. It is now well-established that all cells, from bacteria to human, have a common response to stress that protect them from injury. HSPs, also known as stress proteins and molecular chaperones, play a crucial role in protecting cellular homeostatic processes from environmental and physiologic insult by preserving the structure of normal proteins and repairing or removing damaged ones. An understanding of the interplay between HSPs and cell stress tolerance will provide new tools for treatment and drug design that enhance preservation or restoration of health. For example, the increased vulnerability of tissues to injury in some conditions, such as aging, diabetes mellitus, and menopause, or with the use of certain drugs, such as some antihypertensive medications, is associated with an impaired HSP response, leading to induction of CB molecular pathogenesis in the most vulnerable cells. Additionally, diseases that are associated with tissue oxidation, free radical formation, disorders of protein folding, or inflammation, may be improved therapeutically by elevated expression of HSPs. The accumulation of HSPs, whether induced physiologically, pharmacologically, genetically, or by direct administration of the proteins, protect the organism from a variety of pathological conditions by preventing CB induction, augmenting charnolophagy, and by CSs stabilization, including myocardial infarction, stroke, sepsis, viral infection, trauma, NDDs, retinal damage, congestive heart failure, arthritis, sunburn, colitis, gastric ulcer, diabetic complications, and transplanted organ failure. Conversely, lowering HSPs in cancer tissues can amplify the effectiveness of chemo- or radiotherapy. MT and HSPs are induced in MDR malignancies. Treatments and agents that induce HSPs include hyperthermia, heavy metals (Zn^{2+} and Sn^{2+}), salicylates, dexamethasone, cocaine, nicotine, alcohol, α-adrenergic agonists, PPAR-γ agonists, bimoclomol, geldanamycin, geranylgeranylacetone, and cyclopentenone prostanoids. Compounds that suppress HSPs include quercetin (a bioflavinoid), 15-deoxyspergualin (an immunosuppressive agent) and retinoic acid. Researchers who are cognisant of the HSP-related effects of these and other agents will be able to use them to develop new therapeutic paradigms (Tytell and Hooper 2001). I have recently proposed the therapeutic potential of MTs and HSP-70 as CB inhibitors, charnolophagy inducers, and CS stabilizers in NDDs and CVDs. Just like MTs, HSP-70 is also involved in MDR malignancies as CB inhibitors, charnolophagy inducers, and CS stabilizers (Sharma 2017a,b).

Dopamine Transporter in Drug Addiction. The DAT is member of a large family of Na^+/Cl^- dependent neurotransmitter and amino acid transporters. Little is known about the molecular basis for substrate translocation in this class of transporters as well as their tertiary structure remains elusive. Gether et al. (2001) provided insight into the structural organization of the hDAT based on the identification of an endogenous high affinity Zn^{2+} binding site followed by the engineering of an artificial Zn^{2+} binding site. By binding to the endogenous site, Zn^{2+} acts as a potent non-competitive inhibitor of DA uptake mediated by the hDAT transiently expressed in COS-7 cells. Systematic mutagenesis of potential Zn^{2+} coordinating residues lead to the identification of three residues on the predicted extracellular face of the transporter, 193His in the second extracellular loop, 375His at the external end of the putative transmembrane segment (TM) 7, and 396Glu at the external end of TM 8, forming three coordinates in the endogenous Zn^{2+} binding site. The 3 residues are separate in the primary structure but their common participation in binding the small Zn^{2+} ion define their spatial proximity in the tertiary structure of the transporter. Finally, an artificial inhibitory Zn^{2+} binding site was engineered between TM 7 and TM 8. This binding site both verify the proximity between the two domains as wells as it supports an α-helical configuration at the top of TM 8 in the hDAT.

In earlier studies, Loland et al. (1999) described a distance constraint in the unknown tertiary structure of the hDAT by identification of two histidines, His-(193), in the second extracellular loop, and His-(375) at the top of transmembrane (TM) 7, that form two coordinates in an endogenous, high affinity Zn^{2+}-binding site. To achieve further insight into the tertiary organization of hDAT, they set out to identify additional residues involved in Zn^{2+} binding and subsequently to engineer artificial Zn^{2+}-binding sites. Ten aspartic acids and glutamic acids, predicted to be on the extracellular side, were mutated to asparagine and glutamine, respectively. Mutation of Glu-(396) (E396Q) at the top of TM 8 increased the IC_{50} value for Zn^{2+} inhibition of [^{3}H]-DA uptake from 1.1 to 530 μM and eliminated Zn^{2+}-induced potentiation of [^{3}H]-WIN 35,428 binding. These data suggested that Glu-(396) is involved in Zn^{2+} binding to hDAT. Importantly, Zn^{2+} sensitivity was preserved following the substitution of Glu-(396) with histidine, indicating that the effect of mutating Glu-(396) was not an indirect effect because of the removal of a negatively charged residue. The common participation of Glu-(396), His-(193), and His-(375) in binding the small Zn^{2+} ion implies their proximity in the unknown tertiary structure of hDAT. The close association between TM 7 and 8 was further established by engineering of a Zn^{2+}-binding site between His-(375) and a cysteine inserted in position 400 in TM 8. These data defined an important set of proximity relationships in hDAT that should prove an important template for further exploring the molecular architecture of Na^+/Cl^--dependent neurotransmitter transporters.

Fifteen metallic species, Ag, Al, Ca, Cd, Cr, Cu, Fe, K, Mg, Mn, Na, Ni, Pb, Sr, and Zn, were determined in 46 cocaine samples confiscated by the Spanish police in Galicia (northwest Spain). Classification of these cocaine samples according to their geographic origin (Colombia and Venezuela) was achieved by the application of pattern recognition techniques to the metallic content data. Cocaine samples, around 0.5 g, were directly dissolved in 2 mL of 35.0% (v/v) HNO_3, diluted to 10 ml with ultrapure water. The metals were quantified by means of atomic absorption spectrometry (AAS) (Ag, Al, Cd, Cr, Cu, Mn, Ni, Pb, and Sr), flame AAS (Ca, Fe, Mg, and Zn), and flame atomic emission spectrometry (K and Na). Results showed that two geographic origins can be established through the presence of trace and major elements (Bermejo-Barrera et al. 1999).

The molecular basis for substrate translocation in the Na^+/Cl^--dependent neurotransmitter transporters remains elusive. Norregaard et al. (1998) reported novel insight into the translocation mechanism by delineation of an endogenous Zn^{2+}-binding site in the hDAT. In micromolar concentrations, Zn^{2+} served as a potent, non-competitive blocker of DA uptake in COS cells expressing hDAT. In contrast, binding of the cocaine analogue, WIN 35,428, was potentiated by Zn^{2+}. Surprisingly, these effects were not observed in the closely related human NE transporter (hNET). A single non-conserved histidine residue (His193) in the large second extracellular loop (ECL2) of hDAT was responsible for this difference. Thus, Zn^{2+} modulation could be conveyed to hNET by mutational transfer of only this residue. His375 conserved between hDAT and hNET, present in the fourth extracellular loop (ECL4) at the top of transmembrane segment VII, was identified as a second major coordinate for Zn^{2+} binding, providing evidence for spatial proximity between His193 and His375 in hDAT, representing the first experimentally demonstrated proximity relationship in the Na^+/Cl^--dependent transporter. Since Zn^{2+} did not prevent DA binding, but inhibited DA translocation, suggesting that by constraining movements of ECL2 and ECL4, Zn^{2+} can restrict a conformational change for the transport process. Furthermore, Ennulat and Cohen (1997) utilized a multiplex differential display (MDD), a modification of differential display reverse transcriptase polymerase chain reaction (DD-PCR), to identify cocaine-dependent regulation of known and unknown gene products. Direct comparison of the MDD amplification profiles of duplicate, total RNA samples from the caudate putamen of either vehicle or cocaine treated Sprague-Dawley rats indicated that the relative induction of a 240 bp (8G247) product, likely to represent c-fos mRNA, closely paralleled changes in c-fos mRNA as measured by Northern blot analysis. MDD and Northern blot analysis also revealed the repression of another PCR product (8G226) at 1 hr and 1 day after repeated administration of cocaine. Two days after cocaine exposure, the level of 8G226 returned to control levels. The DNA sequence of 8G226 exhibited identity with a mouse Zn^{2+}-finger protein (PZf) and represented a transcriptional regulator. The repression of 8G226 immediately after cocaine treatment was in direct contrast to the cocaine-dependent increase in expression documented for NGFI-A, another Zn^{2+}-finger protein which also functions as a transcriptional regulator. These investigators recommended further characterization of the prolonged reduction in the expression of 8G226 for the identification of additional regulatory pathways that induce changes in cellular response after repeated cocaine exposure.

Norregaard et al. (2003) obtained evidence based on engineering of Zn^{2+} binding sites that the extracellular parts of transmembrane segment 7 (TM7) and TM8 in the human DAT are important for the transporter function. To further evaluate the role of this domain, they employed the substituted cysteine accessibility method and performed 10 single cysteine substitutions at the extracellular ends of TM7 and TM8. The mutants were made in background mutants of the human DAT with either two (E2C) or 5 endogenous cysteines substituted (X5C) that render the transporter largely insensitive to cysteine modification. In two mutants (M371C and A399C), treatment with the -SH-reactive reagent [2-(trimethylammonium)-ethyl]-methanethiosulfonate (*MT*SET) led to the inhibition of [^{3}H]DA uptake. In M371C, this inactivation was enhanced by Na^+ and blocked by DA. Inhibitors such as cocaine did not alter the effect of MTSET in M371C. The protection of M371C inactivation by DA required Na^+. As DA binding is Na^+-independent, suggesting that DA induces a transport-associated conformational change that decreases the reactivity of M371C with MTSET. In contrast to M371C, cocaine decreased the reaction rate of A399C with MTSET, whereas DA had no effect. The protection by cocaine can either reflect that Ala-399 lines of the cocaine binding crevice or that cocaine induces a conformational change that decreases the reactivity of A399C. These findings added new functionality to the TM7/8 region by providing evidence for the occurrence of distinct Na^+, substrate-, and inhibitor-induced conformational changes critical for the proper function of the transporter. Binding of Zn^{2+} to the endogenous Zn^{2+} binding site in the human DAT leads to inhibition of [(^{3})H]DA uptake. Loland et al. (2002) showed that mutation of an intracellular tyrosine to alanine (Y335A) converts this inhibitory Zn^{2+} switch into an activating Zn^{2+} switch, allowing Zn^{2+}-dependent activation of the transporter. The tyrosine is part of a conserved YXX Phi trafficking motif (X is any residue and Phi is a residue with a bulky hydrophobic group), but Y335A did not show alterations in surface targeting or protein kinase C-mediated internalization. Despite wild-type levels of surface expression, Y335A displayed decrease in [³H]-DA uptake velocity (V(max)) to < 1% of the wild type. In addition, Y335A showed up to 150-fold decreases in the apparent affinity for cocaine, mazindol, and related inhibitors whereas the apparent affinity for several substrates was increased. However, the presence of Zn^{2+} in micromolar concentrations increased the V(max) up to 24-fold and restored the apparent affinities. The capability of Zn^{2+} to restore transport was consistent with a reversible, constitutive shift in the distribution of conformational states in the transport cycle upon mutation of Tyr-335. These investigators proposed that this shift was caused by disruption of intramolecular interactions important for stabilizing the transporter in a conformation in which an extracellular substrate can bind and initiate transport, and that Tyr-335 was critical for regulating isomerization between discrete states in the transport cycle.

The different psychomotor-stimulant effects of cocaine, GBR12909, and benztropine may be originated from their different molecular actions on the DAT. To explore this possibility, Chen et al. (2004) examined binding of these inhibitors to mutated DATs with altered Na^+ dependence of DAT activities and with enhanced binding of a cocaine analog, [³H]2 beta-carbomethoxy-3 beta-(4-fluorophenyl)-tropane (CFT). In [³H]-CFT competition assays with intact cells, the mutation-induced change in the ability of Na^+ to enhance the apparent affinity of CFT, cocaine, GBR12909, and benztropine was inhibitor-independent. Thus, for the 4 inhibitors, the curve of Na^+ versus apparent ligand affinity was steeper at W84L compared with wild type, shallower at D313N, and flat at W84LD313N. With each mutant, the apparent affinity of CFT and cocaine was enhanced regardless of whether Na^+ was present. However, the apparent affinity of GBR12909 and benztropine for W84L was reduced in the absence of Na^+ but near normal in the presence of 130 mm Na^+, and that for D313N and W84LD313N was barely changed. With the single mutants, the alterations in Na^+ dependence and apparent affinity of the four inhibitors were comparable between [(³)H]CFT competition assays and [(³)H]DA uptake inhibition assays, indicating that DAT inhibitors producing different behavioral profiles can respond in an opposite way when residues of the DAT protein are mutated. For GBR12909 and benztropine, their cocaine-like changes in Na^+ dependence suggested that they prefer a DAT state as cocaine. However, their cocaine-unlike changes in affinity argued that, through their diphenylmethoxy moiety, they share DAT binding epitopes those are different from cocaine. In earlier studies, Chen et al. (2004) elucidated the role of aspartate 345, a residue conserved in the third intracellular loop of all Na^+/Cl^--dependent neurotransmitter transporters, in conformational changes of the DAT. Asparagine substitution (D345N) resulted in near normal transporter expression on the cell surface but caused extremely low V_{max} and K_m values for DA uptake, converted the inhibitory effect of Zn^{2+} on DA uptake to a stimulatory one, and eliminated reverse transport. The cocaine-like inhibitor 2-β-carbomethoxy-3beta-(4-fluorophenyl)-tropane or the selective DAT inhibitor GBR12935 bound to D345N with a normal affinity and still inhibited DA uptake potently. However, the mutation reduced the binding capacity of the surface transporter for these two inhibitors by 90% or more. Moreover, the binding activity of D345N could be improved by Zn^{2+} but not by Na^+.

These results were consistent with a defect in reorientation of the substrate-binding site to the extracellular side, leading to a loss of the outward-facing conformational state where external DA binds to initiate uptake and the inhibitors bind to initiate uptake inhibition. Alanine or glutamate substitution produced a similar phenotype, suggesting that both the negative charge and the residue volume at position 345 are vital. Furthermore, in intact cells, cocaine potentiated the reaction of the membrane-impermeant –SH reagent methanethiosulfonate ethyltrimethylammonium with the extracellularly-located endogenous cysteines of D345N but not those of wild type, and this potentiation was blocked upon K^+ substitution for Na^+. Thus, cocaine binding to D345N induced a different and Na^+-dependent conformational change, which may contribute to its inhibitory activity.

The biogenic amine transporters belong to the class of Na^+/Cl^--coupled solute carriers and include the transporters for DA (DAT), norepinephrine (NET), and 5-HT (SERT). These transporters are the targets for the action of many psychoactive compounds including antidepressants as well as drugs such as cocaine and amphetamines. Despite their pharmacological importance, little is known about their structural organization and the molecular mechanisms underlying the substrate translocation process. Loland et al. (2003) described how they used Zn^{2+}-binding sites as a tool to probe the structure and function of Na^+/Cl^--coupled biogenic amine transporters with specific focus on the hDAT. This work not only led to the definition of the first structural constraints in the tertiary structure of this class of transporters, but also allowed inferences about conformational changes accompanying substrate translocation and residues critical for regulating the equilibrium between different functional states in the transport cycle. In addition, Loland et al. (2004) showed evidence that mutation of Tyr-335 to Ala (Y335A) in the hDAT alters the conformational equilibrium of the transport cycle. By substituting, one at a time, 16 different bulky or charged intracellular residues, they identified 3 residues, Lys-264, Asp-345, and Asp-436, the mutation of which to alanine produces a phenotype as Y335A. Like Y335A, the mutants (K264A, D345A, and D436A) were characterized by low uptake capacity that was potentiated by Zn^{2+}. Moreover, the mutants displayed lower affinity for cocaine and other inhibitors, suggesting a role for these residues in maintaining the structural integrity of the inhibitor binding crevice. They investigated the conformational state of K264A, Y335A, and D345A by assessing the accessibility to MTSET ([2-(trimethylammonium)-ethyl]-methanethiosulfonate) of a cysteine into position 159 (I159C) in transmembrane segment 3 of the MTSET-insensitive "E2C" background (C90A/C306A). Unlike its effect at the corresponding position in the homologous NET I155C, MTSET did not inhibit uptake mediated by E2C I159C. Furthermore, no inhibition was observed upon treatment with MTSET in the presence of DA, cocaine, or Zn^{2+}. Without Zn^{2+}, E2C I159C/K264A, E2C I159C/Y335A, and E2C I159C/D345A were also not inactivated by MTSET. In the presence of Zn^{2+} (10 μM), however, MTSET (0.5 mm) caused ~ 60% inactivation. As in NET I155C, this inactivation was protected by DA and enhanced by cocaine. These data were consistent with a Zn^{2+}-dependent partial reversal of altered conformational equilibrium in the mutant transporters and suggested that the conformational equilibrium produced by the mutations resembles that of the NET more than that of the DAT. Moreover, the data provided evidence that the cocaine-bound state of both DAT mutants and of the NET was structurally-distinct from the cocaine-bound state of the DAT.

Serotonin Transporter in Drug Addiction. Residues 386–423 of the rat brain 5-HT transporter (SERT) are predicted to form a hydrophilic loop connecting transmembrane spans 7 and 8 (extracellular loop 4 or EL4). EL4 plays a role in conformational changes associated with substrate translocation. To further investigate EL4 structure and function, Mitchell et al. (2004) performed cysteine-scanning mutagenesis and methanethiosulfonate (MTS) accessibility studies on 38 residues. Four EL4 mutants (M386C, R390C, G402C, and L405C) showed very low transport activities, low cell surface expression, and strong inhibition by MTS reagents, indicating high structural and functional importance. Twelve mutants were sensitive to very low MTS concentrations, indicating positions highly exposed to the aqueous environment. Eleven mutants were MTS-insensitive, indicating positions that were either buried in the EL4 structure or functionally unimportant. The patterns of sensitivity to mutation and MTS reagents were used to produce a structural model of EL4. Positions 386–399 and 409–421 were proposed to form α-helices, connected by 9 consecutive MTS-sensitive positions, within which 4 positions, 402–405, may form a turn or hinge. The presence of 5-HT changed the MTS accessibility of cysteines at 9 positions, while cocaine, a non-transportable blocker, did not affect accessibility. 5-HT-induced accessibility changes required both Na^+ and Cl^-, indicating that they were associated with active substrate translocation. Except a single mutant, F407C, neither mutation to cysteine nor treatment with MTS reagents affected SERT affinities for 5-HT or the cocaine analog β-CIT, suggesting the role of EL4 in conformational changes occurring during translocation and that it does not play a direct role in 5-HT binding.

Development of Cocaine Antagonists as Zn^{2+}-mediated DAT Modulators. It is known that Zn^{2+} plays a major role in the modulation of neurotransmission because it modulates membrane receptors and channels. Recent literature has shown that Zn^{2+} inhibits DA transport through DAT, the main target of cocaine and some other drugs of abuse. Cocaine inhibits DAT and modulation of the DAT by Zn^{2+} may alter effects of cocaine on DAergic neurotransmission. Bjorklund et al. (2007) investigated how Zn^{2+} changes DAT kinetics and its inhibition by cocaine. Steady-state and pre-steady-state kinetics of DAT activity were investigated using rotating disk electrode voltammetry. Values of KM and Vmax in hDAT and effects of cocaine matched those in the literature. Zn^{2+} inhibited transport in the human DAT (hDAT) with a KI = 7.9 +/– 0.42 μM. Removal of endogenous Zn^{2+} with penicillamine in hDAT increased transport values. In contrast, Zn^{2+} did not alter transport by rat DAT (rDAT), with KM and V_{max} values of 1.2 +/– 0.49 μM and 15.7 +/– 2.57 pmol/(sx10(6) cells), respectively, and removal of Zn^{2+} did not increase DA transport values. Zn^{2+} allosterically reduced the inhibition by cocaine in hDAT. Results demonstrated that Zn^{2+} increases the second order binding rate constant for DA to hDAT. In rat striatal homogenates, Zn^{2+} increased initial DA transport velocity and decreased cocaine inhibition providing evidence for differences in sensitivity to Zn^{2+} between the 3 different preparations. Based on these findings, these investigators proposed that modulation of the DAT by Zn^{2+} needs to be assessed further in the development of cocaine antagonists.

To synthesize new analogs of the DA uptake inhibitor methylphenidate, a synthetic methodology based on the Blaise reaction was developed in a study. The reaction between α-bromophenylacetic acid esters, Zn^{2+}, and α-cyano-omega-mesylates gave stable primary enamines. After reduction of the enamines with cyanoborohydride, the amines could be cyclized to methylphenidate analogs in which the amine ring size and aromatic ring were varied. These compounds were tested for inhibitory potency against [³H] WIN 35,428 binding to the cocaine recognition site and [³H]DA uptake using rat striatal tissue. When the heterocyclic ring size was varied, the six-membered ring of methylphenidate appeared to be the optimum ring size. When the aryl ring was varied, the 4-trifluoromethylphenyl analog was less potent than methylphenidate, the β-naphthyl congener was more potent, whereas the α-naphthyl congener was less potent. Most of the compounds tested had ratios of uptake to binding inhibition (discrimination ratio) that were like cocaine and were therefore not lead compounds for the development of cocaine antagonists (Deutsch et al. 2001).

DA receptor genes are under complex transcription control, determining their unique regional distribution in the brain. Huang et al. (2001) described a Zn²⁺ finger type transcription factor, designated DA receptor regulating factor (DRRF), which binds to GC and GT boxes in the D1A and D2 DA receptor promoters and displaces Sp1 and Sp3 from these sequences. Consequently, DRRF can modulate the activity of these DA receptor promoters. Highest DRRF mRNA levels are found in the brain with a specific regional distribution including olfactory bulb and tubercle, nucleus accumbens, striatum, hippocampus, amygdala, and frontal cortex, which express abundant levels of various DA receptors. *In vivo*, DRRF itself can be regulated by manipulations of DAergic neurotransmission. Mice treated with drugs that increase extracellular striatal DA levels (cocaine), block DA receptors (haloperidol), or destroy DA terminals (MPTP), show significant alterations in DRRF mRNA, providing a basis for DA receptor regulation after these manipulations. Based on these findings, these investigators suggested that DRRF is important for modulating DAergic neurotransmission in the brain.

Monoclonal Antibody 15A10 for the Treatment of Cocaine Addiction. Earlier reports have shown that anti-cocaine catalytic monoclonal antibody 15A10 reduces the toxic effect of cocaine by increasing its breakdown to systemically inert products ecgonine methylester and benzoic acid. Therefore, Homayoun et al. (2003) reported the microencapsulation of antibody 15A10 using biodegradable poly (lactic-glycolic) acid (PLGA) by double emulsion technique. Formulation parameters such as protein loading, polymer molecular weight, and the presence of zinc carbonate were studied for their effects on *in vitro* release of antibody from microspheres. The initial burst release was decreased by the reduction of the protein in the formulation. Although changing the polymer molecular weight did not cause a reduction in initial burst release, it was effective in improving the release rate. The inclusion of zinc carbonate in microsphere preparation resulted in increase in initial burst release. An *in vivo* study in mice revealed the presence of antibody in blood up to 10 days following s.c. injections. These data demonstrated a potential role for a sustained-release formulation of monoclonal antibody 15A10 for the treatment of cocaine addiction.

Protective Role of MTs in Alcohol Liver Disease (ALD). Alcoholic liver disease (ALD) is associated with decrease in Zn²⁺ and its major binding protein, MT, in the liver. Studies using animal models showed that Zn²⁺ supplementation prevents alcohol-induced liver injury under both acute and chronic alcohol exposure. There were hepatic and extra hepatic actions of Zn²⁺ in the prevention of alcoholic liver injury. Zn²⁺ supplementation attenuated ethanol-induced hepatic Zn²⁺ depletion and suppressed ethanol-induced CYP2E1 activity, but increased alcohol dehydrogenase activity in the liver; an action that was responsible for Zn^{2+} suppression of alcohol-induced oxidative stress. Zn^{2+} also enhanced glutathione-related antioxidant capacity in the liver and inhibited alcohol-induced apoptosis through suppression of the Fas/FasL-mediated pathway. Zn^{2+} supplementation preserved intestinal integrity and prevented endotoxemia, leading to inhibition of endotoxin-induced TNF-α production in the liver. Zn^{2+} also inhibited the signaling pathway involved in endotoxin-induced TNF-α production. These hepatic and extrahepatic effects of Zn^{2+} were independent of MT. However, low levels of MT in the liver sensitized the organ to alcohol-induced injury, and elevation of MT enhanced the endogenous Zn^{2+} and made Zn^{2+} available when oxidative stress was imposed. Hence, Zn^{2+} may be effective in the prevention and treatment of ALD (Kang and Zhou 2006). In addition, Zhou et al. (2005) examined whether dietary Zn^{2+} supplementation could provide protection from alcoholic liver injury. MT_{dko} and wild-type 129/Sv mice were pair-fed an ethanol-containing liquid diet for 12 weeks, and the effects of Zn^{2+} supplementation on ethanol-induced liver injury were analyzed. Zn^{2+} attenuated ethanol-induced hepatic Zn^{2+} depletion and liver injury as measured by histopathological and ultrastructural analyses, serum alanine transferase activity, and hepatic TNF-α in MT_{dko} and wild-type mice, indicating MTs-independent Zn^{2+} protection. Zn^{2+} inhibited accumulation of ROS, as indicated by dihydroethidium fluorescence, and oxidative damage, as assessed by immune-histochemical detection of 4-hydroxynonenal, nitrotyrosine, and malondialdehyde and protein carbonyl in the liver. Zn^{2+} suppressed ethanol-induced CYP2E1 activity but increased the activity of alcohol dehydrogenase in the liver, without affecting the rate of blood ethanol elimination. Zn^{2+} also prevented ethanol-induced decreases in glutathione and glutathione peroxidase activity and increased glutathione reductase activity, suggesting that Zn^{2+} prevents alcoholic liver injury in MTs-independent manner by inhibiting the generation of ROS (CYP2E1) and enhancing antioxidant pathways. It is now known that intestinal-derived endotoxins are involved in alcohol-induced liver injury. Disruption of intestinal barrier function and endotoxemia are common features associated with liver inflammation and injury due to acute ethanol exposure. Zn^{2+} inhibited acute alcohol-induced liver injury. Lambert et al. (2004) determined the inhibitory effect of Zn^{2+} on alcohol-induced endotoxemia and whether the inhibition is mediated by MTs or is independent of MT. MT_{dko} mice were administered 3 oral doses of zinc sulfate (2.5 mg zinc ion/kg body weight) every 12 hrs before being administered a single dose of ethanol (6 g/kg body weight) by gavage. Ethanol caused liver injury as determined by increased serum transaminases, parenchymal fat accumulation, necrotic foci, and an elevation of TNF-α. Increased plasma endotoxin levels were detected in ethanol-treated animals whose small intestinal structural integrity was compromised as determined by microscopic examination. Zn^{2+} inhibited acute ethanol-induced liver injury and suppressed hepatic TNF-α in association with decreased circulating endotoxin and a significant protection of small intestine structure. MT remained undetectable in the MT_{dko} mice by Zn^{2+} treatment suggesting that Zn^{2+} preservation of intestinal structural integrity is associated with suppression of endotoxemia and liver injury induced by acute exposure to ethanol and the Zn^{2+} protection is independent of MTs (Lambert et al. 2004).

cDNA MicroArray Analyses of Alcohol Liver Disease. The molecular pathogenesis of alcoholic liver disease (ALD) is not well understood. Gene expression profiling has the potential to identify new pathways and altered molecules in ALD. Therefore, Seth et al. (2003) compared the gene expression profiles of ALD in a baboon model and humans using cDNA microarrays. The analysis revealed differential expression of several genes and pathways in addition to genes involved in ALD pathogenesis. Overall gene expression profiles were similar in both species, with majority of genes involved in fibrogenesis and xenobiotic metabolism, as well as inflammation, oxidative stress, and cell signaling. Genes associated with stellate cell activation (collagens, matrix metalloproteinases, and tissue inhibitors of matrix metalloproteinase) were up-regulated. Decreased expression of several MTs was unexpected. Fourteen molecules related to the annexin family were up-regulated, including annexin A1 and A2. Immunofluorescence revealed a marked overexpression of annexin A2 in proliferating bile duct cells, hepatocyte cell surface, and selective co-localization with CD14-positive cells in human ALD. The gene expression profile of ALD was dominated by alcohol metabolism and inflammation and differed from other liver diseases, suggesting that annexins may play a central role in the progression of fibrosis in ALD.

Maotai-induced MTs Prevents Hepatic Fibrosis. Epidemiology investigation showed that no worker drunk Maotai liquor for nearly 30 years died of hepatic diseases, and no obvious hepatic fibrosis and/or cirrhosis were found in 99 workers who had drunk Maotai for a long period by epidemiology investigation and needle biopsy. The same finding was detected in rats that were administered Maotai. Cheng et al. (2003) explored the protective effect of Kweichow Moutai (Maotai) on hepatic fibrosis. Male SD rats were provided with Maotai for 56 days. MTs and MDA were estimated in the liver. Cultured rat hepatocytes (HSC) and human HSC were employed to study the effect of Maotai on HSC's proliferation and collagen synthesis. Histopathological evaluation was conducted after 14 weeks of Maotai ingestion. MTs were 22X induced, whereas lipid peroxidation and MDA levels were significantly decreased in Maotai-treated rats exposed to CCL_4. A concentration-dependent inhibition in HSC proliferation was noticed in Maotai-treated rats. Motai attenuated genes involved in cell proliferation and collagen synthesis. Alcohol-treated control group demonstrated typical liver cirrhosis. Although, fatty degeneration and hepatocyte and mild fibrosis of intestitium were observed, no overt hepatic fibrosis and/or cirrhosis was identified in Maotai-treated group, indicating that it provides protection through MTs induction, inhibition in HSC proliferation, and collagen synthesis. Furthermore, Cheng et al. (2004) investigated the effects of Maotai on the liver and its mechanism of hepatic fibrosis prevention in rats. MTs and malondialdehyde (MDA) were estimated in liver. Hepatic stellate cells (HSCs) and human HSCs were cultured to observe the effect of Maotai on HSCs proliferation and collagen synthesis. After ingestion of Maotai for 14 weeks, the livers of male SD rats were harvested for histopathological examination. The level of MTs in the liver of Maotai-treated rats increased by 22 folds, whereas lipid peroxide and MDA were decreased in Maotai-treated animals exposed to CCl_4. Inhibition in HSCs proliferation was noticed with Maotai treatment. In the alcoholic group, typical liver cirrhosis was observed. However, fatty degeneration of hepatocytes and mild fibrosis were observed, without any evidence of hepatic fibrosis and cirrhosis in Maotai-treated group. Thus, Maotai induced MTs, and inhibited HSCs proliferation and collagen synthesis to prevent hepatic fibrosis. Earlier studies on MTs-over-expressing transgenic mice demonstrated that MT protects liver from alcohol-induced oxidative injury. MTs bind to Zn^{2+} under physiological conditions and releases Zn^{2+}

under oxidative stress and Zn^{2+}, as an antioxidant, mediates the protective action of MT.

Antioxidants are potential pharmaceutical agents for the treatment of alcoholic liver disease. MTs are cysteine-rich proteins and function as an antioxidant. Zhou et al. (2002) determined the role of Zn^{2+} in hepatic protection from alcoholic injury. MT-1/2-knockout (MT-KO) mice along with their wild-type controls were treated with three gastric doses of ethanol at 5 g/kg at 12-hrs intervals. Zinc sulfate was injected i.p. in a dosage of 5 mg/kg/day for 3 days before an ethanol treatment. MTs in MT-KO mice were very low and Zn^{2+} content in MT-KO mice was lower than in wild-type mice. Zn^{2+} treatment elevated hepatic MTs only in wild-type mice and increased Zn^{2+} in both MT-KO and wild-type mice. Ethanol treatment caused degenerative morphological changes and necrosis in the livers of MT-KO mice. Micro-vesicular steatosis was observed only in the liver of wild-type mice. Ethanol treatment decreased glutathione and increased lipid peroxidation. Lipid peroxide products were lower in the wild-type mice as compared to MT-KO mice. The toxic effects of alcohol were attenuated by Zn^{2+} treatment in both MT-KO and wild-type mouse livers, suggesting that Zn^{2+}, independent of MT, is involved in alleviating alcoholic liver injury. However, MT is required to maintain adequate levels of Zn^{2+}, and that the protective action of MT is mediated through Zn^{2+}. In a similar study, Zhou et al. (2002) determined whether MTs confer resistance to acute alcohol-induced hepatotoxicity and explored the association between oxidative stress and alcoholic liver injury. MT-over-expressing transgenic and wild-type mice were administrated 3 doses of alcohol at 5 g/kg. These investigators determined liver injury, oxidative stress, and ethanol metabolism-associated changes. Acute ethanol caused microvesicular steatosis, hepatic necrosis, and elevation of serum alanine aminotransferase in the wild-type mice. Ultrastructural changes in the hepatocytes included glycogen and fat accumulation, organelle abnormality, and focal cytoplasmic degeneration in control wild-type mice. This acute hepatotoxicity was inhibited in the MT-transgenic mice. Ethanol decreased reduced glutathione and increased oxidized glutathione, lipid peroxidation, protein oxidation, and superoxide ions in the wild-type mice. These biomarkers of oxidative stress were significantly attenuated in the MT_{trans} mice. However, MTs did not influence ethanol-induced reduction in NAD(+)/NADH ratio or increase in CYP2E1, suggesting that these Zn^{2+}-binding proteins are effective in cytoprotection against alcohol-induced liver injury by inhibiting alcohol-induced oxidative stress. The reduction of malondialdehyde (MDA) in mouse blood plasma and liver 1 hr^{-1} day after the acute ethanol intoxication (3 g/kg) was determined by Koterov and Shilina (1995). Rat liver zinc-MT in a dose 2 mg/kg inoculated before the alcohol intoxication restored the MDA level to normal; simultaneously the mixture which modulated this protein (albumin, cysteine and Zn^{2+}) had only the tendency to normalize the MDA level. On the 3rd day after the poisoning in all cases, the 2–2.5 times increase of the plasma MDA level was noticed, but the liver MDA did not change as compared to control. It was proposed that Zn^{2+}-MT influence is associated with its ability to inactivate acetaldehyde. Cabre et al. (1995) investigated hepatic lipid peroxidation, MTs, collagen, and proline hydroxylase activity in 16 ethanol-fed rats and in 16 control animals. The rats were divided into 3 groups to receive either, a standard diet, a Zn^{2+}-deficient diet, or a Zn^{2+}-supplemented diet. The animals were sacrificed at week 12 for histological and biochemical assessments. Hepatic tissue examination indicated that oral Zn^{2+} decreases lipid peroxidation, collagen deposition, and proline hydroxylase activity together with an increase in MTs in alcoholic rats. No significant differences in lipid peroxidation in the control group was observed in relation to the diet. Zn^{2+} increased hepatic MTs and decreased proline-hydroxylase and collagen but to a lesser degree than in alcoholic animals, indicating that it is an efficient hepato-protective agent against lipid peroxidation in alcoholic rats and its effect may be mediated by MTs induction. Also, lipid peroxidation may be related to changes in hepatic collagen synthesis.

In a study, MTs levels were determined in the livers (MT-L) and the kidneys (MT-K) of 145 deceased persons. The individual values showed marked variations, average levels were 154.9 +/– 151.4 mg/kg liver wet wt and 160.5 +/– 150.4 mg/kg total kidney wet wt. In contrast to MT-L, MT-K increased with age up to a maximum around mid-life and decreased at higher ages. Neither the MT-L nor the MT-K were dependent on sex. The MT content correlated with the macroscopic and histopathologic status of the liver. As compared to normal tissue, livers with fatty degeneration, cirrhosis, and brown atrophy showed MT-L values of 40%, 25%, and 233% respectively. Individuals with a history of alcohol abuse, demonstrated reduced MT-L of 40% of the control values, accompanied with pathological findings. MT-L also responded to the cause of death. Drug-induced suicides reduced MT-L to 62%, whereas "mechanical" suicides increased MTs to 137%. MT-K was independent of the kidney status and was increased to ~ 190% in male smokers (Drasch et al. 1988). Four to 12 weeks of ethanol ingestion in mice decreased *MTs*-like proteins in the liver but not in the kidneys. The Zn^{2+} and Cu concentration also decreased in the liver and remained unaffected in the kidneys (Hopf et al. 1986).

MTs as CB Inhibitors, Charnolophagy Enhancers, and CS Stabilizers in the Cardiovascular System

Although alcohol-induced cardiomyopathy including fibrosis has been recognized for a long time, its pathogenesis remains partially-understood. Studies using experimental animals have not fully duplicated the pathological changes in humans, and animal models of alcoholic cardiac fibrosis are limited. Reduced insulin sensitivity following alcohol intake plays an important role in alcohol-induced organ damage, although its precise mechanism remains unknown. Lee and Ren (2006) examined the effect of cardiac over-expression of the *MTs* on alcohol-induced cardiac contractile dysfunction and post-receptor insulin signaling. Control and *MTs* mice were fed a 4% alcohol diet for 16 weeks. Cardiomyocyte contractile function was evaluated including peak shortening (PS), time-to-PS (TPS), and time-to-re-lengthening (TR-(90)). Post-insulin receptor signaling molecules Akt, mammalian target of rapamycin (mTOR), and ribosomal p70s6 kinase (p70s6k) were evaluated by immunoblotting. Akt1 kinase activity was assayed with a phosphotransferase kit. Alcohol intake attenuated glucose tolerance, depressed PS, shortened TPS, and prolonged TR-(90), which were abrogated by *MTs* except glucose intolerance, indicating reduced expression of total Akt, phosphorylated mTOR, and phosphorylated p70s6k-to-p70s6k ratio as well as Akt1 kinase activity in alcohol consuming FVB mice. Phosphorylated Akt, total mTOR, and phosphorylated p70s6k were unaffected by alcohol. MTs ablation reduced Akt protein and kinase activity without affecting other proteins or their phosphorylation suggesting that chronic alcohol intake interrupts cardiac contractile function and Akt/mTOR/p70s6k signaling and that Akt may contribute to *MTs*-induced cardioprotective response. In a study, Wang et al. (2005) developed a mouse model in which cardiac hypertrophy and fibrosis were produced in MT_{dko} mice fed an alcohol-containing liquid diet for two months. The same alcohol feeding did not produce cardiac fibrosis in the wild-type (WT) control mice, although there was no difference in the alcohol-induced cardiac hypertrophy between the WT controls and the MT_{dko} mice. Zinc prevented cardiac fibrosis but did not affect hypertrophy in the alcohol-fed MT_{dko} mice, suggesting a specific link between Zn^{2+} homeostasis and cardiac fibrosis. Serum creatine phosphokinase activity was significantly higher in the alcohol-administered MT_{dko} mice than in the WT mice, whereas, Zn^{2+} decreased serum creatine phosphokinase activities and eliminated the difference between the groups. Thus, disturbance in Zn^{2+} homeostasis due to the lack of MT associated with alcohol-induced cardiac fibrosis and severe cardiac injury, suggested the MT_{dko} mouse model of an alcohol-induced cardiac fibrosis to investigate specific factors involved in the alcoholic cardiomyopathy.

Ethanol, under certain conditions, alters the metabolism of sulfur amino acids, *MTs* and Zn^{2+}. Chronic ethanol abuse during pregnancy decreases the availability of sulfur amino acids or Zn^{2+}, could contribute to growth retardation of the fetuses in FAS. Therefore, Harris (1990) investigated whether chronic ethanol intoxication to pregnant rats alters glutathione (GSH), MT, or Zn^{2+} of selected tissues of the dams and fetuses. Sprague-Dawley rats were fed from gestational days 5 to 19 either the control diet (AF), the ethanol diet (EF), or the control diet using the pair-feeding technique (PF). On the 19th day of gestation, hepatic GSH was significantly lower in EF and PF dams than for the AF dams. MTs were similar for the AF and EF dams, and were significantly high in PF dams than the AF and EF dams. The 3 groups did not differ in Zn^{2+} content of dams or fetuses. On the 19th day of gestation, chronic ethanol to pregnant rats did not lower the maternal hepatic GSH level below that of PF dams, did not induce hepatic MTs in the dams, and did not prevent fetuses from achieving body weights and hepatic Zn^{2+} equal to those of controls.

MTs Confer Resistance to Anti-Cancer Therapy by Inhibiting CB Formation, Augmenting Charnolophagy, and by CPS/CS Stabilization

It has been shown that smoking is related to breast cancer mortality. One hypothesis is that this association is due to the elevated expression of proteins associated with resistance to cancer therapies. *MTs* are a family of proteins that play a role in conferring resistance to certain cancer therapies. Therefore, Gallicchio et al. (2004) assessed whether smoking was associated with MT expression in breast carcinomas. Breast tissues with clinical and epidemiological information were collected from three different cancer centers for 123 women diagnosed with invasive breast cancer. MT expression was assessed using immunohistochemical procedures using an immunoreactivity score that was obtained by multiplying the percentage of MT-positive tumor cells by MT staining intensity. The results showed that 27.6% of the women were current smokers. Among women whose tissues were collected at the cancer center where enrolled women had primarily early stage, low grade breast cancer, smokers had increased odds, although not significantly, of having a MT-positive tumor compared to non-smokers, independent of cancer stage. This association was not observed among the women whose tissues were collected from the other cancer centers, suggesting that among specific groups of women, smoking at the time of breast cancer diagnosis may be associated with an increase in breast tissue MTs.

It is known that Cd is a toxic metal associated with emphysema and lung cancer, which is present in both air pollution and cigarette smoke. MT is an inducible protein that binds and detoxifies cellular Cd. Grasseschi et al. (2003) conducted a study to determine whether increased concentrations of Cd are present in alveolar macrophages (AMs) of cigarette smokers (CSMs) and to determine whether MT accumulates in response to the presence of Cd. AMs were recovered by BAL from 10 healthy nonsmokers (NSMs) and 10 CSMs. The Cd content of the AMs was determined by ICP-MS, and the MT content was determined using a Cd/hemoglobin radioassay (with ^{109}Cd). Cd was detected in AMs recovered from all subjects, with higher mean (+/− SEM) concentrations in CSMs compared with those in NSMs (3.4 +/− 0.5 vs 1.3 +/− 0.2 ng/10(6) cells). There was a correlation between current smoking history (cigarettes per day) and the AM content of Cd. The mean AM content of MT was similar in NSMs (1.2 +/− 0.2 µg/10(7) cells) and CSMs (1.0 +/− 0.2 µg/10(7) cells), Thus, AMs in CSMs accumulated significant amounts of Cd without a concurrent increase in MT content, indicating greater saturation of MT. Increased Cd burden in alveolar cells could contribute to the development of lung diseases in CSMs.

Thiocyanate is the major toxic metabolite of HCN, a toxic substance the organism may be exposed due to cigarette smoking or industrial pollution. The complex interactions existing between metals and MT induction are well known. However, the possible role of thiocyanate, which is also an anion, has not been established yet. Considering the interactions between metals and the MTs, in a study, Aydin et al. (2002) investigated in rats the relationship between thiocyanate and the *in vivo* distribution of hepatic MTs and Zn, Cu, Fe, Ca, Mg, and Mn. This study indicated that thiocyanate exerts its effect on the *in vivo* expression of MT and endogenous distribution of essential elements in rat liver. Elevated levels of MT and changes in hepatic concentrations of essential elements suggested a role for thiocyanate in cellular metabolism and it might reflect a direct role of thiocyanate on alteration of cellular functional activities.

Abdominal aortic aneurysm is a smoking-related disorder. Cd, inhaled from cigarettes, may accumulate in the aorta and facilitate weakening of the aorta through adverse effects on tooth muscle cell metabolism. Abu-Hayyeh et al. (2001) measured Cd by AAS in infra-renal aortas from 13 patients with abdominal aortic aneurysm and from 17 age- and sex-matched patients with normal-diameter abdominal aorta. Total Cd content was associated with smoking, assessed as pack-years, but was similar in aneurysmal and undilated aortas. The Cd content (mean +/− SE) was higher in the media (3.25 +/− 0.53 ng/mg dry wt, 7 +/− 1.2 µmol/L) than in the intima or adventitia (1.14 +/− 0.24 and 1.87 +/− 0.38 ng/mg dry wt, respectively). There was a significant correlation between medial Cd content and pack-years of smoking. In aortic smooth muscle cells cultured on fibrillar collagen, Cd inhibited DNA and collagen synthesis and diminished cell numbers (IC_{50} 2 µmol/L, 6 µmol/L, and 6 µmol/L, respectively), but higher concentrations of Cd were required for upregulation of MT (EC_{50} 23 µmol/L). The Cd content of the aorta increases in direct proportion to the pack-years of cigarettes smoked, with selective accumulation in the medial layer. However, the Cd content of aneurysmal aortas was not higher than that of nondilated aortas for patients with matched smoking history. In smokers, the level of Cd accumulation was sufficient to impair the viability of cultured smooth muscle cells. Similar mechanisms could underlie the development of degenerative aortic disease in smokers.

Earlier studies have shown that a single s.c. exposure to Cd can induce injection site sarcomas (ISS) in rats. These tumors, though clearly malignant, do not often metastasize or invade subdermal muscle layers because of their location. Recent evidence indicates that when tumorigenic cells chronically exposed to Cd *in vitro* are inoculated into mice, the tumor progression and invasiveness in the mice are enhanced. Thus, Waalkes et al. (2000) studied the effects of repeated Cd exposures on tumor incidence, progression, and metastatic potential in rats. Wistar (WF) and Fischer (F344) rats (30 per group) were injected s.c. in the dorsal thoracic midline with $CdCl_2$ once weekly for 18 weeks with doses of 0, 10, 20, or 30 µmol Cd/kg. This resulted in total doses of 0, 180, 360, or 540 µmol/kg. One other group of each strain received a low, loading dose of Cd (3 µmol/kg) prior to 17 weekly injections of 30 µmol/kg (total dose 513 µmol/kg). Rats were observed for 2 years. Many F344 rats (57%) died within one week after the first injection of the highest dose, but WF rats were not affected. The low loading dose prevented the acute lethality of the high dose in F344 rats. Surprisingly, latency (time to death by tumor) of ISS was the shortest in the groups given the low loading dose in both strains. ISS in these groups also showed the highest rate of metastasis and subdermal muscle layer invasion. Based on ISS incidence in the groups given the lowest total dose of Cd (180 µmoles/kg), F344 rats were more sensitive to tumor induction, showing an incidence of 37% compared to 3% in WF rats. On the other hand, Cd-induced ISS showed a higher overall metastatic rate in WF rats (18 metastatic ISS/68 total tumors in all treated groups; 27%) compared to F344 rats (6%). Immunohistochemically, the primary ISS showed high levels of MT, a Cd-binding protein, while metastases were devoid of MT, indicating that repeated Cd exposures induces ISS. An initial low exposure to Cd further accelerated the appearance and enhanced the metastatic potential and invasiveness of these tumors. The primary and metastatic ISS appeared to have a differing phenotype, at least with MT production. The association between multiple Cd exposures and enhanced metastatic potential of the tumors may have important implications in chronic exposures to Cd, or in cases of co-exposure of Cd with organic carcinogens, as in tobacco smoking.

Milnerowicz (1997) used SDS-PAGE for separation of heat-stable proteins in placenta, amniotic fluid, and milk of women who smoke actively and those exposed to tobacco smoke (passive smokers). In the number of protein bands stained with Coomassie brilliant blue R-250, several bands were stained with silver nitrate. The presence of low-molecular band with molecular weight of 6.5 kDa, corresponding to the mobility of electrophoretic MT-1, was detected in the placenta, amniotic fluid, and milk. The involvement of MT-2 isoform was much lower, although more evident in amniotic fluid and milk of active smokers. In this group of women, an enhanced concentration of the band with molecular weight of 25–30 kDa was observed in placenta, colostrum, and milk on the second day after delivery; several protein bands emerged in the area of the same mobility in amniotic fluid; the presence of the band with molecular weight of 12.5 kDa and the absence of protein bands of 25–30 kDa were found in milk excreted on the third day postpartum. These results showed the apparent differences between proteingrams of placenta, amniotic fluid, and milk of active and passive smokers. In a similar study, these investigators measured the concentration of metals (Zn, Cu, Cd), MT and the activity of n-acetyl-β-glucosaminidase (NAG) in amniotic fluids and milk from smoking mothers and passive smokers, living in areas of higher environmental pollution with heavy metals. In active smokers, a 3X increase in Cd concentration, higher Cu and lower Zn^{2+} concentrations, higher MT level and enhanced NAG activity in amniotic fluids as well as higher Cd, Cu, and Zn^{2+} concentrations and increased MT and NAG in milk were indicated, when compared to passive smokers. Some dynamics in metal and MTs secretion with mother's milk was noted on successive days after delivery. The highest MT level was observed during the first 24 hrs postpartum, whereas Cd concentration was highest on the third day. There were no significant differences in concentrations of Cu and Zn^{2+} secreted with milk on those days. In environmentally exposed women higher Cd and Cu concentrations, enhanced MT level and Nag activity, higher amniotic fluid and lower milk Zn^{2+} concentration were observed in comparison to women living in the Cieplice region.

MDR Proteins and Smoking. Koomagi et al. (1996) analyzed twenty tumoral and peritumoral tissues from patients with lung cancer immunohistochemically for the drug resistance-related proteins P-glycoprotein (P-170), topoisomerase II (Topo-II), glutathione S-transferase-pi (GST-pi), MTs, HSP-70 and the putative regulators of resistance (ErbB1, Fos, and Jun). Protein expression of Topo-II, GST-pi, MT, HSP-70, ErbB1, Fos, and Jun was elevated in tumor tissue in comparison to normal tissue. The different expression of the proteins between tumoral and normal tissues was significant for Topo-II, MT, and HSP-70, whereas ErbB1 demonstrated a borderline significance. The expression of the proteins was frequently increased in smokers in comparison to non-smokers. In general, increase in the proteins of smokers corresponded in tumoral and non-tumoral tissue. Different expression was only found with MT and HSP-70 which were higher in tissues of smokers.

In a study, exposure to Cd was monitored by measurement of the metal in blood or urine, or by observation of excreted compounds such as β-2-microglobulin or N-acetyl-β-D-glucose. Whilst these approaches are useful for the detection of acute exposure to Cd, their applicability in the management of long-term, low-level exposure remains uncertain. MTs are ubiquitous proteins that are synthesized in response to heavy metal ions and may offer themselves as being a biologically sensitive indicator of Cd exposure. Therefore, Stennard et al. (1995) examined both basal and Cd-induced MTs mRNA levels in cultured lymphocytes from groups with different exposures to Cd, to assess their potential as an indicator of Cd exposure and the suitability of such an assay for routine analysis. Induced MTs mRNA levels, rather than basal mRNA levels, increased in groups who received elevated body burdens of Cd, although these increases were not significant between groups. There was, however, a significant correlation between induced MTs mRNA levels and urinary β-2-microglobulin, suggesting that further work on the *in vitro* lymphocyte response to Cd as a diagnostic tool is required. I have proposed that MTs inhibit molecular pathogenesis involving CB induction, charnolophagy inhibition, and CS destabilization by improving CMB to confer protection in drug addiction as potent free radical scavengers.

References

Abeliovich, A., Y. Schmitz, I. Farinas, D. Choi-Lundberg, W.H. Ho, P.E. Castillo, N. Shinsky, J.M. Verdugo, M. Armanini, A. Ryan, M. Hynes, H., Phillips, D. Sulzer and A. Rosenthal. 2000. Mice lacking alpha-synuclein display functional deficits in the nigrostriatal DA system. Neuron 25: 239–252.

Abu-Hayyeh, S., M. Sian, K.G. Jones, A. Maneul and J.T. Powell. 2001. Cadmium accumulation in aortas of smokers. Arterioscler Thromb Vasc Biol 21: 863–867.

Ajjimaporn, A., J. Swinscoe, S. Shavali, P. Govitrapong and M. Ebadi. 2005. Metallothionein provides zinc-mediated protective effects against METH toxicity in SK-N-SH cells. Brain Res Bull 67: 466–475.

Ajjimaporn, A., P. Phansuwan-Pujito, M. Ebadi and P. Govitrapong. 2007. Zinc protects SK-N-SH cells from METH-induced alpha-synuclein expression. Neurosci Lett 419: 59–63.

Aydin, H.H., H.A. Celik and B. Ersoz. 2002. Role of thiocyanate ion in metallothionein induction and in endogenous distribution of essential elements in the rat liver. Biol Trace Elem Res 90: 187–202.

Bermejo-Barrera, P., J. Moreda-Perieiro, A. Bermejo-Barrera and A.M. Bermejo-Barrera. 1999. A study of illicit *Cocaine* seizure classification by pattern recognition techniques applied to metal data. J Forensic Sci 44: 270–274.

Bernhardm, D., A. Rossmann, B. Henderson, M. Kind, A. Seubert and G. Wick. 2006. Increased serum cadmium and strontium levels in young smokers: effects on arterial endothelial cell gene transcription. Arterioscler Thromb Vasc Biol 26: 833–838.

Bjorklund, N.L., T.J. Volz and J.O. Schenk. 2007. Differential effects of Zn^{2+} on the kinetics and *Cocaine* inhibition of DA transport by the human and rat DA transporters. Eur J Pharmacol 565: 17–25.

Bowen, S., N. Chawla, S.E. Collins, K. Witkiewitz, S. Hsu, J. Grow, S. Clifasefi, M. Garner, A. Douglass, M.E. Larimer and A. Marlatt. 2009. Mindfulness-based relapse prevention for substance use disorders: a pilot efficacy trial. Subst Abus 30(4): 295–305.

Cabin, D.E., K. Shimazu, D. Murphy, N.B. Cole, W. Gottschalk, K.L. McIlwain, B. Orrison, A. Chen, C.E. Ellis, R. Paylor, B. Lu and R.L. Nussbaum. 2002. Synaptic vesicle depletion correlates with attenuated synaptic responses to prolonged repetitive stimulation in mice lacking alpha-synuclein. J Neurosci 22: 8797–8807.

Cabre, M., J. Folch, A. Gimenez, C. Matas, A. Pares, J. Caballeria, J.L. Paternain, J. Rodes, G. Joven and J. Camps. 1995. Influence of zinc intake on hepatic lipid peroxidation and metallothioneins in alcoholic rats: relationship to collagen synthesis. Int J Vitam Nutr Res 65: 45–50.

Cadet, J.L., P. Sheng, S. Ali, R. Rothman, E. Carlson and C. Epstein. 1994. Attenuation of METH-induced neurotoxicity in copper/zinc superoxide dismutase transgenic mice. J Neurochem 62: 380–383.

Cadet, J.L., S.F. Ali, R.B. Rothman and C.J. Epstein. 1995. Neurotoxicity, drugs and abuse, and the CuZn-superoxide dismutase transgenic mice. Mol Neurobiol 11: 155–163.

Carmichael, N.G., B.L. Backhouse, C. Winder and P.D. Lewis. 1982. Teratogenicity, toxicity and perinatal effects of cadmium. Hum Toxicol 1: 159–186.

Chen, L., L. Lei, T. Jin, M. Nordberg and G.F. Nordberg. 2006. Plasma metallothionein antibody, urinary cadmium, and renal dysfunction in a Chinese type 2 diabetic population. Diabetes Care 29: 2682–2687.

Chen, N., J. Rickey, J.L. Berfield and M.E. Reith. 2004. Aspartate 345 of the DA transporter is critical for conformational changes in substrate translocation and *Cocaine* binding. J Biol Chem 279: 5508–5519.

Chen, N., J. Zhen and M.E. Reith. 2004. Mutation of Trp84 and Asp313 of the DA transporter reveals similar mode of binding interaction for GBR12909 and Benztropine as opposed to *Cocaine*. J Neurochem 89: 853–864.

Cheng, M.L., J. Wu, W.S. Zhang, H.Q. Wang, C.X. Li, N.H. Huang, Y.M. Yao, L.G. Ren, L. Ye and L. Li. 2003. An experimental study on the effect of Maotai liquor on the liver. Zhonghua Yi Xue Za Zhi 83: 237–241.

Choudhary, B.A. and R.K. Chandra. 1987. Biological and health implications of toxic heavy metal and essential trace element interactions. Prog Food Nutr Sci 11: 55–113.

de Blasi, A., L. Capobianco, L. Iacovelli, P. Lenzi, M. Ferrucci, G. Lazzeri, F. Fornai and A. Picascia. 2003. Presence of beta-arrestin in cellular inclusions in metamphetamine-treated PC12 cells. Neurol Sci 24: 164–165.

Deng, X. and J.L. Cadet. 2000. METH-induced apoptosis is attenuated in the striata of copper-zinc superoxide dismutase transgenic mice. Brain Res Mol Brain Res 83: 121–124.

Deutsch, H.M., X. Ye, Q. Shi, Z. Liu and M.M. Schweri. 2001. Synthesis and pharmacology of site specific *Cocaine* abuse treatment agents: a new synthetic methodology for methylphenidate analogs based on the Blaise reaction. Eur J Med Chem 36: 303–311.

Drasch, G.A., E. Kretschmer, P. Neidlinger and K.H. Summer. 1988. Metallothionein in human liver and kidney: relationship to age, sex, diseases and tobacco and alcohol use. J Trace Elem Electrolytes Health Dis Dec; 2(4): 233–237.

Dong, Z., D.P. Wolfer, H.P. Lipp and H. Bueler. 2005. Hsp70 gene transfer by adeno-associated virus inhibits MPTP-induced nigrostriatal degeneration in the mouse model of Parkinson disease. Mol Ther 11: 80–88.

Ebadi, M., S. Sharma, S. Wanpen and A. Amornpan. 2004. Coenzyme Q_{10} inhibits mitochondrial complex-1 downregulation and nuclear factor-kappa B activation. J Cellular & Molecular Medicine 8: 213–222.

Ennulat, D.J. and B.M. Cohen. 1997. Multiplex differential display identifies a novel zinc-finger protein repressed during withdrawal from *Cocaine*. Brain Res Mol Brain Res 49: 299–302.

Falck, F.Y. Jr, L.J. Fine, R.G. Smith, J. Garvey, A. Schork, B. England, K.D. McClatchy and J. Linton. 1983. Metallothionein and occupational exposure to cadmium. Br J Ind Med 40: 305–313.

Fornai, F., P. Lenzi, M. Gesi, M. Ferrucci, G. Lazzeri, L. Capobianco, A. de Blasi, G. Battaglia, F. Nicoletti, S. Ruggieri and A. Paparelli. 2004. Similarities between METH toxicity and proteasome inhibition. Ann N.Y. Acad Sci 1025: 162–170.

Fornai, F., P. Lenzi, M. Gesi, P. Soldani, M. Ferrucci, G. Lazzeri, L. Capobianco, G. Battaglia, A. de Blasi, F. Nicoletti and A. Paparelli. 2004. METH produces neuronal inclusions in the nigrostriatal system and in PC12 cells. J Neurochem 88: 114–123.

Gallicchio, L., J.A. Flaws, M. Sexton and O.B. Ioffe. 2004. Cigarette smoking and metallothionein expression in invasive breast carcinomas. Toxocol Lett 152: 245–253.

Gether, U., L. Norregaard and C.J. Loland. 2001. Delineating structure-function relationships in the DA transporter from natural and engineered Zn^{2+} binding sites. Life Sci 68: 2187–2198.

Grasseschi, R.M., R.B. Ramaswamy, D.L. Levin, C.D. Klaassen and S. Wesselius. 2003. Cadmium accumulation and detoxification by alveolar macrophages of cigarette smokers. Chest 124: 1924–1928.

Guarscio, P., F. Yentis, U. Cevikbas, B. Portmann and R. Williams. 1983. Value of copper-associated protein in diagnostic assessment of liver biopsy. J Clin Pathol 36: 18–23.

Harris, J.E. 1990. Hepatic glutathione, metallothionein and zinc in the rat on gestational day 19 during chronic ethanol administration. J Nutr 120: 1080–1086.

Hirata, H., B. Ladenheim, R.B. Rothman, C. Epstein and J.L. Cadet. 1995. METH-induced serotonin neurotoxicity is mediated by superoxide radicals. Brain Res 677: 345–347.

Hirato, H., M. Asanuma and J.L. Cadet. 1998. Superoxide radicals are mediators of the effects of METH on Zif268 (Egr-1, NGFI-A) in the brain: evidence from using CuZn superoxide dismutase transgenic mice. Brain Res Mol Brain Res 58: 209–216.

Homayoun, P., T. Mandal, D. Landry and H. Komiskey. 2003. Controlled release of anti-*Cocaine* catalytic antibody from biodegradable polymer microspheres. J Pharm Pharmacol 55: 933–938.

Hopf, G., R. Bocker, G. Kusch and C.J. Estler. 1986. The effect of long-term ethanol treatment on a metal binding protein fraction in liver and kidneys of mice. Acta Pharmacol Toxicol (Copenh) 59: 43–46.

Hwang, C.K., U.M. D' Souza, A.J. Eisch, S. Yajima, C.H. Lammers, Y. Yang, S.H. Lee, Y.M. Kim, E.J. Nestler and M.M. Mouradian. 2001. DA receptor regulating factor, DRRF: a zinc finger transcription factor. Proc Natl Acad Sci U S A 98: 7558–7563.

Imam, S.Z., J. el-Yazal, G.D. Newport, Y. Itzhak, J.L. Cadet, W. Jr Slikker and S.F. Ali. 2001. METH-induced DArgic neurotoxicity: role of peroxynitrite and neuroprotective role of antioxidants and peroxynitrite decomposition catalysts. Ann N Y Acad Sci 939: 366–380.

Imam, S.Z., Y. Itzhak, J.L. Cadet, F. Islam, W. Jr Slikker and S.F. Ali. 2001. METH-induced alteration in striatal p53 and bcl-2 expressions in mice. Brain Res Mol Brain Res 91: 174–178.

Imam, S.Z., G.D. Newport, Y. Itzhak, J.L. Cadet, F. Islam, W. Jr Slikker and S.F. Ali. 2001. Peroxynitrite plays a role in METH-induced DArgic neurotoxicity: evidence from mice lacking neuronal nitric oxide synthase gene or overexpressing copper-zinc superoxide dismutase. J Neurochem 76: 745–749.

Jayanthi, S., B. ladenheim and J.L. Cadet. 1998. METH-induced changes in antioxidant enzymes and lipid peroxidation in copper/zinc-superoxide dismutase transgenic mice. Ann N Y Acad Sci 844: 92–102.

Jones, L.C., K.A. McCarthy, J.L. Beard, C.L. Keen and B.C. Jones. 2006. Quantitative genetic analysis of brain copper and zinc in BXD recombinant inbred mice. Nutr Neurosci 9: 81–92.

Jones, W.K. 2005. A murine model of alcoholic cardiomyopathy: a role for zinc and metallothionein in fibrosis. Am J Pathol 167: 301–304.

Kang, Y.J. and Z. Zhou. 2005. Zinc prevention and treatment of alcoholic liver disease. Mol Aspects Med 26: 391–404.

Keterov, A.N. and N.M. Shilina. 1995. [Effect of zinc-metallothionein on lipid peroxidation in blood plasma and in mouse liver in acute alcoholic intoxication]. Ukr Biokhim Zh 67: 80–87.

Kirik, D., L.E. Annett, C. Burger, N. Muzyczka, R.J. Mandel and A. Bjorklund. 2003. Nigrostriatal alpha-synucleinopathy induced by viral vector-mediated overexpression of human alpha-synuclein: a new primate model of Parkinson's disease. Proc Natl Acad Sci U.S.A. 100: 2884–2889.

Klongpanichapak, S., P. Govitrapong, S.K. Sharma and M. Ebadi. 2006. Attenuation of cocaine and methamphetamine neurotoxicity by coenzyme Q_{10}. Neurochem Res 31(3): 303–311.

Kobayashi, H., S. Ide, J. Hasegawa, H. Ujike, Y. Sekine, N. Ozaki, T. Inada, M. Harano, T. Komiyama, M. Yamada, M. Iyo, H.W. Shen, K. Ikeda and I. Sora. 2004. Study of association between alpha-synuclein gene polymorphism and METH psychosis/dependence. Ann N.Y. Acad Sci 1025: 325–334.

Koomagi, R., G. Stammler, C. Manegold, J. Mattern and M. Volm. 1996. Expression of resistance-related proteins in tumoral and peritumoral tissues of patients with lung cancer. Cancer Lett 110: 129–136.

Korutla, L., R. Degnan, P. Wang and S.A. Mackler. 2007. NAC1, a *Cocaine*-regulated POZ/BTB protein interacts with CoREST. J Neurochem 101: 611–618.

Korutla Wang, P.J. and S.J. Mackler. 2005. The POZ/BTB protein NAC1 interacts with two different histone deacetylases in neuronal-like cultures. J Neurochem 94: 786–793.

Kumar, A., T. Chatopadhya, M. Raziuddin and R. Ralhan. 2007. Discovery of deregulation of zinc homeostasis and its associated genes in esophageal squamous cell carcinoma using cDNA microarray. Int J Cancer 120: 230–242.

Lambert, J.C., Z. Zhou, L. Wang, Z. Song, C.J. McClain and Y.J. Kang. 2004. Preservation of intestinal structural integrity by zinc is independent of metallothionein in alcohol-intoxicated mice. Am J Pathol 164: 1959–1966.

Lee, Q. and J. Ren. 2006. Cardiac overexpression of metallothionein rescues chronic alcohol intake-induced cardiomyocyte dysfunction: role of Akt, mammalian target of rapamycin and ribosomal p70s6 kinase. Alcohol & Alcoholism. 41: 585–592.

Li, L. 2004. Effect of Maotai liquor on the liver: an experimental study. Hepatobiliary Pancreat Dis Int 3: 93–98.

Loland, C.J., L. Norregaard and U. Gether. 1999. Defining proximity relationships in the tertiary structure of the DA transporter. Identification of a conserved glutamic acid as a third coordinate in the endogenous Zn^{2+}-binding site. J Biol Chem 274: 36928–36934.

Loland, C.J., L. Norregaard, T. Litman and U. Gether. 2002. Generation of an activating Zn(2+) switch in the DA transporter: mutation of an intracellular tyrosine constitutively alters the conformational equilibrium of the transport cycle. Proc Natl Acad Sci U S A 99: 1683–1688.

Loland, C.J., K. Norgaard-Nielsen and U. Gether. 2003. Probing DA transporter structure and function by Zn^{2+}-site engineering. Eur J Pharmacol 479: 187–197.

Loland, C.J., C. Granas, J.A. Javitch and U. Gether. 2004. Identification of intracellular residues in the DA transporter critical for regulation of transporter conformation and *Cocaine* binding. J Biol Chem 279: 3228–3238.

Lomonte, J.N., W.T. Lowry and I.C. Stone. 1976. Contaminants in illicit amphetamine preparations. J Forensic Sci 21: 575–582.

Loney, K.D., R.K. Uddin and S.M. Singh. 2006. Analysis of metallothionein brain gene expression in relation to ethanol preference in mice using cosegregation and gene knockouts. Alcohol Clin Exp Res 30: 15–25.

Lotharius, J., S. Barg, P. Wiekop, C. Lundberg, H.K. Raymon and P. Brundin. 2002. Effect of mutant alpha-synuclein on DA homeostasis in a new human mesencephalic cell line. J Biol Chem 277: 38884–38894.

Mackler, S., A. Pacchioni, R. Degnan, Y. Homan, A.C. Conti, P. Kalivas and J.A. Blendy. 2008. Requirement for the POZ/BTB protein NAC1 in acute but not chronic psychomotor stimulant response. Behav Brain Res 187: 48–55.

Mackler, S.A., L. Korutla, X.Y. Cha, M.J. Koebbe, K.M. Fournier, M.S. Bowers and P.W. Kalivas. 2000. NAC-1 is a brain POZ/BTB protein that can prevent *Cocaine*-induced sensitization in the rat. J Neurosci 20: 6210–6217.

Mackler, S.A., Y.X. Homan, L. Korutla, A.C. Conti and J.A. Blendy. 2003. The mouse nac1 gene, encoding a *Cocaine*-regulated Bric-a-brac Tramtrac Broad complex/Pox virus and Zinc finger protein, is regulated by AP1. Neuroscience 121: 355–361.

McAleer, M.F. and R.S. Tuan. 2004. Cytotoxicant-induced trophoblast dysfunction and abnormal pregnancy outcomes: role of zinc and metallothionein. Birth Defects Res C Embryo Today 72: 361–370.

Milnerowicz, H. 1993. Metalloproteins in human placenta and fetal membranes in non-smoking and smoking women. Acta Biochim Pol 40: 179–181.

Milnerowicz, H. 1997. Concentration of metals, ceruloplasmin, metallothionein and activity of N-acetyl-beta-D-glucosaminidase and gamma-glutamyltransferase in pregnant women who smoke and in those environmentally exposed to tobacco and in their infants. II. Influence of environmental exposure in the copper basin. Int J Occup Med Environ Health 10: 273–282.

Milnerowicz, H. 1997. Influence of tobacco smoking on metallothionein isoforms contents in human placenta, amniotic fluid and milk. Int J Occup Med Environ Health 10: 395–403.

Milnerowicz, H. and M. Schmarek. 2005. Influence of smoking on metallothionein level and other proteins binding essential metals in human milk. Acta Pediatr 94: 402–406.

Milnerowicz, H. and E. Darul. 2005. [Effects of exposure to tobacco smoke on the level of low-molecular proteins in human amniotic fluid in pregnancies complicated by oligohydramnios or premature rapture of the membranes]. Przegl Lek 62: 1034–1038.

Mirecki, A., P. Fitzmaurice, L. Ang, K.S. Kalasinsky, F.J. Peretti, S.S. Aiken, D.J. Wickham, A. Sherwin, J.N. Nobrega, H.J. Forman and S.J. Kish. 2004. Brain antioxidant systems in human METH users. J Neurochem 89: 1396–1408.

Mitchell, S.M., E. Lee, M.L. Garcia and M.M. Stephan. 2004. Structure and function of extracellular loop 4 of the serotonin transporter as revealed by cysteine-scanning mutagenesis. J Biol Chem 279: 24089–24099.

Norregaard, L., D. Fredrickson, E.O. Nielson and U. Gether. 1998. Delineation of an endogenous zinc-binding site in the human DA transporter. EMBO J 17: 4266–4273.

Norregaard, L., C.J. Loland and U. Gether. 2003. Evidence for distinct sodium-, DA-, and *Cocaine*-dependent conformational changes in transmembrane segments 7 and 8 of the DA transporter. J Biol Chem 278: 30587–30596.

Peters, M.A. and J.R. Fouts. 1970. The influence of magnesium and some other divalent cations on hepatic microsomal drug metabolism *in vitro*. Biochem Pharmacol 19: 533–544.

Post, C., B. Johansson and S. Allenmark. 1984. Organ distribution and protein binding of cadmium in autopsy material from heavy smokers. Environ Res 34: 29–37.

Richfield, E.K., M.J. Thiruchelvam, D.A. Cory-Slechta, C. Wuertzer, R.R. Gainetdinov, M.G. Caron, D.A. Di Monte and H.J. Federoff. 2002. Behavioral and neurochemical effects of wild-type and mutated human alpha-synuclein in transgenic mice. Exp Neurol 175: 35–48.

Ronco, A.M., G. Arguello, M. Suazo and M. Llanos. 2005. Increased levels of metallothionein in placenta of smokers. Toxicology 208: 133–139.

Ronco, A.M., F. Garrido and M.N. Llanos. 2006. Smoking specifically induces metallothionein-2 isoform in human placenta at term. Toxicology 223: 46–53.

Schluter, O.M., F. Fornai, M.G. Alessandri, S. Takamori, M. Geppert, R. Jahn and T.C. Sudhof. 2003. Role of alpha-synuclein in 1-methyl-4-phenyl-1,2,3,6-tetrahydropyridine-induced parkinsonism in mice. Neuroscience 118: 985–1002.

Seth, D., M.A. Leo, P.H. McGuinness, C.S. Lieber, Y. Brennan, R. Williams, X.M. Wang, G.W. McCaughan, M.D. Gorrel and P.S. Haber. 2003. Gene expression profiling of alcoholic liver disease in the baboon (Papio hamadryas) and human liver. Am J Pathol 163: 2303–2317.

Shaik, Z.A., C. Tohyama and C.V. Nolan. 1987. Occupational exposure to cadmium: effect on metallothionein and other biological indices of exposure and renal function. Arch Toxicol 59: 360–364.

Sharma, S. and M. Ebadi. 2008. SPECT neuroimaging in translational research of CNS disorders. Neurochem Internat 52: 352–362.

Shilina, N.M. and A.N. Keterov. 1995. Level of substances reacting with 2-thiobarbituric acid in murine blood plasma in acute ethanol poisoning during protection with zinc metallothionein. Biull Eksp Biol Med 119: 46–49.

Simonick, T.F. and V.W. Watts. 1992. Preliminary evaluation of the Abbott TDx for screening of D-METH in whole blood specimens. J Anal Toxicol 16: 115–118.

Sorkun, H.C., F. Bir, M. Akbulut, U. Divrkli, J. Erken, H. Demirhan, E. Duzcan, L. Elci, I. Celik and U. Yozgatli. 2007. The effects of air pollution and smoking on placental cadmium, zinc concentration and metallothionein expression. Toxicology 238: 15–22.

Stennard, F.A., T.C. Stewart and A.K. West. 1995. Effect of prior, low-level cadmium exposure *in vivo* on metallothionein expression in cultured lymphocytes. J Appl Toxicol 15: 63–67.

Tytell, M. and P.L. Hooper. 2001. Heat shock proteins: new keys to the development of cytoprotective therapies. Expert Opin Ther Targets 5: 267–287.

Volm, M. and J. Mattern. 1992. Expression of topoisomerase II, catalase, metallothionein and thymidylate-synthase in human squamous cell lung carcinomas and their correlation with doxorubicin resistance and with patients' smoking habits. Carcinogenesis 13: 1947–1950.

Waalkes, M.P., S. Rehm and M.G. Cherian. 2000. Repeated cadmium exposures enhance the malignant progression of ensuing tumors in rats. Toxicol Sci 54: 110–120.

Wang, J.Q., A.J. Smith and J.F. McGinty. 1995. A single injection of amphetamine or METH induces dynamic alterations in c-fos, zif/268 and preprodynorphin messenger RNA expression in rat forebrain. Neuroscience 68: 83–95.

Wang, L., Z. Zhou, T.J. Saari and Y.J. Kang. 2005. Alcohol-induced myocardial fibrosis in metallothionein-null mice: prevention by zinc supplementation. Am J Pathol 167: 337–344.

Xie, T., L. Tong, U.D. McCann, J. Yuan, K.G. Becker, A.O. Mechan, C. Cheadle, D.M. Donovan and G.A. Ricaurte. 2004. Identification and characterization of metallothionein-1 and -2 gene expression in the context of (+/–)3,4-methylenedioxyMETH-induced toxicity to brain DArgic neurons. J Neurosci 24: 7043–7050.

Zhou, Z., X. Sun and Y.J. Kang. 2002. Metallothionein protection against alcoholic liver injury through inhibition of oxidative stress. Exp Biol Med 227: 214–222.

Zhou, Z., X. Sun, J.C. Lambert, J.T. Saari and Y.J. Kang. 2002. Metallothionein-independent zinc protection from alcoholic liver injury. Am J Pathol 160: 2267–2274.

Zhou, Z., L. Wang, Z. Song, J.T. Saari, C.J. McClain and Y.J. Kang. 2005. Zinc supplementation prevents alcoholic liver injury in mice through attenuation of oxidative stress. Am J Pathol 166: 1681–1690.

CHAPTER-21

Charnoly Body in Cardiovascular Diseases

INTRODUCTION

It has been estimated that ~ 40% of the cardiac muscle is composed of only mitochondria. The heart supplies blood against gravity to brain because it requires a constant supply of glucose, oxygen, and numerous trophic factors for normal function. Hence, cardiovascular MB is extremely important for normal health and well-being. Recently, Anupama et al. (2018) highlighted that metabolic syndromes are characterized by obesity, hypertension, dyslipidemia, and diabetes, whereas cardiometabolic syndrome, represented by cardiovascular, renal, metabolic, prothrombotic, and inflammatory abnormalities, occur due to defects in the MB. Several human diseases of CMB have been identified involving defective mtDNA as we reported in the RhO_{mgko} cells as an experimental model of PD, AD, and aging (Sharma et al. 2004). The RhO_{mgko} cells exhibit mitochondrial oxidative and nitrative stress due to ONOO-generation, down-regulation of $\Delta\Psi$, and complex-1, a rate limiting enzyme system involved in oxidative phosphorylation, triggering CB molecular pathogenesis. Although RhO_{mgko} cells become elliptical and de-differentiated, they do not lose their potential to divide because the nuclear DNA remains structurally and functionally intact in these cells. Transfection of RhO_{mgko} cells with complex-1 gene regained neurotigenesis, tubulinogenesis, myelinogenesis, and synaptogenesis as confirmed by multiple fluorochrome comet assay and digital fluorescence confocal microscopic analysis. The CB molecular pathogenesis was significantly diminished in complex-1-transfected RhO_{mgko} cells.

We determined brain regional distribution of CoQ_{10} and mitochondrial complex-1 activity of control-(C57BL/6), MT_{dko}, MT_{trans}, and wv/wv mice; and cultured SK-N-SH neurons to determine the neuroprotective potential of CoQ_{10} in PD. Complex-1 activity as well as CoQ_{10} were significantly higher in the cerebral cortex as compared to the striatum in all the genotypes examined. Complex-1 activity and CoQ_{10} were significantly reduced in wv/wv mice and MT_{dko} mice but were significantly increased in MT_{trans} mice. The reduced complex-1 activity and ^{18}F-DOPA uptake occurred concomitantly with negligible differences in the CoQ_{10} between in the cerebral cortex and striatum of wv/wv mice. Administration of CoQ_{10} increased complex-1 activity and partially improved motoric performance in wv/wv mice. Direct exposure of a potent complex-1 inhibitor, rotenone, also reduced CoQ_{10}, complex-1 activity, and $\Delta\Psi$ in SK-N-SH neurons. Rotenone-induced down-regulation of complex-1 activity was attenuated by CoQ_{10} treatment, suggesting that complex-1 is down-regulated due to depletion of CoQ_{10} in the brain. Therefore, MTs-induced CoQ_{10} synthesis provides neuroprotection by augmenting complex-1 activity (Sharma et al. 2006). We also reported that MTs boost the MB by inhibiting free radical-induced CB formation involved in various NDDs, CVDs, and MDR malignancies. In another series of experiments, we used control-wv/wv mutant, and -heterozygous wv+/− mice to explore the basic molecular mechanism of neurodegeneration and the neuroprotective potential of CoQ_{10}. The wv/wv mice exhibited progressive neurodegeneration in the hippocampus, striatum, and cerebellum, and a reduction in the striatal dopamine and CoQs (Q_9 and Q_{10}) without any significant changes in NE and 5-HT. Mitochondrial complex-1 was down regulated, whereas, the NFκβ was up regulated in wv/wv mice. Rotenone inhibited complex-1, enhanced NFκβ, and caused apoptosis in SK-N-SH neurons; whereas NFκβ antibody suppressed rotenone-induced apoptosis, suggesting that enhancing CoQ_{10} synthesis and suppressing the induction of NFκβ provide neuroprotection by boosting the MB (Ebadi et al. 2004).

Generally, aging is accompanied with biochemical and physiological changes, and increased susceptibility to NDDs, CVDs, and MDR malignancies. As chronic inflammation and oxidative stress are hallmarks of aging, we investigated the cytoprotective role of MTs as potent free radical scavengers, CB inhibitors, charnolophagy agonists, and CS stabilizers to investigate their therapeutic potential in aging. We reported that MTs are low molecular weight, metal-binding, anti-inflammatory, and antioxidant proteins that provide cardioprotection in aging through Zn^2-mediated transcriptional regulation of genes involved in cell growth, proliferation, and differentiation. In addition to Zn^{2+} homeostasis, the antioxidant role of MTs is routed through -SH moieties on cysteine residues. MTs are induced in aging as a defensive mechanism to attenuate oxidative and nitrative stress implicated in diversified CVDs and NDDs. In addition, MTs as free radical scavengers inhibit CB formation to provide protection by boosting the MB. In general, MT-1 and MT-2 induce cell growth and differentiation, whereas MT-3 is a growth inhibitory factor, which is reduced in AD. We reported that MTs are down-regulated in wv/wv mice exhibiting progressive neurodegeneration, early aging, morbidity, and mortality due to CMB. These degenerative changes were attenuated in wv/wv-MTs mice, suggesting the protective role of MTs in aging (Sharma and Ebadi 2014).

Recently, I reported the therapeutic potential of antioxidants in functional foods (which form a part of Mediterranean diet) and MB for sustained energy and enhanced human performance (Sharma 2017). It is now well-established that various biochemical pathways can modulate function involving mitofusin-mediated mitochondrial synthesis and repair, maintenance of $\Delta\Psi$, and generation of free radicals (·OH, CO·, NO·) as a byproduct of oxidative phosphorylation during ATP synthesis in the electron transport chain. Hence, free radical-induced redox imbalance, involving CB formation, charnolophagy, and CS destabilization have been recognized as biomarkers and potential drug discovery targets to develop novel DSST charnolopharmacotherapeutics to accomplish the targeted, safe, and effective

EBPT of diversified CVDs, NDDs, and MDR malignancies, as described elegantly in this book.

This chapter highlights the functional significance of cardiovascular MB for normal health and well-being. More specifically, the chapter describes that cardiac-specific ablation of the E3 ubiquitin ligase Mdm2 results in mitochondrial oxidative stress and mitochondrial depletion resulting in early mortality. In addition, it describes the cardioprotective role of antioxidant, acylcarnitine, involvement of CMB in reduced ejection fraction, functional assessment of the heart by peripheral blood mtDNA analysis, and physiological adaptation of heart with exercise as a booster of MB and ICD for normal cellular function and better quality of life.

Myocardial Oxygen Consumption and Efficiency in Aortic Valve Stenosis Patients with and without Heart Failure. It is known that myocardial oxygen consumption (MVO_2) and its coupling to contractility are fundamentals of cardiac function and may be involved in the transition from compensated left ventricular hypertrophy to failure. Nevertheless, these processes have not been studied previously in patients with aortic valve stenosis (AS). Therefore, Hansson et al. (2017) conducted a study in which participants underwent ^{11}C-acetate PET, cardiovascular MRI, and echocardiography to measure MVO_2 and myocardial external efficiency (MEE) defined as the ratio of left ventricular stroke work and the energy equivalent of MVO_2. They studied 10 healthy controls (group A), 37 asymptomatic AS patients with left ventricular ejection fraction $\geq 50\%$ (group B), 12 symptomatic AS patients with left ventricular ejection fraction $\geq 50\%$ (group C), and 9 symptomatic AS patients with left ventricular ejection fraction $< 50\%$ (group D). MVO_2 did not differ among groups A, B, C, and D (0.105 ± 0.02, 0.117 ± 0.024, 0.129 ± 0.032, and 0.104 ± 0.026 mL/min per gram, respectively), whereas MEE was reduced in group D ($21.0 \pm 1.6\%$, $22.3 \pm 3.3\%$, $22.1 \pm 4.2\%$, and $17.3 \pm 4.7\%$, respectively). Similarly, patients with global longitudinal strain greater than -12% and paradoxical low-flow, low-gradient AS had impaired MEE. The ability to discriminate between symptomatic and asymptomatic patients was superior for global longitudinal strain compared with MVO_2 and MEE (area under the curve 0.98, 0.48, and 0.61, respectively). AS patients displayed a persistent ability to maintain normal MVO_2 and MEE (i.e., the ability to convert energy into stroke work); however, patients with left ventricular ejection fraction $< 50\%$, global longitudinal strain greater than -12%, or paradoxical low-flow, low-gradient AS demonstrated reduced MEE, suggesting that mitochondrial uncoupling contributes to the dismal prognosis in patients with reduced contractile function or paradoxical low-flow, low-gradient AS.

Cardiac-Specific Ablation of E3 Ubiquitin Ligase Mdm2 Leads to Oxidative Stress, Mitochondrial Depletion, and Early Demise. It is known that the maintenance of normal heart function requires proper control of protein turnover. The ubiquitin-proteasome system is a principal regulator of protein degradation. Mdm2 is the main E3 ubiquitin ligase for p[53] in mitotic cells thereby regulating cellular growth, DNA repair, oxidative stress and apoptosis. However, which of these Mdm2-related activities are preserved in differentiated cardiomyocytes remains unknown. Hence, Hauck et al. (2017) investigated the role of Mdm2 in the regulation of normal cardiac function. They observed reduced Mdm2 mRNA accompanied by increased p[53] protein expression in the hearts of wild type mice subjected to myocardial infarction or trans-aortic banding. These investigators generated conditional cardiac-specific Mdm2 gene knockout (Mdm2f/f;mcm) mice. In adulthood, Mdm2f/f;mcm mice developed spontaneous cardiac hypertrophy and left ventricular dysfunction with early mortality post-tamoxifen. A decreased polyubiquitination of myocardial p^{53} was observed, leading to its stabilization and activation, in the absence of acute stress. In addition, transcriptomic analysis of Mdm2-deficient hearts revealed that there is an induction of E2f1 and c-Myc mRNA levels with reduced expression of the Pgc-1a/Ppara/Esrrb/g axis and Pink1, associated with cardiomyocyte apoptosis, and an inhibition of redox homeostasis and MB. All these processes were early Mdm2-associated events and contributed to the development of pathological hypertrophy, indicating the pivotal role for Mdm2 in cardiac growth control through the regulation of p^{53}, the Pgc-1 family of transcriptional coactivators, and the antioxidant Pink1.

Energy Metabolic Changes in Heart Failure with Preserved Ejection Fraction and Heart Failure with Reduced Ejection Fraction. It is known that alterations in cardiac energy metabolism contribute to the severity of heart failure. However, the energy metabolic changes that occur in heart failure are complex and are dependent not only on the severity and type of heart failure present, but also on the coexistence of common comorbidities such as obesity and type 2 diabetes. Recently, De Jong et al. (2017) reviewed the cardiac energy metabolic changes that occur in heart failure. An emphasis was made on distinguishing the differences in cardiac energy metabolism between heart failure with preserved ejection fraction (HFpEF) and heart failure with reduced ejection fraction (HFrEF) and in clarifying the common misconceptions surrounding the fate of fatty acids and glucose in the failing heart. The major key points in this review were: (1) mitochondrial oxidative capacity is reduced in HFpEF and HFrEF; (2) fatty acid oxidation is HFrEF, which still exceeds that of glucose; (3) glucose oxidation is decreased in HFpEF and HFrEF; (4) there is an uncoupling between glucose uptake and oxidation in HFpEF and HFrEF, resulting in an increased rate of glycolysis; (5) ketone body oxidation is increased in HFrEF, which might further reduce fatty acid and glucose oxidation; and eventually, (6) branched chain amino acid oxidation is impaired in HFrEF. Based on these observations, these investigators emphasized the importance of understanding these changes in cardiac energy metabolism in heart failure for the development of metabolic modulators in the treatment of heart failure.

Mitochondria-Targeting Peptide in Heart Failure Treatment: A Randomized, Placebo-Controlled Trial of Elamipretide. It has been realized that mitochondrial dysfunction and energy depletion in the failing heart are innovative therapeutic targets in heart failure management. Elamipretide is a novel tetrapeptide that increases mitochondrial energy; however, its safety, tolerability, and therapeutic effect on cardiac structure and function have not been studied in heart failure with reduced ejection fraction. In this double-blind, placebo-controlled, ascending-dose trial, patients with heart failure with reduced ejection fraction (ejection fraction, $\leq 35\%$) were randomized to either a single 4-hrs infusion of elamipretide (cohort 1 [n = 8], 0.005; cohort 2 [n = 8], 0.05; and cohort 3 [n = 8], 0.25 mg·kg^{-1}·h^{-1}) or placebo control (n = 12). Safety and efficacy were assessed by clinical, laboratory, and echocardiographic assessments performed at pre-, mid-, and end-infusion and 6-, 8-, 12-, and 24-hrs post-infusion start. Peak plasma concentrations of elamipretide occurred at end-infusion and were undetectable by 24 hrs post-infusion. There were no serious adverse events. Blood pressure and heart rate remained stable in all cohorts. Compared with placebo, a significant decrease in left ventricular end-diastolic volume and end-systolic volume occurred at end infusion in the highest dose cohort. This study evaluated elamipretide in heart failure with reduced ejection fraction and demonstrated that a single infusion of elamipretide is safe and well tolerated. High-dose elamipretide resulted in favorable changes in left ventricular volumes that correlated with peak plasma concentrations, supporting a temporal association and dose-effect relationship. These investigators recommended further study of elamipretide to determine its long-term safety and efficacy for the heart failure patients.

Acylcarnitine in Human Heart Failure. Heart failure (HF) is associated with metabolic perturbations, particularly of fatty acids (FAs), which remain to be better understood in humans. Hence, Ruiz et al. (2017) tested the hypothesis that HF patients with reduced ejection fraction display systemic perturbations in levels of energy-related metabolites, especially those having dysregulation of FA metabolism, namely, acylcarnitines (ACs). Circulating metabolites were assessed using mass spectrometry (MS)-based methods in two cohorts. The main cohort consisted of 72 control subjects and 68 HF patients exhibiting depressed left ventricular ejection fraction (25.9 ± 6.9%) and mostly of ischemic etiology with ≥ 2 comorbidities. HF patients displayed marginal changes in plasma levels of TCA-related metabolites or indexes of mitochondrial or cytosolic redox status. They had, however, 22–79% higher circulating ACs, irrespective of chain length (adjusted for sex, age, renal function, and insulin resistance, determined by shotgun MS/MS), which reflected defective mitochondrial β-oxidation, and were associated with levels of NH_2-terminal pro-B-type natriuretic peptide levels, a disease severity marker. Subsequent extended LC-MS analysis of 53 plasma ACs in a subset group from the primary cohort confirmed with lipidomic analysis in a validation cohort revealed in HF patients a more complex circulating AC profile. The latter included dicarboxylic-ACs and dihydroxy-ACs as well as very long chain (VLC) ACs or sphingolipids with VLCFAs (> 20 carbons), which are proxies of dysregulated FA metabolism in peroxisomes. This study identified alterations in circulating ACs in HF patients that were independent of biological traits and associated with disease severity biomarkers. These alterations reflected dysfunctional FA metabolism in mitochondria but also in peroxisomes, suggesting a novel mechanism contributing to global lipid perturbations in human HF. Mass spectrometry-based profiling of circulating energy metabolites, including acylcarnitines, in two cohorts of heart failure versus control subjects revealed multiple alterations in fatty acid metabolism in peroxisomes in addition to mitochondria, thereby highlighting a novel mechanism contributing to global lipid perturbations in heart failure. Podcast at http://ajpheart.podbean.com/e/acylcarnitines-in-human-heart-failure/.

Peripheral Blood mtDNA and Myocardial Function. Recently, Kuznetsova and Knez (2017) described the experimental, clinical, and epidemiological data of the possible impact of mtDNA content on cardiac structure and function. Heart failure is a complex progressive clinical syndrome which is initiated by risk factors (e.g., hypertension, obesity, and diabetes), then proceeds to asymptomatic maladaptive left ventricular remodeling and dysfunction, and finally evolves into clinically overt, symptomatic heart failure, disability, and death. The progression of left ventricular dysfunction is associated with changes in cardiac energy metabolism. Mitochondria play a central role in a variety of cardiomyocytes functions, including oxidative energy production, storage of Ca^{2+} ions, and apoptosis. The mtDNA content correlates with the size and number of mitochondria, which change under different energy demands and oxidative stress. Experimental studies demonstrated that any genetic manipulation resulting in significantly decreased mtDNA could accelerate the aging process and cause adverse myocardial remodeling and dysfunction. On the other hand, preservation of the mtDNA copy number in mouse hearts delays the development of heart failure after myocardial infarction. Recent general population study also demonstrated that echocardiographic indexes of left ventricular structure and function are associated with mtDNA content measured in peripheral blood cells.

Role of Estrogen in Cardiac Metabolism and Diastolic Function. Heart failure with preserved ejection fraction (HFpEF) has similar prevalence and prognosis as HF with reduced EF, but there is no approved treatment for HFpEF. HFpEF is common in post-menopausal women, which suggests that the absence of estrogen (E2) plays a crucial role in its pathophysiology. With the country's growing elderly population, the prevalence of HFpEF is rapidly increasing. This has triggered a renewed urgency in finding novel approaches to preventing and slowing the progression of HFpEF. Recently, Li and Gupta (2017) addressed the role of E2 in left ventricular diastolic function and how it impacts women with HFpEF as well as animal models. These investigators also discussed the potential mechanisms that represent critical nodes in the mechanistic pathways of HFpEF and how new treatments could be developed to target those mechanisms.

Improved Survival in a Long-Term Rat Model of Sepsis is Associated with Reduced Mitochondrial Ca^{2+} Uptake Despite Increased Energy Demand. To investigate the relationship between prognosis, changes in mitochondrial Ca^{2+} uptake, and bioenergetic status in the heart during sepsis, Pinto et al. (2017) performed *in vivo and ex vivo* controlled experimental studies in male adult Wistar rats. Sepsis was induced by i.p. injection of fecal slurry. Sham-operated animals served as controls. Confocal microscopy was used to study functional and bioenergetic parameters in cardiomyocytes isolated after 24-hrs sepsis. E.M. was used to characterize structural changes in mitochondria and sarcoplasmic reticulum. The functional response to dobutamine was assessed *in vivo* by echocardiography. Peak aortic blood flow velocity measured at 24 hrs was a good discriminator for 72-hrs survival and was used in *ex vivo* experiments at 24 hrs to identify septic animals with good prognosis. Measurements from animals with good prognosis showed (1) a smaller increase in mitochondrial Ca^{2+} content and in nicotinamide adenine dinucleotide fluorescence following pacing and (2) increased distance between mitochondria and sarcoplasmic reticulum on E.M., and (3) nicotinamide adenine dinucleotide redox potential and ATP/ADP failed to reach a new steady state following pacing, suggesting mismatching of energy supply and demand. *In vivo*, good prognosis animals had a blunted response to dobutamine with respect to stroke volume and kinetic energy. In situations of higher energetic demand, decreased mitochondrial Ca^{2+} uptake may constitute an adaptive cellular response that confers a survival advantage in response to sepsis at the cost of decreased oxidative capacity.

Physiological Adaptations to Interval Training and the Role of Exercise Intensity.
Interval exercise typically involves repeated bouts of relatively intense exercise
interspersed by short periods of recovery. A common classification scheme subdivides
this method into high-intensity interval training (HIIT; 'near maximal' efforts)
and sprint interval training (SIT; 'supramaximal' efforts). Both forms of interval
training induce the classic physiological adaptations characteristic of moderate-
intensity continuous training (MICT) such as increased aerobic capacity ($\dot{V}O_2$ max)
and mitochondrial content. MacInnis et al. (2017) considered the role of exercise
intensity in mediating physiological adaptations to training, with a focus on the
capacity for aerobic energy metabolism. With respect to skeletal muscle adaptations,
cellular stress and the resultant metabolic signals for mitochondrial biogenesis
depend primarily on exercise intensity, with limited work suggesting that increases
in mitochondrial content are superior after HIIT compared to MICT, at least when
matched-work comparisons are made within the same individual. It is well established
that SIT increases mitochondrial content to a similar extent to MICT despite a reduced
exercise volume. At the whole-body level, $\dot{V}O_2$ max was generally increased more
by HIIT than MICT for a given training volume, whereas SIT and MICT similarly
improved $\dot{V}O_2$ max despite differences in training volume. There was less evidence
available regarding the role of exercise intensity in mediating changes in skeletal
muscle capillary density, maximum stroke volume and cardiac output, and blood
volume. Furthermore, the interactions between intensity and duration and frequency
have not been thoroughly explored. While interval training is a potent stimulus for
physiological remodeling in humans, the integrative response to this type of exercise
warrants further attention, especially in comparison to traditional endurance training
as highlighted by these researchers.

References

Anupama, N., G. Sindhu and K.G. Raghu. 2018. Significance of mitochondria on cardiometabolic
     syndromes. Fundam Clin Pharmacol Feb 17 (in press).
De Jong, K.A. and G.D. Lopaschuk. 2017. Complex energy metabolic changes in heart failure with
     preserved ejection fraction and heart failure with reduced ejection fraction. Can J Cardiol
     33: 860–871.
Ebadi, M., S.K. Sharma, S. Wanpen and A. Amornpan. 2004. Coenzyme Q_{10} inhibits mitochondrial
     complex-1 down-regulation and nuclear factor-kappa B activation. J Cell Mol Med 8: 213–222.
Hansson, N.H., J. Sörensen, H.J. Harms, W.Y. Kim, R. Nielsen, L.P. Tolbod, J. Frøkiær,
     K. Bouchelouche, K.K. Dodt, I. Sihm, S.H. Poulsen and H. Wiggers. 2017. Myocardial oxygen
     consumption and efficiency in aortic valve stenosis patients with and without heart failure. J Am
     Heart Assoc 6: pii: e004810.
Hauck, L., S. Stanley-Hasnain, A. Fung, D. Grothe, V. Rao, T.W. Mak and F. Billia. 2017.
     Cardiac-specific ablation of the E3 ubiquitin ligase Mdm2 leads to oxidative stress,
     broad mitochondrial deficiency and early death. PLoS One 12: e0189861.
Kuznetsova, T. and J. Knez. 2017. Peripheral blood mitochondrial DNA and myocardial function. Adv
     Exp Med Biol 982: 347–358.
Li, S. and A.A. Gupte. 2017. The role of estrogen in cardiac metabolism and diastolic function.
     Methodist Debakey Cardiovasc J 13: 4–8.
MacInnis, M.J. and M.J. Gibala. 2017. Physiological adaptations to interval training and the role of
     exercise intensity. J Physiol 595: 2915–2930.
Pinto, B.B., A. Dyson, M. Umbrello, J.E. Carré, C. Ritter, I. Clatworthy, M.R. Duchen and
     M. Singer. 2017. Improved survival in a long-term rat model of sepsis is associated with

reduced mitochondrial calcium uptake despite increased energetic demand. Crit Care Med 45: e840–e848.

Ruiz, M., F. Labarthe, A. Fortier, B. Bouchard, J. Thompson Legault, V. Bolduc, O. Rigal, J. Chen, A. Ducharme, P.A. Crawford, J.C. Tardif and C. Des Rosiers. 2017. Circulating acylcarnitine profile in human heart failure: a surrogate of fatty acid metabolic dysregulation in mitochondria and beyond. Am J Physiol Heart Circ Physiol 313: H768–H781.

Sharma, S., M. Kheradpezhou, S. Shavali, H.El. Refaey, J. Eken, C. Hagen and M. Ebadi. 2004. Neuroprotective actions of coenzyme Q10 in Parkinson's disease. Methods Enzymol 382: 488–509.

Sharma, S. and M. Ebadi. 2014. Significance of metallothioneins in aging brain. Neurochem Int 65: 40–48.

Sharma, S. 2017. Antioxidants and Mitochondrial Bioenergetics. Sustained Energy & Enhanced Human Functions and Activity. Ed. D. Bagchi. Chapter 5. pp. 81–102. Elsevier Science Publishers, Netherlands.

Sharma, S.K., H.El. Refaey and M. Ebadi. 2006. Complex-1 activity and ^{18}F-DOPA uptake in genetically engineered mouse model of Parkinson's disease and the neuroprotective role of coenzyme Q10. Brain Res Bull 70: 22–32.

CHAPTER-22

Charnoly Body in Stroke

INTRODUCTION

An acute ischemic stroke (AIS) is one of the most prevalent cause of disability in the entire world. Stroke either kills or renders a victim crippled for the rest of his/her life depending on the severity of the brain regional ischemic attack. Stroke is an emergency and requires prompt theranostic management. It has been shown that mitochondrial disorders result from dysfunctional mitochondria that are unable to generate sufficient energy to meet the needs of various organs. Mitochondrial encephalomyopathy, lactic acidosis, and stroke-like episodes (MELAS) syndrome is one of the most frequent maternally-inherited mitochondrial disorders. There is growing evidence to suggest that NO deficiency occurs in MELAS which results in impaired blood perfusion that contributes to several complications in this disease. NO is synthesized from arginine by NOS, which catalyzes the conversion of arginine to NO and citrulline. Citrulline can be recycled into arginine, and therefore, both arginine and citrulline support NO synthesis. The use of $^{15}N_2$-arginine and ^{13}C-, $^2H_4$-citrulline stable isotope infusion allows measuring arginine flux, citrulline flux, citrulline-to-arginine flux (which represents the *de novo* arginine synthesis rate), and arginine-to-citrulline flux, which represents the NO production rate. El-Hattab and Jahoor (2017) recently highlighted the utility of the stable isotope tracer infusion technique in providing additional evidence for NO deficiency in MELAS, adding more insight into the potential mechanisms of NO deficiency in this syndrome for the assessment of the effects of supplementation with the NO donors, arginine and citrulline, on improving NO production in MELAS.

It is now well-established that preconditioning of the brain induces tolerance to the damaging effects of ischemia and prevents cell death in ischemic penumbra. The development of this phenomenon is mediated by mitochondrial ATP-sensitive K^+ channels and NO signaling. Hence, Deryagin et al. (2017) investigated molecular changes in mitochondria after ischemic preconditioning (IP) and the effect of pharmacological preconditioning (PhP) with the channel opener diazoxide on NO levels after ischemic stroke in rats. Immunofluorescence-histochemistry and laser-confocal microscopy were applied to evaluate the cortical expression of electron transport chain enzymes, mitochondrial-channels, neuronal and iNOS, as well as the dynamics of nitrosylation and nitration of proteins during early and delayed phases of IP. The cerebral NO was studied employing electron paramagnetic resonance

(EPR) spectroscopy using spin trapping. These investigators found that 24 hrs after IP, there was a 2-fold decrease in the expression of cerebral mitochondrial-channels, a comparable increase in the expression of cytochrome c oxidase, and a decrease in intensity of protein S-nitrosylation and nitration. PhP led to a 56% reduction of free NO concentration 72 hrs after AIS. They attributed these results to the restructuring of tissue energy metabolism (namely the provision of increased catalytic sites to mitochondria), and increased elimination of NO, which prevented a decrease in cell sensitivity to oxygen during subsequent periods of severe ischemia.

This chapter describes the basic molecular mechanism of neurodegeneration in AIS involving CB molecular pathogenesis and its possible prevention and/or treatment by improving the MB with antioxidants and novel charnolopharmacotherapeutics.

Mitochondrial Mechanisms of Neuronal Cell Death: Potential Therapeutics. It is now known that mitochondria lie at the crossroads of neuronal survival and cell death. They play a pivotal role in cellular bioenergetics, intracellular Ca^{2+} homeostasis, and in metabolic pathways. Mutations in genes involved in mitochondrial quality control cause a myriad of NDDs. Mitochondria have evolved strategies to kill cells when they are unable to continue their vital functions. Dawson and Dawson (2017) recently provided an overview of the role of mitochondria in neurological diseases and the cell death pathways that are mediated through mitochondria, including their role in accidental cell death, the regulated cell death pathways of apoptosis and parthanatos, and programmed cell death. These investigators described the current state of parthanatic cell death and discussed potential therapeutic strategies targeting initiators and effectors of mitochondrial-mediated cell death in NDDs, as illustrated in this book.

Effects of Ghrelin in Brain Diseases. Ghrelin, a peptide released by the stomach that plays a major role in regulating energy metabolism, has recently been shown to have effects on neurobiological behaviors. Jiao et al. (2017) reported that ghrelin enhances neuronal survival by inhibiting apoptosis, alleviating inflammation and oxidative stress, and by improving mitochondrial function. Ghrelin also stimulates the proliferation, differentiation, and migration of NPCs. Additionally, ghrelin is beneficial for the improvement of memory, mood, and cognitive performance following AIS or traumatic brain injury (TBI). Because of its neuroprotective and neurogenic roles, ghrelin may be used as a therapeutic agent to combat NDDs. These investigators highlighted the pre-clinical evidence and proposed mechanism underlying the role of ghrelin in physiological and pathological brain function. However, the exact role of ghrelin in CB molecular pathogenesis and NDDs currently remains uncertain.

Adaptive Responses of Neuronal Mitochondria to Bioenergetic Challenges. Recently, Raefsky and Mattson (2017) highlighted that an important concept in neurobiology is "neurons that fire together, wire together", that is, the formation and maintenance of synapses is promoted by activation of those synapses. Similar to the effects of the stress of exercise on muscle cells, emerging findings suggest that neurons respond to activity by enhancing signaling pathways (e.g., Ca^{2+}, CREB, PGC-1α, NF-κB) that stimulate mitochondrial biogenesis and cellular stress resistance. These pathways are also activated by aerobic exercise and food deprivation, two bioenergetic challenges of fundamental importance in the evolution of the brains of all mammals, including humans. The metabolic 'switch' in fuel source from liver glycogen store-derived glucose to adipose cell-derived fatty acids and their ketone metabolites during fasting and sustained exercise, appears to be a pivotal trigger of both brain-intrinsic and peripheral organ-derived signals that enhance learning and memory and underlying synaptic plasticity and neurogenesis. Brain-intrinsic extracellular signals include the excitatory neurotransmitter glutamate and the neurotrophic factor BDNF, and peripheral signals may include the liver-derived ketone 3-hydroxybutyrate and the muscle cell-derived protein irisin. Emerging findings suggest that fasting, exercise, and an intellectually-challenging lifestyle can protect neurons against the dysfunction and degeneration that they would otherwise suffer in acute brain injuries (AIS and TBI) and NDDs including AD, PD, and HD. Among the prominent intracellular responses of neurons to these bioenergetic challenges are up-regulation of antioxidant defenses, charnolophagy, and DNA repair. A better understanding of such fundamental hormesis-based adaptive neuronal response mechanisms may result in the development and implementation of novel interventions to promote normal brain function and healthy brain aging.

Role of Mitochondria in Neuronal Differentiation and Synaptic Plasticity. As a neuron differentiates from a stem cell and begins to elaborate undifferentiated neurites (pre-polarization stage), mitochondria congregate at the base of one of the neurites; that neurite then grows rapidly and differentiates into the axon and the remaining neurites differentiate into dendrites, thus establishing cell polarity. Mitochondria also play important roles in synaptic plasticity as they provide energy (ATP) necessary for restoration of transmembrane ion gradients in the presynaptic neurons after it fires an action potential, and in the postsynaptic neuron after glutamate-induced depolarization of the postsynaptic dendrite. By virtue of their ability to sequester and release Ca^{2+}; mitochondria influence the cytoskeletal dynamics involved in neurotransmitter release and in structural adaptations of dendritic spines during learning and memory. Interestingly, the activation of a synapse can result in the selective movement of mitochondria in the dendrite to a position at the base of the spine of the activated synapse to provide additional energy and Ca^{2+}-buffering to support synaptic activity. Mechanisms by which physiological bioenergetic challenges improve mitochondrial health and thereby promote neuroplasticity and resistance to brain injury and disease are yet to be explored.

Activity in neuronal circuits increase in response to exercise, fasting/dietary energy restriction, and cognitive challenges. Such excitatory synaptic activity is mediated by the neurotransmitter glutamate, which binds to ionotropic receptors in the plasma membrane resulting in Ca^{2+} influx/and activation of kinases such as Ca^{2+}/calmodulin-dependent kinase IV (CaMKIV). CaMKIV in turn activates the transcription factor cAMP response element-binding protein (CREB) which induces the expression of multiple genes that encode proteins that influence mitochondrial function and stress resistance. These genes include BDNF, sirtuin 3 (SIRT3), peroxisome proliferator-activated receptor γ coactivator 1α (PGC-1α), and mitochondrial transcription factor A (TFAM). BDNF, which is generated by enzymatic cleavage of the precursor protein proBDNF, is released from neurons and activates specific high affinity cell surface receptors (trkB) on adjacent neurons or the same neuron. TrkB, in turn engages intracellular signaling pathways that include the kinases Akt and extracellular signal-regulated kinase (ERK) and downstream transcription factors, including CREB. SIRT3 is a mitochondrial NAD^+-dependent protein deacetylase that plays important roles in mitochondrial function and stress resistance in neurons. Two protein substrates of SIRT3 in mitochondria are SOD2 and cyclophilin D; deacetylation by SIRT3 increases the enzyme activity of SOD2 to reduce mitochondrial superoxide levels, while deacetylation of cyclophilin D prevents the opening of mitochondrial membrane permeability transition pores, thereby preventing apoptosis. PGC-1α and TFAM regulate multiple nuclear (PGC-1α) and mitochondrial (TFAM) genes that are required for mitochondrial biogenesis. PGC-1α also promotes the transcription of genes that are responsive to the nuclear transcription factors, nuclear regulatory factors 1 and 2 (NRF1/2), and peroxisome proliferator-activated receptor γ (PPARγ). The latter two transcription factors induce the expression of genes encoding proteins that protect the mitochondria against stress including antioxidant enzymes, uncoupling proteins, and anti-apoptotic Bcl-2 family members. Via similar pathways involving synaptic activity and BDNF, *exercise, fasting, and cognitive stimulation* can enhance the clearance of CB through a process known as charnolophagy in which the damaged mitochondrial membranes are phagocytosed by the lysosomes. In the metabolically unchallenged state (i.e., sedentary and fed), neurons utilize mainly glucose as an energy source which is transported into the neurons by the cell surface glucose transporter (GLUT3). By depleting liver glycogen stores and mobilizing fatty acids from adipose cells, fasting and vigorous exercise also cause the production of ketone body 3-hydroxybutyrate (3OHB), which is transported into neurons via the activity of the monocarboxylic acid transporter 2 (MCT2). In addition, 3OHB can induce the production of BDNF in neurons by a mechanism involving mitochondrial ROS production, and activation of the transcription factor NF-κB. Altogether, neuronal circuits respond to intermittent bioenergetic challenges in ways that enhance synaptic plasticity and neurogenesis, improve cognitive function, and increase neuronal resistance to metabolic, oxidative, and excitotoxic stresses.

Role of Mitochondrial Bioenergetics in Age-related Decline in Brain Function and NDDs. Unfavorable changes in the body and brain that occur during normal aging (oxidative molecular damage, impaired mitochondrial function, accumulation of molecular waste involving CB molecular pathogenesis, and chronic inflammation) are amplified by a lifestyle that includes little or no exercise, excessive energy intake, and few cognitive challenges. In the periphery, such adverse changes induce a chronic positive energy balance with hyperglycemia, low amounts of ketones, insulin resistance, and inflammation in many organs. In the brain, there is reduced neuronal activity, and so, reduced levels of activation of signaling pathways involved in neuroplasticity and stress resistance. Consequently, neurons experience excessive oxidative stress and accumulation of CB and CS destabilization, secondary to impaired function or overload of lysosome and proteasome-induced *charnolophagy*. As synapses and neurons begin to degenerate due to CS destabilization, brain tissue inflammation accelerates. Neuronal demise may occur due to destabilized CS-induced excitotoxicity, apoptosis, and/or necroptosis.

Mitochondrial Function in Hypoxic Ischemic Injury and Influence of Aging. Mitochondria are a major target in hypoxic/ischemic injury. Mitochondrial impairment increases with age leading to dysregulation of molecular pathways linked to mitochondria. The perturbation of mitochondrial homeostasis and cellular bioenergetics worsens the outcome following hypoxic-ischemic insults in elderly individuals. In response to acute DPCI, cellular machinery relies on rapid adaptations by modulating miRNA-mediated post-translational modifications. Therefore, post-translational regulation of molecular mediators such as hypoxia-inducible factor 1α (HIF-1α), peroxisome proliferator-activated receptor γ coactivator α (PGC-1α), c-MYC, SIRT1, and AMPK play a critical role in the control of the glycolytic-mitochondrial energy axis in response to hypoxic-ischemic conditions (Ham et al. 2017). The deficiency of oxygen and nutrients leads to decreased energetic reliance on mitochondria, promoting glycolysis. The combination of pseudohypoxia, declining charnolophagy, and dysregulation of stress responses with aging adds to impaired host response to hypoxic-ischemic injury. Furthermore, intermitochondrial signal propagation and tissue wide oscillations in mitochondrial metabolism in response to oxidative stress are emerging as vital to cellular bioenergetics. Recently-reported intercellular transport of mitochondria through tunneling nanotubes also play a role in the response to and treatments for ischemic injury. These investigators provided an overview of some of the molecular mechanisms and potential therapies involved in the alteration of cellular energetics with aging and injury with a neurobiological perspective.

Control of Mitochondrial Physiology and Cell Death by the Bcl-2 Family Proteins Bax and Bok. Neuronal cell death is often triggered by events that involve intracellular increases in Ca^{2+}. Under resting conditions, the $[Ca^{2+}]_i$ concentration is controlled by numerous extrusion and sequestering mechanisms involving the plasma membrane, mitochondria, and ER. These mechanisms prevent a disruption of neuronal ion homeostasis. As these processes require ATP, excessive Ca^{2+} overloading may cause energy depletion, mitochondrial dysfunction, CMB, and may eventually lead to Ca^{2+}-dependent cell death. Excessive Ca^{2+} entry though glutamate receptors (excitotoxicity) has been implicated in several neurologic and chronic NDDs, including AIS, epilepsy, and AD. Recent evidence revealed that excitotoxic cell death is regulated by the Bcl-2 family of proteins. Bcl-2 proteins, comprising of both pro-apoptotic and anti-apoptotic members, mediate the apoptotic pathway by controlling outer membrane integrity, and control neuronal Ca^{2+} homeostasis and MB. D'Orsi et al. (2017) recently highlighted the role of Bcl-2 family proteins in the regulation of apoptosis, their expression in the CNS, and how they control Ca^{2+}-dependent neuronal injury. They reviewed the current knowledge on Bcl-2 family proteins in the regulation of mitochondrial function and bioenergetics, including the fusion and fission machinery, and their role in Ca^{2+} homeostasis in the mitochondria and ER. Specifically, they discussed how the 'pro-apoptotic' Bcl-2 family proteins, Bax and Bok, physiologically-expressed in the CNS, regulate such non-apoptotic functions.

Accumulating evidence suggests that altered cellular metabolism is systemic in pulmonary hypertension (PH) and central to disease pathogenesis. However, MB changes in PH patients and their association with disease severity remain uncertain. It was hypothesized that alteration in the bioenergetic function is present in platelets from PH patients and correlates with clinical parameters of PH. Platelets isolated from controls and PH patients ($n = 28$) were subjected to extracellular flux analysis to determine O_2 consumption and glycolytic rates. Platelets from PH patients showed greater glycolytic rates than controls. Surprisingly, this was accompanied by significant increases in the maximal capacity for O_2 consumption, leading to enhanced respiratory reserve capacity in PH platelets. This increased platelet reserve capacity correlated with mean pulmonary artery pressure, pulmonary vascular resistance, and right ventricular stroke work index in PH patients and was abolished by the inhibition of fatty acid oxidation (FAO). Consistent with a shift to FAO, PH platelets showed augmented enzymatic activity of carnitine palmitoyltransferase-1 and electron transport chain complex II. These data extended the observation of a metabolic alteration in PH from the pulmonary vascular axis to the hematologic compartment and suggested that the measurement of platelet MB is useful in assessment of disease progression and severity.

Mitochondrial Metabolism and Oxidative Stress in Ischemic Stroke: An Epigenetic Connection. Recently, Narne et al. (2017) presented an update on various aspects linking mitochondrial energy metabolism, oxidative stress, and epigenetic modifications in the pathological setting of AIS. The advent of epigenetics brought a shift in the understanding of molecular basis of complex diseases like AIS. Substantial scientific inquiry into the epigenetic basis of NDDs has bolstered the idea that altered carbon flux into central carbon metabolism and disturbed redox states govern the transcriptional profiles through stochastic epigenetic changes. In view of an increasing understanding of the link between MB, oxidative stress, and epigenetics in AIS, 'neuroenergetics' is gaining sustained attention. Defined metabolic transitions during AIS are a function of transiently altered abundance of critical metabolic substrates of TCA and other pathways viz. acetyl-CoA, citrate, 2-oxo-glutarate, succinate, fumarate, S-adenosyl methionine, β-hydroxybutyrate, and cofactors (NAD^+, FAD, ATP, vitamin C) in neuronal mitochondria. These changes impinge on the cellular transcriptome by regulating the activity of several chromatin modifying enzymes that bring about epigenomic transition through alteration in DNA methylation and histone post translational modifications through acetylation. This triggers downstream signaling cascades that evoke adaptive and cell death responses during AIS. Indeed, they also prevail on the functionality of the neuronal network, brain plasticity, and neurogenesis during post stroke recovery. Indeed! Understanding the epigenetic mechanisms that alter the brain transcriptomes through impaired charnolosomics could provide the targeted, safe, and effective personalized theranostics of stroke and other chronic diseases as described in this book.

Sex Differences in Brain Mitochondrial Metabolism: Influence of Endogenous Steroids and Stroke. It is well established that steroids are neuroprotective, and a growing body of evidence indicates that mitochondria are a potential target of their effects. The mitochondria are the site of cellular energy synthesis, regulate oxidative stress, and play a key role in cell death after brain injury and NDDs. After an extensive search of the literature on the general functions of mitochondria and the effects of sex steroid administrations on mitochondrial metabolism, Gaignard et al. (2017) summarized and discussed their recent findings concerning sex differences in brain mitochondrial function in physiological and pathological conditions. To analyze the influence of endogenous sex steroids, oxidative phosphorylation system, mitochondrial oxidative stress, and brain steroid levels were compared between male and female mice, either intact or gonadectomized. Their results showed that females had higher mitochondrial respiration and lower oxidative stress as compared to males and these differences were suppressed by ovariectomy but not by orchidectomy. These investigators also showed that the decrease in brain MB induced by ischemia/reperfusion is different according to sex. In both sexes, treatment with progesterone reduced the ischemia/reperfusion-induced mitochondrial alterations, indicating sex differences in brain mitochondrial function under physiological conditions and after stroke, and identify mitochondria as a target of the neuroprotective properties of progesterone. Thus, it is highly prudent to investigate sex specificity in brain physio-pathological mechanisms, especially when CB molecular pathogenesis is involved.

Inflexibility of AMPK-Mediated Metabolic Reprogramming in Mitochondrial Disease. It has been identified that mitochondrial encephalomyopathy, lactoacidosis, and stroke-like episodes (MELAS) syndrome is commonly caused by the A3243G mutation of mtDNA. The capacity to utilize fatty acid or glucose as a fuel source and how such dynamic switches of metabolic fuel preferences and transcriptional modulation of adaptive mechanism in response to energy deficiency in MELAS syndrome have not been fully elucidated. Recently, Lin et al. (2017) reported that the fibroblasts from patients with MELAS syndrome demonstrated a remarkable deficiency of electron transport chain complexes I and IV, an impaired cellular biogenesis under glucose deprivation, and a decreased ATP synthesis. The analysis of the MB of MELAS cells demonstrated an attenuated fatty acid oxidation that occurred with impaired mitochondrial respiration, while energy production was primarily dependent on glycolysis. Furthermore, the transcriptional modulation was mediated by the AMP-activated protein kinase (AMPK) signaling pathway, which activated its downstream modulators leading to increase in glycolytic flux through activation of pyruvate dehydrogenase. In contrast, the activities of carnitine palmitoyltransferase for fatty acid oxidation and acetyl-CoA carboxylase-1 for fatty acid synthesis were reduced and transcriptional regulation factors for the biogenesis remained unaltered, indicating that MELAS cells lack the adaptive mechanism to switch the fuel source from glucose to fatty acid, as the rate of glycolysis increases in response to CMB. These investigators indicated that aberrant secondary cellular responses to disrupted metabolic homeostasis mediated by the AMPK signaling pathway may contribute to the development of the clinical phenotype.

UCP2-866G/A Polymorphism as a Genetic Biomarker of Prognosis in AIS. Recent studies based on experimental animal models of stroke suggested that an inner mitochondrial membrane uncoupling protein (UCP2), regulates energy metabolism, reduces ROS generation, and provides protection against reperfusion damage. Díaz-Maroto Cicuéndez et al. (2017) investigated whether -866G/A polymorphism in the promoter of the UCP-2 gene, which enhances its transcriptional activity, is associated with better prognosis in patients with embolic ischemic stroke after early recanalization. They investigated a hospital-based prospective cohort of patients with AIS due to middle cerebral artery occlsion (MCAO) diagnosed by transcranial Doppler who obtained a partial/complete recanalization 24 hrs after administration of i.v. thrombolysis. The main focus of the study was functional independence defined as modified Rankin Scale 0–2 on day 90 in 80 patients. The UCP-2-866G/A polymorphism was determined by the polymerase chain reaction-restriction fragment length polymorphism technique (14 genotype A/A (18%), 45 genotype A/G (56%), and 21 genotype G/G (26%)). The percentage of patients with good functional outcome at 3 months was higher in patients harboring the A/A genotype than in those with A/G or G/G genotypes (85 vs 41%, p = 0.01). The A/A genotype was found to be a biomarker of good prognosis after adjustment for secondary variables (age, sex, glucose level, NIHSS score at baseline, complete recanalization, and early neurological improvement) in a logistic regression analysis, suggesting that the AA genotype of UCP-2-866 may predict a better functional outcome in AIS after recanalization of the proximal MCAO.

Significance of Mitochondrial Protein in Post-Translational Modifications and Pathophysiology of Brain Injury. Mitochondria are complex organelles that undergo constant fusion and fission to adapt to the ever-changing cellular environment. The fusion/fission proteins, localized in the inner and outer mitochondrial membrane, play critical roles under pathological conditions such as acute brain injury and NDDs. Post-translational modifications of these proteins regulate their function and activity, impacting mitochondrial dynamics, and their efficiency to generate ATP. The miRNA-mediated post-translational modifications that are known to affect MB include SUMOylation, ubiquitination, phosphorylation, S-nitrosylation, acetylation, O-linked N-acetyl-glucosamine glycosylation, ADP-ribosylation, and proteolytic cleavage. Under stress or pathologic conditions, these modifications are activated and shifts the state of the mitochondrial network involving CB molecular pathogenesis. Hence, Klimova et al. (2017) recommended that we need to accommodate and adapt the MB to the energy demand of the new extra- and/or intracellular environment. Understanding the complex relationship between these modifications on fusion and fission proteins particularly pathologic stress or diseases, can provide promising theranostic targets and therapeutic options. These investigators discussed the specific post-translational modifications of mitochondrial fusion/fission proteins under pathologic conditions and their impact on mitochondrial dynamics in AIS.

Reverse Electron Transfer Induces Loss of Flavin from Mitochondrial Complex I: Mechanism for Brain Ischemia Reperfusion Injury. The major brain tissue damage in AIS takes place upon the reperfusion of ischemic tissue. Energy failure due to alterations in mitochondrial metabolism and the elevated production of ROS is one of the main causes of brain ischemia-reperfusion (IR) injury. Ischemia results in the accumulation of succinate in tissues, which favors reverse electron transfer (RET) when a fraction of electrons derived from succinate is directed to mitochondrial complex-I for the reduction of matrix NAD^+. Stepanova et al. (2017) demonstrated that in intact brain mitochondria oxidizing succinate, complex-I, was down-regulated and was unable to contribute to the physiological respiration. This process was associated with a decline in ROS release and a dissociation of the enzyme's flavin, representing a major molecular mechanism of injury in stroke and induction of oxidative stress after reperfusion and that the origin of ROS during RET was flavin of mitochondrial complex-I. This study highlighted a novel target for neuroprotection against IR brain injury and provided a sensitive biomarker for this process.

Neurotoxicity of Zinc. Zinc-induced neurotoxicity is known to play a role in neuronal damage and death associated with TBI, stroke, seizures, and NDDs. Morris and Levenson (2017) reported that during normal firing of "zinc-ergic" neurons, vesicular free Zn^{2+} is released into the synaptic cleft where it modulates numerous postsynaptic neuronal receptors. However, excess Zn^{2+}, released after injury or disease, leads to excitotoxic neuronal death. The mechanisms of Zn^{2+}-mediated neurotoxicity include not only neuronal signaling but also regulation of MB as well as other mechanisms such as an aggregation of amyloid-β peptides in AD. However, recent data raised concerns about assumptions about the mechanisms of Zn^{2+} in neurotoxicity.

Epilepsy in POLG Related Disease. It is known that epilepsy is common in the polymerase gamma (POLG) related disease and is associated with high morbidity and mortality. Epileptiform discharges affect the occipital regions initially and focal seizures, evolving to bilateral convulsive seizures which are the most common seizures in both adults and children. Hikmat et al. (2017) showed that mtDNA depletion—i.e., the quantitative loss of mtDNA-in neurones is the earliest and most important factor of the cellular dysfunction. Loss of mtDNA leads to loss of mitochondrial respiratory chain (MRC) components that, in turn, compromises MB. This critically balanced neuronal energy metabolism leads to both chronic and progressive neurodegeneration and leaves the neurons unable to cope with an increased demand that can trigger a potentially catastrophic cycle that results in acute focal necrosis. These investigators believed that it is the onset of epilepsy that triggers the cascade of neurodegeneration involving CMB and CB molecular pathogenesis to enhance intracellular toxicity. These events can be identified by characteristic clinical symptoms, EEG, neuro-imaging, and neuropathological findings. Hence, early recognition with prompt and aggressive seizure management is vital and may play a crucial role in modifying the epileptogenic process and improving survival.

Targeting of Transcription and Metabolism in Glioblastoma. It is known that glioblastoma (GBM) is highly resistant to treatment, due to disease heterogeneity and resistance mechanisms. Recently, Su et al. (2017) investigated a promising drug that can inhibit multiple aspects of cancer cell survival mechanisms and become effective therapeutics for GBM patients. To investigate TG02, an agent with known penetration of the blood-brain barrier, they examined the effects as single agent and in combination with temozolomide, a commonly used chemotherapy in GBM. They utilized human GBM cells and a syngeneic mouse orthotopic GBM model, evaluating survival and pharmacodynamics of TG02. These studies included TG02-induced transcriptional regulation, apoptosis, and RNA sequencing in treated GBM cells as well as the investigation of MB and glycolytic function assays. TG02 inhibited cell proliferation, induced cell death, and synergized with temozolomide in GBM cells with different genetic background but not in astrocytes. TG02-induced cytotoxicity was blocked by the overexpression of phosphorylated CDK9, suggesting a CDK9-dependent cell killing. TG02 suppressed transcriptional progression of anti-apoptotic proteins, and induced apoptosis in GBM cells. They further demonstrated that TG02 caused mitochondrial dysfunction and glycolytic suppression and ultimately ATP depletion in GBM. A prolonged survival was observed in GBM mice receiving a combined treatment of TG02 and temozolomide. The TG02-induced decrease of CDK9 phosphorylation was observed in the brain tumor tissue, suggesting that TG02 inhibits multiple survival mechanisms and decreases energy production with temozolomide synergistically, representing a therapeutic strategy in GBM.

Antiapoptotic Effects of MGV-1 in the Thalamus and Hippocampus and Cognitive Deficits Following Cortical Infarct in Rats. Focal cortical infarction causes neuronal apoptosis in the ipsilateral nonischemic thalamus and hippocampus, associated with poststroke cognitive deficits. The translocator protein (TSPO) is critical in regulating mitochondrial apoptotic pathways. Chen et al. (2017) examined the effects of the novel TSPO ligand 2-(2-chlorophenyl) quinazolin-4-yl dimethylcarbamate (2-Cl-MGV-1) on post-stroke cognitive deficits, neuronal mitochondrial apoptosis, and secondary damage in the ipsilateral thalamus and hippocampus after cortical infarction. One hundred fourteen hypertensive rats underwent distal MCAO (n = 76) or sham procedures (n = 38). 2-Cl-MGV-1 or dimethyl sulfoxide as vehicle was administrated 2 hrs after distal MCAO and then for 6 or 13 days (n = 19 per group). Spatial learning and memory were tested using the Morris water maze. Secondary degeneration and mitochondrial apoptosis in the thalamus and hippocampus were assessed using Nissl staining, immunohistochemistry, TUNEL, JC-1 staining, and immunoblotting 7 and 14 days after surgery. Infarct volumes did not significantly differ between the vehicle and 2-Cl-MGV-1 groups. There were more neurons and fewer glia in the ipsilateral thalamus and hippocampus in the vehicle groups than in the sham-operated group 7 and 14 days post-distal MCAO. 2-Cl-MGV-1 ameliorated spatial cognitive impairment and decreased neuronal demise and glial activation when compared with vehicle treatment. The $\Delta\Psi$ collapse, cytoplasmic release of AIF, and Cyt-C was prevented within the thalamus. Caspase cleavage and the numbers of TUNEL and Nissl atrophic cells were reduced within the thalamus and hippocampus. This was accompanied by upregulation of BCl-2 and downregulation of Bax. Thus, 2-Cl-MGV-1 reduced neuronal apoptosis via mitochondrial-dependent pathways and attenuated secondary damage in the nonischemic thalamus and hippocampus, contributing to ameliorated cognitive deficits after cortical infarction.

microRNA-434-3p Regulates Age-related Apoptosis Through eIF5A1 in the Skeletal Muscle. It is known that increased activation of catabolic pathways, including apoptosis causes sarcopenia. However, the precise molecular mechanism that initiates apoptosis during aging is not well understood. Pardo et al. (2017) reported that aging alters miRNA expression profile in mouse skeletal muscle as evidenced by miRNA microarray and real-time PCR. They identified miR-434-3p as a highly downregulated miRNA in the skeletal muscle of aging mice. Myocytes transfected with miR-434-3p mimic prevented apoptosis induced by various apoptotic stimuli, and co-transfection of miR-434-3p antagomir eliminated the inhibitory role of miR-434-3p. miR-434-3p inhibited apoptosis by targeting the eukaryotic translation initiation factor 5A1 (eIF5A1). Overexpression of miR-434-3p in myocytes reduced the loss of $\Delta\Psi$, and activation of caspases-3, -8 and -9 by suppressing eIF5A1 in response to various apoptotic stimuli whereas inhibition of miR-434-3p reversed the scenario. Skeletal muscles from aging mice exhibited low levels of miR-434-3p and high levels of eIF5A1, suggesting a possible role for miR-434-3p in the initiation of apoptosis in aging muscle. These results identified that miR-434-3p is an anti-apoptotic miRNA that may be therapeutically beneficial for treating muscle atrophy in various pathophysiological conditions, including sarcopenia.

Mitochondrial Bioenergetics and Theranostic Potential of Antioxidants in Stroke

Extracellular Mitochondria in CSF and Neurological Recovery after Subarachnoid Hemorrhage. Recent studies suggest that extracellular mitochondria may be involved in the pathophysiology of stroke. In a study, Chou et al. (2017) assessed the functional relevance of endogenous extracellular mitochondria in CSF in rats and humans after subarachnoid hemorrhage (SAH). They used a standard rat model of SAH, where an intraluminal suture was used to perforate a cerebral artery, thus leading to blood extravasation into subarachnoid space. At 24 and 72 hrs after SAH, neurological outcomes were measured, and the standard JC-1 (5,5',6,6'-tetrachloro-1,1',3,3'-tetraethyl-benzimidazolylcarbocyanineiodide) assay was used to determine CSF mitochondrial $\Delta\Psi$. To further support the rat model experiments, CSF samples were obtained from 41 patients with SAH and 27 control subjects. $\Delta\Psi$ were measured with the JC1 assay, and correlations with clinical outcomes were assessed at 3 months. In the standard rat model of SAH, extracellular mitochondria were detected in CSF at 24 and 72 hrs after injury. JC-1 assays demonstrated that $\Delta\Psi$ in CSF was decreased after SAH compared with sham-operated controls. In human CSF samples, extracellular mitochondria were also detected and JC-1 levels were also reduced after SAH. Furthermore, higher $\Delta\Psi$ in the CSF were correlated with better clinical prognosis at 3 months after a SAH onset, suggesting that extracellular mitochondria may provide a biomarker-like glimpse into brain integrity and recovery after injury.

Edaravone Ameliorates Compression-induced Damage in Rat Nucleus Pulposus Cells. Edaravone is a potent free radical scavenger used for treating AIS. In a study, Lin et al. (2017) investigated the protective effects and underlying mechanisms of edaravone on compression-induced damage in rat nucleus pulposus (NP) cells. Cell viability was determined using MTT assay methods. NP cell apoptosis was measured by Hoechst 33,258 staining and Annexin V/PI double staining. Intracellular ROS, $\Delta\Psi$, and $[Ca^{2+}]_i$ were determined by fluorescent probes DCFH-DA, JC-1, and Fluo-3/AM, respectively. Apoptosis-related proteins (cleaved caspase-3, cytosolic cytochrome c, Bax and Bcl-2) and extracellular matrix proteins (aggrecan and collagen II) were analyzed by immunoblotting. Edaravone attenuated the compression-induced decrease in viability of NP cells in a dose-dependent manner. Hoechst 33,258 and Annexin V/PI double staining showed that edaravone protected NP cells from compression-induced apoptosis. Further studies confirmed that edaravone protects NP cells against compression-induced mitochondrial pathway of apoptosis by inhibiting overproduction of ROS, $\Delta\Psi$ collapse, and $[Ca^{2+}]_i$ overload. In addition, edaravone promoted aggrecan and collagen-II expression in compression-treated NP cells, indicating that it ameliorates compression-induced damage in rat nucleus pulposus cells and could be a potential new drug for the treatment of IDD.

Edaravone Protects Against Hyperosmolarity-induced Oxidative Stress and Apoptosis in Primary Human Corneal Epithelial Cells. An increase in the osmolarity of tears induced by excessive evaporation of the aqueous tear phase is a major pathological mechanism behind xerophthalmia. Exposure of epithelial cells on the surface of the human eye to hyperosmolarity leads to oxidative stress, mitochondrial dysfunction, and apoptosis. Edaravone, a hydroxyl radical scavenging agent, is clinically used to reduce neuronal damage following AIS. In a recent study, Li et al. (2017) found that treatment with hyperosmotic media at 400 and 450 mOsM increased the levels of ROS and mitochondrial oxidative damage, which were ameliorated by edaravone treatment. They also found that edaravone could improve MB in HCEpiCs by increasing the levels of ATP and $\Delta\Psi$. MTT and LDH assays indicated that edaravone could attenuate hyperosmolarity-induced cell death. Edaravone prevented apoptosis by decreasing cleaved caspase-3 and by attenuating the release of Cyt-C involving CB molecular pathogenesis. Furthermore, these investigators found that edaravone augments the expression of Nrf2 and its target genes, such as HO-1, GPx-1, and GCLC.

Knockingout Mitochondrial Sirtuin Protects Neurons from Degeneration in Caenorhabditis Elegans. Sirtuins are NAD$^+$-dependent deacetylases, lipoamidases, and ADP-ribosyltransferases that link cellular metabolism to multiple intracellular pathways that influence cell survival, longevity, and cancer growth. Sirtuins influence the extent of neuronal demise in stroke. However, different sirtuins appear to have opposite roles in neuroprotection. In C. elegans, Sangaletti et al. (2017) found that knocking out mitochondrial sirtuin sir-2.3, homologous to mammalian SIRT4, was protective in both chemical ischemia and hyperactive channel induced necrosis. The protective effect of sir-2.3 knock-out was enhanced by blocking glycolysis and abolished by a null mutation in daf-16/FOXO transcription factor, supporting the involvement of the insulin/IGF pathway. However, data in the C. elegans cell culture suggested that the effects of sir-2.3 knock-out act downstream of the DAF-2/IGF-1 receptor. Analysis of ROS in sir-2.3 knock-out revealed that ROS are elevated in this mutant under ischemic conditions in dietary deprivation (DD), but to a lesser extent than in the wild type, suggesting robust activation of a ROS scavenging system in this mutant in the absence of food and a deleterious role of SIRT4 during ischemia in mammals that warrent further investigations and revealed a novel pathway that could be targeted for the design of therapies aimed at protecting neurons from death in ischemic conditions.

Therapeutic Effect of Curcumin in Stroke. Recently, Zhang et al. (2017) conducted a study to understand the therapeutic benefit of curcumin (CUR) against stroke in the experimental animal model. These investigators investigated the healing effect of CUR on mitochondrial dysfunction and inflammation. They used male albino Wistar strain rats for the induction of MCAO and reperfusion. ELISA was used to determine IL-6 and TNF-α in the brain region and immunoblotting to determine the protein expression levels of Bax, Bcl-2, p53, and Sirt1. The water level was determined in the brain region by using the standard method. CUR significantly reduced brain regional edema and water content, significantly reduced IL-6 and TNF-α, and normalized $\Delta\Psi$. Protein expression of p^{53} and Bax were significantly reduced, whereas Bcl-2 and Sirt1 were increased following CUR treatment, suggesting its potential therapeutic role for the treatment of stroke as rejuvenator of MB and attenuator of CB molecular pathogenesis involving CS destabilization and toxic metabolites release.

Progesterone Induces Neuroprotection Following Reperfusion-Promoted Mitochondrial Dysfunction after Focal Cerebral Ischemia. Organelle damage and increased mitochondrial permeabilization are key events in the development of cerebral ischemic tissue injury because they cause both modifications in ATP turnover and cellular apoptosis/necrosis via CB molecular pathogenesis. Early restoration of blood flow and improvement of mitochondrial function might reverse the situation and help in recovery following an onset of stroke. Hence, MB can be effectively used as a pharmacological target. Andrabi et al. (2017) reported that progesterone (P4), one of the promising neurosteroids, has been found to be neuroprotective in various models of neurological diseases, through numerous mechanisms. This motivated these investigators to investigate the role of P4 in the mitochondria-mediated neuroprotection in an AIS model of a rat. They demonstrated the positive effect of P4 on behavioral deficits and MB in an AIS injury model of transient middle cerebral artery occlusion (tMCAO). After induction of tMCAO, the rats received an initial ip injection of P4 (8 mg/kg body weight) or vehicle at 1 hr post-occlusion followed by sc injections at 6, 12, and 18 hrs. Behavioral assessment for functional deficits included grip strength, motor coordination, and gait analysis. A significant improvement with P4 treatment was noticed in tMCAO animals. Staining of isolated brain slices from P4-treated rats with 2,3,5-triphenyltetrazolium chloride (TTC) exhibited a reduction in the infarct area in comparison to the vehicle group, indicating the presence of an increased number of viable mitochondria. P4 treatment also attenuated mitochondrial ROS production, as well as blocked the mitochondrial permeability transition pore (mPTP) in the tMCAO model. In addition, it ameliorated the altered $\Delta\Psi$ and respiration ratio in the ischemic animals, suggesting that P4 has amiliorative effect on MB. These findings demonstrated that P4 treatment is beneficial in preserving the mitochondrial functions that are altered in cerebral ischemic injury and thus can help in defining better therapies.

Dexpramipexole Improves Mitochondrial Bioenergetics in the Experimental Stroke Model. Dexpramipexole, a drug recently tested in patients with ALS can bind F1Fo ATP synthase and increase mitochondrial ATP production. Therefore, Muzzi et al. (2017) investigated its effects on experimental ischemic brain injury. The effects of dexpramipexole on bioenergetics, Ca^{2+} fluxes, electrophysiological functions, and death were evaluated in primary neural cultures and hippocampal slices exposed to oxygen-glucose deprivation (OGD). Effects on infarct volumes and neurological functions were also evaluated in mice following proximal or distal MCAO. Distribution of dexpramipexole within the ischemic brain was evaluated by mass spectrometry imaging. Dexpramipexole improved MB by increasing ATP production in cultured neurons or glia and reduced energy failure, prevented $[Ca^{2+}]_i$ overload, and conferred cytoprotection in OGD cultures. This compound also recovered ATP depletion, mitochondrial swelling, anoxic depolarization, loss of synaptic activity and neuronal death in OGD hippocampal slices. Post-ischemic treatment with dexpramipexole, at doses consistent with those already used in ALS patients, reduced brain infarct size and ameliorated neuroscore in mice subjected to transient or permanent MCAO. The concentrations of dexpramipexole reached within the ischemic penumbra as those found neuroprotective *in vitro*. Dexpramipexole increased mitochondrial F1Fo ATP-synthase activity and reduced ischemic brain injury. These findings, together with the excellent brain penetration and favorable safety profile in humans, made dexpramipexole a drug with translational potential for the treatment of stroke as a potent CB inhibitor and CS stabilizer.

Mitochondrial SIRT3 and Neurodegenerative Brain Disorders. Recently, Anamika et al. (2017) summarized findings on (1) the implication of SIRT3 in NDDs and (2) whether SIRT3 modulation could ameliorate neuropathologies in relevant models. Sirtuins are highly conserved NAD^+ dependent class III histone deacetylases and catalyze deacetylation and ADP ribosylation of non-histone proteins. Since, they require NAD^+ for their activity, the cellular level of sirtuins represents redox status of the cells and thus serves as metabolic stress sensors. Out of 7 homologues of sirtuins identified in mammals, SIRT3, 4, and 5 were localized and active in mitochondria.

Clusters of protein substrates for SIRT3 have been identified in mitochondria and thereby advocating SIRT3 as the main mitochondrial sirtuin which could be involved in protecting stress-induced mitochondrial integrity and energy metabolism. As mitochondrial dysfunction underlies the pathogenesis of almost all NDDs, a role of SIRT3 becomes speculation in such brain disorders. Some recent findings demonstrate that SIRT3 over-expression could prevent neuronal derangements in certain *in vivo* and *in vitro* models of aging and NDDs like AD, HD, and stroke. Similarly, loss of SIRT3 accelerated neurodegeneration in the brain challenged with excitotoxicity. Therefore, SIRT3 could be a relevant target to understand pathogenesis of NDDs involving CB molecular pathogenesis.

Neuroprotective Effect of 3-(Naphthalen-2-Yl(Propoxy)Methyl) Azetidine Hydrochloride on Brain Ischaemia/Reperfusion Injury. Because ischemic stroke is one of the most common brain disorders, diverse effective therapies are urgently needed. Recent studies reported a variety of azetidine-based scaffolds for the development of CNS-focused lead-like libraries. However, their mechanisms of action and *in vivo* functions remain uncertain. Hence, Kim et al. (2017) investigated the mechanism and beneficial effects of 3-(naphthalen-2-yl(propoxy)methyl) azetidine hydrochloride (KHG26792), a novel azetidine derivative, on ischemia/reperfusion (I/R) brain injury. They employed a mouse brain ischemia model induced by 2 hrs of MCAO followed by 24 hrs of reperfusion. They measured apoptotic cell death, inflammatory mediators, free radical generation, and anti-oxidative enzymes activities. They also measured the mitochondrial ATP level and Na^+, K^+-ATPase, and Cyt-C oxidase activities to assess the MB. By immunoblotting, they analyzed the protein levels of iNOS, hypoxia-upregulated protein 1, PTEN-induced putative kinase, uncoupling protein 2, p-Akt, MMP-3, and full-length receptor for advanced glycation end-products (RAGE). KHG26792 improved neurological deficits and brain edema and suppressed I/R-induced apoptosis. KHG26792 attenuated I/R-induced inflammation and oxidative stress by upregulating SOD and catalase activity, GSH, p-Akt, ATP, Na^+, K^+-ATPase, Cyt-c oxidase, and soluble RAGE and downregulating iNOS, HYOUP1, and MMP-3, suggesting an anti-inflammatory and antioxidant role of KHG26792. This was the first study to demonstrate that KHG26792 can protect mouse brains against I/R injury by inhibiting apoptotic damage, modulating inflammation, scavenging free radicals, ameliorating oxidative stress, and improving the MB of the brain; although the clinical relevance of these findings remains unknown.

CB Molecular Pathogenesis in AIS. The pathological triad of extrasynaptic NMDA receptor signaling has been proposed as a common molecular mechanism in neurodegenerative conditions. This pathological triad is induced due to increased extrasynaptic NMDA receptor signaling which triggers (a) structural disintegration, (b) transcriptional desregulation, and (b) mitochondrial dysfunction. The structural disintegration and transcriptional deregulation induce impairments in cognitive functions. The transcriptional deregulation induces mitochondrial dysfunction to cause CMB resulting in CB molecular pathogenesis leading to neurodegenerative apoptosis due to charnolophagy and release of toxic metabolites from the destabilized CS. This pathological triad leads to impaired cognitive performance, bioenergetics failure, and neuronal cell death in AIS.

Therapeutic Targeting of the Pathological Triad of Extrasynaptic NMDA Receptor Signaling in Neurodegenerations. It is known that activation of extrasynaptic NMDA receptors cause neurodegeneration and cell death. The disease mechanism involves a pathological triad consisting of mitochondrial dysfunction, loss of integrity of neuronal structures and connectivity, and disruption of excitation-transcription coupling caused by CREB (cAMP-responsive element-binding protein) shut-off and nuclear accumulation of class IIa histone deacetylases. Interdependency within the triad fuels an accelerating disease progression that culminates in failure of mitochondrial energy production and cell loss. Both acute and slowly progressive NDDs, including stroke, AD, ALS, and HD, share increased death signaling by extrasynaptic NMDA receptors caused by elevated extracellular glutamate concentrations or relocalization of NMDA receptors to extrasynaptic sites. Six areas of therapeutic objectives were defined, based on which a broadly applicable combination therapy was proposed to combat the pathological triad of extrasynaptic NMDA receptor signaling that was common to many NDDs. There is antagonism by extrasynaptic NMDA receptors of both local signaling and synapse-to-nucleus signaling activated by synaptic NMDA receptors. Not depicted, for simplicity, is the contribution of back-propagating action potential firing and opening of L-type voltage-gated Ca^{2+} channels to activity-driven, synaptic NMDA receptor–dependent gene expression (Bading 2013). Synapse-to-nucleus signaling is mediated by a propagating Ca^{2+} signal but in addition can involve protein-based communication pathways including the ERK-MAPK cascade, Jacob, and TORC1/2 (Hagenston and Bading 2011; Panayotis et al. 2015). NMDA receptor–interacting protein (NIP) indicates extrasynaptic NMDA receptor–interacting protein that may be part of the death-signaling complex. Local signaling and plasticity refers particularly to dendritic mRNA translation, AMPA receptor trafficking, and control of synaptic efficacy (Steward and Schuman 2001; Kelleher et al. 2004; Kim et al. 2005; Costa-Mattioli et al. 2009; Bading 2017).

Survival of Stem Cells after their Injection in Ischemic Neural Tissue. High post-transplantation cell mortality is the main limitation of various approaches that are aimed at improving regeneration of injured neural tissue by an injection of neural stem cells (NSCs) and mesenchymal stromal cells (MStroCs) in and/or around the lesion. Therefore, it is important to identify efficient ways to increase cell transplant viability. Therefore, Sandvig et al. (2017) proposed the "evolutionary stem cell paradigm," which explains the association between stem cell anaerobic/microerophilic metabolic set-up and stem cell self-renewal and inhibition of differentiation. These investigators identified the main critical point in the collection and preparation of these cells for experimental therapy: exposure of the cells to atmospheric O_2, that is, to oxygen concentrations that are several times higher than the physiologically relevant ones. In this way, the primitive anaerobic cells become either inactivated or adapted, through commitment and differentiation, to highly aerobic conditions (20%–21% O_2 in atmospheric air). This compromises the cells' survival once they are transplanted into normal tissue, especially in the hypoxic/anoxic/ischemic environment, which is typical of CNS lesions. In addition to the findings suggesting that stem cells can shift to glycolysis and can proliferate in anoxia, recent studies also proposed that stem cells can proliferate in completely anaerobic or ischemic conditions by relying on anaerobic mitochondrial respiration. These investigators proposed strategies to enhance the survival of NSCs and MStroCs that are implanted in hypoxic/ischemic neural tissue by harnessing their anaerobic nature and maintaining as well as enhancing their anaerobic properties via appropriate *ex vivo* conditioning.

Longer-Term Impact of Hemiparetic Stroke on Skeletal Muscle Metabolism. Hemiparetic stroke leads to structural and metabolic alterations of skeletal muscle tissue, thereby contributing to functional impairment associated with stroke. *In situ* metabolic processes in skeletal muscle have not been investigated. Klaer et al. (2017) hypothesized that muscular metabolic capacity is limited after hemiparetic stroke, and that changes affect rather the paretic than non-paretic limb. Nine male hemiparetic stroke survivors (age, 62 ± 8 years; BMI, 28 ± 4 kg/m^2; median stroke latency, 23 months ranging from 7 to 34 months poststroke) underwent dynamic *in situ* measurements of carbohydrate and lipid metabolism at fasting condition and during oral glucose tolerance testing, using bilateral microdialysis. Results were compared to 8 healthy male subjects of similar age and BMI. Tissue perfusion, fasting, and postprandial profiles of interstitial metabolites glucose, pyruvate, lactate, and glycerol did not differ between paretic and non-paretic muscle. Patients displayed higher fasting and postprandial dialysate glycerol levels compared to controls with elevated plasma FFA. Glycolytic activity was higher in patients vs controls, with increased lactate production upon glucose load. An elevated lipolytic and glycolytic activity suggested an impaired substrate metabolism with blunted oxidative metabolism in bilateral skeletal muscle in patients after hemiparetic stroke involving CMB and CB molecular pathogenesis. Muscular metabolic properties did not differ between the paretic and non-paretic leg. These investigators suggested further work to investigate the clinical significance of this impaired muscular metabolic capacity in post-stroke patients.

Fluorescence-based ATG8 Sensors Monitor Localization and Function of LC3/ GABARAP Proteins. It is well-established that autophagy is a cellular surveillance pathway that balances metabolic and energy resources and transports specific cargos, including damaged mitochondria (CB), other broken organelles, or pathogens for degradation to the lysosome through energy (ATP) driven charnolophagy and CS exocytosis. Central components of autophagosomal biogenesis are 6 members of the LC3 and GABARAP family of ubiquitin-like proteins (mATG8s). Stolz et al. (2017) used phage display to isolate peptides that possessed bona fide LIR (LC3-interacting region) properties and were selective for individual mATG8 isoforms. Sensitivity of the developed sensors was optimized by multiplication, charge distribution, and fusion with a membrane recruitment (FYVE) or an oligomerization (PB1) domain. These investigators demonstrated the use of the engineered peptides as intracellular sensors that recognized specifically GABARAP, GABL1, GABL2, and LC3C, as well as a bispecific sensor for LC3A and LC3B. By using an LC3C-specific sensor, they could monitor recruitment of endogenous LC3C to Salmonella during xenophagy, as well as to mitochondria during charnolophagy and suggested that sensors are general tools to monitor the fate of mATG8s and will be valuable in decoding the biological functions of the individual LC3/GABARAPs.

Global Ablation of the Mitochondrial Ca^{2+} Uniporter Increases Glycolysis in Cortical Neurons Subjected to Energetic Stressors. Nichols et al. (2017) investigated the effects of global mitochondrial Ca^{2+} uniporter (MCU) deficiency on hypoxic-ischemic (HI) brain injury, neuronal Ca^{2+} handling, MB, and hypoxic preconditioning (HPC).

Forebrain mitochondria isolated from global MCU nulls displayed reduced Ca^{2+} uptake and Ca^{2+}-induced opening of the membrane permeability transition pore. Despite evidence that these effects should be neuroprotective, global MCU nulls, and wild-type (WT) mice suffered comparable HI brain damage. Energetic stress enhanced glycolysis and depressed complex-I activity in global MCU null, relative to WT, cortical neurons. HI reduced forebrain NADH levels more in global MCU nulls than WT mice suggesting that increased glycolytic consumption of NADH suppressed complex-I activity. Compared to WT neurons, pyruvate dehydrogenase (PDH) was hyper-phosphorylated in MCU nulls at several sites that lower the supply of substrates for the TCA cycle. Elevation of cytosolic Ca^{2+} with glutamate or ionomycin decreased PDH phosphorylation in MCU null neurons suggesting the use of alternative mitochondrial Ca^{2+} transport. Under basal conditions, global MCU nulls showed similar increases of Ca^{2+} handling genes in the hippocampus as WT mice subjected to HPC. These investigators proposed that long-term adaptations, common to HPC, in global MCU nulls compromise resistance to HI brain injury and disrupt HPC.

Glutamate Dehydrogenase as a Neuroprotective Target in Brain Ischemia and Reperfusion. It is now well established that deregulation of glutamate homeostasis is associated with NDDs. Glutamate dehydrogenase (GDH) is important for glutamate metabolism and plays a central role in expanding the pool of TCA cycle intermediate α-ketoglutarate (α-KG), which improves MB. Under high energy demand, maintenance of ATP production results in functionally active mitochondria. Therefore, Kim et al. (2017) tested whether the modulation of GDH activity can rescue ischemia/reperfusion-induced neuronal demise in an *in vivo* mouse model of MCAO and in an *in vitro* oxygen/glucose depletion model. Iodoacetate, an inhibitor of glycolysis, was also used in a model of energy failure, remarkably depleting ATP and α-KG. To stimulate GDH activity, the GDH activator 2-aminobicyclo-(2,2,1)-heptane-2-carboxylic acid and potential activator β-lapachone were used. The GDH activators restored α-KG and ATP levels in the injury models and provided neuroprotection. They also found that β-lapachone increased glutamate utilization, accompanied by a reduction in extracellular glutamate. Thus, their hypothesis that mitochondrial GDH activators increase α-KG production as an alternative energy source in the TCA cycle under energy-depleted conditions was confirmed and suggested that increasing GDH-mediated glutamate oxidation represents a novel therapeutic intervention for NDDs, including stroke.

Stimulation of Astrocyte Fatty Acid Oxidation by Thyroid Hormone is Protective Against AIS-induced Damage. Sayre et al. (2017) demonstrated that stimulation of astrocyte mitochondrial ATP production via P2Y₁ receptor agonists was neuroprotective after cerebral AIS. Another mechanism that increases ATP production is fatty acid oxidation (FAO). These investigators showed that in primary human astrocytes, FAO and ATP production are stimulated by 3,3,5 triiodo-l-thyronine (T3). They tested whether T3-stimulated FAO enhances neuroprotection and showed that T3 increases astrocyte survival after either H_2O_2 exposure or OGD. T3-mediated ATP production and protection were both eliminated with etomoxir, an inhibitor of FAO. T3-mediated protection *in vitro* was also dependent on astrocytes expressing HADHA (hydroxyacyl-CoA dehydrogenase/3-ketoacyl-CoA thiolase/enoyl-CoA hydratase) was critical for T3-mediated FAO in fibroblasts. T3-treatment decreased stroke volumes in mice.

While T3 decreased stroke volume in etomoxir-treated mice, T3 had no protective effect on stroke volume in HADHA +/– mice or in mice unable to upregulate astrocyte-specific energy production. *In vivo*, 95% of HADHA co-localized with glial-fibrillary acidic protein, suggesting the effect of HADHA is astrocyte-mediated, and that astrocyte-FAO modulates lesion size and is required for T3-mediated neuroprotection after post. This was the first report of a neuroprotective role for FAO in the brain.

Post-Stroke Depression: Mechanisms and Pharmacological Treatment. It is known that depression, the most frequent psychiatric disorder following ischemic stroke, negatively affects survivals' functional outcome, response to rehabilitation, and quality of life. Approximately, one-third of them are affected by post-stroke depression (PSD), making it a serious social and public health problem and anti-depressant preventive and curative therapies worth investigating. However, a two-way association between depression and stroke has been also established: stroke increases the risk of PSD, but depression is an independent risk factor for stroke. Villa et al. (2017) reported multifactorial pathophysiology of PSD, involving a combination of diversified ischemia-induced neurobiological dysfunctions in the context of psychosocial distress. The damage of frontal-basal ganglia brainstem pathway suggested alterations of monoaminergic neurotransmitter systems. Several lines of evidence point to a relationship between neuroinflammatory response to AIS, stress activation of the hypothalamic-pituitary-adrenal (HPA) axis, and the impairment of adaptive response (neurogenesis) within a background of altered MB. The complexity of PSD mechanisms makes its biologically-based prevention and treatment a difficult task. So far, especially the selective serotonin (5-HT) reuptake inhibitors (SSRIs) have proved clinically effective in preventing and treating PSD, although their effects have not been demonstrated unequivocally and they may cause female genital tract bleeding, GIT bleeding, and intracerebral hemorrhage. Besides the primary pharmacological activity of SSRIs their pleiotropic mechanisms of action: anti-inflammatory and enhanced neurogenesis through the up-regulation of neurotrophins supported by the stimulation of MB. In the future, novel developments might point at anti-cytokine modulators which can improve symptoms of depression, especially in subjects affected by inflammation. These investigators addressed various areas of epidemiology, pathophysiology, preventive, and therapeutic strategies for PSD. The activity of SSRIs in clinical trials, as well as their pharmacology, pharmacokinetics, safety and mechanisms of action, in addition to the effect of depression as risk factor for stroke. I have described hippocampal sclerosis due to depletion of BDNF due to CB formation and CS destabilization in major depressive disorders (MDDs) and MTs as potent free radical scavengers and antagonists of CB. Hence, any pharmacological or physiological intervention to enhance brain regional MTs can alleviate diversified clinical symptoms of MDDs accompanied with or without AIS (Sharma 2015). For further details, please refer to my books" Beyond Diet and Depression" Vol-1 and Vol-2, and "Alleviating Stress of the Soldier & Civilian" published by Nova Science Publishers, New York, U.S.A.

References

Anamika, K.A, P. Acharjee, A. Acharjee and S.K. Trigun. 2017. Mitochondrial SIRT3 and neurodegenerative brain disorders. J Chem Neuroanat Nov 9. pii: S0891-0618(17)30123-0.

Andrabi, S.S., S. Parvez and H. Tabassum. 2017. Progesterone induces neuroprotection following reperfusion-promoted mitochondrial dysfunction after focal cerebral ischemia in rats. Dis Model Mech 10: 787–796.

Bading, H. 2017. Therapeutic targeting of the pathological triad of extrasynaptic NMDA receptor signaling in neurodegenerations. J Exp Med 214: 569–578.

Chen, Y., L. Veenman, S. Singh, F. Ouyang, J. Liang, W. Huang, I. Marek, J. Zeng and M. Gavish. 2017. 2-Cl-MGV-1 ameliorates apoptosis in the thalamus and hippocampus and cognitive deficits after cortical infarct in rats. Stroke 48: 3366–3374.

Chou, S.H., J. Lan, E. Esposito, M. Ning, L. Balaj, X. Ji, E.H. Lo and K. Hayakawa. 2017. Extracellular mitochondria in cerebrospinal fluid and neurological recovery after subarachnoid hemorrhage. Stroke 48: 2231–2237.

Costa-Mattioli, M., W.S. Sossin, E. Klann and N. Sonnenberg. 2009. Translational control of long-lasting synaptic plasticity and memory. Neuron 61: 10–26.

Daubert, M.A., E. Yow, G. Dunn, S. Marchev, H. Barnhart, P.S. Douglas, C. O'Connor, S. Goldstein, J.E. Udelson and H.N. Sabbah. 2017. Novel mitochondria-targeting peptide in heart failure treatment: a randomized, placebo-controlled trial of elamipretide. Circ Heart Fail 10: pii: e004389.

Dawson, T.M. and V.L. Dawson. 2017. Mitochondrial mechanisms of neuronal cell death: potential therapeutics. Annu Rev Pharmacol Toxicol 57: 437–454.

Deryagin, O.G., S.A. Gavrilova, K.L. Gainutdinov, A.V. Golubeva, V.V. Andrianov, G.G. Yafarova, S.V. Buravkov and V.B. Koshelev. 2017. Molecular bases of brain preconditioning. Front Neurosci 11: 427.

Díaz-Maroto Cicuéndez, I., E. Fernández-Díaz, J. García-García, J. Jordán, I. Fernández-Cadenas, J. Montaner, G. Serrano-Heras and T. Segura. 2017. The UCHARNOLOPHAGY2-866G/A polymorphism could be considered as a genetic marker of different functional prognosis in ischemic stroke after recanalization. Neuromolecular Med 19: 571–578.

D'Orsi, B., J. Mateyka and J.H.M. Prehn. 2017. Control of mitochondrial physiology and cell death by the Bcl-2 family proteins Bax and Bok. Neurochem Int 109: 162–170.

El-Hattab, A.W. and F. Jahoor. 2017. Assessment of nitric oxide production in mitochondrial encephalomyopathy, lactic acidosis, and stroke-like episodes syndrome with the use of a stable isotope tracer infusion technique. J Nutr 147: 1251–1257.

Gaignard, P., M. Fréchou, P. Liere, P. Thérond, M. Schumacher, A. Slama and R. Guennoun. 2017. Sex differences in brain mitochondrial metabolism: influence of endogenous steroids and stroke. J Neuroendocrinol Jun 26.

Hagenston, A.M. and H. Bading. 2011. Calcium signaling in synapse-to-nucleus communication. Cold Spring Harb Perspect Biol Nov 1; 3(11): a004564.

Ham, P.B. 3rd and R. Raju. 2017. Mitochondrial function in hypoxic ischemic injury and influence of aging. Prog Neurobiol 157: 92–116.

Hikmat, O., T. Eichele, C. Tzoulis and L.A. Bindoff. 2017. Understanding the epilepsy in POLG related disease. Int J Mol Sci 18: pii: E1845.

Jiao, Q., X. Du, Y. Li, B. Gong, L. Shi, T. Tang and H. Jiang. 2017. The neurological effects of ghrelin in brain diseases: Beyond metabolic functions. Neurosci Biobehav Rev 73: 98–111.

Kelleher, R.J. 3rd, A. Govindarajan and S. Tonegawa. 2004. Translational regulatory mechanisms in persistent forms of synaptic plasticity. Neuron 44(1): 59–73.

Khanna, A., P. Acharjee, A. Acharjee and S.K. Trigun. 2017. Mitochondrial SIRT3 and neurodegenerative brain disorders. J Chem Neuroanat pii: S0891-0618(17)30123-0.

Kim, A.Y., K.H. Jeong, J.H. Lee, Y. Kang, S.H. Lee and E.J. Baik. 2017. Glutamate dehydrogenase as a neuroprotective target against brain ischemia and reperfusion. Neuroscience 340: 487–500.

Kim, M.J., A.W. Dunah, Y.T. Wang and M. Shang. 2005. Differential role of NR2A and NR2B-containing NMDA receptors in RAS-ERK signaling and AMPA receptor trafficking. Neuron 46: 745–760.

Kim, E.A., J.M. Na, J. Kim, S.Y. Choi, J.Y. Ahn and S.W. Cho. 2017. Neuroprotective effect of 3-(Naphthalen-2-Yl(Propoxy)Methyl)Azetidine hydrochloride on brain ischaemia/reperfusion injury. J Neuroimmune Pharmacol 12: 447–461.

Klaer, J., A. Mähler, N. Scherbakov, L. Klug, S. von Haehling, M. Boschmann and W. Doehner. 2017. Longer-term impact of hemiparetic stroke on skeletal muscle metabolism—A pilot study. Int J Cardiol 230: 241–247.

Klimova, N., A. Long and T. Kristian. 2017. Significance of mitochondrial protein post-translational modifications in pathophysiology of brain injury. Transl Stroke Res Sep 21.

Li, Y., H. Liu, W. Zeng and J. Wei. 2017. Edaravone protects against hyperosmolarity-induced oxidative stress and apoptosis in primary human corneal epithelial cells. PLoS One 12: e0174437.

Lin, D.S., S.H. Kao, C.S. Ho, Y.H. Wei, P.L. Hung, M.H. Hsu, T.Y. Wu, T.J. Wang, Y.R. Jian, T.H. Lee and M.F. Chiang. 2017. Inflexibility of AMPK-mediated metabolic reprogramming in mitochondrial disease. Oncotarget 8: 73627–73639.

Lin, H., X. Ma, B.C. Wang, L. Zhao, J.X. Liu, F.F. Pu, Y.Q. Hu, H.Z. Hu and Z.W. Shao. 2017. Edaravone ameliorates compression-induced damage in rat nucleus pulposus cells. Life Sci 189: 76–83.

Morris, D.R. and C.W. Leverson. 2017. Neurotoxicity of zinc. Advances in Neurobiology 18: 303–312.

Muzzi, M., E. Gerace, D. Buonvicino, E. Coppi, F. Resta, L. Formentini, R. Zecchi, L. Tigli, D. Guasti, M. Ferri, E. Camaioni, A. Masi, D.E. Pellegrini-Giampietro, G. Mannaioni, D. Bani, A.M. Pugliese and A. Chiarugi. 2017. Dexpramipexole improves bioenergetics and outcome in experimental stroke. Br J Pharmacol Mar 20.

Narne, P., V. Pandey and P.B. Phanithi. 2017. Interplay between mitochondrial metabolism and oxidative stress in ischemic stroke: An epigenetic connection. Mol Cell Neurosci 82: 176–194.

Nguyen, Q.L., C. Corey, P. White, A. Watson, M.T. Gladwin, M.A. Simon and S. Shiva. 2017. Platelets from pulmonary hypertension patients show increased mitochondrial reserve capacity. JCI Insight 2: e91415.

Nichols, M., P.A. Elustondo, J. Warford, A. Thirumaran, E.V. Pavlov and G.S. Robertson. 2017. Global ablation of the mitochondrial calcium uniporter increases glycolysis in cortical neurons subjected to energetic stressors. J Cereb Blood Flow Metab 37: 3027–3041.

Panayotis, N., A. Karpova, M.R. Kreutz and M. Fainzilber. 2015. Macromolecular transport in synapse to nucleus communication. Trends Neurosci 38(2): 108–116.

Pardo, P.S., A. Hajira, A.M. Boriek and J.S. Mohamed. 2017. microRNA-434-3p regulates age-related apoptosis through eIF5A1 in the skeletal muscle. Aging (Albany NY) 9: 1012–1029.

Raefsky, S.M. and M.P. Mattson. 2017. Adaptive responses of neuronal mitochondria to bioenergetic challenges: Roles in neuroplasticity and disease resistance. Free Radic Biol Med 102: 203–216.

Sandvig, I., I. Gadjanski, M. Vlaski-Lafarge, L. Buzanska, D. Loncaric, A. Sarnowska, L. Rodriguez, A. Sandvig and Z. Ivanovic. 2017. Strategies to enhance implantation and survival of stem cells after their injection in ischemic neural tissue. Stem Cells Dev 26: 554–565.

Sangaletti, R., M. D'Amico, J. Grant, D. Della-Morte and L. Bianchi. 2017. Knock-out of a mitochondrial sirtuin protects neurons from degeneration in Caenorhabditis elegans. PLoS Genet 13: e1006965.

Sayre, N.L., M. Sifuentes, D. Holstein, S.Y. Cheng, X. Zhu and J.D. Lechleiter. 2017. Stimulation of astrocyte fatty acid oxidation by thyroid hormone is protective against ischemic stroke-induced damage. J Cereb Blood Flow Metab 37: 514–527.

Stepanova, A., A. Kahl, C. Konrad, V. Ten, A.S. Starkov and A. Galkin. 2017. Reverse electron transfer results in a loss of flavin from mitochondrial complex I: Potential mechanism for brain ischemia reperfusion injury. J Cereb Blood Flow Metab 37: 3649–3658.

Steward, O. and E.M. Schuman. 2001. Protein synthesis at synaptic sites on dendrites. Annu Rev Neurosci 24: 299–325.

Stolz, A., M. Putyrski, I. Kutle, J. Huber, C. Wang, V. Major, S.S. Sidhu, R.J. Youle, V.V. Rogov, V. Dötsch, A. Ernst and I. Dikic. 2017. Fluorescence-based ATG8 sensors monitor localization and function of LC3/GABARAP proteins. EMBO J 36: 549–564.

Su, Y.T., R. Chen, H. Wang, H. Song, Q. Zhang, L.Y. Chen, H. Lappin et al. 2017. Novel targeting of transcription and metabolism in glioblastoma. Clin Cancer Res pii: 2032.2017.

Villa, R.F., F. Ferrari and A. Moretti. 2017. Post-stroke depression: Mechanisms and pharmacological treatment. Pharmacol Ther pii: S0163-7258(17)30289-9.

Zhang, Y., Y. Yan, Y. Cao, Y. Yang, Q. Zhao, R. Jing, J. Hu and J. Bao. 2017. Potential therapeutic and protective effect of curcumin against stroke in the male albino stroke-induced model rats. Life Sci 183: 45–49.

CHAPTER-23

Charnoly Body in Traumatic Brain Injury and Post Traumatic Stress Disorder

INTRODUCTION

TBI is a common combat injury, which can occur through explosive blast, and produces brain changes due to various mechanisms of injury. Although mild traumatic brain injury (mTBI) is the most common, it is extremely difficult to diagnose and is the least understood. Some mTBIs have progressive, long-term debilitating consequences. A single TBI can produce gray and white matter atrophy, accelerate age-related progressive neurodegeneration, and increase the risk of developing AD, PD, and motor neuron disease later in life. TBI is the common cause of PTSD among people of all ages (Jaffee and Meyer 2009). TBI can also occur in children due to parental neglect, among adolescents due to impaired drunk-driving, vehicle over-speeding, and in soldiers during blast injury in the war theater.

Conflicts in Afghanistan and Iraq are responsible for > 1.2 million deployed soldiers every year. At present the number of PTSD victims in US is ~ 13 million and is increasing alarmingly. Sibner et al. (2014) recently reported that by 2050, > 13 million Americans of all ages will be living with AD, and the costs of care will expand to ~ $1.2 trillion. The rapidly rising number of those affected with AD includes aging military veterans who may have increased risk as consequence of TBI, PTSD, and/or service-related injuries. The increasing number of individuals, the long duration of disability, and the rising cost of care for AD and other dementia are public health challenges augmented by increasing veteran population that is much younger, with an increased risk of AD and other dementia, and who may experience disability, emphasizing the immediate need for AD cure and related war-related dementia.

mTBI is the primary cause of PTSD among war-wounded soldiers. Hence, this topic is of universal importance for both soldiers as well as civilians and their families and friends. The quality of life of soldiers suffering from PTSD is compromised due to remarkable psychological and physical stress a soldier and veteran experience during war operation. It has been demonstrated that organization of resting-state cortical functional connectivity is severely impaired following concussive mTBI (Han et al. 2014). However, all these studies had cross-sectional designs, which resulted in low quality ratings and limited the conclusions. Bahraini et al. (2014) reviewed recent literature to explore the epidemiology, pathophysiology, evaluation, and treatment of TBI-related PTSD. Cognitive difficulties were reported by OEF/OIF soldiers. Cooper et al. (2014) examined factors that may contribute to cognitive difficulties in post-deployment clinical settings. A total of 84 soldiers who sustained a mild or moderate TBI and cognitive difficulties underwent neurocognitive testing. Regression analyses were used to determine the variance in neurocognitive performance by the predictor variables (demographic, mechanism of injury, time since injury, headache severity, combat stress, postconcussive complaints, and effort/performance validity). The predictor variables accounted for 51.7% of the variance in cognitive performance. The most significant predictor of cognitive function was performance validity/effort, accounting for 16.3% of the variance. Symptom severity, including postconcussive complaints, combat stress, and headache, accounted for 7.2% of the variance. Demographic factors and injury characteristics, such as time since injury and mechanism of injury, were not significant predictors of cognitive performance. This study emphasized the need to include post-deployment settings for the evaluation of mTBI-induced cognitive impairments.

Recent research has explored the cognitive and psychiatric sequelae of blast-related mTBI. A meta-analysis evaluated the chronic effects of mTBI on cognitive performance. Karr et al. (2014) identified 9 studies reporting 12 samples meeting eligibility criteria. The overall posterior mean effect size and highest density interval (HDI), verbal delayed memory, and processing speed were the most sensitive cognitive domains to blast-related mTBI. When dividing executive function into diverse sub-constructs (i.e., working memory, inhibition, and set-shifting), presented the largest effect size. PTSD symptoms did not predict cognitive effects, indicating chronic cognitive impairment following mTBI, especially in set-shifting, a relevant aspect of executive attention consistent with meta-analyses on multiple mTBI and neuroimaging on the cognitive correlates of white matter damage.

This chapter describes an overview of the war-related TBI co-morbidities including blast injuries and mental health of soldiers. Military-related mild (mTBIs) and pregressive neurodegeneration, association of TBIs/PTSDs with AD in Veterans and CB molecular pathogenesis in TBI-related NDDs and its attenuation by antioxidants. The chapter also highlights screening of TBI and PTSD in soldiers, impact of blast-plus impact TBI on PTSD, MRI, and MRSI evaluation of military-related TBI, blast-related mTBI with a loss of consciousness (LOC) verses without LOC, post-deployment binge drinking, impact of blast-plus impact TBI on PTSD and its impact on learning, academic performance, and mental health of US soldiers.

TBI Screening: Sensitivity, Specificity, and Predictive Value. Zollman et al. (2014) recently reported that TBI is referred to as the signature injury of the wars in Iraq and Afghanistan. Given the prevalence of TBI in soldiers, there is a need for instruments to screen for TBI in this population. A sum of 300 soldiers or veterans underwent a screen and a comprehensive diagnostic assessment to identify the occurrence of TBI and/or the presence of PTSD. Negative predictive value, positive predictive value, sensitivity, and specificity were calculated. This screening tool for TBI yielded 96% sensitivity, 64% specificity, 95% negative predictive, and 69% predictive value. The

Rehabilitation Institute of Chicago Military TBI Screening Instrument has a high negative predictive value and sensitivity for TBI. This tool identifies individuals likely to have sustained a TBI. Moreover, it detects those who are likely not to have sustained such an injury and can be reassured in this regard. Because such distinction can be made with a high degree of accuracy in cost-effective fashion, it represents an important contribution to the TBI screening program.

Blast Injuries and Mental Health of Soldiers. Blast injury has been identified as primary cause of mental health problems including PTSD among soldiers in the conflicts in Iraq and Afghanistan. However, it remains uncertain whether basic differences exist between blast-related TBI and TBI due to other mechanisms. To determine similarities and differences between clinical outcomes in US soldiers with blast-related vs non-blast-related concussive TBI and to identify impairment that correlates with disability, MacDonald et al. (2014) conducted a study involving US soldiers from Iraq or Afghanistan to Landstuhl Regional Medical Center, Germany. Four groups of participants were enrolled from 2010–2013: (1) blast plus impact complex TBI (n = 53), (2) non-blast related TBI with injury due to other mechanisms (n = 29), (3) blast-exposed controls evacuated for other medical reasons (n = 27), and (4) non-blast-exposed controls evacuated for other medical reasons (n = 69). All patients with TBI met inclusion criteria for concussive (mild) TBI. The participants were evaluated 6–12 months after injury at Washington University in St Louis. In total, 255 subjects were enrolled in the study, and 183 participated in follow-up. Clinical evaluation included for disability, a neurological exam, headache questionnaires, neuropsychological test battery, combat exposure and alcohol use, and interview for PTSD and depression. Global outcomes, headache severity, neuropsychological performance, and PTSD severity and depression were indistinguishable between the two TBI groups, independent of mechanism of injury. Both TBI groups had higher rates of moderate to severe disability than the control groups: 77% of blast plus impact TBI and 79% of nonblast TBI vs 59% of blast-exposed controls and 41% of non-blast-exposed controls. In addition, blast-exposed controls had severe headaches and PTSD symptoms as compared to the non-blast-exposed controls. Combat exposure intensity was higher in the blast plus impact TBI group than in nonblast TBI group and was higher in blast-exposed controls than in non-blast-exposed controls. However, combat exposure intensity did not correlate with PTSD severity in the TBI groups; a modest correlation was observed in the controls. Overall outcomes were correlated with depression, headache, and other abnormalities on neuropsychological testing, suggesting that TBI itself, independent of injury mechanism and combat exposure intensity, is responsible for the poor prognosis. Many other factors are unexplored, and poor prognosis following war-time injuries are difficult to explain at present.

Impact of Blast-Plus Impact TBI on PTSD. Several questions remain unresolved about the impact of blast-plus-impact TBI from wars in Iraq and Afghanistan. MacDonald et al. (2014) measured clinical outcome in US soldiers to Landstuhl Regional Medical Center (LRMC) in Germany after "blast-plus" concussive TBIs. Glasgow Outcome Scale-Extended assessments completed in 6–12 months indicated a moderate disability in 41/47 (87%) blast-plus TBI subjects and a smaller number of similar US military controls without TBI for other medical reasons. Cognitive function assessed with neuropsychological tests was similar between blast-plus TBI subjects and controls; performance of both groups was normal without any evidence of focal neurological deficits. However, 29/47 (57%) of blast-plus subjects with TBI met all criteria for PTSD versus 5/18 (28%) of controls. PTSD was associated with overall disability; 31/34 patients with PTSD versus 19/31 patients who did not meet full PTSD criteria had moderate to severe disability. Symptoms of depression were also severe in the TBI group, and correlated with PTSD severity, suggesting that high rates of PTSD and depression but not cognitive impairment or focal neurological deficits are observed after concussive blast-plus-impact TBI. Overall disability was greater than civilian non-blast concussive ("mild") patients with TBI, even with polytrauma. The exact relationship between these clinical outcomes and specific blast-related brain injuries versus other combat-related factors remains unknown.

Blast-Related mTBI with a Loss of Consciousness (LOC) vs without LOC. Norris et al. (2014) compared symptoms with a blast-related mTBI with LOC to those without LOC in US soldiers within 72 hrs of sustaining a blast-related mTBI and at a follow-up visit 48–72 hrs later (n = 210). Demographics, post-concussive symptoms, diagnosis of acute stress reaction (ASR), and simple reaction time data from the Automated Neuropsychological Assessment Metric (ANAM) were collected. ASRs were more severe in patients reporting LOC versus patients reporting no LOC. At the first post-injury visit, LOC was associated with difficulty sleeping, hearing loss, memory impairments, and severe symptoms. A follow-up explored if symptomatic differences were influenced by ASR. Adjusting for ASR, the statistical relationships between LOC and symptoms were weaker. At the follow-up visit, difficulty sleeping was associated with LOC before and after adjusting for ASR. Patients with both ASR and LOC had the slowest simple reaction times suggesting that ASR may partially mediate symptoms and cognitive dysfunction in the acute phase following blast-related mTBI requiring further research.

Mild TBI and Progressive Neurodegeneration. Mild TBI includes concussion, subconcussion, and exposures to explosive blasts from explosive devices. Repetitive mTBIs can provoke tauopathy and chronic traumatic encephalopathy (CTE). McKee and Robinson (2014) found early changes of CTE in four young veterans of the Iraq and Afghanistan conflict who were exposed to an explosive blast and in another young veteran who was repetitively concussed. Four of the five veterans with early-stage CTE were also diagnosed with PTSD. Advanced CTE has been found in veterans who experienced repetitive neurotrauma while in service and in others who were athletes. CTE is associated with behavioral changes, executive dysfunction, memory loss, and cognitive impairments that progress slowly over decades. CTE produces atrophy of the frontal and temporal lobes, thalamus, and hypothalamus; septal abnormalities; and deposits of hyperphosphorylated tau as neurofibrillary tangles and disordered neurites throughout the brain. The incidence and prevalence of chronic traumatic encephalopathy and the genetic risk factors involved in its development are presently unknown. CTE has clinical and pathological features that overlap with postconcussion syndrome and PTSD, suggesting that these disorders might share some molecular biological mechanisms involving CB pathogenesis.

Effect of TBI and PTSD on Learning and Academic Achievement. A study was conducted to delineate the effects of self-reported TBI or PTSD on self-regulated learning and academic achievement for university-enrolled soldiers (Ness et al.

2014). Students (N = 192) from 8 universities, representing an estimated 6% of soldiers enrolled across schools. Public universities that were members of the soldier opportunity college consortium participated in this study. A cross-sectional study was performed to evaluate the relationships between self-reported TBI, PTSD, and learning variables and their contribution to academic achievement. Self-report of military service symptoms of TBI and PTSD included self-regulation strategies including effort, time/environment regulation, and academic self-efficacy and grade point average (GPA). There was no effect of self-reported TBI or PTSD on GPA, effort regulation, or time/environment regulation strategies; however, participants with TBI or PTSD reported lower academic self-efficacy. Self-efficacy was the most powerful predictor of GPA among all participants, followed by military rank. The sample consisted of high achieving students responsive to a university administrator, which raised the possibility of sampling bias. Because of the low recruitment rate for this study and lack of published research, further confirmation is necessary before drawing generalized conclusions.

TBI Among Soldiers. mTBI is common among soldiers who served in OEF/OIF/OND. O'Neil et al. (2014) described the cognitive, mental health, physical health, functional, social, and cost consequences of mTBI in veterans and soldiers. Of 2668 reviewed abstracts, 31 provided low evidence for the questions of interest. Cognitive, physical, and mental health symptoms were reported by Veterans/soldiers with a history of mTBI. These symptoms were not common in those with a history of mTBI than in those without, although a lack of differences did not rule out the possibility that some individuals could experience PTSD related to mTBI. The evidence of potential risk or protective factors moderating mTBI outcomes was unclear. Although the overall evidence was low, these findings were consistent with civilian studies. Hence re-integration services are needed to address comorbid conditions, such as treatment for PTSD, substance use disorders, headaches, and other disorders that Veterans and soldiers may experience after deployment regardless of mTBI history.

TBI and PTSD Screening in Soldiers. A study was performed to identify latent classes of soldiers according to persistent post-concussive symptom patterns and to characterize the classes relative to other post-deployment variables including PTSD and mTBI screening results. Such comparisons may inform policy regarding these assessments and translate to improved treatment decisions. Aralis et al. (2014) obtained a data for 12,581 combat-exposed male U.S. Navy and Marine soldiers who returned from deployment in 2008–2009 and completed a Post-Deployment Health Assessment (PDHA) and an associated Post-Deployment Health Reassessment (PDHRA). Persistent post-concussive symptoms indicated on the PDHRA were used in a latent class analysis yielding 4 distinct classes: systemic, cognitive/behavioral, comorbid, and nonpresenting. Although the non-presenting class endorsed few or no post-concussive symptoms, the systemic and cognitive/behavioral classes displayed elevated likelihoods of neurological and mental health symptoms, respectively. Members of the comorbid class had an increased probability of reporting a wide range of symptoms across both domains. Characterization of classes suggested that membership may indicate the presence or absence of persistent conditions resulting from head injury and/or mental health issues. Under this assumption, estimated class membership probabilities implied a rate of neurological injury to be 17.9%, whereas the assessments identifying repercussions of mild TBI reported 13.1% positive rate, suggesting that PDHA and PDHRA underestimate the prevalence of soldiers experiencing post-deployment health problems. Supplemental items or an alternative screening algorithm incorporating persistent post-concussive symptoms may enable identification.

MRI of Military-related TBI with Compromized Neurocircuitry. Whether the vulnerability of white matter differs between blast and impact injury, and the consequences of morphological changes on neuropsychological function are poorly understood in TBI patients. Yeh et al. (2014) used diffusion tensor imaging (DTI) to assess the neurocircuitry in 37 U.S. soldiers (29 mild, 7 moderate, 1 severe, 17 blast, and 20 nonblast), who sustained a TBI while deployed, compared to 14 nondeployed controls. High-dimensional deformable registration of DTI data was followed by fiber tracking and tract-specific analysis along with region-of-interest (ROI) analysis. DTI results were examined in relation to post-concussion and PTSD symptoms. The most prominent white matter microstructural injury for both blast and nonblast patients was in the frontal fibers within the fronto-striatal (corona radiata, internal capsule) and fronto-limbic circuits (fornix, cingulum), the fronto-parieto-occipital association fibers, in brainstem fibers, and in callosal fibers. Subcortical superior-inferiorly oriented tracts were more vulnerable to blast injury than nonblast injury, while direct impact force had more deleterious effects on anterio-posteriorly oriented tracts, which caused heterogeneous left and right hemispheric asymmetries of white matter connectivity. The tractography using diffusion anisotropy deficits revealed the cortico-striatal-thalamic-cerebellar-cortical (CSTCC) networks, where increased post-concussion and PTSD symptoms were associated with low fractional anisotropy in the major nodes of compromised CSTCC neurocircuitry, and the consequences on cognitive dysfunction.

MRSI to Determine TBI. Explosive blast mTBI is associated with memory impairment and PTSD. Explosive shock waves can cause hippocampal injury in a large animal model. de Lanerolle et al. (2014) recently reported a method for detecting brain injury in soldiers with explosive blast mTBI using MRSI in veterans exposed to blast. The hippocampus of 25 veterans with explosive blast mTBI, 20 controls, and 12 subjects with PTSD but without exposure to explosive blast were studied using MRSI at 7 Tesla. Psychiatric and cognitive assessments were made to characterize the neuropsychiatric deficits and compared with findings from MRSI. Significant reductions in the ratio of *N*-acetyl aspartate to choline (NAA/Ch) and *NAA* to creatine (NAA/Cr) were observed in the anterior hippocampus with explosive blast mTBI in comparison to controls and were more pronounced in the right hippocampus, which was 15% smaller in volume. Decreased NAA/Ch and NAA/Cr were not influenced by comorbidities—PTSD, depression, or anxiety. Soldiers with PTSD without blast had lesser injury, which tended to be in the posterior hippocampus. Explosive blast mTBI subjects had a reduction in visual memory compared to PTSD without blast, suggesting that the region of the hippocampus injured differentiates explosive blast mTBI from PTSD. Hence, MRSI is quite sensitive in detecting and localizing regions of neuronal injury from explosive blast associated with memory impairment.

TBI and Post-Deployment Binge Drinking. Adams et al. (2016) examined whether experiencing a TBI on a combat deployment was associated with post-deployment binge drinking, independent of PTSD. Using the 2008 Department of Defense Survey of Health-Related Behaviors among Active Duty Soldier, a survey completed by 28546 soldiers, the study included 6824 soldiers who had a combat deployment in the past year. Path analysis was used to examine whether PTSD accounted for the association between TBI and binge drinking. The dependent variable, binge drinking days, was an ordinal measure capturing the number of times personnel drank 5+ drinks on one occasion (4+ for women). TBI level captured the severity after a combat injury exposure: TBI-AC (altered consciousness only), TBI-LOC of 20 or less (loss of consciousness up to 20 minutes), and TBI-LOC (loss of consciousness > 20 minutes). A PTSD-positive screen relied on the diagnostic cutoff of 50+ on the PTSD Checklist-Civilian. While the direct effect of TBI on binge drinking was smaller than that of PTSD, both were significant, ~ 70% of the total effect of TBI on binge drinking was from the direct effect; only 30% represented the indirect effect through PTSD, suggesting that further research is needed to confirm these findings and to understand the basic molecular mechanisms that explain the relationship between TBI and increased post-deployment drinking.

Prognosis of TBI in Soldiers. WHO Collaborating Centre Task Force on mTBI published its findings on the prognosis of mTBI in 2004. This review focused on deployed soldiers. Literature published between January 2001 and February 2012 listed in MEDLINE and four other databases was reviewed. Boyle et al. (2014) selected controlled-trials and cohort and case-control studies according to predefined criteria. After 77,914 titles and abstracts were screened, 13 articles were eligible for this review and 3 (23%) with a low risk of bias were accepted. Two independent reviewers evaluated eligible studies using a modification of the Scottish Intercollegiate Guidelines Network criteria. The reviewers extracted data from eligible studies and produced evidence tables. The evidence was synthesized and presented in evidence tables. These findings were based on three studies of U.S. soldiers who were deployed in Iraq or Afghanistan. Soldiers with mTBI reported PTSD and postconcussive symptoms. In addition, postconcussive symptoms differed based on combat stress, suggesting a slight decline in neurocognitive function after mTBI, which was in the normal range of brain functioning. There was limited evidence that combat stress, PTSD, and postconcussive symptoms affect recovery and prognosis of mTBI in soldiers. Further research is needed to precisely assess the prognosis of mTBI in soldiers.

TBI and PTSD in US Soldiers. Many researchers are interested in investigating veterans from recent conflicts in Afghanistan and Iraq with TBI and/or PTSD. Such studies may experience problems in recruiting sufficient numbers unless effective strategies are implemented. Currently, there is limited information on recruitment strategies for individuals with TBI and/or PTSD. It is likely that patients with medical conditions may be less likely to volunteer for clinical research. This study investigated the feasibility of recruiting veterans returning from recent military conflicts—OEF and OIF. Bayley et al. (2014) selected soldiers from an epidemiological study. Three study sites focused on survey respondents (n = 445) who lived within a 60-mile radius. The successful recruitment of veterans using a population-based sampling method was dependent on the ability to contact participants. Study enrollment of participants with TBI and/or PTSD had a recruitment yield of 5.4%. Twenty-four veterans were enrolled. The population-based sampling method for recruitment of recent combat veterans demonstrated the challenges, particularly in contacting and screening participants. These data can help guide recruitment for future studies using population-based studies.

TBI and PTSD in Marines. Whether TBI is a risk factor for PTSD has been difficult to determine because of the prevalence of comorbid conditions, overlapping symptoms, and cross-sectional samples. Yurgil et al. (2014) examined the extent to which self-reported predeployment and deployment-related TBI confers increased risk of PTSD when accounting for combat intensity and predeployment mental health symptoms. As part of the Marine Resiliency Study, clinical interviews and assessments were administered ~ 1 month before a 7-month deployment to Iraq or Afghanistan and again 3–6 months after deployment. The study was conducted on a Marine Corps base in southern California or at Veterans Affairs San Diego Medical Center. Participants for the final analytic sample were 1648 Marine and Navy servicemen who completed predeployment and postdeployment assessments. The exclusion criteria were non-deployment (n = 34), missing data (n = 181), and rank of noncommissioned and commissioned officers (n = 66). The primary outcome was the total score on the Clinician-Administered PTSD Scale (CAPS), three months after deployment. At the predeployment assessment, 56.8% of the participants reported prior TBI; at postdeployment assessment, 19.8% reported sustaining TBI between predeployment and postdeployment assessments (i.e., deployment-related TBI). Approximately 87.2% of deployment-related TBIs were mild; 250 of 287 participants (87.1%) who reported < 24 hrs of posttraumatic amnesia (37 reported ≥ 24 hours), and 111 of 117 of those who lost consciousness (94.9%) reported < 30 minutes of unconsciousness. Predeployment CAPS score and combat intensity score increased predicted 3-month postdeployment CAPS scores by factors of 1.02 per unit increase. Deployment-related mTBI raised predicted CAPS scores by a factor of 1.23, and moderate/severe TBI raised predicted scores by a factor of 1.71. Probability of PTSD was highest for participants with severe predeployment symptoms, high combat intensity, and deployment-related TBI. TBI doubled the PTSD rates for participants with less severe predeployment PTSD symptoms. Even while accounting for predeployment symptoms, prior TBI, and combat intensity, TBI during the most recent deployment was the strongest predictor of postdeployment PTSD symptoms.

PTSD and TBI Co-morbidity and Therapeutic Strategies. Both PTSD and TBI occur in the civilian population, share pathophysiological characteristics, and are associated with sleep disruption and cognitive impairment. PTSD and TBI present with overlapping symptoms can lead to over-diagnosis or misdiagnosis and are associated with co-morbidities relevant to diagnosis and treatment. Further research is needed to elucidate more effective treatments of PTSD and TBI co-morbidity and on factors predictive of better prognosis. To summarize the literature on PTSD and TBI and their co-morbidity, on diagnosis, clinical symptoms, and treatment issues, Tanev et al. (2014) performed Pubmed searches using the terms PTSD, TBI, sleep, cognitive, depression, anxiety, treatment, and combinations of these terms. This study presented pathophysiological, neuroimaging, and clinical data on co-morbid PTSD and TBI and associated disorders, emphasizing the impact of cognitive and sleep problems. It summarized the treatment for co-morbid PTSD and TBI, including psychotherapy, pharmacotherapy, and cognitive rehabilitation. Note: For further details please refer to my recently published book "Alleviating Stress of the Soldier & Civilian" Nova Science Publishers, New York, U.S.A. (2015).

References

Adams, R.S., M.J. Larson, J.D. Corrigan, G.A. Ritter, C.M. Horgan, R.M. Bray and T.V. Williams. 2016. Combat-acquired traumatic brain injury, posttraumatic stress disorder, and their relative associations with post-deployment binge drinking. J Head Trauma Rehabil 31: 13–22.

Aralis, H.J., C.A. Macera, M.J. Rauh and A.J. Macgregor. 2014. Traumatic brain injury and PTSD screening efforts evaluated using latent class analysis. Rehabil Psychol 59: 68–78.

Bahraini, N.H., R.E. Breshears, T.D. Hernández, A.L. Schneider, J.E. Forster and L.A. Brenner. 2014. Traumatic brain injury and posttraumatic stress disorder. Psychiatr Clin North Am 37: 55–75.

Bayley, P.J., J.Y. Kong, D.A. Helmer, A. Schneiderman, L.A. Roselli, S.M. Rosse, J.A. Jackson, J. Baldwin, L. Isaac, M. Nolasco, M.R. Blackman, M.J. Reinhard, J.W. Ashford and J.C. Chapman. 2014. MIND Study Group. Challenges to be overcome using population-based sampling methods to recruit veterans for a study of post-traumatic stress disorder and traumatic brain injury. BMC Med Res Methodol 14: 48.

Boyle, E., C. Cancelliere, J. Hartvigsen, L.J. Carroll, L.W. Holm and J.D. Cassidy. 2014. Systematic review of prognosis after mild traumatic brain injury in the military: results of the international collaboration on mild traumatic brain injury prognosis. Arch Phys Med Rehabil 95(3 Suppl): S230–237.

Cooper, D.B., R.D. Vanderploeg, P. Armistead-Jehle, J.D. Lewis and A.O. Bowles. 2014. Factors associated with neurocognitive performance in OIF/OEF soldiers with postconcussive complaints in postdeployment clinical settings. J Rehabil Res Dev 51: 1023–1034.

de Lanerolle, N.C., H. Hamid, J. Kulas, J.W. Pan, R. Czlapinski, A. Rinaldi, G. Ling, F.A. Bandak and H.P. Hetherington. 2014. Concussive brain injury from explosive blast. Ann Clin Transl Neurol 1: 692–702.

Han, K., C.L. Mac Donald, A.M. Johnson, Y. Barnes, I. Wierzechowski, D. Zonies, J. Oh, S. Flaherty, R. Fang, M.E. Raichle and D.L. Brody. 2014. Disrupted modular organization of resting-state cortical functional connectivity in U.S. military personnel following concussive 'mild' blast-related traumatic brain injury. Neuroimage 4: 76–96.

Jaffee, M.S. and K.S. Meyer. 2009. A brief overview of traumatic brain injury (TBI) and post-traumatic stress disorder (PTSD) within the Department of Defense. Clin Neuropsychol 23: 1291–1298.

Karr, J.E., C.N. Areshenkoff, E.C. Duggan and M.A. Garcia-Barrera. 2014. Blast-related mild traumatic brain injury: a Bayesian random-effects meta-analysis on the cognitive outcomes of concussion among military personnel. Neuropsychol Rev 24: 428–444.

Mac Donald, C.L., M. Ann, A.M. Johnson, L. Wierzechowski, E. Kassner, T. Stewart, E.C. Nelson, N.J. Werner, D. Zonies, J. Oh, R. Fang and D.L. Brody. 2014. Prospectively assessed clinical outcomes in concussive blast vs nonblast traumatic brain injury among evacuated US military personnel. JAMA Neurology E1–E9.

MacDonald, C.L., A.M. Johnson, E.C. Nelson, N.J. Werner, R. Fang, S.F. Flaherty and D.L. Brody. 2014. Functional status after blast-plus-impact complex concussive traumatic brain injury in evacuated United States soldier. J Neurotrauma 31: 889–898.

McKee, A.C. and M.E. Robinson. 2014. Military-related traumatic brain injury and neurodegeneration. Alzheimers Dement 10: S242–253.

Ness, B.M., M.R. Rocke, C.J. Harrist and K.G. Vroman. 2014. College and combat trauma: an insider's perspective of the post-secondary education experience shared by service members managing neurobehavioral symptoms. NeuroRehabilitation 35: 147–158.

Norris, J.N., R. Sams, P. Lundblad, E. Frantz and E. Harris. 2014. Blast-related mild traumatic brain injury in the acute phase: Acute stress reactions partially mediate the relationship between loss of consciousness and symptoms. Brain Inj 28: 1052–1062.

O'Neil, M.E., K.F. Carlson, D. Storzbach, L.A. Brenner, M. Freeman, A.R. Quiñones, M. Motu'apuaka and D. Kansagara. 2014. Factors associated with mild traumatic brain injury in veterans and soldier: a systematic review. J Int Neuropsychol Soc 20: 249–261.

Sibener, L., I. Zaganjor, H.M. Snyder, L.J. Bain, R. Egge and M.C. Carrillo. 2014. Alzheimer's Disease prevalence, costs, and prevention for soldiers and veterans. Alzheimers Dement 10(3 Suppl): S105–110.

Tanev, K.S., K.Z. Pentel, M.A. Kredlow and M.E. Charney. 2014. PTSD and TBI co-morbidity: scope, clinical presentation and treatment options. Brain Inj 28: 261–270.

Yeh, P.H., B. Wang, T.R. Oakes, L.M. French, H. Pan, J. Graner, W. Liu and G. Riedy. 2014. Postconcussional disorder and PTSD symptoms of military-related traumatic brain injury associated with compromised neurocircuitry. Hum Brain Mapp 35: 2652–2673.

Yurgil, K.A., D.A. Barkauskas, J.J. Vasterling, C.M. Nievergelt, G.E. Larson, N.J. Schork, B.T. Litz, W.P. Nash and D.G. Baker. 2014. Marine Resiliency Study Team. Association between traumatic brain injury and risk of posttraumatic stress disorder in active-duty Marines. JAMA Psychiatry 71: 149–157.

CHAPTER-24

Charnolopharmacotherapy of Neurodegenerative and Other Diseases

INTRODUCTION

Charnoly body (CB) was discovered for the first time in the developing UN rat Purkinje neurons due to nutritional stress-induced free radical overproduction (Sharma et al. 1986; Sharma et al. 1987). CB is a highly unstable, pleomorphic, quasi-crystalline, multi-lamellar, electron-dense membrane stack that is formed due to mitochondrial degeneration in response to nutritional stress and/or toxic exposure (Sharma et al. 1986; Sharma et al. 1987; Sharma et al. 1993). Free radical-induced CMB triggers CB formation in the most vulnerable cell as a primary event in the etiopathogenesis of intra-neuronal inclusions in various NDDs, including AD, PD, major depressive disorders (MDDs), and chronic drug addiction. Free radical-induced mitochondrial $\Delta\Psi$ collapse triggers oxidation of mtDNA to cause 8-OH, 2dG accumulation, and CB formation, which is the initial step in the etio-pathogenesis of progressive NDDs (Sharma et al. 2003; Sharma et al. 2004). MTs prevent CB formation by serving as potent free radical scavengers to provide neuroprotection by regulating Zn^{2+}-mediated transcriptional activation of genes involved in growth, proliferation, differentiation, and development (Sharma et al. 2013a; Sharma et al. 2013b). Non-specific induction of CB formation causes GIT stress, myelosuppression, and alopecia as noticed in MDR malignancies and major depressive disorders, Parkinsonism, and schizophrenia (Sharma 2014).

Depending on the type of neurons involved, MAO-A or MAO-B specific CBs is formed in the soma as well as in the synaptic regions of DA-ergic, 5-HTergic, NE-ergic, GABAergic, glutamatergic, or other neurons. Hence, novel drugs may be developed to prevent and/or eradicate MAO-A or MAO-B specific CB formation to provide neuroprotection (Sharma 2015, 2016). Particularly, charnolophagy is the most efficient early molecular mechanism of ICD during acute phase of neurotoxicity and/or nutritional insult in the developing or aging brain (Sharma and Ebadi 2014a; Sharma and Ebadi 2014b). CB sequestration during chronic phase releases MAOs as well as Cyt-C to cause not only depletion of synaptic NE, 5-HT, and DA, but also apoptosis to enhance atherosclerotic plaque rupture and progressive NDDs (Sharma 2016). Accumulation of CB at the junction of the axon hillock can impair normal axoplasmic flow of various ions, enzymes, neurotropic factors (BDNF, IGF-1, NGF), and mitochondria to cause abnormal axoplasmic flow and hence, degeneration of synaptic terminals to cause abnormal synaptic neurotransmission and cognitive impairments in AD and aging. MAOIs such as selegiline and rasagiline augment brain regional MTs to provide neuroprotection by inhibiting CB formation and by serving as potent free radical scavengers (Sharma 2016). Hence novel MAOIs or other mitochondrially-targeted drugs may be developed to prevent DSST tissue-specific CB formation, enhance charnolophagy, and/or prevent CB sequestration for the treatment of PD, AD, drug addiction, and MDDs, and vice versa for the EBPT of MDR malignancies with minimum or no adverse effects. Free radicals ($\cdot$OH, NO$\cdot$)-induced α-synuclein index (SI) triggers mitochondrial degeneration to enhance CB formation and eventually Lewy body formation, amyloid-β deposition, and aggregation of several other proteins, implicated in diversified NDDs. Similarly, brain region-specific protein nitration is involved in CB formation and eventually, accumulation of lysosomal-resistant intra-neuronal inclusions in various NDDs particularly in HD, AD, and ALS. I discovered CB as an early, pre-apoptotic biomarker of CMB in progressive NDDs which can be detected at an earlier stage of neuronal impairment (Sharma et al. 2013a; Sharma et al. 2013b; Sharma 2014, 2015).

Hypothesis. I proposed that stress (nutritional/environmental)-induced cortisol release augments, whereas MTs, IGF-1, and BDNF inhibit hippocampal CB formation to prevent progressive neurodegeneration, and hence, early morbidity and mortality in progressive neurodegenerative and other diseases. Hence, DSST-CB inhibitors, charnolophagy-agonists, and CS-stabilizers may be developed for the targeted, safe, and effective EBPT of NDDs, CVDs, and MDR malignancies.

We have shown that specific MAOI-B inhibitors, selegiline and rasagiline, provide mitochondrial protection through MTs-mediated CB inhibition by serving as potent free radical scavengers (Sharma et al. 2003; Sharma and Ebadi 2013a; Sharma et al. 2013; Sharma 2014). Several antioxidants including: MTs, melatonin, sirtuins, resveratrol, and CoQ$_{10}$ may also serve as CB inhibitors to provide neuroprotection. Exactly similar molecular mechanism of mitochondrial neuroprotection might be afforded by other MAOIs for better patient care, treatment of diseases, promotion of health, and better quality of life by preventing DSST-CB formation. Based on two types of MAOs localized on the outer mitochondrial membranes, we proposed two types of CBs: (a) MAOI-A-Specific CB and (b) MAOI-B-Specific CB as novel drug discovery targets for the personalized treatment of PD, AD, chronic drug addiction, PTSD, and treatment resistant MDDs, which could serve as a unique platform for future research and development of novel drugs. Hence, future development of MAO-specific CB antagonists will have superior pharmacological profile, enhanced margin of safety, maximum therapeutic index, and minimum or no adverse effects (Sharma 2015).

^{18}F-DOPA and ^{18}FdG Neuroimaging in Experimental Model of Neurodegeneration. MicroPET imaging was performed employing Siemens Medical Solutions microPET imaging system equipped with microPET Manager for the data acquisition and AsiPro for image reconstruction as described in our publications (Sharma and Ebadi 2005; Sharma et al. 2006; Ebadi and Sharma 2006). MicroPET imaging of ^{18}FdG in C57BL/6J mouse exhibited maximum localization in the CNS, heart, lungs and the adipose tissue. ^{18}FdG (250 μCi) was injected in the caudal vein after 350 mg/kg, i.p. tribromoethane anesthesia. After 20 min, the imaging data was acquired by microPET Manager and analyzed by Asi-Pro computer software. ^{18}F-DOPA (250 μCi) was injected in the caudal vein after anesthesia. MicroPET neuroimaging exhibited significantly reduced striatal ^{18}F-DOPA uptake in wv/ wv mouse as compared to control and wv/+ mice. Ethanol augmented cocaine and METH-induced neurotoxicity in the CNS and other body parts such as heart and lungs of C57BL/6J mouse. MicroPET neuroimages of C57BL/6J mice were acquired which were intoxicated with cocaine, cocaine+METH, and cocaine+METH+ethanol for 21 days. MicroPET images were acquired after injecting ^{18}F-DOPA or ^{18}FdG in these animal models of multiple drug abuse. ^{18}F-DOPA uptake was significantly reduced in cocaine-treated mice. Coadministration of METH induced further reduction in the striatal ^{18}F-DOPA uptake. A more severe reduction in the striatal ^{18}F-DOPA uptake was noticed in mice intoxicated with cocaine+METH, and ethanol in combination, suggesting that ethanol serves as a gateway to multiple drug abuse. Cocaine in combination with ethanol, forms a highly toxic metabolite, coca-ethylene, which induces severe loss of striatal DA-ergic neurons. ^{18}FdG uptake was also significantly reduced in the myocardium and lungs as observed in the sagittal and coronal sections of these experimental animals. These experiments demonstrated that brain regional DA-ergic as well as myocardial and pulmonary MB are significantly compromised to cause early morbidity and mortality in multiple drug abuse due to accumulation of lysosomal-resistant CB formation in the most vulnerable neurons. Recently we reported that multiple drug abuse triggers progressive neurodegeneration due to free radical-induced CB formation, involved in apoptosis and pro-inflammatory cascade, causing cognitive impairment, early morbidity, and mortality, whereas antioxidants such as MTs prevent CB formation and hence prevention of progressive NDDs by acting as free radical scavengers (Sharma S. Charnoly body as a universal biomarker of multiple drug addiction, 3rd International Conference on drug Addiction, Orlando, FL, U.S.A. Aug 3–5, 2015) [Invited Speaker and Chairperson].

Described below are the distinct cellular, subcellular, and molecular events involved in CB pathogenesis and their prevention/inhibition in progressive NDDs including PD, AD, MDD, schizophrenia, and chronic drug addiction by developing specific CB inhibitors or charnolophagy agonists/antagonists.

The oxidation of the mtDNA generates 8-OH, 2dG, which is significantly increased in the plasma, serum, and urine samples of PD, AD, and aging subjects. 8-OH 2dG causes impairments in the normal epigenetics needed for the normal body functions and can cause impaired DNA methylation and histone acetylation. We developed multiple fluorochrome comet assay to detect 8-OH, 2dG in the cultured SK-N-SH neurons in response to overnight exposure of MPP$^+$ (10 μM), by employing FITC-conjugated 8-OH, 2dG antibody (Ebadi and Sharma 2003). It is now well established that hyper-methylation of the promoter region: of IGF-1 causes insulin-resistant type-2 diabetes, of BDNF causes major depression, and of VEGF causes stroke. Chronic ethanol consumption can induce global hypo-methylation and promoter region hyper-methylation to cause hepato-encaphalopathy. Hence, it is highly prudent to avoid ethanol consumption particularly during 3rd trimester of pregnancy as it is associated with deleterious craniofacial abnormalities as noticed in FASD victims. Furthermore, an efficient charnolophagy is required during the pre-zygotic phase to escape from the deleterious consequences of FASD (Sharma et al. 2014). 8-OH-2dG also interferes with the normal function of microRNAs involved in various aspects of health and disease as described in this chapter.

α-Synuclein Index (SI). α-Synuclein is a synaptic protein and is involved in normal DA-ergic neurotransmission. During oxidative and nitrative stress, α-synuclein is converted to nitrated α-synuclein. The nitrated α-synuclein can easily aggregate to form Lewy bodies in PD. We discovered α-synuclein index (SI), which is a ratio of the native α-synuclein vs nitrated α-synuclein. The SI can be estimated from the biological fluids including CSF, serum, plasma, and saliva of a PD and AD patient as a sensitive diagnostic biomarker of severity of NDDs (Sharma et al. 2003). We estimated SI by performing double radio-immunoprecipitation of native and nitrative α-synuclein, and by immunofluorescence microscopic analyses in saline control and MPP+-treated SK-N-SH neurons. Currently, SI can be easily determined by LC-MS analyses, capillary electrophoresis, FRET analyses SPR spectroscopy, magnetic resonance spectroscopy (MRS), immunoblotting, ELISA, RT-PCR, and by microPET neuroimaging with ^{13}N-labeled α-synuclein.

Charnolophagy Index. Charnolophagy index is a ratio of charnolophagy vs autophagy, which can also be determined by afore-mentioned biotechnology. The simplest method to determine charnolophagy index is by digital fluorescence imaging or confocal microscopy. We need to have lysotrackers to determine autophagy and mitotracker to determine charnolophagy.

RhO$_{mgko}$ Cells as Experimental Model of Aging. The mitochondrial genome is highly susceptible to nutritional and environmental toxic insult as it is an introne-less, low molecular weight (34 Kb) GC-rich, uncoiled, double-stranded macromolecule. The mitochondrial genome is downregulated in PD, AD, and other chronic NDDs. We prepared the RhO$_{mgko}$ SK-N-SH neurons by using 5 ng/l ethidium bromide in the cultured DMEM, glucose, and glutamine, and NaHCO$_3$ for 8 weeks. At this concentration of ethidium bromide, the nuclear DNA remains structurally and functionally intact; however, the functional ability of the mtDNA to generate mitochondrial complex-1 is compromised. Consequently, RhO$_{mgko}$ cells become de-differentiated and their tubulinogenesis, myelinogenesis, axonogenesis, synaptogenesis, and neuritogenesis is compromised. However, RhO$_{mgko}$ cells can divide as observed in aging. We authenticated these cells by RT-PCR of complex-1 gene, which was down-regulated in these cells. The RhO$_{mgko}$ cell synthesized significantly high amounts of 8-OH-2dG as compared to normal aging cells and had significantly stunted growth and neuritogenesis. Transfection of RhO$_{mgko}$ cells with complex-1 gene triggered axonogenesis, tubulinogenesis, myelinogenesis, synaptogenesis, and neuritogenesis involved in the structural and functional integrity of the developing brain regional neurocircuitry (Sharma et al. 2004). These cells were differentiated to perform normal biochemical and physiological functions. CB formation was triggered when the mitochondrial genome was knocked in these neurons. SI was significantly increased in RhO$_{mgko}$ cells and ran parallel with the induction of CB molecular pathogenesis. The incidence of CB formation increased as a function of aging in RhO$_{mgko}$ neurons, suggesting that mitochondrial bio-energetics is compromised in aging to cause cognitive impairments in PD, AD, and aging. Since mtNA is G-C rich, it is highly susceptible to oxidation and epigenetic modulation, pharmacological and nonpharmacological interventions to preserve the structural and functional integrity of mtDNA and inhibition of free radical generation will be highly significant to sustain MB. These interventions will minimize SI and inhibit CB formation for the targeted, safe, and effective theranostic management of PD, AD and other progressive NDDs of aging.

Therapeutic Potential of Antioxidants. Recently, we described in detail the therapeutic potential of various antioxidants in progressive NDDs (Sharma and Ebadi 2013). These antioxidants are resveratrol, lycopene, catechin, polyphenols, flavonoids, sirtuins, and rutins, which can be derived from natural sources and from functional foods as described in this chapter. We highlighted that CB is a universal biomarker of cell injury and is induced in a highly vulnerable cell in response to genetic, environmental, and/or toxic insult due to free radical-mediated damage to mitochondrial membranes and mtDNA in a highly vulnerable cell. Free radicals are highly reactive, ultra-short-lived ($t_{1/2}$: 10^{-13}–10^{-14} Sec) reactive oxygen and nitrogen species ($\cdot$OH, CO$\cdot$, and NO$\cdot$) and induce lipid peroxidation, which triggers the structural and functional breakdown of PUFA in the plasma membranes to cause neuronal cell damage through CB formation. In addition, omega-3 fatty acids (eicosapentonic acid: EPA, docosopentenoic acid, and hexosapentoic acid: HPA) are also down-regulated during CB molecular pathogenesis. Hence, supplementation of PUFA and omaga-3 fatty acids can prevent CB molecular pathogenesis to a certain extent.

CB appears as highly unstable, pleomorphic, electron-dense, multi-lamellar membrane stacks in the perinuclear region or adjacent to the desmosomes or degenerating membranes as a hallmark of CMB. It is important to emphasize that free radicals induce differential damage to the plasma membrane as well as DNA. The desmosomal regions (cell attachments sites) are highly resistant to free radical-induced lipid peroxidation as compared to other regions of the plasma membranes. Similarly, free radicals induce selective damage to mtDNA as compared to nDNA. The damage to mtDNA is more severe as compared to nDNA.

The aggregation of CB at the junction of the axon hillock can impair the normal axoplasmic flow of various ions, neurotransmitters, hormones, neurotrophic growth factors, and mitochondria to cause cognitive impairment (Sharma and Ebadi 2014; Henchcliffe 2015; Zhang et al. 2015). CB formation in the hippocampal region may cause AD, in the NS-DAergic region it may cause PD, and in the mediobasal hypothamalic region it may cause bulimia. CB formation may also be utilized as an early and sensitive biomarker of NDDs and MDDs. Nonspecific induction of CB formation in MDR malignancies, causes GIT distress, myelosuppression, and alopecia (Sharma et al. 2013; Sharma 2014; Li et al. 2014). Hence, (i) novel CB antagonists as synthetic or natural antioxidants in functional foods and natural herbs may be investigated to promote health and prevent the earlier phase of disease progression, (ii) charnolophagy agonists during intermediate phase as intracellular detoxifiers, and (iii) CB sequestration inhibitors during the chronic phase as therapeutic agents in various NDDs, and CVDs, and vice versa for the eradication of MDR malignancies with minimum or no adverse effects. We reported that during the chronic phase, lysosomal resistant CB develops. Hence, CB sequestration during the chronic phase may induce neurodegeneration due to the uncontrolled intracellular release of Cyt-C, iron, and free radicals, which can be prevented by developing novel CB sequestration antagonists.

Two main hypotheses have been proposed in the etiopathogenesis of AD. These are (a) Amyloid-β (Aβ-1-42) Hypothesis and (b) Mitochondrial hypothesis. According to amyloid hypothesis, AD occurs due to abnormal accumulation of Aβ-1-42 in the senile plaques in the cortical ribbon. This hypothesis was confirmed by detecting the Aβ-1-42 senile plaques in the autopsy AD samples using Congo-Red and by immune-histochemical analyses using specific Aβ-1-42 antibody in the senile plaques of AD patients. The senile plaques can be detected *in vivo* by performing ^{18}F-PiB (^{18}F-Florbetapir) PET neuroimaging in AD patients. The Aβ-1-42 hypothesis was further confirmed by observing the progression of neurobehavioral symptoms with neurodegeneration and the cognitive impairment was proportional to the number of amyloid-β 1-42 containing senile plaques. Nevertheless, several AD patients do not exhibit amyloid-β senile plaques in the brain yet exhibit progressive cholinergic and other neurodegeneration as a function of time. Hence, the MB can be evaluated by performing [18]FdG PET neuroimaging. AD patients exhibit distinct loss of glucose metabolism in the fronto-temporal regions, ventriculomegaly, and hippocampal atrophy accompanied with callosal and cerebral atrophy. Early manifestation of CB formation can be evaluated by estimating fluid biomarkers such as 8-OH, 2DG, lactate, glutamate, choline, and N-acetyl apartate (NAA) as rudiments of CB formation and sensitive indicators of NDDs molecular pathogenesis. Platelets, lymphocytes, buccal cells, and skin cells can be cultured and used to examine ΔΨ collapse and CB molecular pathogenesis, using sensitive fluorescent indicators, such as JC-1, dihydrofluorescein, rhodamine, or mitoTracker, lysoTracker, and ER Tracker. In general, the mitochondrial hypothesis relies on the structural and functional integrity of the mitochondrial bioenergetics which may be compromised due to oxidative and nitrative stress.

We proposed MAOIs-mediated neuroprotection through CB inhibition which has been described in greater detail in one of my recently published books (Sharma 2015). Currently there is considerable scientific evidence in support of the proposed hypotheses. Although free radical theory of mitochondrial neurodegeneration is well established, we discovered for the first time the basic molecular mechanism of MAOIs-induced mechanism of neuroprotection through MTs-mediated CB inhibition. Hence, this chapter is primarily based on original discoveries and unique compared to already existing publications because of the following considerations:

Since currently there is no immediate and promising option of neuronal replacement therapy and/or radical surgery in the CNS, neuro-restorative therapies with either endogenous antioxidants (such as MTs, glutathione, SOD, and catalase) or exogenous antioxidant derived from functional foods containing flavonoids, polyphenols, sirtuins, rituins, reseveratrol, catechin, and other inhibitors of lysine deacetylases (LSDs) will have significant therapeutic potential to preserve the MB, inhibit CB formation, augment charnolophagy, sustain CS stabilization, and hence, prevent progressive NDDs. The distinct advantage of functional foods is that these are rich in antioxidants and can easily cross through blood brain barrier, without causing any deleterious central or peripheral adverse effects. However, their reduced potency necessitates bulk consumption. Moreover, these cannot enter through the blood brain barrier quite easily. Hence, future development of ROS scavenging antioxidant (such as curcumin) loaded NPs will improve the EBPT of NDDs, CVDs, and MDR malignancies.

MTs as CB Inhibitors. MTs are zinc-binding, anti-inflammatory, and anti-apoptotic, free radical scavenging proteins, involved in the Zn^{2+}-mediated transcriptional activation of genes involved in the regulation of DNA synthesis, growth, proliferation, differentiation, and development. MTs store, donate, buffer, and/or sequester Zn^{2+} and are 30 times more potent as compared to glutathione in the mitochondria and nucleus (Sharma and Ebadi 2014), whereas mitochondria release and sequester Ca^{2+} ions depending on the inducers and microenvironment surrounding these energy (ATP) synthesizing power houses. Hence, any therapeutic intervention inducing MTs would inhibit CB formation to provide mitochondrial neuroprotection in progressive NDDs such as PD, AD, MDD, schizophrenia, and multiple drug abuse. CB pathogenesis in the developing and/or aging brain supports the mitochondrial hypothesis of progressive NDDs as we have now proposed. Hence, drugs may be developed to prevent and/or inhibit CB formation, enhance charnolophagy, and/or inhibit CB sequestration as a basic molecular mechanism of ICD and MB in the developing and aging brain to cure AD and other NDDs of unknown etiopathogenesis.

Mitochondrial Bioenergetics and ICD. DPCI including, malnutrition, toxins, and microbial infections induce free radical overproduction by inducing mitochondrial oxidative and nitritive stress. Free radicals are generated as a byproduct of oxidative phosphorylation in the electron transport chain. Free radicals induce lipid peroxidation of the mitochondrial membranes. These fragmented mitochondrial membranes condense to contain toxic metabolites in the microenvironment to cause CB formation. CB is recognized as foreign substance in a living cell and is readily phagocytosed by lysosomes to form charnolophagosome (CPS). The CPS is transformed to CS when the phagocytosed CB is hydrolyzed by the lysosomes. CS is structurally and functionally highly labile and is exocytosed by an energy (ATP) dependent process in the circulation. CS destabilization release highly toxic mitochondrial metabolites as described in this book. Early free radical attack may induce the formation of CS bodies, which pinch off from the CS and fuse with the plasm membrane to cause the formation of apoptotic bodies. When apoptotic bodies disintegrate and the entire cytoplasmic constituents are released out of the cell to cause non-DNA dependent cellular demise. Hence, DDST charnolosomics along with conventional omics (genomic, proteomic, metabilmic, lipidomic, glycomic) analysis employing correlative and combinatorial bioinformatics can facilitate targeted, safe, and effective EBPT of NDDs, CVDs, and MDR malignancies. It is also impotant to highlight that a healthy life-style involving diet control, antioxidants, and moderate exercise can also influence our quality of life in addition to combating CB molecular pathogenesis as highlighted in Fig. 50.

CB Pleomorphism in Response to Domoic Acid (DOM). Recently, I examined the effect of domoic acid (DOM) on cultured NPCs. The cells were exposed to increasing concentration of DOM overnight and were examined under the light and EM level. The DNA was extracted to evaluate DOM-induced apoptosis. The results of this study are presented in Fig. 51. Low concentration of DOM (1–10 nM) induced apoptosis

Mitochondrial Bioenergetics and Intracellular Detoxification

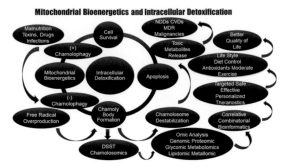

Fig. 50: Mitochondrial bioenergetics and ICD.

CB Pleomorphism in Neuronal Progenitor Cells
(Domoic Acid)

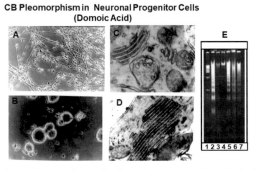

Fig. 51: (A) Cultured neural progenitor cells from the mouse embryonic brain; (B) Domoic acid (DOM)-exposed cultured neuronal progenitor cells after 24 hrs at the light microscopic level; (C) DOM-induced formation of pleomorphic CB due to CMB at the E.M. level. The inner mitochondrial membrane was destroyed first as it remains constantly in a hostile microenvironment of free radicals generated as a byproduct of oxidative phosphorylation in the electron transport chain; (D) Formation of a mature multilamellar CB due to the aggregation of degenerated mitochondrial membranes to contain toxic metabolites such as Cyt-C for intracellular detoxification. (E) DNA Analysis: Lanes: 1: 1 kB DNA Ladder, 2: 100 nM DOM, 3: Control, 4: 10 nM DOM, 5: 20 nM DOM, 6: 30 nM DOM, 7: 50 nM DOM.

represented by internucleosomal DNA fragmentation of 180–200 bp; medium concentrations (10–50 nM) induced necro-apoptosis, whereas higher concentrations (> 100 nM) induced necrosis represented by a smear in the DNA gel. These data suggest that CB molecular pathogenesis can be utilized for the environmental monitoring of toxicity as well as for the targeted, safe, and effective EBPT of chronic MDR diseases.

CB Index (CBI) as a Novel Biomarker of CMB. CBI can be determined in blood, serum, plasma, saliva, nasal discharge, tear, sweat, urine, cultured cells, and in diseased tissue spectrofluorometrically by employing the following equation: *CBI = Mitotracker Fluorescence/2,3 Dihydroxy Nonenal Fluorescence+8-OH, 2dG Fluorescence.* It will be more appropriate to determine CBI from a C.S.F. sample to accomplish EBPT of progressive NDDs.

CB Molecular Pathogenesis and Theranostic Significance of DSST Charnolopharmacotherapeutics in Chronic MDR Diseases. Based on the experimental evidence from genetically-engineered mouse models *in vivo*, and cultured cell lines *in vitro*, CB can be classified as (i) micro-CB (2–4 lamellae, 250–500 nm); (ii) medium CB (5–7 lamellae, 750–100 nm); and (iii) mega-CB (8–15 lamellae, 1.5–2.5 μm or more). A micro-CB can form in any metabolically-active and physiologically normal cell under any physico-chemical stress and is readily eliminated by energy (ATP)-deriven charnolophagy due to lysosomal activation and CS exocytosis as a basic molecular mechanism of ICD. The elimination of medium-sized CB requires mitochondrial energy (ATP) and lysosomes to enhance charnolophagy. Various endogenous as well as exogenous antioxidants stabilize CS and facilitate its exocytosis for ICD as observed in Fig. 51 (upper right panel). A severe physico-chemical injury can induce massive production of free radicals due to oxidative and nitrative stress to cause lipid peroxidation characterized by the structural and functional breakdown of PUFA to cause fragmentation of the mitochondrial membranes. The inner mitochondrial membrane is destroyed first because it is directly exposed to free radicals, generated as a byproduct of oxidative phosphorylation. The formation of electron-dense membrane stacks (CB) occurs to contain toxic mitochondrial metabolites (i.e., Cyt-C, iron, Ca^{2+}, lactate, aceate, ceramide, acetate, ammonia, H_2O_2, superoxide, CO·, NO·, ·OH radicals, $ONOO^-$, GAPDH, 8-OH, 2dG, AIF, caspases, 2,3 dihydroxy nonenal to name a few). The elimination of mega-CB is highly challenging due to limited number of lysosomes and energy (ATP) required to execute successful charnolophagy as observed in Fig. 51 (lower right panel). The persistence of lysosomal-insensitive or resistant mega-CB induces severe pathophysiological complications. Moreover, increased intracellular acidity enhances CS destabilization characterized by increased permeabilization, sequestration, and fragmentation to cause AgNOR inactivation involved in ribosomal production for protein synthesis involved in normal biological activity, cellular growth, and development. CS destabilization also triggers genetic and epigenetic impairments to cause mtDNA, mtRNA, and mt-microRNA down-regulation to cause degenerative apoptosis and chronic MDR diseases.

α-*Synuclein Index (SI) and Charnolophagy-Index in CB Molecular Pathogenesis.* The induction or repression of SI and charnolophagy index depends on the intensity and frequency of DPCI to the most vulnerable cell. (i) The SI is significantly low, whereas, the charnolophagy index is significantly high in a cell possessing micro-CB as it is efficiently eliminated by energy (ATP)-driven CS exocytosis to sustain normal mitochondrial bioenergetics (MB) and ICD. (ii) The SI is elevated, whereas, the charnolophagy index is reduced in a cell possessing medium CB. The exogenous as well as endogenous antioxidants stabilizes CS and facilitate its exocytosis as a basic molecular mechanism of ICD to sustain MB and ICD. (iii) The SI is significantly increased and the charnolophagy index is significantly reduced in a cell possessing mega-CB. The endogenous, exogenous, and synthetic antioxidants stabilize CS and facilitate its exocytosis to a certain extent to sustain MB and ICD for a normal cellular function. The formation of mega-CB and its destabilization and sequestration releases toxic mitochondrial metabolites as describe above to form intracellular or extracellular protein aggregates (as inclusion bodies) as observed in various neurodegenerative and chronic MDR diseases. Hence, a novel discovery of DSST charnolopharmacotherapeutics to prevent/inhibit CB molecular pathogenesis and a precise understanding of CS-antioxidant interaction will confer better understanding of environmental protection and the targeted, safe, and effective EBPT of chronic interactable diseases for a better quality of life (BQL) as highlighted in this book.

Conclusion

The basic understanding of complex diseases such as sporadic AD has been a major challenge. Unlike the familial forms of AD, the genetic and environmental risks factors for sporadic AD are extensive. AD is the most common form of dementia, but the identification of reliable, early, and non-invasive biomarkers remains a major challenge. I proposed a novel CB-based signature for detecting AD from peripheral cells including: skin cells, buccal mucosa cells, platelets, and lymphocytes and highlighted that CMB triggers CB formation involved in AD, PD, Pick's disease, alcoholism, schizophrenia, chronic drug addiction (cocaine, and METH), Down's syndrome, autism, Prion's disease, HD, ALS, MS, AIDs dementia, and several other chronic conditions of unknown etiopathogenesis. Nutritional stress, environmental toxins, and microbes can induce hippocampal atrophy, callosal atrophy, fronto-temporal cortical atrophy, ventriculomegaly, cerebral hyperthermia, dehydration, cerebral ischemia, stroke, and epilepsy due to free radical-induced CB formation, which can be ameliorated to a certain extent by supplementation of antioxidant-rich functional foods in old age to prevent progressive neurodegeneration in AD and other NDDs. The basic advantage of antioxidants derived from functional foods (including resveratrol, lycopenes, sirtuins, rutins, catechin, flavonoids, LSDs, and polyphenols) is that these can easily pass through blood brain barrier and do not produce adverse effects as other standard pharmaceutical agents. Presently, we have limited scope of removing any degenerating brain region because of its limited regenerative potential and serious impairment in the sensory modality due to somatotropic representation of specific brain regions. Hence, the importance of antioxidants in EBPT becomes highly significant. The main limitation of antioxidants derived from functional foods and Mediterranean diets is that they have significantly reduced potency; their therapeutic potential is also limited at this moment. Hence, novel drugs targeted to prevent or inhibit CB formation during the early phase of disease progression, charnolophagy inducers during the intermediate phase, and CB sequestration inhibitors and CS stabilizers during the chronic phase will go a long way in the targeted, safe, and effective EBPT of chronic NDDs, CVDs, and MDR malignancies as described in this chapter.

References

Chen, Y., W.D. Parker, H. Chen and K. Yang. 2013. Aberrant mitochondrial RNA in the role of aging and aging associated diseases. Medical Hypotheses 85: 178–182.

Duarte, F.V., C.M. Palmeira and A.P. Rolo. 2015. The emerging role of mitomirs in the pathophysiology of human disease. Adv Exp Med Biol 888: 123–154.

DuBoff, B., J. Götz and M.B. Feany. 2012. Tau promotes neurodegeneration via DRP1 mis-localization *in vivo*. Neuron 75: 618–632.

Ebadi, M., H. Brown-Borg, S. Sharma, S. Shavali, H.El ReFaey and E.C. Carlson. 2006. Therapeutic efficacy of selegiline in *NDDs* and neurological diseases. Current Drug Targets 7: 1–17.

García-Escudero, V., P. Martín-Maestro, G. Perry and J. Avila. 2013. Deconstructing mitochondrial dysfunction in Alzheimer disease. Oxidative Medicine and Cellular Longevity 2013: 1–13.

Hayashi, H., H. Nakagami, M. Takeichi, M. Shimamura, N. Koibuchi, E. Oiki, N. Sato, H. Koriyama, M. Mori, R. Gerardo Araujo, A. Maeda, R. Morishita, K. Tamai and Y. Kaneda. 2012. HIG1, a novel regulator of mitochondrial γ-secretase, maintains normal mitochondrial function. FASEB J 26: 2306–2317.

Henchcliffe, C. 2015. Blood and cerebrospinal fluid markers in Parkinson's disease: current biomarker findings. Current Biomarker Findings 5: 1–11.

Kandimalla, R. and P.H. Reddy. 2016. Multiple faces of dynamin-related protein 1 and its role in Alzheimer's disease pathogenesis. Biochim Biophys Acta 1862: 814–828.

Leidinger, P., C. Backes, S. Deutscher, K. Schmitt, S.C. Mueller, K. Frese, J. Haas, K. Ruprecht, F. Paul et al. 2013. A blood based 12-miRNA signature of Alzheimer disease patients. Genome Biology 201314: R78.

Li, Z., Q. Lin, Q. Ma, C. Lu and C.M. Tzeng. 2014. Genetic predisposition to Parkinson's disease and cancer. Curr Cancer Drug Targets 14: 310–321.

Logue, S.E., P. Cleary, S. Saveljeva and A. Samali. 2013. New directions in ER stress-induced cell death. Apoptosis 18: 537–546.

Lykhmus, O., N. Mishra, L. Koval, O. Kalashnyk, G. Gergalova, K. Uspenska, S. Komisarenko, H. Soreq and M. Skok. 2016. Molecular mechanisms regulating LPS-induced inflammation in the brain. Front Mol Neurosci 9: 19.

Maes, O.C., H.M. Chertkow, E. Wang and H.M. Schipper. 2009. microRNA: Implications for Alzheimer disease and other human CNS disorders. Curr Genomics 10: 154–168.

Moreira, P.I., C. Carvalho, X. Zhu, M.A. Smith and G. Perry. 2010. Mitochondrial dysfunction is a trigger of Alzheimer's disease pathophysiology. Biochimica et Biophysica Acta (BBA)— Molecular Basis of Disease 1802: 2–10.

Schonrock, N., M. Matamales, L.M. Ittner and J. Götz. 2012. microRNA networks surrounding APP and amyloid-β metabolism—implications for Alzheimer's disease. Exp Neurol 235: 447–454.

Sharma, S. and M. Ebadi. 2005. Distribution kinetics of ^{18}F-DOPA in weaver mutant mice. Molecular Brain Research 139: 23–30.

Sharma, S., H.El Refaey and M. Ebadi. 2006. Complex-1 activity and ^{18}F-DOPA uptake in genetically engineered mouse model of Parkinson's disease and the neuroprotective role of coenzyme Q_{10}. Brain Res Bull 70: 22–32.

Sharma, S. and M. Ebadi. 2008. SPECT neuroimaging in translational research of CNS disorders. Neurochem Internat 52: 352–362.

Sharma, S. and M. Ebadi. 2008. Therapeutic potential of metallothioneins in Parkinson's disease. pp. 1–41. In: Hahn, T.M. and Julian Werner (eds.). New Research on Parkinson's Disease. Chapter-1. Nova Science Publishers USA.

Sharma, S. and M. Ebadi. 2008. Therapeutic potential of metallothioneins in PD. pp. 1–28. In: Timothy F. Hahn and Julian Werner (eds.). New Research on PD. Nova Science Publishers, New York.

Sharma, S. and M. Ebadi. 2011. Metallothioneins as early & sensitive biomarkers of redox signaling in neurodegenerative disorders. Journal of Institute of Integrative Omics & Applied Biotechnology (IIOAB Journal) 2: 98–106.

Sharma, S. and M. Ebadi. 2011. Therapeutic potential of metallothioneins as anti-inflammatory agents in polysubstance abuse. Journal of Institute of Integrative Omics & Applied Biotechnology (IIOAB Journal) 2: 50–61.

Sharma, S. and M. Ebadi. 2013. Antioxidant Targeting in Neurodegenerative Disorders. Ed. I. Laher, Springer Verlag. Germany. Chapter 85, pp. 1–30.

Sharma, S., C.S. Moon, A. Khogali, A. Haidous, A. Chabenne, C. Ojo, M. Jelebinkov, Y. Kurdi and M. Ebadi. 2013. Biomarkers of PD (Recent Update). Neurochemistry International 63: 201–229.

Sharma, S., C.S. Moon, A. Khogali, A. Haidous, A. Chabenne, C. Ojo, M. Jelebinkov, Y. Kurdi and M. Ebadi. 2013a. Biomarkers of Parkinson's disease (Recent Update). Neurochemistry International 63: 201–229.

Sharma, S., A. Rais, R. Sandhu, W. Nel and M. Ebadi. 2013b. Clinical significance of metallothioneins in cell therapy and nanomedicine. International Journal of Nanomedicine 8: 1477–1488.

Sharma, S. and M. Ebadi. 2013c. In vivo molecular imaging in Parkinson's disease. pp. 787–80. In: Pfeiffer, R.F.. Z.K. Wszolek and M. Ebadi (eds.). Parkinson's Disease. IInd Edition, Chapter 58, CRC Press Taylor & Francis Group. Boca Rotan, FL, USA.

Sharma, S. 2014. Beyond Diet and Depression *(Volume-1)*. Book Nova Sciences Publishers, New York, U.S.A.

Sharma, S. 2014. Beyond Diet and Depression (*Volume-2*). Book Nova Science Publishers, New York, U.S.A.

Sharma, S. 2014. Nanotheranostics in evidence based personalized medicine. Current Drug Targets 15: 915–930.

Sharma, S. 2014. Molecular pharmacology of environmental neurotoxins. *In*: Kainic Acid: Neurotoxic Properties, Biological Sources, and Clinical Applications. Nova Science Publishers. New York. pp. 1–47.

Sharma, S. and M. Ebadi. 2014. Charnoly body as a universal biomarker of cell injury. Biomarkers and Genomic Medicine 6: 89–99.

Sharma, S. and M. Ebadi. 2014. Significance of metallothioneins in aging brain. Neurochemistry International 65: 40–48.

Sharma, S. and M. Ebadi. 2014. Antioxidant Targeting in Neurodegenerative Disorders. Ed. I. Laher, Springer Verlag. Germany. Chapter 85, pp. 1–30.

Sharma, S. and M. Ebadi. 2014. Charnoly body as a universal biomarker of cell injury. Biomarkers and Genomic Medicine 6: 89–98.

Sharma, S. and M. Ebadi. 2014b. Significance of metallothioneins in aging brain. Neurochemistry International 65: 40–48.

Sharma, S. 2015. Synthetic and herbal monoamine oxidase inhibitors. monoamine oxidase inhibitors. Cinical Pharmacology, Benefits, and Potential Health Risks. Nova Science Publishers, New York, U.S.A. Chapter 2, pp. 33–78.

Sharma, S. 2015. Alleviating Stress of the Soldier and Civilian. Nova Science Publishers, New York, U.S.A.

Sharma, S., S. Gawande, A. Jagtap, R. Abeulela and Z. Salman. 2015. Fetal alcohol syndrome; prevention, diagnosis, & treatment. pp. 39–94. *In*: Jeffrey Raines (ed.). Alcohol Abuse: Prevalence, Risk Factors. Nova Science Publishers, New York, U.S.A. Chapter 3.

Sharma, S. 2016a. Charnoly body as a novel biomarker of *ZIKV* induced *microcephaly*. Proceedings of the Drug Discovery and Therapy World Congress (Track: CNS Drug Discovery & Therapy) 22nd to 25th August. Boston, USA.

Sharma, S. 2016b. Monoamine Oxidase Inhibitors: Clinical Pharmacology, Therapeutic Applications, and Adverse Effects. Nova Science Publishers, New York.

Shi, Q. and G.E. Gibson. 2011. Up-regulation of the mitochondrial malate dehydrogenase by oxidative stress is mediated by miR-743a. J Neurochem 118: 440–448.

Tomasetti, M., J. Neuzil and L. Dong. 2014. microRNAs as regulators of mitochondrial function: Role in cancer suppression. Biochimica et Biophysica Acta (BBA)—General Subjects. Frontiers of Mitochondrial Research 1840: 1441–1453.

Zhang, S., C. Lei, P. Liub, M. Zhang, W. Taoa, H. Liud and M. Liu. 2015. Association between variant amyloid deposits and motor deficits in FAD-associated presenilin-1 mutations: A systematic review. Neuroscience and Biobehavioral Reviews 56: 180–192.

Index

About the Author

Dr. Sushil Sharma is Academic Dean at the American International School of Medicine, Guyana, South America. He was Professor and Course Director of Pharmacology of the Saint James School of Medicine, Saint Vincent and Bonaire (Netherlands). He received Ph.D. in Neuropharmacology from A.I.I.M.S., New Delhi; Radiopharmaceutical Trainings from B.A.R.C., Bombay, GE, Siemens, Agilent Technologies, and Cardinal Health in USA; Served as Research Officer in A.I.I.M.S.: 1979–88; was awarded Royal Society Fellowship (UK: 1988–89); MHRC Post-doctoral Fellowship (Canada: 1989–91); Research Officer (University of Montreal: 1993–94); Research Associate (McGill University: 1994–95); Offered Deputy Director (Scientist-E) Position in Defense Research Institute (New Delhi: 1993–97); Senior Scientific Officer (Clinical Research Institute of Montreal: 1995–97); Research Scientist (University of Manitoba: 1997–99); Assistant Professor 2000–04; Associate Professor & Director (Research) UND School of Medicine, Grand Forks: 2004–08; Associate Professor and Director (Methodist Hospital) and Research Scientist (University Texas Medical Center: 2008–11). He organized and chaired several World Conferences; was awarded 5 Gold Medals; Certificate of Honor at I.T. Nano-2014 Conference, Boston (Original Discoveries: Electromicroinjector; CB in Purkinje Neurons, IL-10 Receptors on Cortical Neurons, & MTs-Gene-Manipulated Mice). Author: 265 publications; Books: "Beyond Diet & Depression" (Vol. 1 & Vol. 2) Nova Sciences Publishers, N.Y. U.S.A.; "Alleviating Stress of the Soldier & Civilian" Nova Science Publishers, N.Y. U.S.A., Monoamine Oxidase Inhibitors (Clinical Pharmacology, Benefits, and Potential Health Risks), Nova Science Publishers, New York, U.S.A.; Personalized Medicine (Beyond PET Biomarkers) Nova Science Publishers, New York, U.S.A.; Progress in PET RPs (Quality Control and Therapeutics) Nova Science Publishers, New York, U.S.A.; ZIKV Disease (Prevention and Cure) Nova Sciences Publishers, New York, U.S.A.; Fetal Alcohol Spectrum Disorders (Concepts, Mechanisms, and Cure) Nova Science Publishers, New York, U.S.A.; Nicotinism and Emerging Role of E-Cigarettes (With Special Reference to Adolescents (Volume 1–4), Nova Science Publishers, New York, U.S.A.

He has guided many M.D./Ph.D. students. He is invited as scientific consultant, chairperson, and invited speaker in international conferences. He serves as the expert reviewer of international research proposals and senior editorial consultant of international journals.